Decision Making in Vascular Surgery

Decision Making in Vascular Surgery

Jack L. Cronenwett, MD
Professor of Surgery
Dartmouth Medical School
Chief, Section of Vascular Surgery
Dartmouth Hitchcock Medical Center
Lebanon, New Hampshire

Robert B. Rutherford, MD
Emeritus Professor of Surgery
University of Colorado School of Medicine
Denver, Colorado

W.B. Saunders Company
A Harcourt Health Sciences Company
Philadelphia • London • New York • St. Louis • Sydney • Toronto

W.B. SAUNDERS COMPANY
A Harcourt Health Sciences Company

The Curtis Center
Independence Square West
Philadelphia, Pennsylvania 19106

Library of Congress Cataloging-in-Publication Data

Cronenwett, Jack L.
  Decision making in vascular surgery / Jack L. Cronenwett, Robert B. Rutherford.
    p. ; cm.
  ISBN 0-7216-8684-2
  1. Blood-vessels—Surgery. 2. Arteries—Surgery. 3. Decision making.
    I. Rutherford, Robert B., II. Title. [DNLM: 1. Vascular Surgical
    Procedures. 2. Decision Making. WG 170 C947d 2001]
  RD598.5 .C76 2001   617.4'13—dc21

  DNLM/DLC   2001020323

Acquisitions Editor: Richard Lampert
Manuscript Editor: Carol J. Robins
Production Manager: Norman Stellander
Illustration Specialists: Walt Verbitski and John Needles
Book Designer: Steven Stave

DECISION MAKING IN VASCULAR SURGERY   ISBN 0-7216-8684-2

Copyright © 2001 by W.B. Saunders Company

All rights reserved. No part of this publication may be reproduced or transmitted in any form or by any means, electronic or mechanical, including photocopy, recording, or any information storage and retrieval system, without permission in writing from the publisher.

Printed in the United States of America.

Last digit is the print number: 9   8   7   6   5   4   3   2   1

CONTRIBUTORS

Ahmed M. Abou-Zamzam, MD
Assistant Professor, Division of Vascular Surgery, Department of Surgery, Loma Linda University School of Medicine, Loma Linda, California
Deep Vein Insufficiency: Evaluation and Conservative Management

Ali F. Aburahma, MD
Professor and Chief of Vascular Surgery, Department of Surgery, West Virginia University School of Medicine. Medical Director, Vascular Laboratory, Charleston Area Medical Center, Charleston, West Virginia
Post-traumatic Pain Syndrome

Farzin Adili, MD
Assistant Professor, Department of Vascular Surgery, Johann Wolfgang Goethe University, Frankfurt, Germany
Carotid Body Tumors

Joseph P. Archie, PhD, MD
Clinical Professor of Surgery, University of North Carolina at Chapel Hill School of Medicine, Chapel Hill. Adjutant Professor of Mechanical Engineering, North Carolina State University, Raleigh, North Carolina
Carotid Endarterectomy

Dennis F. Bandyk, MD
Professor of Surgery, University of South Florida College of Medicine, Tampa, Florida
Infrainguinal Graft Surveillance

Ramon Berguer, MD, PhD
Professor of Surgery, Wayne State University School of Medicine. Chief, Division of Vascular Surgery, Detroit Receiving Hospital and University Medical Center, Detroit, Michigan
Vertebral Artery Disease

Thomas Bilfinger, MD, ScD
Professor of Clinical Surgery, State University of New York at Stony Brook School of Medicine, Stony Brook, New York. Research Associate, Neuroscience Institute, State University of New York at Old Westbury, Old Westbury, New York. Senior Research Scientist, Mind Body Medical Institute, Beth Israel Deaconess Medical Center, Boston, Massachusetts
Carotid Plus Coronary Disease

Fred S. Bongard, MD
Professor of Surgery, University of California, Los Angeles, School of Medicine. Chief, Division of Trauma and Critical Care, Harbor–UCLA Medical Center, Torrance, California
Abdominal Vascular Trauma

David C. Brewster, MD
Clinical Professor of Surgery, Harvard Medical School. Senior Attending Surgeon, Division of Vascular Surgery, Department of Surgery, Massachusetts General Hospital, Boston, Massachusetts
Aortic Graft Limb Thrombosis

Keith D. Calligaro, MD
Chief, Section of Vascular Surgery, Pennsylvania Hospital, Philadelphia, Pennsylvania
Infrainguinal Prosthetic Graft Infection

Richard P. Cambria, MD
Professor of Surgery, Harvard Medical School. Chief, Division of Vascular Surgery, Massachusetts General Hospital, Boston, Massachusetts
Thoracoabdominal Aortic Aneurysm

Robert E. Carlin, MD
Vascular Surgery Resident, University of North Carolina Hospitals, Chapel Hill, North Carolina
Amputation Level

Kathleen Chaimberg, MD
Assistant Professor, Department of Anesthesiology, Dartmouth Medical School, Hanover, New Hampshire. Staff Anesthesiologist, Dartmouth Hitchcock Medical Center, Lebanon, New Hampshire
Perioperative Care and Anesthesia

Kenneth J. Cherry, Jr., MD
Professor of Surgery, Mayo Medical School. Consultant, Division of Vascular Surgery, Mayo Clinic, Rochester, Minnesota
Brachiocephalic Arterial Occlusive Disease

G. Patrick Clagett, MD
Jan and Bob Pickens Professor of Medical Science and Chairman, Division of Vascular Surgery, Department of Surgery, University of Texas Southwestern Medical Center at Dallas Southwestern Medical School, Dallas, Texas
Aortic Graft Infection

Anthony J. Comerota, MD
Professor of Surgery, Temple University School of Medicine. Chief, Vascular Surgery, Temple University Hospital, Philadelphia, Pennsylvania
Iliofemoral Deep Vein Thrombosis

Jack L. Cronenwett, MD
Professor of Surgery, Dartmouth Medical School. Chief, Section of Vascular Surgery, Dartmouth Hitchcock Medical Center, Lebanon, New Hampshire
Symptomatic Carotid Artery Stenosis; Asymptomatic Carotid Artery Stenosis; Abdominal Aortic Aneurysm; Aortoiliac Disease

Ralph G. DePalma, MD
Professor of Surgery, University of Nevada School of Medicine, Reno, Nevada. National Director of Surgery, Department of Veterans Affairs, VA Central Office, Washington, District of Columbia
Erectile Dysfunction

Tina R. Desai, MD
Assistant Professor of Surgery, University of Chicago Pritzker School of Medicine, Chicago, Illinois
Acute Mesenteric Ischemia

Anthony W. DiScipio, MD
Chief Resident, Department of Cardiothoracic Surgery, Boston Medical Center, Boston, Massachusetts
Aortic Dissection

M. C. Donaldson, MD
Associate Professor of Surgery, Harvard Medical School. Attending Surgeon, Division of Vascular Surgery, Brigham and Women's Hospital, Boston, Massachusetts
Infrainguinal Occlusive Disease

Kim A. Eagle, MD
Albion Walter Hewlett Professor of Internal Medicine, University of Michigan Medical School. Interim Chief, Division of Cardiology, and Chief of Clinical Cardiology, University of Michigan Health System, Ann Arbor, Michigan
Preoperative Cardiac Risk Assessment

R. David Edrington, MD
Clinical Professor of Surgery, University of North Carolina at Chapel Hill School of Medicine, Chapel Hill. Staff, Wake Medical Center, Raleigh, North Carolina
Carotid Endarterectomy

Bo Eklof, MD, PhD
Clinical Professor of Surgery, University of Hawaii at Mānoa John A. Burns School of Medicine. Vascular Surgeon, Straub Clinic and Hospital, Honolulu, Hawaii
Deep Vein Insufficiency: Surgical Treatment

Calvin B. Ernst, MD
Professor of Surgery and Chairman, Department of Vascular Surgery, MCP Hahnemann University, Philadelphia, Pennsylvania
Aortoenteric Fistula

Alik Farber, MD
Attending Vascular Surgeon, Cedars-Sinai Medical Center, Los Angeles, California
Symptomatic Carotid Artery Stenosis; Asymptomatic Carotid Artery Stenosis

Mark Fillinger, MD
Associate Professor of Surgery, Dartmouth Hitchcock Medical Center, Lebanon, New Hampshire
Endovascular Abdominal Aortic Aneurysm Repair

Lisa Flynn, MD
Staff Vascular Surgeon, Department of Surgery, St. John's Hospital and Medical Center, Detroit, Michigan
Vertebral Artery Disease

James B. Froehlich, MD
Assistant Professor of Medicine, Harvard Medical School. Director, Vascular Medicine, Beth Israel Deaconess Medical Center, Boston, Massachusetts
Preoperative Cardiac Risk Assessment

Bruce L. Gewertz, MD
Dallas B. Phemister Professor and Chairman, Department of Surgery, and Chief, Section of Vascular Surgery, University of Chicago Pritzker School of Medicine, Chicago, Illinois
Acute Mesenteric Ischemia

Joseph M. Giordano, MD
Professor and Chairman, Department of Surgery, George Washington University School of Medicine, Washington, District of Columbia
Takayasu's Disease

Peter Gloviczki, MD
Professor of Surgery, Mayo Medical School. Chair, Division of Vascular Surgery, Mayo Clinic, Rochester, Minnesota
Lymphedema

Jerry Goldstone, MD
Professor of Surgery, Case Western Reserve University School of Medicine. Chief, Vascular Surgery, University Hospitals of Cleveland, Cleveland, Ohio
Carotid Artery Aneurysm

Yara Gorski, MD
Academic Clinical Instructor and Vascular Fellow, State University of New York at Stony Brook, Stony Brook, New York
Carotid Plus Coronary Disease

Lazar J. Greenfield, MD
Frederick A. Coller Distinguished Professor and Chairman, Department of Surgery, University of Michigan Medical School. Surgeon-in-Chief, University of Michigan Hospitals, Ann Arbor, Michigan
Pulmonary Embolism

John W. Hallett, Jr., MD
Professor of Surgery and Associate Dean of Faculty Affairs, Mayo Medical School. Staff Surgeon, Division of Vascular Surgery, Mayo Clinic, Rochester, Minnesota
Ruptured Abdominal Aortic Aneurysm

Sharon L. Hammond, MD
Adjunct Assistant Professor of Surgery, Uniformed Services University of the Health Sciences F. Edward Hébert School of Medicine, Bethesda, Maryland. Attending Vascular Surgeon, Rose Medical Center, Denver, Colorado
Neurogenic Thoracic Outlet Syndrome

Kimberley J. Hansen, MD
Professor of Surgery, Wake Forest University School of Medicine, Winston-Salem, North Carolina
Renovascular Occlusive Disease: Evaluation

Peter K. Henke, MD
Assistant Professor, Section of Vascular Surgery, Department of Surgery, University of Michigan Medical School. Staff Surgeon, University of Michigan Hospital, and Chief, Section of Vascular Surgery, Ann Arbor Veterans Administration Medical Center, Ann Arbor, Michigan
Hypercoagulable Syndrome

William R. Hiatt, MD
Novartis Professor of Cardiovascular Research, University of Colorado School of Medicine, Denver, Colorado
Management of Hyperlipidemia

Robert W. Hobson II, MD
Professor and Director, Division of Vascular Surgery, Department of Surgery, University of Medicine and Dentistry of New Jersey–New Jersey Medical School, Newark, New Jersey
Stroke Following Carotid Endarterectomy

Douglas B. Hood, MD
Assistant Professor of Surgery, Keck School of Medicine of the University of Southern California, Los Angeles, California
Extremity Vascular Trauma

Thomas S. Huber, MD, PhD
Associate Professor, Department of Surgery, University of Florida College of Medicine. Staff Surgeon, Shands Teaching Hospital at the University of Florida, Gainesville, Florida
Transfusion Strategies

Scott Hurlbert, MD
Private Practice, Colorado Springs, Colorado
Subclavian-Axillary Vein Thrombosis

Mark R. Jackson, MD
Associate Professor of Surgery, University of Texas Southwestern Medical Center at Dallas Southwestern Medical School, Dallas, Texas
Aortic Graft Infection

Kaj H. Johansen, MD, PhD
Professor of Surgery, University of Washington School of Medicine. Director of Surgical Education, Swedish Medical Center–Providence Campus, Seattle, Washington
Portal Hypertension

K. Wayne Johnston, MD
Professor of Surgery and R. Fraser Elliott Chair in Vascular Surgery, Division of Vascular Surgery, University of Toronto Faculty of Medicine. Division Head, Vascular Surgery, Toronto General Hospital, Toronto, Ontario, Canada
Sigmoid Ischemia After Aortic Surgery

Peter G. Kalman, MD
Associate Professor, Department of Surgery, University of Toronto Faculty of Medicine. Attending Surgeon, Toronto East General Hospital, Toronto, Ontario, Canada
Sigmoid Ischemia After Aortic Surgery

Jeffrey L. Kaufman, MD
Associate Professor of Surgery, Tufts University School of Medicine, Boston. Surgeon, Baystate Medical Center and Mercy Hospital, Springfield, Massachusetts
Atheroembolism

Blair A. Keagy, MD
Professor and Chief, Division of Vascular Surgery, Department of Surgery, University of North Carolina at Chapel Hill School of Medicine, Chapel Hill, North Carolina
Amputation Level

Robert L. Kistner, MD
Clinical Professor of Surgery, University of Hawaii at Mānoa John A. Burns School of Medicine. Vascular Surgeon, Straub Clinic and Hospital, Honolulu, Hawaii
Deep Vein Insufficiency: Surgical Treatment

William C. Krupski, MD
Professor of Surgery, University of Colorado School of Medicine. Chief, Division of Vascular Surgery, University of Colorado Health Sciences Center, Denver, Colorado
Iliac Artery Aneurysm; Femoral Artery Aneurysm

S. Ram Kumar, MD
Resident in Surgery, Keck School of Medicine at the University of Southern California, Los Angeles, California
Extremity Vascular Trauma

Brajesh K. Lal, MD
Vascular Surgery Fellow, University of Medicine and Dentistry of New Jersey–University Hospital, Newark, New Jersey
Vascular Access for Hemodialysis

Glenn M. La Muraglia, MD
Associate Professor of Surgery, Harvard Medical School. Associate Visiting Surgeon, Division of Vascular Surgery, Massachussets General Hospital, Boston, Massachusetts
Carotid Body Tumors

Gregory J. Landry, MD
Assistant Professor, Division of Vascular Surgery, Department of Surgery, Oregon Health Sciences University School of Medicine, Portland, Oregon
Raynaud's Syndrome

James T. Lee, MD
Clinical Instructor, University of California, Los Angeles, School of Medicine, Los Angeles. Fellow, Peripheral Vascular Surgery and Endovascular Surgery, Harbor–UCLA Medical Center, Torrance, California
Abdominal Vascular Trauma

Lewis Levien, MB, BCh, PhD(Med)
Vascular Surgeon, Milpark Hospital, Parktown, Johannesburg, South Africa
Popliteal Artery Entrapment Syndrome and Popliteal Cystic Adventitial Disease

William C. Mackey, MD
Professor of Surgery, Tufts University School of Medicine. Chief of Vascular Surgery, New England Medical Center, Boston, Massachusetts
Acute Stroke

M. Ashraf Mansour, MD
Assistant Professor of Surgery, Loyola University Stritch School of Medicine, Maywood, Illinois
Aortovenous Fistula

Martha McDaniel, MD
Professor of Surgery, Community-Family Medicine, and Anatomy, Dartmouth Medical School, Hanover, New Hampshire
Patients with Leg Pain While Walking

Kenneth E. McIntyre, Jr., MD
Professor of Surgery, University of Texas Southwestern Medical Center at Dallas Southwestern Medical School. Chief of Vascular Surgery, St. Paul Medical Center, Dallas, Texas
Brachiocephalic Vascular Trauma

Mark H. Meissner, MD
Associate Professor, Department of Surgery, University of Washington School of Medicine, Seattle, Washington
Lower Extremity Deep Vein Thrombosis

Louis M. Messina, MD
Professor of Surgery and Chief of Vascular Surgery, University of California, San Francisco, School of Medicine, San Francisco, California
Carotid Dissection

Gregory L. Moneta, MD
Professor and Chief, Divison of Vascular Surgery, Department of Surgery, Oregon Health Sciences University School of Medicine. Staff Surgeon, Portland Department of Veterans Affairs Hospital, Portland, Oregon
Deep Vein Insufficiency: Evaluation and Conservative Management

Mark D. Morasch, MD
Assistant Professor of Surgery, Northwestern University Medical School. Clinical Practice Director, Northwestern Medical Faculty Foundation, Chicago, Illinois
Upper Extremity Ischemia

Mark R. Nehler, MD
Assistant Professor, Division of Vascular Surgery, Department of Surgery, University of Colorado School of Medicine, Denver, Colorado
Management of Hyperlipidemia; Iliac Artery Aneurysm; Femoral Artery Aneurysm

Peter R. Nelson, MD
Fellow in Vascular Surgery, Dartmouth Hitchcock Medical Center, Lebanon, New Hampshire
Chronic Mesenteric Ischemia

Audra A. Noel, MD
Assistant Professor of Surgery, Mayo Medical School. Senior Associate Consultant, Mayo Clinic, Rochester, Minnesota
Brachiocephalic Arterial Occlusive Disease; Lymphedema

Sean P. O'Brien, MD
Vascular Surgery Fellow, MCP Hahnemann University Hospital, Philadelphia, Pennsylvania
Aortoenteric Fistula

Kenneth Ouriel, MD
Professor, Department of Surgery, Ohio State University College of Medicine and Public Health, Columbus. Chairman, Department of Vascular Surgery, Cleveland Clinic Foundation, Cleveland, Ohio
Intraoperative Hemorrhage and Bleeding Diathesis

Laura K. Pak, MD
Vascular Surgery Fellow, University of California, San Francisco, School of Medicine, San Francisco, California
Carotid Dissection

William H. Pearce, MD
Professor of Surgery, Northwestern University Medical School. Chief, Division of Vascular Surgery, Northwestern Memorial Hospital, Chicago, Illinois
Upper Extremity Ischemia

Bruce A. Perler, MD
Professor of Surgery, Johns Hopkins University School of Medicine. Director of Vascular Surgery Fellowship and Noninvasive Vascular Laboratory, Johns Hopkins Hospital, Baltimore, Maryland
Subclavian Artery Occlusive Disease

Malcolm O. Perry, MD
Professor Emeritus, University of Texas Southwestern Medical Center at Dallas Southwestern Medical School, Dallas, Texas
Brachiocephalic Vascular Trauma

John M. Porter, MD
Professor, Division of Vascular Surgery, Department of Surgery, Oregon Health Sciences University School of Medicine, Portland, Oregon
Raynaud's Syndrome

Richard J. Powell, MD
Assistant Professor of Surgery, Attending Surgeon, Section of Vascular Surgery, Dartmouth Hitchcock Medical Center, Lebanon, New Hampshire
Popliteal Artery Aneurysm

Mary C. Proctor, MS
Senior Research Associate, Department of Surgery, University of Michigan Hospitals, Ann Arbor, Michigan
Pulmonary Embolism

Todd E. Rasmussen, MD
Instructor in Surgery, Mayo Medical School, Rochester, Minnesota. Assistant Professor of Surgery, Uniformed Services, University of the Health Sciences F. Edward Hébert School of Medicine, Bethesda, Maryland
Ruptured Abdominal Aortic Aneurysm

Daniel J. Reddy, MD
Head, Division of Vascular Surgery, Henry Ford Hospital, Detroit, Michigan
Femoral Artery Pseudoaneurysm from Trauma

Thomas F. Rehring, MD
Clinical Assistant Professor, Division of Vascular Surgery, Department of Surgery, University of Colorado School of Medicine. Chief, Endovascular Surgery, Colorado Permanente Medical Group, and St. Joseph's Hospital, Denver, Colorado
Aortic Graft Limb Thrombosis

Michael A. Ricci, MD
Roger H. Allbee Professor of Surgery, University of Vermont College of Medicine, Burlington, Vermont
Evaluating Cerebrovascular Symptoms

John J. Ricotta, MD
Professor and Chair, Department of Surgery, State University of New York at Stony Brook School of Medicine. Chief of Surgery, University Hospital, Stony Brook, New York
Carotid Plus Coronary Disease

Thomas S. Riles, MD
Professor and Chairman, Department of Surgery, New York University School of Medicine, New York, New York
Recurrent Carotid Stenosis

Caron Rockman, MD
Assistant Professor of Medicine and Director of Clinical Research, Division of Vascular Surgery, Department of Surgery, New York University School of Medicine. Attending Surgeon, Division of Vascular Surgery, Tisch Hospital, Bellevue Hospital, and Manhattan VA Hospital, New York, New York
Recurrent Carotid Stenosis

Sean P. Roddy, MD
Assistant Professor of Surgery, Albany Medical College. Attending Surgeon, Institute for Vascular Health and Disease, Albany, New York
Acute Stroke

James H. Rothstein, MD
Vascular Surgeon, National Naval Medical Center, Bethesda, Maryland
Carotid Artery Aneurysm

Robert B. Rutherford, MD
Emeritus Professor of Surgery, University of Colorado School of Medicine, Denver, Colorado
Acute Limb Ischemia; Subclavian-Axillary Vein Thrombosis; Varicose Veins; Congenital Vascular Malformations

Richard J. Sanders, MD
Clinical Professor of Surgery, University of Colorado School of Medicine. Attending Surgeon, Rose Medical Center, Denver, Colorado
Neurogenic Thoracic Outlet Syndrome

Marc L. Schermerhorn, MD
Assistant Professor of Surgery, Dartmouth Hitchcock Medical Center, Lebanon, New Hampshire
Abdominal Aortic Aneurysm

Peter A. Schneider, MD
Vascular and Endovascular Surgeon and Chief, Division of Vascular Therapy, Hawaii Permanente Medical Group, Honolulu, Hawaii
Fibromuscular Disease of the Carotid Artery

James M. Seeger, MD
Professor and Associate Chairman, Department of Surgery, University of Florida School of Medicine. Chief, Division of Vascular Surgery, J. Hillis Miller Health Center, Gainesville, Florida
Transfusion Strategies

Cynthia C. Shortell, MD
Associate Professor of Surgery and Hematology, University of Rochester School of Medicine and Dentistry, Rochester, New York
Intraoperative Hemorrhage and Bleeding Diathesis

Michael B. Silva, Jr., MD
Professor and Chief, Vascular Surgery and Vascular Interventional Radiology, Department of Surgery, Texas Tech University Health Sciences Center School of Medicine, Lubbock, Texas
Vascular Access for Hemodialysis

Donald Silver, MD
Professor Emeritus of Surgery, University of Missouri–Columbia School of Medicine. Staff Surgeon, University of Missouri Health Care, Columbia, Missouri
Heparin-Induced Complications

Gregory T. Simonian, MD
Clinical Instructor II, Department of Surgery, UMDNJ–New Jersey Medical School, Newark. Chief, Division of Endovascular Studies, Hackensack University Medical Center, Hackensack, New Jersey
Stroke Following Carotid Endarterectomy

John J. Skillman, MD
Professor of Surgery, Harvard Medical School. Surgeon, Division of Vascular Surgery, Beth Israel Deaconess Medical Center, Boston, Massachusetts
Superficial Phlebitis

James C. Stanley, MD
Professor of Surgery, University of Michigan Medical School. Head, Section of Vascular Surgery, University Hospital, Ann Arbor, Michigan
Renovascular Occlusive Disease: Treatment

Yaron Sternbach, MD
Assistant Professor, Division of Vascular Surgery, Department of Surgery, University of Rochester School of Medicine. Attending Surgeon, Strong Memorial Hospital, Rochester, New York
Subclavian Artery Occlusive Disease

Lars G. Svensson, MD, PhD
Professor, Division of Cardiothoracic Surgery, Department of Surgery, Tufts University School of Medicine, Boston. Director, Center for Aortic Surgery, Lahey Clinic, Burlington, Massachusetts
Aortic Dissection

Jonathan B. Towne, MD
Professor and Chairman of Vascular Surgery, Department of Surgery, Medical College of Wisconsin. Staff Surgeon, Froedtert Memorial Lutheran Hospital, Milwaukee, Wisconsin
Diabetic Foot Infections

William D. Turnipseed, MD
Professor of Surgery, University of Wisconsin Medical School. Chief, Vascular Surgery, University Health Hospital and Clinics, Madison, Wisconsin
Compartment Syndromes

Gilbert R. Upchurch, Jr., MD
Assistant Professor of Surgery, University of Michigan Medical School. Attending Surgeon, Section of Vascular Surgery, University Hospital, Ann Arbor, Michigan
Renovascular Occlusive Disease: Treatment

Scott Van Duzer, MD
Surgical Resident, Department of Surgery, Temple University Hospital, Philadelphia, Pennsylvania
Chronic Critical Limb Ischemia

Angela Vouyouka, MD
Resident Physician in Vascular Surgery, University of Missouri–Columbia School of Medicine, Columbia, Missouri
Heparin-Induced Complications

Thomas W. Wakefield, MD
Professor, Section of Vascular Surgery, Department of Surgery, University of Michigan Medical School. Staff Surgeon and Director, Noninvasive Vascular Laboratory, University of Michigan Hospital and Ann Arbor Veterans Administration Medical Center, Ann Arbor, Michigan
Hypercoagulable Syndrome

Daniel B. Walsh, MD
Professor of Surgery and Vice Chair, Department of Surgery, Dartmouth Hitchcock Medical Center, Lebanon, New Hamphire
Infrainguinal Graft Thrombosis

Fred A. Weaver, MD
Professor of Surgery, Keck School of Medicine of the University of Southern California, Los Angeles, California
Extremity Vascular Trauma

John V. White, MD
Chairman, Department of Surgery, Lutheran General Hospital, Park Ridge, Illinois
Chronic Critical Limb Ischemia

Anthony D. Whittemore, MD
Professor of Surgery, Harvard Medical School. Chief, Division of Vascular Surgery, Brigham and Women's Hospital, Boston, Massachusetts
Infrainguinal Occlusive Disease

James M. Wong, MD
Vascular Fellow, Department of General Surgery, Wake Forest University School of Medicine, Winston-Salem, North Carolina
Renovascular Occlusive Disease: Evaluation

Gerald B. Zelenock, MD
Chairman, Department of Surgery, and Chief, Surgical Services, William Beaumont Hospital, Royal Oak, Michigan
Hepatic and Renal Artery Aneurysms

Robert M. Zwolak, MD, PhD
Professor of Surgery, Dartmouth Hitchcock Medical Center, Lebanon, New Hampshire
Chronic Mesenteric Ischemia

PREFACE

Correct decision making is central to good surgical outcome. It is, arguably, more difficult to master than surgical technique. Nowhere is this truer than in vascular surgery because of the complexity and diversity of the treatment options available and the associated co-morbidity of the affected patients. Recent developments in endovascular surgery have further increased the difficulty of decision making.

This book codifies decision making in vascular surgery and represents this in stepwise algorithms that are broadly applicable. This is a difficult process that exposes the gaps in our underlying data and reflects the biases that result from our own experience. Furthermore, the application of these algorithms to individual patients is sufficiently imprecise that they cannot be applied in an absolute manner because of unique aspects that cannot be included in a generic algorithm. These concerns notwithstanding, we believe that explicit decision-making algorithms, written by experts in this field, can be quite useful. To the extent that they point out missing data and different opinions, they highlight areas for future study. We hope that they will provide both a resource for vascular practitioners and a source of instruction for vascular trainees.

We have selected 75 topics for this book that require decision making in vascular surgery. Authors with extensive experience in each area have been asked to analyze and codify their decision-making process in algorithm form and to annotate it with commentary and references that explain the basis for their decisions. When there is not a clear-cut choice between options, this has been indicated and the options discussed. We are grateful for the effort of each contributor and acknowledge the difficulty involved in the preparation of these unique chapters.

Surgical decision making is a fascinating aspect of patient management, one that requires precise thinking, careful data analysis, and considerable experience. We have been stimulated and influenced by the pioneering textbook *Surgical Decision Making,* originally published in 1978, by Drs. Ben Eiseman and Roger S. Wothyns, with subsequent editions by Norton, Steele, and Eiseman. We also acknowledge the publication *Decision Making in Vascular Surgery,* by Drs. Scribner, Brown, and Tawes, in 1987. In the intervening years, vascular surgery has expanded to become a distinct surgical discipline, with even more complex decision making. For this reason, we were stimulated to develop the current text. We are grateful for the assistance of the editorial staff at W.B. Saunders Company for their careful rendering of these complex algorithms.

JACK L. CRONENWETT

ROBERT B. RUTHERFORD

NOTICE

Medicine is an ever-changing field. Standard safety precautions must be followed, but as new research and clinical experience broaden our knowledge, changes in treatment and drug therapy may become necessary or appropriate. Readers are advised to check the most current product information provided by the manufacturer of each drug to be administered to verify the recommended dose, the method and duration of administration, and contraindications. It is the responsibility of the treating physician, relying on experience and knowledge of the patient, to determine dosages and the best treatment for each individual patient. Neither the Publisher nor the editor assumes any liability for any injury and/or damage to persons or property arising from this publication.

THE PUBLISHER

CONTENTS

GENERAL TOPICS, 1

1
Preoperative Cardiac Risk Assessment, 2
JAMES B. FROEHLICH, MD
KIM A. EAGLE, MD

2
Management of Hyperlipidemia, 6
WILLIAM R. HIATT, MD
MARK R. NEHLER, MD

3
Hypercoagulable Syndrome, 8
PETER K. HENKE, MD
THOMAS W. WAKEFIELD, MD

4
Perioperative Care and Anesthesia, 12
KATHLEEN CHAIMBERG, MD

5
Transfusion Strategies, 14
THOMAS S. HUBER, MD, PhD
JAMES M. SEEGER, MD

CEREBROVASCULAR DISEASE, 21

6
Evaluating Cerebrovascular Symptoms, 22
MICHAEL A. RICCI, MD

7
Symptomatic Carotid Artery Stenosis, 28
ALIK FARBER, MD
JACK L. CRONENWETT, MD

8
Asymptomatic Carotid Artery Stenosis, 34
ALIK FARBER, MD
JACK L. CRONENWETT, MD

9
Carotid Endarterectomy, 38
JOSEPH P. ARCHIE, PhD, MD
R. DAVID EDRINGTON, MD

10
Recurrent Carotid Stenosis, 44
CARON ROCKMAN, MD
THOMAS S. RILES, MD

11
Acute Stroke, 50
SEAN P. RODDY, MD
WILLIAM C. MACKEY, MD

12
Carotid Artery Aneurysm, 54
JAMES H. ROTHSTEIN, MD
JERRY GOLDSTONE, MD

13
Carotid Dissection, 58
LAURA K. PAK, MD
LOUIS M. MESSINA, MD

14
Fibromuscular Disease of the Carotid Artery, 62
PETER A. SCHNEIDER, MD

15
Carotid Body Tumors, 66
GLENN M. LA MURAGLIA, MD
FARZIN ADILI, MD

16
Stroke Following Carotid Endarterectomy, 70
GREGORY T. SIMONIAN, MD
ROBERT W. HOBSON II, MD

17
Vertebral Artery Disease, 74
LISA FLYNN, MD
RAMON BERGUER, MD, PhD

18
Subclavian Artery Occlusive Disease, 76
BRUCE A. PERLER, MD
YARON STERNBACH, MD

19
Brachiocephalic Arterial Occlusive Disease, 80
AUDRA A. NOEL, MD
KENNETH J. CHERRY, JR., MD

20
Carotid Plus Coronary Disease, 84
JOHN J. RICOTTA, MD
THOMAS BILFINGER, MD, ScD
YARA GORSKI, MD

ANEURYSMS, 89

21
Abdominal Aortic Aneurysm, 90
MARC L. SCHERMERHORN, MD
JACK L. CRONENWETT, MD

22
Thoracoabdominal Aortic Aneurysm, 98
RICHARD P. CAMBRIA, MD

23
Ruptured Abdominal Aortic Aneurysm, 104
JOHN W. HALLETT, JR., MD
TODD E. RASMUSSEN, MD

24
Aortovenous Fistula, 108
M. ASHRAF MANSOUR, MD

25
Aortoenteric Fistula, 112
SEAN P. O'BRIEN, MD
CALVIN B. ERNST, MD

26
Sigmoid Ischemia After Aortic Surgery, 118
PETER G. KALMAN, MD
K. WAYNE JOHNSTON, MD

27
Endovascular Abdominal Aortic Aneurysm Repair, 120
MARK FILLINGER, MD

28
Aortic Dissection, 128
ANTHONY W. DiSCIPIO, MD
LARS G. SVENSSON, MD, PhD

29
Iliac Artery Aneurysm, 132
WILLIAM C. KRUPSKI, MD
MARK R. NEHLER, MD

30
Femoral Artery Aneurysm, 136
MARK R. NEHLER, MD
WILLIAM C. KRUPSKI, MD

31
Femoral Artery Pseudoaneurysm from Trauma, 142
DANIEL J. REDDY, MD

32
Popliteal Artery Aneurysm, 146
RICHARD J. POWELL, MD

33
Hepatic and Renal Artery Aneurysms, 150
GERALD B. ZELENOCK, MD

EXTREMITY OCCLUSIVE DISEASE, 155

34
Patients with Leg Pain While Walking, 156
MARTHA McDANIEL, MD

35
Chronic Critical Limb Ischemia, 162
JOHN V. WHITE, MD
SCOTT VAN DUZER, MD

36
Acute Limb Ischemia, 168
ROBERT B. RUTHERFORD, MD

37
Atheroembolism, 172
JEFFREY L. KAUFMAN, MD

38
Aortoiliac Disease, 176
JACK L. CRONENWETT, MD

39
Aortic Graft Limb Thrombosis, 180
THOMAS F. REHRING, MD
DAVID C. BREWSTER, MD

40
Aortic Graft Infection, 186
MARK R. JACKSON, MD
G. PATRICK CLAGETT, MD

41
Infrainguinal Occlusive Disease, 192
M. C. DONALDSON, MD
ANTHONY D. WHITTEMORE, MD

42
Infrainguinal Graft Surveillance, 198
DENNIS F. BANDYK, MD

43
Infrainguinal Graft Thrombosis, 204
DANIEL B. WALSH, MD

44
Infrainguinal Prosthetic Graft Infection, 208
KEITH D. CALLIGARO, MD

45
Diabetic Foot Infections, 212
JONATHAN B. TOWNE, MD

46
Amputation Level, 218
ROBERT E. CARLIN, MD
BLAIR A. KEAGY, MD

47
Compartment Syndromes, 222
WILLIAM D. TURNIPSEED, MD

48
Popliteal Artery Entrapment Syndrome and Popliteal Cystic Adventitial Disease, 228
LEWIS LEVIEN, MB, BCh, PhD(Med)

49
Upper Extremity Ischemia, 232
MARK D. MORASCH, MD
WILLIAM H. PEARCE, MD

RENOVASCULAR DISEASE, 237

50
Renovascular Occlusive Disease: Evaluation, 238
JAMES M. WONG, MD
KIMBERLEY J. HANSEN, MD

51
Renovascular Occlusive Disease: Treatment, 242
JAMES C. STANLEY, MD
GILBERT R. UPCHURCH, JR., MD

52
Acute Mesenteric Ischemia, 250
TINA R. DESAI, MD
BRUCE L. GEWERTZ, MD

53
Chronic Mesenteric Ischemia, 256
PETER R. NELSON, MD
ROBERT M. ZWOLAK, MD, PhD

VENOUS DISEASE, 261

54
Subclavian-Axillary Vein Thrombosis, 262
ROBERT B. RUTHERFORD, MD
SCOTT HURLBERT, MD

55
Superficial Phlebitis, 268
JOHN J. SKILLMAN, MD

56
Lower Extremity Deep Vein Thrombosis, 272
MARK H. MEISSNER, MD

57
Iliofemoral Deep Vein Thrombosis, 282
ANTHONY J. COMEROTA, MD

58
Pulmonary Embolism, 286
LAZAR J. GREENFIELD, MD
MARY C. PROCTOR, MS

59
Varicose Veins, 290
ROBERT B. RUTHERFORD, MD

60
Deep Vein Insufficiency: Evaluation and Conservative Management, 294
AHMED M. ABOU-ZAMZAM, MD
GREGORY L. MONETA, MD

61
Deep Vein Insufficiency: Surgical Treatment, 298
ROBERT L. KISTNER, MD
BO EKLOF, MD, PhD

MISCELLANEOUS TOPICS, 305

62
Portal Hypertension, 306
KAJ H. JOHANSEN, MD, PhD

63
Lymphedema, 312
AUDRA A. NOEL, MD
PETER GLOVICZKI, MD

64
Brachiocephalic Vascular Trauma, 318
MALCOLM O. PERRY, MD
KENNETH E. McINTYRE, JR, MD

65
Abdominal Vascular Trauma, 324
JAMES T. LEE, MD
FRED S. BONGARD, MD

66
Extremity Vascular Trauma, 332
S. RAM KUMAR, MD
DOUGLAS B. HOOD, MD
FRED A. WEAVER, MD

67
Post-traumatic Pain Syndrome, 336
ALI F. ABURAHMA, MD

68
Neurogenic Thoracic Outlet Syndrome, 340
RICHARD J. SANDERS, MD
SHARON L. HAMMOND, MD

69
Raynaud's Syndrome, 342
GREGORY J. LANDRY, MD
JOHN M. PORTER, MD

70
Erectile Dysfunction, 346
RALPH G. DePALMA, MD

71
Congenital Vascular Malformations, 350
ROBERT B. RUTHERFORD, MD

72
Vascular Access for Hemodialysis, 354
MICHAEL B. SILVA, JR., MD
BRAJESH K. LAL, MD

73
Takayasu's Disease, 360
JOSEPH M. GIORDANO, MD

74
Intraoperative Hemorrhage and Bleeding Diathesis, 364
CYNTHIA C. SHORTELL, MD
KENNETH OURIEL, MD

75
Heparin-Induced Complications, 370
DONALD SILVER, MD
ANGELA VOUYOUKA, MD

Index, 375

GENERAL TOPICS

Chapter 1 Preoperative Cardiac Risk Assessment

JAMES B. FROEHLICH, MD • KIM A. EAGLE, MD

(A) Perioperative cardiac complications are a major source of morbidity and mortality for patients undergoing vascular surgery. Accurate assessment of the severity of cardiac disease and perioperative cardiac risk is therefore critical in this patient population. Furthermore, cardiac disease is the leading cause of late death with peripheral vascular disease. Preoperative cardiac assessment, therefore, offers an important opportunity for evaluation and intervention to prevent not only perioperative but also long-term cardiac complications. This is not a process of "clearing" patients for surgery but, rather, a process of assessing risk by employing selective stress testing or cardiac catheterization in high-risk patients to identify patients for whom coronary revascularization or medical intervention carries long-term benefit. This information can be used to optimize perioperative risk and to facilitate informed surgical decision making. This algorithm for cardiac risk assessment is based on the American College of Cardiology/American Heart Association Guidelines.[1]

(B) Assessment of perioperative risk is superfluous if the patient's need for surgery is emergent. Otherwise, assessment of cardiac risk may carry important long-term prognostic implications.

(C) Patients who have had adequate coronary revascularization within the previous 5 years, without any recurrent angina symptoms, have been shown in previous studies to have a low risk of perioperative complication.[2-4] Data from the Cleveland Clinic revealed a very low complication rate after vascular surgery in patients who had undergone previous coronary artery bypass surgery regardless of their clinical risk.[2] Another study, looking at registry data from the Coronary Artery Surgery Study (CASS), also showed a protective effect from previous coronary artery bypass surgery for patients undergoing vascular surgery.[4]

(D) As patients often present repeatedly for vascular procedures, a recent (within the previous 2 years), adequate, unremarkable functional assessment should suffice for cardiac evaluation. It is incumbent upon the consultant to ascertain that this stress test has been adequate and that there have been no changes in the patient's clinical status.

(E) An accurate and rigorous clinical evaluation of the patient is the keystone to effective cardiac risk assessment.[10] Early studies identified those clinical factors that carry significant risk of perioperative complications, including (1) severe aortic stenosis, (2) active congestive heart failure, (3) unstable angina, and (4) recent acute myocardial infarction.[5] Patients with these unstable or uncompensated cardiac conditions represent sufficiently prohibitive risk that consideration should be given to cancellation of the planned surgery and cardiac catheterization to accurately define cardiac physiology and coronary anatomy.

Several groups have identified clinical markers of perioperative risk.[6-9] Excluding markers of severe risk, the most consistent clinical risk factors include age older than 70 years and a history of the following:

- Angina
- Myocardial infarction (as shown by either history or electrocardiogram)
- Congestive heart failure (either on examination or by history)
- Diabetes

The absence of all of these markers of risk has correlated with a very low clinical risk, comparable to that associated with a normal functional study.[7] This suggests that further functional analysis in this group is unnecessary. The presence of one or two of these factors correlates clinically with moderate risk of perioperative coronary events[7] and with an intermediate (~50%) incidence of angiographically significant coronary disease.[6] The presence of three or more of these factors has been associated with a high incidence of perioperative clinical events and a high likelihood of angiographically significant coronary disease.[6,7] The benefit of stress testing in the "high-risk" subset may be at times debatable, because there is such a high pretest probability of significant coronary disease that even a negative stress test result is associated with significant risk.[7,14] Therefore, selected high-risk patients should undergo cardiac catheterization.

(F) Functional capacity by history, or patients' ability to exert themselves, is a useful adjunct to the clinical evaluation. An important element of the clinical evaluation is the presence or absence of angina. If the patient reports a very low functional capacity, this renders the assessment of anginal symptoms unreliable. For this reason, patients with a poor exercise capacity cannot truly be said to be angina-free; they should therefore be considered for noninvasive testing before surgery unless no other clinical markers of risk are present and the contemplated surgery is low risk. Several studies corroborate a favorable risk associated with a high functional capacity.[11,12]

Daily activities can be used to estimate functional capacity.[13] Some of these are as follows:

- Dressing without stopping or without symptoms, 2 METs (metabolic equivalents)
- Walking 2.5 mph, 3 METs
- Bowling or taking a shower, 4 METs
- Stripping and making the bed, 4 to 5 METs
- Gardening, dancing, having sexual intercourse, 5 to 6 METs
- Walking 4 mph or walking up stairs, 5 to 6 METs
- Participating in recreational sports (squash, tennis) 7 to 10 METs
- Running 5 mph, 9 METs

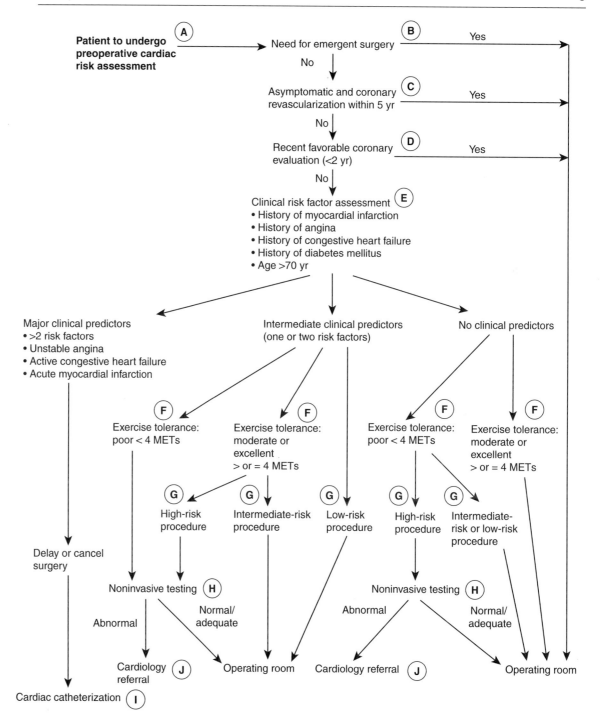

G The type of anticipated surgery also confers risk for cardiovascular complications. Most of this attendant risk is the result of increased likelihood of co-morbid coronary disease, such as in patients with peripheral vascular disease undergoing vascular surgery. Some surgical procedures impart greater cardiovascular stress as well.

High-risk surgery includes procedures with reported cardiac event rates greater than 5%. Among vascular operations, higher cardiac stress is associated with aortic clamping (especially supraceliac) and procedures associated with extensive blood loss.

Intermediate-risk surgery includes procedures with cardiac event risk generally reported between 1% and 5% and comprises most elective vascular surgery procedures.

Low-risk surgery, associated with cardiac event rates below 1%, includes only minor vascular procedures.

H The preferred screening modality is exercise electrocardiography, with or without an imaging modality, such as echocardiography or thallium nuclear scanning. Exercise testing offers additional prognostic information by determining achievable heart rate and workload capacity. Many patients with peripheral vascular disease, however, cannot undergo exercise testing.

Dobutamine echocardiography and adenosine thallium functional testing generally have excellent negative predictive value and high sensitivity for identifying patients at risk for cardiac complications of surgery. The specificity and positive predictive value, however, are quite low. Selective testing using this clinical screening algorithm improves these values.

At many institutions, dobutamine echocardiography and adenosine thallium are equally effective tools for evaluating cardiac ischemia. If an institutional strength exists, one should consider this fact when choosing between them. Dobutamine echocardiography offers the advantage of evaluating ventricular function as well as cardiac valvular anatomy and function. It may be limited when images are inadequate, such as in chronic obstructive pulmonary disease or obesity. Adenosine thallium nuclear scanning may be preferable when heart rate response is compromised, such as with a pacemaker or β blocker dependency. It may fail to detect balanced multivessel coronary artery disease.

Patients with evidence of coronary ischemia on stress testing should be referred for cardiology consultation before surgery. Consideration should be given to cardiac catheterization in patients whose functional assessment suggests the presence of symptomatic or multivessel coronary artery disease or left ventricular dysfunction with coronary ischemia.[15] Specifically, catheterization should be considered in those patients with ischemia documented at less than 7 METS on exercise testing, ischemia with left ventricular dilation and/or increased lung uptake of tracer on thallium testing, ischemia with left ventricular dilation on echocardiographic assessment, left ventricular dysfunction, or ischemia documented in multiple coronary vessel territories.[15]

(I) The results of cardiac catheterization usually clarify subsequent management. Patients with *one-vessel* or *two-vessel* disease and a normal left ventricular (LV) ejection fraction may undergo percutaneous transluminal angioplasty (PTA) and stenting at the discretion of the cardiologist, or they may simply be managed by β blockade. Patients with *three-vessel* or left main disease and those with *two-vessel* disease involving the left anterior descending artery or with a low ejection fraction are at higher risk. If revascularization is feasible, coronary artery bypass is recommended; if not, one should reconsider the indications to perform major vascular surgery, the severity of its physiologic challenge to the patient, and whether there are less stressful methods of managing the problem.

(J) The cardiologist, after reviewing the dobutamine echocardiogram or adenosine thallium scan, LV function, and exercise tolerance together with the clinical picture, should advise the patient regarding the best strategy. For example, patients with ischemia in a two-vessel territory, with a lower ejection fraction and symptoms at less than 7 METs would probably need cardiac catheterization, whereas patients with normal LV function, good exercise tolerance (>10 METs) and single-vessel distribution ischemia would probably undergo the planned surgery with metoprolol or bisoprolol β blockade.

REFERENCES

1. Eagle KA, Brundage BH, Chaitman BR, et al: Guidelines for perioperative cardiovascular evaluation for noncardiac surgery: Report of the American College of Cardiology/American Heart Association Task Force on Practice Guidelines: Committee on Perioperative Cardiovascular Evaluation for Noncardiac Surgery. Circulation 1996;93(6):1278–1317.
2. Paul SD, L'Italien GJ, Hendel RC, et al: Influence of prior heart disease on morbidity and mortality after vascular surgery: Role of coronary artery bypass grafting. J Am Coll Cardiol 1994;1A–484A.
3. Mahar LJ, Steen PA, Tinker JH, et al: Perioperative myocardial infarction in patients with coronary artery disease with and without aorto-coronary artery bypass grafts. J Thorac Cardiovasc Surg 1978;76:533–537.
4. Eagle KA, Rihal CS, Mickel MC, et al: Cardiac risk of noncardiac surgery: Influence of coronary disease and type of surgery in 3368 operations. Circulation 1997;96:1882–1887.
5. Goldman L, Caldera DL, Nussbaum SR, et al: Multifactorial index of cardiac risk in noncardiac surgical procedures. N Engl J Med 1977;297:845–850.
6. Paul S, Eagle KA, Young JR, Hertzer NR: Coronary heart disease/myocardial infarction: Concordance of preoperative clinical risk with angiographic severity of coronary artery disease in patients undergoing vascular surgery. Circulation 1996;94:1561–1566.
7. Eagle KA, Coley CM, Newell JB, et al: Combining clinical and thallium data optimizes preoperative assessment of cardiac risk before major vascular surgery. Ann Intern Med 1989;110:859–866.
8. Detsky AS, Abrams HB, McLaughlin JR, et al: Predicting cardiac complications in patients undergoing non-cardiac surgery. J Gen Intern Med 1986;1:211–219.
9. Mangano DT, Browner WS, Hollenberg M, et al: Association of perioperative myocardial ischemia with cardiac morbidity and mortality in men undergoing noncardiac surgery: The Study of Perioperative Ischemia Research Group. N Engl J Med 1990;323:1781–1788.
10. Hubbard BL, Gibbons RJ, Lapeyre AC III, et al: Identification of severe coronary artery disease using simple clinical parameters. Arch Intern Med 1992;152:309–312.
11. Cutler BS, Wheeler HB, Paraskos JA, Cardulla PA: Applicability and interpretation of electrocardiographic stress testing in patients with peripheral vascular disease. Am J Surg 1981;141:501–506.
12. McPhail N, Clavin JE, Shariatmadar A, et al: The use of preoperative exercise testing to predict cardiac complications after arterial reconstruction. J Vasc Surg 1988;7:60–68.
13. Goldman L, Hashimoto B, Cook EF, Loscalzo A: Comparative reproducibility and validity of systems for assessing cardiovascular functional class: Advantages of a new specific activity scale. Circulation 1981;64(6):1227–1234.
14. L'Italien GJ, Paul SD, Hendel RC, et al: Development and validation of a Bayesian model for perioperative cardiac risk assessment in a cohort of 1081 vascular surgical candidates. J Am Coll Cardiol 1996;27(4):799–802.
15. Scanlon PJ, Faxon DP, Faxon Audet A, et al: ACC/AHA guidelines for coronary angiography: A report of the American College of Cardiology/American Heart Association Task Force on Practice Guidelines (Committee on Coronary Angiography) developed in collaboration with the Society for Cardiac Angiography and Interventions. J Am Coll Cardiol 1999;33:1756–1824.

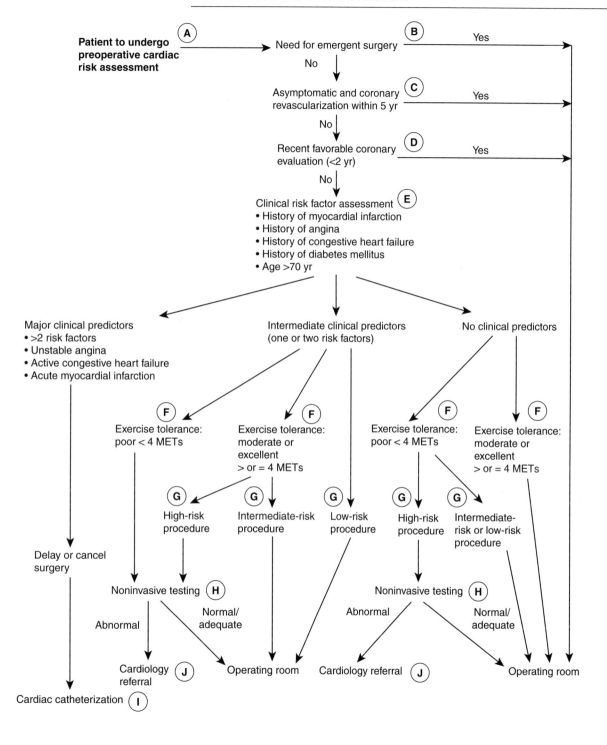

Chapter 2 Management of Hyperlipidemia

WILLIAM R. HIATT, MD • MARK R. NEHLER, MD

(A) Patients with clinically apparent atherosclerotic peripheral arterial disease (PAD) should undergo testing for hyperlipidemia. This commonly includes (1) patients with an abnormal ankle/brachial index (ABI < 0.90) or history of previous peripheral bypass surgery or angioplasty and (2) patients with internal carotid artery stenosis on duplex scanning or a history of previous carotid surgery. Obviously, these criteria apply to patients with known coronary artery disease as well.

(B) Accurate testing for hyperlipidemia requires a 12-hour fast prior to blood sampling. The measured values include total cholesterol, *high-density* lipoprotein (HDL) cholesterol, and triglycerides. The *low-density* lipoprotein (LDL) cholesterol (chol) concentration is calculated as follows:

LDL chol = total chol − (triglycerides/5 + HDL chol)

This correlates well with direct measurement of LDL cholesterol in both diabetic and nondiabetic patients without hypertryglyceridemia.[1] If the triglyceride concentration is above 400 mg/dL, LDL cholesterol should be measured directly.[2]

(C) HDL cholesterols are favorable lipoproteins for protection from atherosclerosis, and therapy is only indicated for *low* values (in contrast to *high* values for triglycerides and LDL cholesterol). Low levels of HDL cholesterol are associated with increased risk for coronary artery disease events.[3] The National Cholesterol Education Program (NCEP) guidelines for instituting therapy for low levels of HDL cholesterol are as shown for men and women.[4] Elevated triglycerides and low HDL cholesterol levels are the two most common lipid abnormalities in diabetic patients.[5–8] Therapy includes diet, aerobic exercise, and medication.

(D) Aerobic exercise (20 to 40 minutes/day, 5 days/week) is the initial therapy for low HDL cholesterol levels. If these measures are unsuccessful, drug therapy with niacin starting at 500 mg/day, up to 1500 to 2000 mg/day, and/or fibrates (gemfibrozil 600 mg PO twice a day) is the treatment of choice.[9] Lipid levels are monitored every 4 weeks to guide therapy until target levels are achieved.

(E) LDL cholesterol is the lipid subgroup considered to pose the greatest atherogenic risk.[10] In multiple epidemiologic studies, elevated LDL cholesterol levels (>130 mg/dL) in patients with cardiovascular disease has been shown to increase the cardiovascular mortality by 3-fold to 6-fold.[7,11] The ability of statin drugs to effectively reduce LDL cholesterol has been the basis of multiple clinical trials examining efficacy in LDL cholesterol reduction to lower cardiovascular morbidity and mortality.[12,13]

(F) Patients with LDL cholesterol levels below 100 mg/dL require no specific therapy. Evaluation should be repeated periodically, depending on other risk factors and potential progression of atherosclerosis. Only a small percentage of the population of patients with vascular disease has baseline LDL cholesterol levels below 100 mg/dL.[14]

(G) The American Diabetes Association recommends aggressive intervention to bring the LDL cholesterol level to below 100 mg/dL in diabetic patients.[15] This is in part related to the greater incidence of reduced HDL cholesterol and elevated triglycerides in these patient populations, with only modest LDL cholesterol elevation.[16] In nondiabetic patients, the efficacy of such strict guidelines is currently unproven, but diet therapy seems prudent as initial treatment in such instances. The diet would feature low fat content with restriction of high-cholesterol foods (e.g., eggs, cheese, organ meats).

(H) NCEP guidelines recommend drug therapy for patients with PAD and LDL cholesterol levels above 130 mg/dL.[4] As stated earlier in E., the statins are the lipid-lowering drug of choice for this indication.[17–19] Simvastatin, starting at 5 mg/day and doubling the dose every 4 weeks up to 80 mg/day based on the results of repeated lipid testing, is appropriate. Pravastatin, atorvastatin, and other statins are also acceptable agents. Bile resin–binding agents (cholestyramine) and fibrates (gemfibrozil) are considered second-line drugs because of the increased incidence of side effects (i.e., gastrointestinal and myositis, respectively).

(I) As stated earlier, elevated triglyceride levels are frequently observed in diabetic patients.[16] Large epidemiologic studies of diabetes mellitus demonstrate triglyceride levels above 150 mg/dL in more than 10%.[16,20] One meta-analysis has demonstrated increased cardiac mortality for women and men (76% and 31%, respectively), with elevated triglyceride levels.[21]

(J) The initial therapy for elevated triglyceride levels includes weight reduction and aerobic exercise (see HDL therapy). Initial drug therapy is gemfibrozil 600 mg twice a day. Patients taking gemfibrozil need to be monitored for symptoms of myositis. A second-line agent is niacin 500 mg/day, increased to 1500 to 2000 mg/day. Patients taking niacin should be monitored for worsening glucose control and hepatic function. Many of these patients also need statin therapy to treat an elevated LDL cholesterol level.

REFERENCES

1. Branchi A, Rovellini A, Torri A, Sommariva D: Accuracy of calculated serum low-density lipoprotein cholesterol for the assessment of coronary heart disease risk in NIDDM patients. Diabetes Care 1998;21:1397–1402.
2. McNamara JR, Cohn JS, Wilson PW, Schaefer EJ: Calculated values for low-density lipoprotein cholesterol in the assessment of lipid abnormalities and coronary disease risk. Clin Chem 1990;36:36–42.
3. Rader DJ: Pathophysiology and management of low high-density lipoprotein cholesterol. Am J Cardiol 1999;83:22F–24F.
4. Summary of the second report of the National Cholesterol Education Program (NCEP) expert panel on detection,

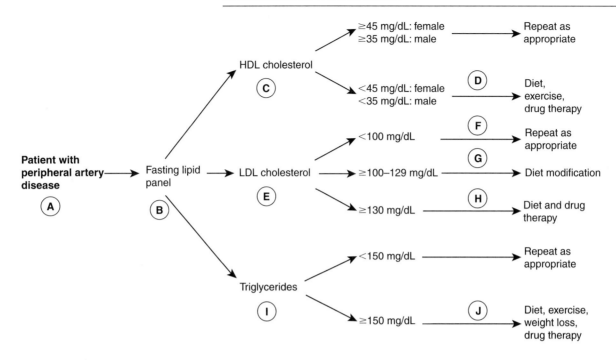

evaluation, and treatment of high blood cholesterol in adults (Adult Treatment Panel II). JAMA 1993;329:3015–3023.
5. Laakso M: Lipids and lipoproteins as risk factors for coronary heart disease in non–insulin-dependent diabetes mellitus. Ann Med 1996;28:341–345.
6. Feingold KR, Grunfeld C, Pang M, et al: LDL subclass phenotypes and triglyceride metabolism in non–insulin-dependent diabetes. Arterioscler Thromb 1992;12:1496–1502.
7. Austin MA, Breslow JL, Hennekens CH, et al: Low-density lipoprotein subclass patterns and risk of myocardial infarction. JAMA 1988;260:1917–1921.
8. Fontbonne A, Eschwege E, Cambien F, et al: Hypertriglyceridaemia as a risk factor of coronary heart disease mortality in subjects with impaired glucose tolerance or diabetes: Results from the 11-year follow-up of the Paris Prospective Study. Diabetologia 1989;32:300–304.
9. Sposito AC, Caramelli B, Serrano CVJ, et al: Effect of niacin and etofibrate association on subjects with coronary artery disease and serum high-density lipoprotein cholesterol <35 mg/dl. Am J Cardiol 1999;83:98–100, A8.
10. Nielsen LB: Atherogenicity of lipoprotein(a) and oxidized low density lipoprotein: Insight from in vivo studies of arterial wall influx, degradation and efflux. Atherosclerosis 1999;143:229–243.
11. LaRosa JC: Cholesterol and cardiovascular disease: How strong is the evidence? Clin Cardiol 1992;15:III2–III7.
12. Kong SX, Crawford SY, Gandhi SK, et al: Efficacy of 3-hydroxy-3-methylglutaryl coenzyme a reductase inhibitors in the treatment of patients with hypercholesterolemia: A meta-analysis of clinical trials. Clin Ther 1997;19:778–797.
13. Waters D, Higginson L, Gladstone P, et al: Design features of a controlled clinical trial to assess the effect of an HMG CoA reductase inhibitor on the progression of coronary artery disease: Canadian Coronary Atherosclerosis Intervention Trial Investigators, Montreal, Ottawa, and Toronto, Canada. Control Clin Trials 1993;14:45–74.
14. McDermott MM, Mehta S, Ahn H, Greenland P: Atherosclerotic risk factors are less intensively treated in patients with peripheral arterial disease than in patients with coronary artery disease. J Gen Intern Med 1997;12:209–215.
15. American Diabetes Association: Management of dyslipidemia in adults with diabetes [see comments]. Diabetes Care 1998;21:179–182.
16. Connelly PW, Petrasovits A, Stachenko S, et al: Prevalence of high plasma triglyceride combined with low HDL-C levels and its association with smoking, hypertension, obesity, diabetes, sedentariness and LDL-C levels in the Canadian population: Canadian Heart Health Surveys Research Group. Can J Cardiol 1999;15:428–433.
17. Gould AL, Rossouw JE, Santanello NC, et al: Cholesterol reduction yields clinical benefit: Impact of statin trials. Circulation 1998;97:946–952.
18. Grundy SM: Statin trials and goals of cholesterol-lowering therapy. Circulation 1998;97:1436–1439.
19. Scandinavian Simvastatin Survival Study Group: Randomised trial of cholesterol lowering in 4444 patients with coronary heart disease: The Scandinavian Simvastatin Survival Study (4S). Lancet 1994;344:1383–1389.
20. MacGregor AS, Price JF, Hau CM, et al: Role of systolic blood pressure and plasma triglycerides in diabetic peripheral arterial disease: The Edinburgh Artery Study. Diabetes Care 1999;22:453–458.
21. Austin MA: Epidemiology of hypertriglyceridemia and cardiovascular disease. Am J Cardiol 1999;83:13F–16F.

Chapter 3 Hypercoagulable Syndrome

PETER K. HENKE, MD • THOMAS W. WAKEFIELD, MD

A Potential indications for evaluation of possible hypercoagulable syndrome include (1) deep vein thrombosis (DVT) (see G), (2) some preoperative vascular surgery patients (see B), and (3) patients who have experienced postoperative graft thrombosis (see E).

B For patients undergoing any vascular intervention, their family history and past history of thrombosis should be assessed. Basic coagulation tests to be obtained are prothrombin time (PT), activated partial thromboplastin time (aPTT), and a complete blood count (CBC), including platelet count.

C A prolonged aPTT with otherwise normal coagulation test results suggests the possibility of a lupus anticoagulant, a factor deficiency, or the presence of a coagulation inhibitor (such as an antibody to one of the coagulation factors).[1] Antiphospholipid antibodies are not uncommon (26%) in the vascular surgery patient.[2] This aPTT prolongation is a laboratory artifact; in the presence of an antiphospholipid antibody, phospholipid is antagonized and the aPTT is prolonged. Mixing studies should be performed for this abnormality and can differentiate a factor deficiency or inhibitor from the presence of an antiphospholipid antibody.

D Patients with a familial thrombotic history, recurrent graft thromboses, or a history of multiple idiopathic DVTs should undergo a full hypercoagulable screen. Additionally, young individuals with severe atherosclerotic disease should undergo evaluation.[3]

E After postoperative graft thrombosis, the cause must be determined. The most common causes include coagulation problems, technical defects, a poor conduit, and inadequate inflow or runoff.[4] A hypercoagulable evaluation is usually not needed when either a technical defect or a runoff problem is identified. Postoperative anticoagulation therapy is usually not indicated (with the exception of an antiplatelet agent) unless a coagulation disorder is identified or strongly suspected, although this is controversial.

F Besides the basic coagulation parameters (see B), the full laboratory evaluation of a potential hypercoagulable disorder includes:

- Antithrombin III activity and antigen
- Free and total protein C
- Free protein S
- Mixing studies (if aPTT is prolonged)
- Anticardiolipin antibody
- Factor V Leiden functional test with or without genetic analysis
- Genetic analysis for prothrombin gene 20210 polymorphism
- Homocysteine level
- Some measure of fibrinolysis, such as functional plasminogen
- Platelet aggregation testing if available

If heparin-induced thrombocytopenia is suspected, a ^{14}C-serotonin release assay or ELISA assays for the heparin-dependent antibody or platelet factor 4 (PF-4), are indicated. Most of these tests, except for the genetic analyses, are best performed with the patient not taking any anticoagulants and not during the acute thrombotic process.

G If a definable, transient risk factor is found for a first-time DVT, no further evaluation is indicated. Such risk factors include:

- A history of prolonged immobilization
- Recent major surgery under general anesthesia (e.g., orthopedic or abdominal)
- Pregnancy
- Older age
- Medications such as estrogen

Cancer is a well-known risk factor, and idiopathic DVT may be a harbinger of an occult malignancy. If no definable risk factor can be found, suspicion should be raised for the presence of a hypercoagulable disorder. Besides recurrent DVT, young age, a positive family history, or an unusual presenting anatomic site such as mesenteric or cerebral venous thrombosis should prompt a workup for a hypercoagulable disorder.

H In patients with a first-time DVT and a well-documented transient cause, anticoagulation therapy with a vitamin K antagonist, such as sodium warfarin (Coumadin), is indicated. Coumadin can be started once the patient is therapeutic on heparin and should be given 4 to 5 days concurrently with heparin to allow full inhibition of vitamin K–dependent clotting factors. The optimal duration is between 3 and 6 months and the patient's International Normalized Ratio (INR) should be kept between 2.0 and 3.0.[1, 5, 6] The risk of recurrence is less than 5% once therapeutic anticoagulation has been achieved.

I Overall, before the discovery of factor V Leiden, a defined hypercoagulable syndrome accounted for only about 5% to 10% of all cases of DVT whereas its direct role in graft failure was much less.[7] Factor V Leiden mutation is now the most common disorder; it is present in 20% to 40% of all cases of DVT. It may be homozygous or heterozygous and the risk for DVT varies directly.[7, 8] Prothrombin 20210 polymorphism is also being found more frequently with DVT (5% to 6%).

Antithrombin III and protein C and S deficiencies are the next most common disorders, accounting for 1% to 3% of DVTs. Hyperhomocysteinemia not only is a risk factor for accelerated atherosclerosis but also may increase DVT incidence 2.5 times and may account for 10% to 20% of patients with DVT. Folate and vitamins B_{12} and B_6 may help reduce the thrombotic risk, although these measures are speculative at present. Defects that have been identified with arterial thrombosis include antithrombin III, proteins C and S, presence of factor V Leiden, presence of antiphos-

HYPERCOAGULABLE SYNDROME

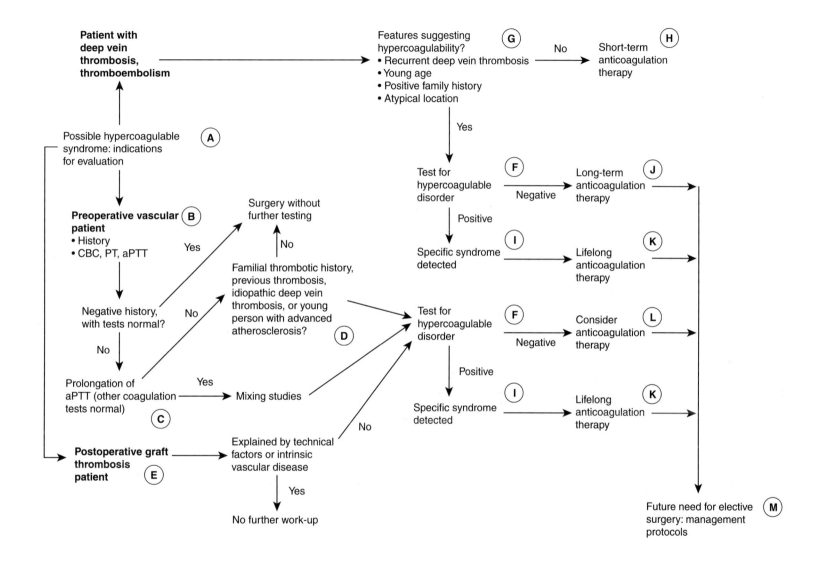

Hypercoagulable Syndrome *(continued)*

pholipid antibodies, heparin-induced thrombocytopenia, and abnormal platelet aggregation.[2,3,9,10,11]

(J) In patients with one recurrence of DVT and an identified risk factor or a primary idiopathic DVT, duration of anticoagulation is less well studied. Our practice is to keep these patients on a regimen of Coumadin with an INR between 2.0 and 3.0 for 1 year and then, if indicated, to re-screen for a hypercoagulable disorder (especially if the patient is young). New data suggest that with idiopathic DVT, a prolonged course of oral anticoagulation therapy may be indicated.[12] Close follow-up for the interim development of a malignancy is also important.

(K) Once a diagnosis of venous thrombosis and a hypercoagulable disorder (including homozygous factor V Leiden, deficiencies of antithrombin III or protein C or S, antiphospholipid syndrome or recurrent idiopathic DVT) is confirmed, lifelong anticoagulation therapy with Coumadin is indicated. The INR is adjusted to 2 to 3 times control except for the antiphospholipid syndrome, in which a higher INR (between 3.0 and 4.0) may be more efficacious. Tests that may have been affected by the acute phase of clotting (such as antithrombin III, protein C or S, or antiphospholipid antibody status) may need to be repeated after a period of anticoagulation. In patients with a noncontrolled malignancy and DVT, anticoagulation therapy should also be continued indefinitely or until the malignancy is cured. Patients with recurrent graft thromboses without an anatomic origin should also continue taking Coumadin indefinitely. The use of lifelong oral anticoagulation agents must always depend on an evaluation of the risk of bleeding to the benefit of thrombosis prevention. Patients who are heterozygous for factor V Leiden with one thrombotic episode should be treated for 3 to 6 months. In patients with a defined hypercoagulable syndrome but no prior DVT (e.g., as shown by familial screening), Coumadin prophylaxis is controversial and is probably indicated only when the patient is at high risk for DVT.[7]

(L) In general, patients undergoing a vascular procedure who do not have a defined hypercoagulable state should not receive anticoagulation prophylactic therapy unless there is a very strong clinical suspicion of a hypercoagulable state combined with a procedure that carries a high risk of thrombosis (e.g., a distal bypass with marginal conduit). However, patients without a defined hypercoagulable state who have already experienced unexplained graft thrombosis and who require a new graft may be candidates for long-term anticoagulation therapy. This judgment depends on the potential risk of anticoagulation and the probability that an undefined hypercoagulable state exists.

(M) The patient who has undergone anticoagulation and who requires a surgical procedure presents a challenging balancing act in terms of need for hemostasis and prevention of recurrent thrombosis.[13] Clearly, the risk of recurrent thrombosis diminishes with time as the clot resolves. Before surgery, hospitalization with Coumadin cessation (normal PT) and institution of intravenous (IV) heparin is indicated only in patients with a recent DVT or arterial thromboembolism (<1 month). Heparin is stopped 6 hours before surgery and is restarted approximately 12 hours after the operative procedure is complete. Two to 3 months after the thrombotic episode, a patient need not be hospitalized before the procedure and can be covered preoperatively with subcutaneous (or low-molecular-weight) heparin and postoperatively with IV heparin and subsequent Coumadin. Patients with a history of a nonacute, recurrent DVT or patients who are more than 3 months after the thrombotic episode need be covered only postoperatively with subcutaneous heparin. The addition of mechanical DVT prophylaxis, such as pneumatic compression stockings, is recommended for high-risk patients.

REFERENCES

1. Hirsh J, Hoak J: Management of deep vein thrombosis and pulmonary embolism: A statement for healthcare professionals. Circulation 1996;93:2212–2245.
2. Lee RW, Taylor LM Jr, Landry GJ, et al: Prospective comparison of infrainguinal bypass grafting with and without antiphospholipid antibodies. J Vasc Surg 1996;24:524–533.
3. Eldrup-Jorgenson J, Flanigan DP, Brace L, et al: Hypercoagulable states and lower limb ischemia in young adults. J Vasc Surg 1989;9:334–341.
4. Stept LL, Flinn WR, McCarthy WJ, et al: Technical defects as a cause of early graft failure after femorodistal bypass. Arch Surg 1987;122:599–604.
5. Ginsberg JS: Management of venous thromboembolism. N Engl J Med 1996;335:1816–1828.
6. Hyers TM, Agnelli G, Hull RD, et al: Antithrombotic therapy for venous thromboembolic disease. Chest 1998;114:561S–578S.
7. Thomas DP, Roberts HR: Hypercoagulability in venous and arterial thrombosis. Ann Intern Med 1997;126:638–644.
8. Lensing AW, Prandoni P, Prins MH, et al: Deep-vein thrombosis. Lancet 1999;353:479–485.
9. Towne JB, Bernhard VM, Hussey C, et al: Antithrombin deficiency—a cause of unexplained thrombosis in vascular surgery. Surgery 1981;89:735–742.
10. Sampram E, Lindblad B, Dahlback B: Activated protein C resistance in patients with peripheral vascular disease. J Vasc Surg 1998;28:624–629.
11. Donaldson MC, Weinberg DS, Belkin M, et al: Screening for hypercoagulable states in vascular surgical practice: A preliminary study. J Vasc Surg 1990;11:825–831.
12. Kearon C, Gent M, Hirsh J, et al: A comparison of three months of anticoagulation with extended anticoagulation for a first episode of idiopathic venous thromboembolism. N Engl J Med 1999;340:901–907.
13. Kearon C, Hirsh J: Management of anticoagulation before and after elective surgery. N Engl J Med 1997;336:1506–1511.

HYPERCOAGULABLE SYNDROME

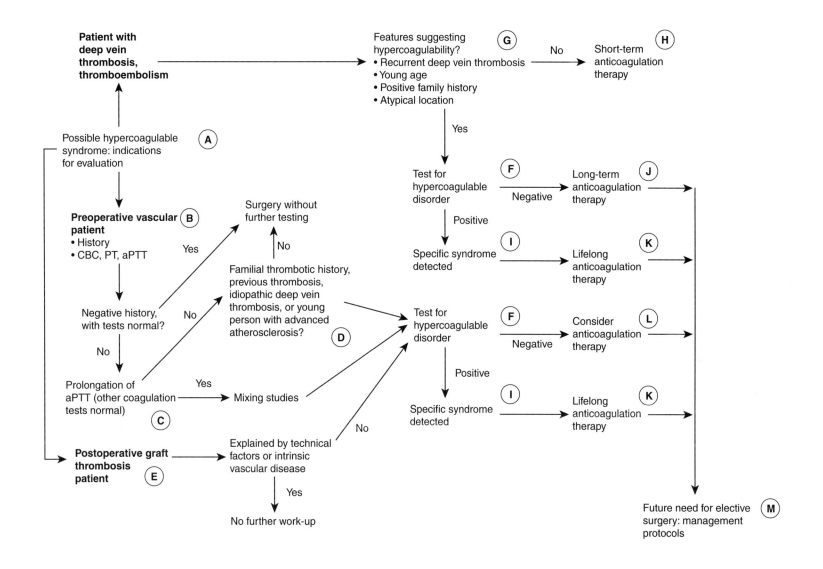

Chapter 4 Perioperative Care and Anesthesia

KATHLEEN CHAIMBERG, MD

(A) Given the systemic nature of the atherosclerotic process, patients presenting with symptomatic peripheral vascular disease are assumed to be at risk for coronary artery disease (CAD). In fact, CAD is the most common cause of death in long-term follow-up of patients undergoing vascular surgery.[1] In addition, these patients tend to be older, to have had an extensive smoking history with concomitant chronic obstructive pulmonary disease, and may also be diabetic, either with or without renal insufficiency. Other less common co-morbidities may exist, particularly in those with nonatherosclerotic disease (e.g., recent deep vein thrombosis with or without pulmonary embolism, coagulopathies, congenital or inflammatory diseases of the vascular system).

(B) Good communication between the anesthesiologist and the surgeon is essential for the optimal management of these medically complex patients. Preoperative evaluation may identify a patient at high risk for perioperative cardiac or pulmonary complications who might be better served by a less invasive procedure than the one originally scheduled. A thorough understanding of the surgical plan will ensure that the extent of intravenous access and level of monitoring are appropriate to the anticipated complexity of the case.

(C) The focus of the preoperative evaluation should be to determine the extent of preexisting chronic neurologic disease as well as to identify any recent acute exacerbations (e.g., new-onset transient ischemic attacks). Patients who are to undergo regional anesthesia must be examined, and any neurologic deficit must be well documented in order to avoid diagnostic confusion in the postoperative period.

(D) Cardiovascular morbidity remains the single most important determinant of overall operative outcome in the vascular surgical population.[2] Preoperative cardiac risk assessment is covered in depth in Chapter 1. Preoperative admission for invasive monitoring and optimization toward predetermined hemodynamic endpoints has not been shown to significantly reduce cardiac complications or to improve outcome and cannot be routinely recommended.[3] Control of the heart rate should be the goal of a well-conducted anesthetic in the patient with a known risk for ischemia. β Blockers may be effective in reducing overall cardiac mortality when they are used throughout the perioperative period.[4]

(E) General anesthesia with the patient supine results in decreases in functional residual capacity, vital capacity, and expiratory flows.[5] Rapid, shallow breathing seen in the immediate postoperative period leads to alveolar collapse, the development of atelectasis, and ventilation-perfusion mismatch. PaO_2 may decrease by 10% to 30%. Although such alterations may go undetected in the patient with normal baseline respiratory function, these changes can result in significant pulmonary compromise in patients with marginal pulmonary reserve. Factors associated with an increased risk for postoperative pulmonary complications include:

- Upper abdominal or thoracic incision
- Morbid obesity
- Long-term and current smoking
- Productive cough and wheezing[6]

Epidemiologic evidence suggests that a significantly reduced 1-second forced expiratory volume is usually associated with symptoms.[7] Therefore, routine preoperative spirometry is not indicated in asymptomatic patients. The more risk factors a patient has, the more likely preoperative pulmonary function tests (including a baseline arterial blood gas analysis and response to bronchodilators) would help to assess severity of dysfunction and to guide perioperative management.

(F) In the patient at risk for renal dysfunction who has undergone preoperative angiographic evaluation with contrast media, it is important to determine that adequate time and hydration have allowed creatinine concentrations to return to baseline levels before the scheduled surgery date.

(G) The need for, and extent of, invasive monitoring is assessed as a function of three variables:

- The severity of the patient's co-morbidities
- The complexity of the surgical procedure
- The experience and training of the personnel who will be caring for the patient perioperatively

In patients with baseline abnormalities (left bundle branch block, pacemaker dependency, left ventricular hypertrophy with strain pattern) that make electrocardiographic monitoring for cardiac ischemia unreliable, use of alternative modalities, such as regional anesthesia with an awake patient, pulmonary artery catheter, or transesophageal echocardiography, should be considered. When the decision is made to monitor central venous pressure, placement of an introducer will allow for easy conversion to a pulmonary artery catheter if necessary later. Pulmonary artery catheters are most useful for monitoring patients with known left ventricular dysfunction or severe valvular disease.

(H) When carefully conducted, regional or general anesthetic techniques are associated with comparable rates of cardiac and most other morbidity in patients undergoing lower extremity peripheral vascular surgery.[8] Some studies have suggested an increased incidence of early graft failure requiring reoperation in patients who receive general rather than epidural anesthesia.[8, 9] Other studies, however, have not verified this finding.[10, 11] Similarly, it is a clinical perception that vascular patients who are at higher risk from a cardiac standpoint tolerate a regional technique

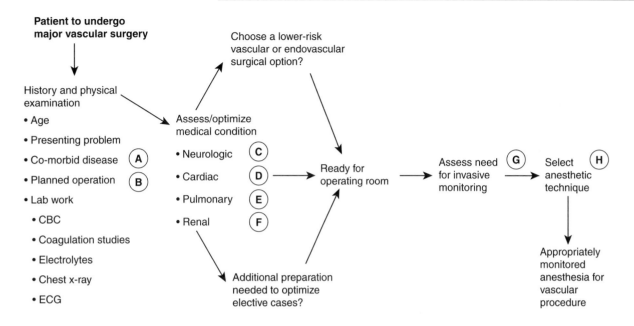

better than a general anesthetic. Although the scientific literature remains inconclusive on these points, we favor regional anesthesia for most patients undergoing infrainguinal bypass for these potential benefits. In aortic surgery, multiple outcome studies have demonstrated decreased pulmonary complications when high-risk patients receive general anesthesia with postoperative epidural analgesia rather than general anesthesia with intravenous opioid analgesia.[12, 13, 14] The choice of regional versus general anesthesia for carotid endarterectomy remains a matter for debate with valid arguments on either side. Factors to consider should include:

1. The anatomy of the lesion.
2. Airway evaluation.
3. The impact of a potential local anesthetic-induced phrenic nerve palsy on the patients respiratory mechanics.
4. The ability of a patient to cooperate (e.g., in the presence of chronic irritative cough or claustrophobia).
5. Patient or surgeon preference.

REFERENCES

1. Bry JDL, Belkin M, O'Donnell TF: An assessment of the positive predictive value and cost-effectiveness of dipyridamole myocardial scintigraphy in patients undergoing vascular surgery. J Vasc Surg 1994;19:112–124.
2. Yeager MP: Regional anesthesia for vascular surgery. In Yeager MP, Glass DD (eds): Anesthesiology and Vascular Surgery. Norwalk, Conn, Appleton & Lange, 1990.
3. Ziegler DW, Wright JG, Choban PS, et al: A prospective randomized trial of preoperative "optimization" of cardiac function in patients undergoing elective peripheral vascular surgery. Surgery 1997;122:584–592.
4. Mangano DT, Layug EL, Wallace A, et al: Effect of atenolol on mortality and cardiovascular morbidity after noncardiac surgery. N Engl J Med 1996;335:1713–1720.
5. Nunn JF: Respiratory aspects of anesthesia. In Nunn's Applied Respiratory Physiology, 4th ed. Oxford, Butterworth-Heinemann, 1993.
6. Celli BR: What is the value of preoperative pulmonary function testing? Med Clin North Am 1993;77:309–325.
7. Zibrak JD, O'Donnell CR: Indications for preoperative pulmonary function testing. Clin Chest Med 1993;14:227–236.
8. Christopherson R, Beattie C, Frank SM, et al: Perioperative morbidity in patients randomized to epidural or general anesthesia for lower extremity vascular surgery. Anesthesiology 1993;79:422–434.
9. Tuman KJ, McCarthy RJ, March RJ, et al: Effects of epidural anesthesia and analgesia on coagulation and outcome after major vascular surgery. Anesth Analg 1991;73: 696–704.
10. Schunn CD, Hertzer NR, O'Hara PJ, et al: Epidural versus general anesthesia: Does anesthetic management influence early infrainguinal graft thrombosis? Ann Vasc Surg 1998; 12:65–69.
11. Pierce ET, Pomposelli FB, Stanley GD, et al: Anesthesia type does not influence early graft patency or limb salvage rates of lower extremity bypass. J Vasc Surg 1997;2:226–232; discussion 232–233.
12. Yeager MP, Glass DD, Neft RK, et al: Epidural anesthesia and analgesia in high risk surgical patients. Anesthesiology 1987;66:729–736.
13. Major CP, Greer MS, Russell WL, et al: Postoperative pulmonary complications and morbidity after abdominal aneurysmectomy: A comparison of postoperative epidural versus parenteral opioid analgesia. Am Surg 1996;62: 45–51.
14. Ballantyne JC, Carr DB, DeFarranti S, et al: The comparative effects of postoperative analgesia therapies on pulmonary outcome: Cumulative meta-analysis of randomized controlled trials. Anesth Analg 1998;86:598–612.

Chapter 5 Transfusion Strategies

THOMAS S. HUBER, MD, PhD • JAMES M. SEEGER, MD

(A) The optimal transfusion strategy for patients undergoing major vascular surgical procedures involves the complementary approaches of blood conservation therapy and appropriate transfusion.

(B) The preoperative history and physical examination should identify abnormal bleeding or thrombotic events. Transfusion history and responses to iatrogenic and incidental trauma should be obtained and a family history of bleeding or thrombotic events sought. Platelet abnormalities are suggested by petechiae or excessive bleeding after incidental trauma. Coagulation disorders are suggested by hemarthroses or hematomas. Medication history should include the use of aspirin, nonsteroidal anti-inflammatory agents, anticoagulants, and oral contraceptives.

The normal ranges for the standard hematologic studies are as follows:

- Red blood cells (RBCs), male: hemoglobin > 14 g/dL or hematocrit > 42%
- Red blood cells, female: hemoglobin > 12 g/dL or hematocrit > 36%
- Platelets: 150,000 to 400,000/μL
- Prothrombin time (PT): 11 to 14 seconds
- Partial thromboplastin time (PTT): 22 to 36 seconds

Routine preoperative coagulation studies are of questionable value as a screening tool but may be helpful in the vascular patient population because of the large magnitude of the operative procedures and the underlying co-morbidities.

(C) The medical evaluation and treatment of patients with hematologic disorders is beyond the scope of the algorithm presented in this chapter. Patients with abnormalities that cannot be explained by antiplatelet agents or anticoagulants merit further aggressive investigation. This may require the assistance of either an internist or a hematologist.

(D) The indications for the antiplatelet and anticoagulant medications should be examined. Antiplatelet agents are usually continued throughout the perioperative period because of their cardiac protective effects, but they may be stopped 5 to 7 days preoperatively in patients undergoing aortic reconstruction if bleeding problems are anticipated. The management of patients who have received chronic anticoagulation therapy with warfarin is contingent upon the indication. Warfarin therapy is stopped 3 to 5 days before the operative procedure in patients at low risk for thrombotic or embolic events (i.e., chronic atrial fibrillation). Patients at higher risk are admitted to the hospital, and the warfarin anticoagulation therapy is reversed with either vitamin K (2.5 to 10.0 mg SC or IV) or fresh frozen plasma (FFP) (2 to 4 units) with the choice contingent upon the urgency. Patients are simultaneously started on IV heparin (80 units/kg bolus with 18 units/kg continuous drip).

Red blood cell transfusions are indicated for the treatment of anemia in patients who require increased oxygen-carrying capacity and red blood cell mass. The decision to transfuse red blood cells to a patient is based on a variety of factors that collectively comprise clinical judgment and include (1) the duration of anemia, (2) intravascular volume, (3) extent of operation, (4) likelihood of massive blood loss, and (5) the presence of co-morbid conditions.

Transfusion guidelines have been issued by several consensus panels, including those from the National Institutes of Health,[1] the American College of Physicians,[2] and the American Society of Anesthesiologists.[3] Collectively, they recommend that red blood cells should not be transfused prophylactically and that a transfusion threshold for a hemoglobin of 7 to 8 mg/dL is appropriate in patients who are not critically ill.

The applicability of these findings to patients with peripheral vascular disease and concomitant coronary artery disease is confounded by a 1998 study showing that elderly patients undergoing elective, noncardiac surgery were at risk for intraoperative and postoperative myocardial ischemia with a hematocrit below 28%.[4] A hemoglobin of 8 mg/dL is an appropriate transfusion threshold for noncritically ill vascular patients without coronary artery disease, whereas a hemoglobin of 10 mg/dL is appropriate for patients at risk for myocardial ischemia.[5] One unit of packed red blood cells should increase the hemoglobin by approximately 1 mg/dL (3% hematocrit) in an adult.

Platelets are required in the perioperative period to correct both quantitative and qualitative platelet deficiencies. A platelet count above 100,000/μL is sufficient for most operative procedures; counts between 50,000/μL and 100,000/μL are sufficient for procedures when significant blood loss is not anticipated. Platelets are administered at 1 unit/10 kg, and each unit should increase the platelet count by 5,000/μL in an adult. Patients alloimmunized from repeated platelet transfusions and patients with platelet-destructive disorders (e.g., immune thrombocytopenic purpura) may become refractory to platelet transfusions and may require human leukocyte antigen (HLA)–matched or crossmatched platelets.

FFP transfusions are indicated in the perioperative period to correct known coagulation factor deficiencies when concentrates are not available and to rapidly reverse warfarin anticoagulation therapy. FFP is not indicated to correct minor abnormalities (<1.5 control values) in the PT or PTT, since clinically significant abnormalities in coagulation should not occur unless these values exceed 1.5 to 1.8 times control values.[3] Indeed, factor levels above 25% to 35% and fibrinogen levels above 100 mg/dL should be sufficient to prevent major bleeding.[6] FFP at a dosage of 10 to 15 mL/kg is sufficient to restore more than 30% of the circulating factor levels.

Cryoprecipitate transfusions are indicated in the perioperative period to correct deficiencies of factor XIII, fibrinogen, and von Willebrand's factor

TRANSFUSION STRATEGIES

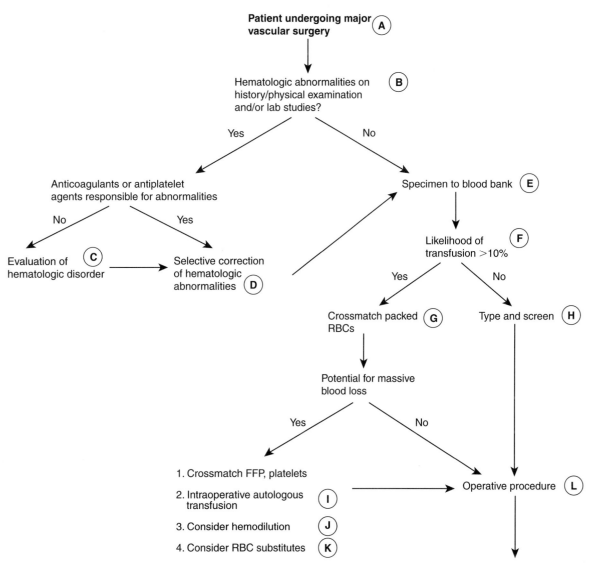

Illustration continued on page 19

unresponsive to desmopressin (DDAVP). One unit of cryoprecipitate should increase the fibrinogen concentration by 5 mg/dL in an adult.

(E) Jehovah's Witnesses and others who object to allogenic blood transfusions based on their religious beliefs constitute an important subset of patients. Acceptable practices should be established with each patient, and liaison committees composed of informed congregation members are available in most institutions. Most Jehovah's Witnesses do not accept allogenic blood products or autologous products that have been separated from the body but do accept cardiopulmonary bypass, hemodialysis, and intraoperative autologous transfusion. An extensive discussion should be conducted with the patient as part of the informed consent process outlining the consequences of refusing a transfusion. If the risks are deemed prohibitive, transfer to a Bloodless Surgical Center or to other institutions with more experience should be considered. The consequences of violating the transfusion policy for a Jehovah's Witness should not be underestimated. These potentially include excommunication from the church, loss of eternal life, and severance of one's relationship with God.[7]

(F) The risks associated with allogenic blood transfusions have markedly decreased within the past two decades as a result of increased awareness and improvement in the ability to screen for the various viral agents. The current risk of death from a blood transfusion is as likely related to bacterial contamination, transfusion reaction, or acute lung injury as to viral illnesses.[5] Furthermore, the risk of transfusion-related viral diseases should decrease further when polymerase chain reaction–based techniques are used to screen donors. Goodnough and colleagues have summarized the current risk of blood transfusion.[5]

(G) The utility of *preoperative* autologous donation for patients undergoing elective vascular surgery remains unresolved. This measure potentially places patients with coronary artery disease at risk for ischemic events because of the induced anemia, and it does not prevent transfusion-associated complications from ABO incompatibility due to human error, bacterial contamination, and volume overload. Furthermore, preoperative autologous donation is not cost-effective. The handling and processing costs exceed those for allogenic transfusions,[8] and a large percentage of the autologous units collected are discarded because it is recommended that surplus units not be transfused to patients other than the donor. These increased costs are compounded by the reduction in the viral transmission risks associated with allogenic blood that provided a major impetus for preoperative autologous donation. Indeed, autologous transfusion of 2 units prior to coronary artery bypass has been reported to cost $500,000 per quality adjusted life-years saved and is far in excess of the standard $50,000 per quality-adjusted life-year threshold generally accepted as cost-effective.[9]

Directed donation is not recommended because the transfusion-associated risks are comparable to those with first-time volunteer donors.[10]

The maximal surgical blood order schedule (MSBOS) is an effective strategy to reduce the number of unnecessarily crossmatched units.[11] The MSBOS represents the maximum number of units that would be crossmatched for a specific procedure on the basis of historical operative transfusion requirements (i.e., aortobifemoral bypass: 4 units of packed red blood cells). The rationale for the schedule is that surgeons and anesthesiologists commonly crossmatch more units than they will transfuse intraoperatively. Both the surgeons and the anesthesiologists may override the MSBOS if greater blood losses are expected.

(H) Only a blood type and screen is required if the probability of a blood transfusion is less than 10%.[12] The type and screen establishes the ABO and Rh types and screens for unexpected antibodies. Appropriate units may be crossmatched quickly as needed, since most of the screening has been accomplished. Whenever clinically significant antibodies are identified by the screen, units of blood lacking the appropriate antigen are crossmatched to ensure availability.

(I) *Intraoperative* autologous transfusion provides a readily available source of blood when significant blood loss is encountered, conserves blood bank resources, and provides a source of blood that is acceptable to most individuals who object to allogenic transfusion on the basis of religious principles. Intraoperative autologous transfusion is useful in selected cases when significant blood loss is anticipated, including ruptured aneurysms and complex aortic reconstructions such as suprarenal aneurysms, thoracoabdominal aortic aneurysms, and aortocaval fistulae. Routine use during elective, infrarenal aortic reconstruction has not been shown to reduce the number of allogenic transfusions[13] or to be cost-effective.[14] The reported salvage volume necessary to achieve cost effectiveness has ranged from 2 to 6 salvaged units.[14,15,16]

(J) The utility of acute, normovolemic hemodilution in patients undergoing vascular surgery remains unresolved. Whole blood is removed immediately prior to surgery and stored in standard blood bags in the operating room. The removed blood is simultaneously replaced with either crystalloid or colloid and is subsequently reinfused during the operative procedure as necessary. Red blood cell volume is theoretically preserved, since the blood lost during the operation has a lower hematocrit. Recent guidelines have suggested that hemodilution should be considered in patients without severe myocardial disease and a hemoglobin greater than 10 mg/dL when the operative blood loss is expected to exceed 20% of the blood volume.[17]

TRANSFUSION STRATEGIES

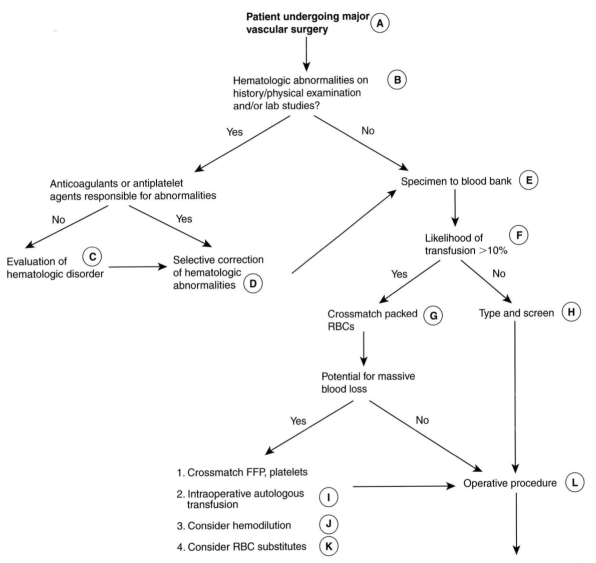

Illustration continued on page 19

Transfusion Strategies (continued)

(K) Red blood cell substitutes should be considered experimental. A variety of compounds are in clinical trials and include cell-free hemoglobin solutions and perfluorocarbon emulsions. These compounds afford the potential advantages of prolonged shelf life, universal biocompatibility, and minimal viral transmission rates. Disadvantages include interference with standard plasma laboratory assays and limited serum half-lives. In 1999, a multicenter trial reported that use of a bovine-hemoglobin solution during elective, infrarenal aortic aneurysm repair resulted in a reduction in the need for allogenic blood transfusions without untoward effects.[18]

(L) Surgical technique designed to limit blood loss is the standard of care, and the adage that "blood that is not lost does not have to be replaced" is the cornerstone of the blood conservation and transfusion strategy.

(M) The indications for red blood cell transfusions within the operating room are identical to those throughout the perioperative period (see D).

(N) Patients undergoing elective vascular procedures are routinely given systemic anticoagulation therapy with heparin (100 units/kg IV) prior to vascular occlusion. A baseline activated clotting time is performed before application of the clamp, and adequacy of anticoagulation is confirmed by a doubling of the baseline value. The activated clotting time is repeated at half-hour intervals throughout the procedure, and supplemental heparin is administered as needed.

Systemic anticoagulation is not used in patients with ruptured abdominal aortic aneurysms or uncontrolled hemorrhage, although it is used selectively in patients with thoracoabdominal aortic aneurysms. Admittedly, withholding systemic anticoagulation increases the risk of thrombotic events. These untoward events can be minimized by local administration of heparin and balloon catheter thromboembolectomy of the major occluded vessels prior to reperfusion.

(O) Heparin anticoagulation is reversed with protamine sulfate routinely after all intra-abdominal procedures and selectively after both carotid and infrainguinal procedures, depending on the quantity of microvascular bleeding (small vessel bleeding within the surgical field). The protamine dose is based upon the activated clotting time and both the total amount of heparin and its time course. The plasma half-life of heparin is between 60 to 90 minutes, and 1 mg of protamine neutralizes 100 units of heparin. Roughly, a dose of 0.5 mg of protamine per 100 units of heparin is given to reverse a bolus of heparin given 30 to 60 minutes earlier. Protamine should be infused slowly over approximately 5 minutes to prevent any untoward hemodynamic compromise.

(P) The assessment of intraoperative bleeding and the need for blood products is a dynamic, ongoing process that requires communication between the anesthetic and surgical teams.

(Q) The indications for platelet and FFP transfusions (see D) have been summarized. Platelet transfusions are indicated for patients with evidence of significant bleeding and platelet counts below 50,000/μL. They also may be indicated for patients with evidence of microvascular bleeding and platelet counts below 100,000/μL or in patients with known platelet dysfunction. FFP transfusions are indicated for patients with evidence of bleeding and coagulation studies above 1.5 times control values. Massive blood loss (>100% blood volume) may result in a dilutional coagulopathy and prolongation of PT and PTT. Transfusions of FFP are indicated in patients with massive blood losses and evidence of microvascular bleeding. FFP at a dosage of 10 to 15 mL/kg is sufficient to restore more than 30% of the circulating factor levels.

(R) Detecting ongoing bleeding in the immediate postoperative period may be difficult. Hemodynamic changes may not be evident until there is a significant decrease in the intravascular volume. Additionally, fluid shifts and third-space losses may confound the clinical picture. A pulmonary artery catheter should be inserted if the intravascular volume status is uncertain.

REFERENCES

1. Consensus Conference: Perioperative red blood cell transfusion. JAMA 1988;260:2700–2703.
2. American College of Physicians: Practice strategies for elective red blood cell transfusion. Ann Intern Med 1992;116:403–406.
3. American Society of Anesthesiologists Task Force: Practice guidelines for blood component therapy. Anesthesiology 1996;84:498–501.
4. Hogue CW, Goodnough LT, Monk TG: Perioperative myocardial ischemic episodes are related to hematocrit level in patients undergoing radical prostatectomy. Transfusion 1998;38:924–931.
5. Goodnough LT, Brecher ME, Kanter MH, AuBuchon JP: Transfusion medicine: First of two parts. N Engl J Med 1999;340:438–447.
6. Lane TA (ed): Blood Transfusion Therapy: A Physician's Handbook, 5th ed. Bethesda, Md, American Association of Blood Banks, 1996, p 91.
7. Spence RK: Surgical red blood cell transfusion practice policies. Am J Surg 1995;170(Suppl):3S–15S.
8. Etchason J, Petz L, Keeler E, et al: The cost effectiveness of preoperative autologous blood donations. N Engl J Med 1995;332:719–724.
9. Birkmeyer JD, AuBuchon JP, Littenberg B, et al: Cost-effectiveness of preoperative autologous donation in coronary artery bypass grafting. Ann Thorac Surg 1994;57:161–169.
10. Dodd R: The risk of tranfusion-transmitted infection. N Engl J Med 1992;327:419–421.
11. Friedman BA, Oberman HA, Chadwick AR, Kingdon KI: The maximum surgical blood order schedule and surgical blood use in the United States. Transfusion 1976;16:380–387.
12. Lane TA (ed): Blood Transfusion Therapy: A Physician's Handbook, 5th ed. Bethesda, Md, American Association of Blood Banks, 1996, p 117.
13. Clagett GP, Valentine RJ, Jackson MR, et al: A randomized trial of intraoperative autotransfusion during aortic surgery. J Vasc Surg 1999;29:22–31.

TRANSFUSION STRATEGIES

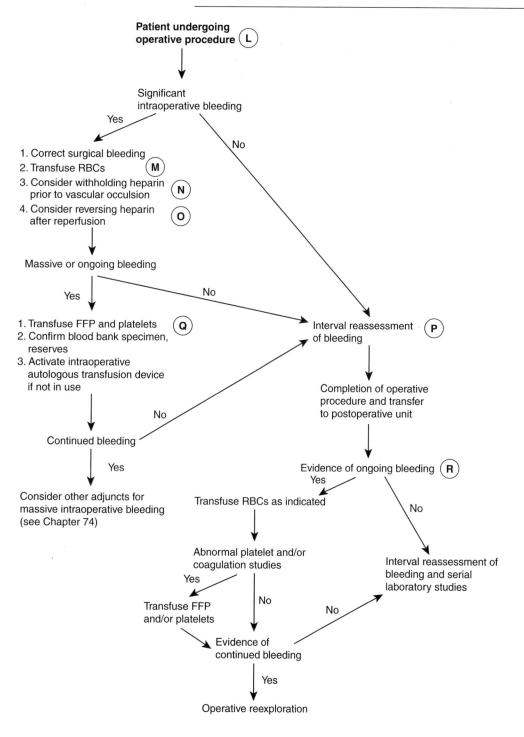

Transfusion Strategies (continued)

14. Huber TS, McGorray SP, Carlton LC, et al: Intraoperative autologous transfusion during elective infrarenal aortic reconstruction: A decision analysis model. J Vasc Surg 1997;25:984–994.
15. Bovill DF, Moulton CW, Jackson WS, et al: The efficacy of intraoperative autologous transfusion in major orthopedic surgery: A regression analysis. Orthopedics 1986;9:1403–1407.
16. Goodnough LT, Monk TG, Sicard G, et al: Intraoperative salvage in patients undergoing elective abdominal aortic aneurysm repair: An analysis of cost and benefit. J Vasc Surg 1996;24:213–218.
17. Napier JA, Bruce M, Chapman J, et al: Guidelines for autologous transfusion: II. Perioperative haemodilution and cell salvage. Br J Anaesth 1997;78:768–771.
18. LaMuraglia GM, O'Hara PJ, Baker WH, et al: Reduction of transfusion requirement in aortic aneurysm surgery using a hemoglobin solution. Presented at the 53rd Society for Vascular Surgery Annual Meeting, June 6, 1999, Washington, DC.

CEREBROVASCULAR DISEASE

Chapter 6 Evaluating Cerebrovascular Symptoms

MICHAEL A. RICCI, MD

(A) Symptoms of cerebrovascular disease may be caused by hemorrhage, thrombosis, embolism, diffuse or regional low blood flow, intense vessel spasm, or even arterial obstruction related to neck position. This chapter considers the evaluation of significant extracranial cerebrovascular disease (ECD), a frequent cause of symptoms and the focus of vascular surgeons and diagnostic vascular laboratories. Subsequent decisions concerning management of specific clinical scenarios are covered in Chapters 7 to 19 (see also the algorithm).

Initial evaluation begins with a stratification of symptoms by (1) duration (transient or permanent), (2) temporal pattern (isolated or recurrent, recent or remote), and (3) likely cerebrovascular territory (carotid, vertebral, or global).

Transient ischemic attacks (TIAs) by definition resolve within 24 hours; however, the median time for a carotid territory TIA is 14 minutes, and for a vertebrobasilar (VB) TIA it is 8 minutes. In fact, if an initial symptom persists more than 1 hour, only 14% resolve by 24 hours.[1] The medical history may provide a clue to the cause, with particular regard to symptoms of systemic diseases, such as atherosclerosis, nonspecific aortoarteritis, giant cell arteritis, and cardiac arrhythmias.

Carotid territory symptoms should be localized to one hemisphere; otherwise, a cardiac source should be suspected. These include hemiparesis, hemiparalysis, hemiparesthesia, or monocular blindness (see F).

Vertebrobasilar insufficiency can present with a variety of symptoms, including ataxia/disequilibrium, orthostatic dizziness, drop attacks, vertigo, blurred vision, hemianopsia, diplopia, cortical blindness, dysarthria, and distal paresthesias (see G).

Global symptoms are primarily those of syncope or near-syncope (dizziness, dimmed vision, weakness, loss of mental function), but reductions in cerebral perfusion pressure can, in the presence of focal cerebrovascular occlusive disease, cause localized symptoms.

Physical examination should include:
- Assessment of pulses for diminution
- Auscultation of neck for bruit
- Retinal evaluation and visual field check
- A directed neurologic examination
- A cardiac evaluation

Pulse deficits in the neck or arms are important indicators of great vessel disease that are often overlooked initially.

(B) Duplex ultrasound surveillance is now accepted as the first diagnostic test in evaluating patients with symptoms suggestive of ECD. Duplex scanning of the extracranial neck arteries has had extensive study and validation. Indications for duplex scanning for ECD, established by both medical experts and State Medicare Boards[2-4] are limited to the following:
- Cervical bruit in an asymptomatic patient
- Amaurosis fugax, focal TIA, stroke in a potential candidate for intervention
- Drop attacks (rare indication)
- Follow-up of known stenoses (>20%) in asymptomatic patient and after carotid endarterectomy

Strandness[2] has defined criteria for the ultrasound diagnosis of carotid artery stenosis. With increasing degrees of stenosis, one observes first, a loss of reversed flow in the carotid bulb (0% to 15% diameter stenosis), then additively, in sequence, spectral broadening (15% to 49%), the peak systolic velocity (PSV) exceeding 125 meters/sec (50% to 79%) and the end-diastolic velocity (EDV) exceeding 140 meters/sec (80% to 99%). With these criteria, Strandness[2] has reported a sensitivity of 99% and a specificity of 84%; other authors[5] have reported 96% accuracy using these criteria to detect stenosis greater than 50% with 97% accuracy in the detection of occlusion.

Because of the importance of a 70% internal carotid artery (ICA) stenosis established by NASCET,[14] Moneta and coworkers[15] developed duplex criteria to determine this degree of stenosis. Although this group measured several criteria, the maximum accuracy to determine 70% to 99% ICA stenosis was 88% with PSV ≥ 325 cm/sec or ICA/CCA [common carotid artery] ratio ≥ 4.0. Of these, they recommended the use of the ICA/CCA ratio ≥ 4.0 as the best predictor of 70% to 99% arteriographic stenosis because of the greater sensitivity (91% versus 83%). It is important that these criteria be validated in each vascular laboratory in which they are used, since various laboratories and even different machines may require different criteria for accuracy.[6,7]

Severe contralateral disease may result in increased flow through the ipsilateral carotid artery, such that modification of standard diagnostic criteria may be required.[8] In addition to carotid bifurcation disease, the CCA and the vertebral arteries can be studied by duplex scans, and, although with less specificity, one may draw inferences regarding stenoses or occlusions in these vessels.

(C) For patients with acute symptoms of stroke or crescendo TIAs, brain computed tomography (CT) or magnetic resonance imaging (MRI) is warranted to identify cerebral infarcts (new, old, multiple, bilateral) and to rule out intracranial hemorrhage. Patients with atypical symptoms also merit brain imaging to exclude other causes of symptoms (e.g., tumor, arteriovenous malformation [AVM], lacunar stroke). This includes patients who have pure sensory or pure motor strokes, since they more frequently represent "small vessel disease" and a lacunar infarct. Patients with hypertension or diabetes appear to be at greatest risk for this type of event. For patients with typical symptoms, well localized to a discrete territory, routine CT or MRI is not cost-effective. Patients with an acute stroke are managed as discussed in Chapter 11. Patients with other, non-ECD disease are beyond the scope of this chapter.

EVALUATING CEREBROVASCULAR SYMPTOMS

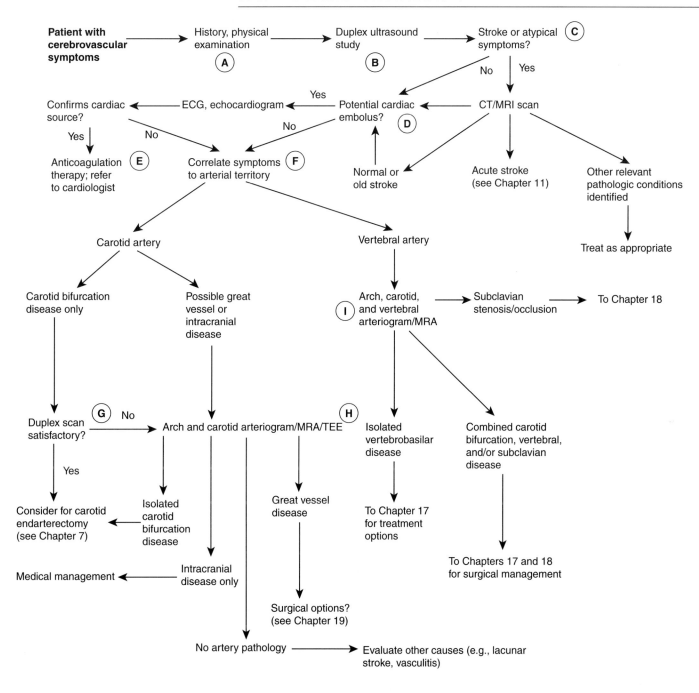

Evaluating Cerebrovascular Symptoms (continued)

(D) Patients who possibly have cardiac emboli as the source of their symptoms (bilateral symptoms or infarcts, focal symptoms of atypical distribution, arrhythmias, history of emboli elsewhere, history of myocardial infarction or ventricular aneurysm, minimal or no carotid disease) should undergo electrocardiography and echocardiography. For some patients, transesophageal echocardiography (TEE) is required for a good definition of cardiac pathology. TEE is also helpful in demonstrating potential atheroembolic plaque in the aortic arch.

(E) Patients identified as having a cardiac embolic source should receive anticoagulation therapy immediately and should be referred to a cardiologist for definitive care.

(F) It is important to localize cerebrovascular symptoms to the brain territory involved in order to determine further diagnosis and treatment. Of patients with carotid artery TIAs, symptoms that occurred in more than 20% included ipsilateral loss of vision, contralateral motor or sensory complaints, and dysphasia for left-sided disease.[9] Of patients with VB TIAs, ataxia, diplopia, blurred vision, and dizziness were most common. Dysarthria was common for both carotid and VB TIAs and did not discriminate well between them. Loss of consciousness and confusion were most often not associated with TIAs.

Combinations of symptoms are particularly useful for localizing the brain territory involved. Ipsilateral blindness and contralateral motor-sensory loss was well localized to the carotid disease, dysphasia and right motor-sensory loss to the left carotid, and the combination of diplopia, bilateral decreased vision, ataxia, and dizziness to VB disease.[9]

(G) Only vascular laboratories that have adequate, regular quality assurance programs and proven accuracy should attempt to use duplex scanning as the sole test for planning treatment of carotid artery disease.[2, 8, 10] This requires vascular technologists who undergo regular quality assurance reviews, as suggested by the Intersocietal Commission for the Accreditation of Vascular Laboratories.

A suggested alternative approach is the combination of duplex scanning and magnetic resonance angiography (MRA).[11–13] This approach may be an accurate means of selecting patients for appropriate treatment, especially surgery. It is less expensive than arteriography but is more expensive than duplex scanning alone. Quality assurance should be carried out for both duplex scanning and MRA if this approach is selected.

Because arteriography carries a stroke risk between 1% and 6%, eliminating it should reduce the overall risk of treatment for symptomatic carotid stenosis. Pitfalls include the possibility of missing disease of the arch vessels, carotid siphon stenosis, intracranial aneurysms, or brain tumors; fortunately, however, these conditions coexisting with severe carotid stenosis are uncommon. Furthermore, duplex scanning and careful history and physical examination often disclose other pathologic conditions, especially proximal great vessel disease.

Carotid endarterectomy without arteriography can be safely performed if:
1. The accuracy of duplex scanning in the laboratory is known.
2. The duplex scan is technically adequate.
3. Vascular anomalies, kinks, or loops are not present.
4. The CCA is free of significant disease.
5. The distal ICA is visualized and is free of significant disease.[16]

Management of symptomatic patients with carotid bifurcation disease is discussed in Chapter 7.

(H) Patients who may have carotid artery disease other than at the bifurcation warrant additional arterial imaging. This recommendation also applies to patients with carotid bifurcation disease that does not appear sufficient to explain symptoms that are atypical in distribution and character. In such patients, disease in the proximal brachiocephalic vessels or in the distal intracranial vessels should be sought. In some cases, these possibilities are apparent from clinical, duplex, CT, and MRI findings, as previously discussed. In our practice, we have used TEE for initial evaluation of potential aortic arch and proximal great vessel disease in order to possibly eliminate the need for arteriography. If severe atherosclerotic plaque is found after this minimally invasive examination, arch arteriography is then selected.

In patients with carotid artery disease at more than one level, it is important to visualize all segments and to attribute the symptoms to the most probable anatomic source. In such patients, carotid and arch arteriography with intracranial views is required. The choice between conventional arteriography and MRA depends on the institutional experience and the particular anatomic region in question. Although MRA is noninvasive, it may not provide sufficient detail for planning arch reconstruction. MRA generally provides excellent intracranial imaging.

Management of patients with proximal brachiocephalic disease is discussed in Chapter 19. Patients with only intracranial disease are generally managed medically. If no carotid disease can be found, other sources for apparent carotid TIAs must be sought, such as lacunae and arteritis.

(I) Because duplex scanning does not provide sufficient anatomic information to plan treatment, patients with VB symptoms generally undergo four-vessel and arch arteriography. Again, MRA can be used in institutions with good results with this technique, but most surgeons have used conventional arteriography when planning vertebral surgery.

Management of patients with VB disease is discussed in Chapter 17. Patients with VB symptoms due to proximal subclavian artery disease with associated "subclavian steal" are discussed in Chapter 18. Patients with combined carotid, vertebral, and subclavian disease are complex (see Chapters 17 and 18).

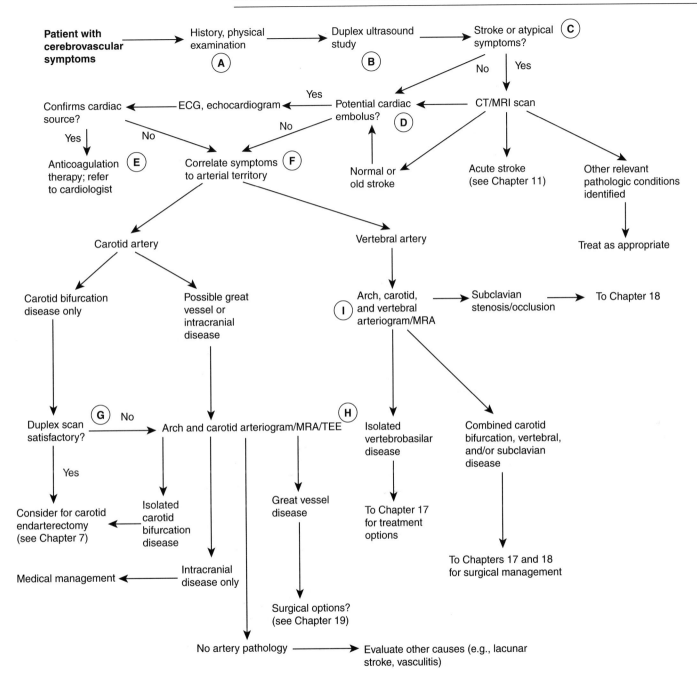

Evaluating Cerebrovascular Symptoms (continued)

REFERENCES

1. Feinberg WM, Albers GW, Barnett HJ, et al: Guidelines for the management of transient ischemic attacks. From the Ad Hoc Committee on Guidelines for the Management of Transient Ischemic Attacks of the Stroke Council of the American Heart Association. Circulation 1994;89:2950-2965.
2. Strandness DE Jr (ed): Extracranial arterial disease. In Duplex Scanning in Vascular Disorders, 2nd ed. New York, Raven Press, 1993, pp 113-158.
3. Providers' News, Medicare Services, Louisiana, April 1, 1993.
4. Strandness DE Jr: Indications for and frequency of noninvasive testing. Semin Vasc Surg 1994;7:245.
5. Bandyk DF, Levine AW, Pohl L, Towne JB: Classification of carotid bifurcation disease using quantitative Doppler spectrum analysis. Arch Surg 1985;120:306.
6. Alexandrov AV, Vital D, Brodie DS, et al: Grading carotid stenosis with ultrasound: An interlaboratory comparison. Stroke 1997;28:1208.
7. Fillinger MF, Baker RJ, Zwolak RM, et al: Carotid duplex criteria for a 60% or greater angiographic stenosis: Variation according to equipment. J Vasc Surg 1996;24:856.
8. Ricci MA: The changing role of duplex scan in the management of carotid bifurcation disease and endarterectomy. Semin Vasc Surg 1998;11:3-11.
9. Futty DE, Conneally M, Dyken ML, et al: Cooperative study of hospital frequency and character of transient ischemic attacks: V. Symptom analysis. JAMA 1977;238:2386-2390.
10. Hachinski V: The issue is standards, not techniques. Arch Neurol 1995;52:834.
11. Lee KS: What workup should be required for a patient who has one TIA and demonstrates 80% carotid stenosis? J Neurosurg Anesth 1996;8:305.
12. Lustgarten JH, Soloman RA, Quest DO, et al: Carotid endarterectomy after noninvasive evaluation by duplex ultrasonography and magnetic resonance angiography. Neurosurg 1994;34:612.
13. Turnipseed WD, Kennell TW, Turski PA, et al: Combined use of duplex imaging and magnetic resonance angiography for evaluation of patients with symptomatic ipsilateral high-grade stenosis. J Vasc Surg 1993;17:832.
14. North American Symptomatic Carotid Endarterectomy Trial Collaborators: Beneficial effect of carotid endarterectomy in symptomatic patients with high-grade carotid stenosis. N Engl J Med 1991;325:445.
15. Moneta GL, Edwards JM, Chitwood RW, et al: Correlation of North American Symptomatic Carotid Endarterectomy Trial (NASCET) angiographic definition of 70% to 99% internal carotid artery stenosis with duplex scanning. J Vasc Surg 1993;17:152.
16. Strandness DE Jr: Angiography before carotid endarterectomy—no. Arch Neurol 1995;52:832.

Chapter 7 begins on the following page

Chapter 7 Symptomatic Carotid Artery Stenosis

ALIK FARBER, MD • JACK L. CRONENWETT, MD

(A) Patients presenting with a neurologic deficit pertaining to the territory of the carotid artery should undergo a careful history, general physical examination, detailed neurologic examination, routine laboratory evaluation, and an electrocardiogram (ECG). Further workup may include a head computed tomography (CT) scan or magnetic resonance imaging (MRI) to evaluate the presence, type, and extent of infarction or to rule out other intracranial sources of the patient's symptoms, particularly if they are atypical (see Chapter 6).

(B) Because extracranial carotid artery (ECA) disease is responsible for up to 50% of ischemic strokes, all patients who have suffered a transient ischemic attack (TIA) or a stroke need to be evaluated for the presence of carotid stenosis. Duplex ultrasound surveillance has supplanted arteriography as the primary modality to assess the presence and degree of carotid stenosis and to monitor patients for progression of disease.[1]

(C) The North American Symptomatic Carotid Endarterectomy Trial (NASCET) found that patients with less than 50% internal carotid artery (ICA) stenosis who were treated with aspirin versus aspirin plus endarterectomy showed no statistically significant difference in ipsilateral stroke rate after 5 years (19% versus 15%).[2] In such patients, it is highly likely that another etiologic mechanism is responsible, and a careful evaluation of the source of symptoms is thus warranted.

(D) In addition to general evaluation (see A), patients with apparent carotid symptoms but an absence of significant carotid stenosis should undergo a complete blood count (CBC) to look for polycythemia or thrombocytosis. The erythrocyte sedimentation rate (ESR) and antinuclear antigen analysis may identify vasculitis or other autoimmune disorders. A coagulation profile may be particularly useful in younger patients and in those with a history of thrombosis (see Chapter 3). ECG, echocardiography, and Holter monitoring may suggest a source of cardiac emboli. Head CT or MRI may identify intracranial tumor, arteriovenous malformation, aneurysm, or other abnormality.

(E) Patients with less than 50% ICA stenosis by duplex scan, in whom no obvious etiology for their symptoms is present and in whom symptoms persist despite medical therapy, should be evaluated with aortic arch and cerebral arteriography. This imaging modality can identify possible sources of atheroemboli that can be missed by duplex scanning, including ulceration of the carotid bulb, proximal great vessel disease, or intracranial disease.

(F) Medical therapy for the patient with a TIA and stroke includes smoking cessation and control of atherosclerotic risk factors, such as hyperlipidemia, hypertension, and diabetes. The mainstay of medical treatment, however, is antiplatelet therapy.

Aspirin reduces the relative risk of stroke by nearly one third and is the first-line drug of choice.[3] Ticlopidine further decreases the risk of stroke and death by 12% compared with aspirin, but carries a 2.4% incidence of reversible neutropenia.

Clopidogrel, a new ticlopidine analogue that does not cause neutropenia, provides a 7% to 24% relative risk reduction of stroke, myocardial infarction, or vascular death compared with aspirin but is substantially more expensive.[3] Patients with carotid symptoms who are already taking aspirin but who are not appropriate candidates for surgery are candidates for clopidogrel treatment. Patients who present with frequent or progressive TIAs while receiving aspirin therapy (crescendo TIAs) are usually hospitalized for heparin anticoagulation therapy and expeditious preoperative evaluation.

(G) Patients with isolated intracranial atherosclerosis without more proximal disease are usually treated with aggressive medical therapy. Although some centers are developing experience with balloon angioplasty of symptomatic intracranial carotid lesions,[4] a careful comparison with medical treatment is needed. Fortunately, the presence of intracranial disease in conjunction with a significant extracranial carotid stenosis does not adversely affect stroke rates in patients undergoing carotid endarterectomy.[5] In fact, such patients benefited more from carotid endarterectomy in the NASCET trial because they had a higher stroke rate under medical management.[6]

(H) Although the severity of ICA stenosis correlates well with stroke risk, patients with less than 50% ICA stenosis may have carotid bulb ulceration that is a source of atheroemboli and symptoms. Arteriography may detect ulceration not apparent on the duplex scan.[7] Patients with carotid ulceration and less than 50% ICA stenosis who do not respond to aggressive antiplatelet therapy and for whom there is no other source of emboli should be evaluated for carotid endarterectomy in the same fashion as patients with more severe ICA stenosis (see L).

(I) Arteriography in the setting of less than 50% carotid stenosis may be helpful in the diagnosis of less common extracranial carotid disease, including proximal common carotid artery or innominate artery ulceration or stenosis, Takayasu's or temporal arteritis, carotid fibromuscular dysplasia, dissection, carotid body tumor, carotid kink or coil, and extracranial carotid artery aneurysm (see Chapters 12 to 15, 18–19, and 73).

(J) The NASCET and the European Carotid Surgery Trial (ECST) both demonstrated a significant benefit of carotid endarterectomy over aspirin treatment for patients with more than 50% ICA stenosis, defined as the stenosis diameter compared to the distal, normal ICA diameter.[2, 8, 9] However, the benefit for surgery was most pronounced in patients with more severe stenosis

SYMPTOMATIC CAROTID ARTERY STENOSIS

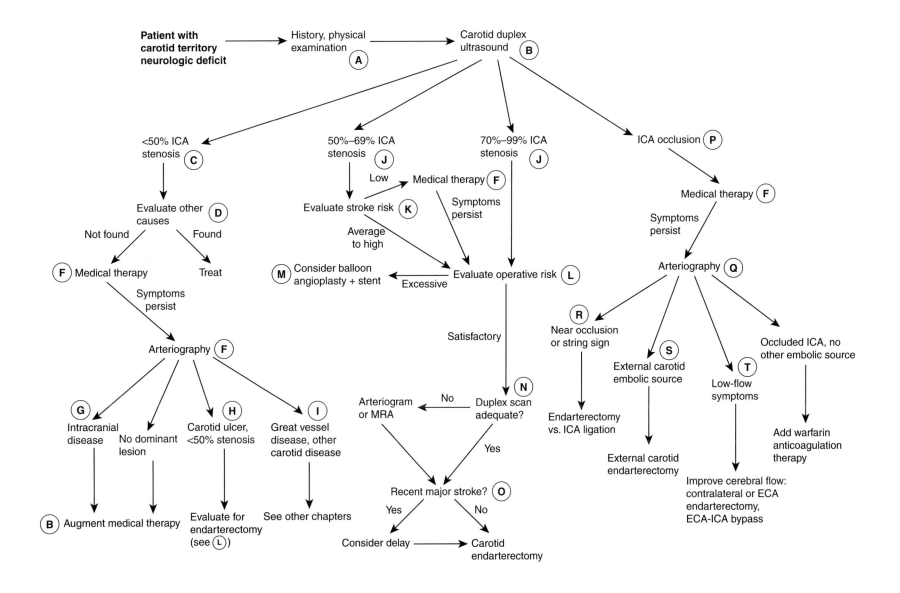

Symptomatic Carotid Artery Stenosis (continued)

because the risk of stroke in these patients was much higher without surgery. In the NASCET, patients with 70% to 99% stenosis had a 2-year ipsilateral stroke rate of 26% in the medical group; the rate was only 9% in the surgical group.[1] However, the reduction in stroke risk for patients with 50% to 69% stenosis was less striking. The 5-year ipsilateral stroke rate was only 22% in the medical group but 16% in the surgical group.[2]

Thus, for patients with 70% ICA stenosis, the risk of stroke is high and evaluation for endarterectomy is appropriate (see L). For patients with 50% to 69% ICA stenosis, however, evaluation of other risk factors for stroke is appropriate to select a high-risk group in whom surgery would be most beneficial (see K).

(K) The severity of ICA stenosis appears to be the most important predictor of ipsilateral stroke risk, so that patients with more severe stenoses benefit most from endarterectomy. For patients with less severe (50% to 69%) stenosis, other factors that affect stroke risk should be considered in evaluating the potential benefit of surgery. Factors known to increase stroke risk in such patients[2, 10, 11] include:

- Male gender
- Stroke (versus TIA)
- Hemispheric TIA (versus retinal TIA)
- Plaque surface irregularity (ulceration)

The time interval since the last neurologic symptom is also important, since stroke risk returns to baseline values after 6 to 12 months following a TIA, and 1 to 2 years following the initial stroke. From an assessment of individual patients with 50% to 69% ICA stenosis according to these risk factors, those patients with lower stroke risk can be identified for medical treatment and those at higher risk can be evaluated for surgery.

(L) The cardiologist must consider operative risk of stroke, death, and other complications in determining patient suitability for carotid endarterectomy. Factors shown to increase operative risk[2, 11, 12] include:

- Female gender
- Peripheral vascular disease
- Hypertension
- Contralateral carotid occlusion
- Ipsilateral stroke on brain imaging
- Diabetes
- Renal insufficiency

Determination of perioperative risk from coronary artery disease needs to be stratified (see Chapters 1 and 20). Low surgeon or hospital volume are also important determinants of poor outcome after carotid surgery.[13] Occasionally, factors such as previous neck irradiation may increase the morbidity of surgical exposure. In patients with multiple risk factors for operative stroke, medical treatment may be more appropriate. In selected patients with high operative mortality or morbidity, nonsurgical treatment with balloon angioplasty and stenting may be considered. For most symptomatic patients, however, carotid endarterectomy is the best treatment.

(M) Carotid angioplasty with stenting is being used in some centers to treat selective cases of symptomatic carotid stenosis. Initial experience suggests that the rate of stroke after angioplasty/stenting is higher than that after surgical endarterectomy.[14] A randomized clinical trial is under way to compare these treatment modalities. Until this comparison is completed, we reserve angioplasty with stenting for proximal great vessel stenosis, in which the procedural stroke risk appears lower. Some have used angioplasty with stenting for (1) very-high-risk patients with carotid bifurcation disease, (2) patients who could not tolerate endarterectomy because of uncorrectable cardiac disease, or (3) patients in whom surgical exposure was hazardous because of previous irradiation or head and neck surgery.

(N) Carotid duplex scanning has been very accurate in the diagnosis of carotid stenosis and is used at an increasing number of centers as the sole preoperative study before carotid endarterectomy to avoid the stroke risk of cerebral arteriography.[1] Even in laboratories known for their high rates of accuracy, however, sometimes preoperative duplex evaluation alone is not adequate. The most important situation is evidence of disease in the proximal common carotid or in the distalmost visualized portion of the ICA. Each of these circumstances may significantly alter the conduct of the operation. In addition, severe calcification may obscure accurate stenosis determination, and a loop or kink in the ICA may be difficult to interpret. In these instances, selective carotid arteriography or magnetic resonance angiography (MRA) is often beneficial.

(O) Patients with a recent, large stroke (depressed level of consciousness, large lesion on CT scan) are at increased risk for worsening of their neurologic deficit after early carotid endarterectomy. It is best to treat this group of patients conservatively and withhold operation for 2 to 6 weeks until symptoms begin to improve or stabilize. Recent experience suggests that patients with less severe strokes and with minimal neurologic deficit may safely undergo early carotid endarterectomy when symptoms have stabilized or abated. Early operation may avoid the risk of stroke recurrence and may be particularly important in patients with severe ICA stenosis.[15]

(P) When an ICA stenosis progresses to occlusion, approximately 25% of patients experience a TIA, 25% have an ipsilateral stroke, and 50% remain asymptomatic.[16] Most do not continue to experience new ipsilateral symptoms from continued embolization or ischemia except for symptoms relating to the residual stroke. Thus, in the absence of ongoing TIAs, patients with ICA occlusion are treated with medical therapy and careful attention to future surveillance of the contralateral carotid artery.

(Q) If ipsilateral carotid symptoms persist despite medical therapy in a patient with ICA occlusion, as determined by duplex scanning, several

SYMPTOMATIC CAROTID ARTERY STENOSIS

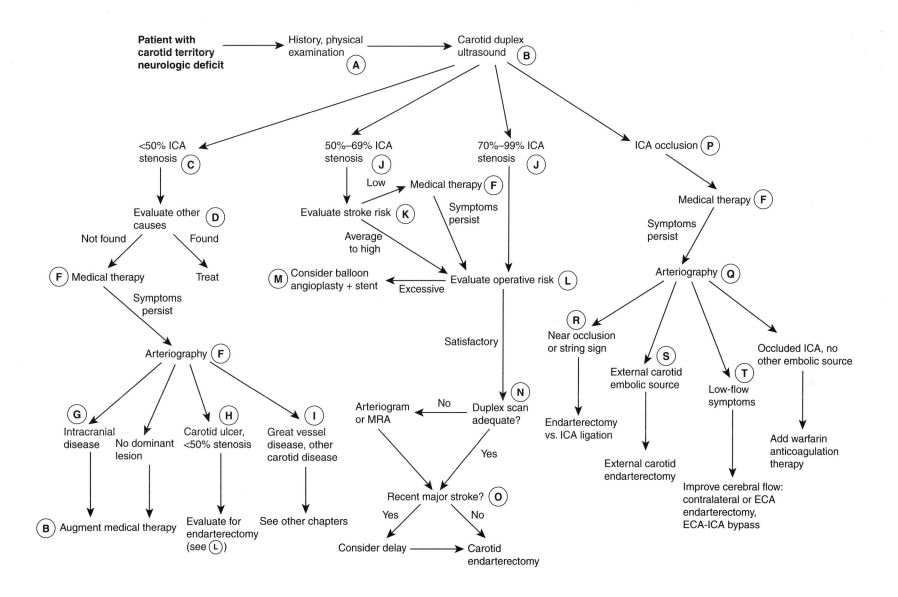

clinical scenarios may exist. The ipsilateral ICA may not be occluded, other sources of embolization may be present (such as the distal end of the occluded ICA), or cerebral symptoms may be a result of hypoperfusion from inadequate collateral circulation. In these cases, detailed cerebral arteriography is helpful to define the specific cause of ongoing symptoms and to select optimal therapy.

(R) In a patient with apparent ICA occlusion but ongoing symptoms, arteriography may reveal persistent patency of the nearly occluded ICA, which has been misinterpreted by duplex ultrasound surveillance. In this case, there may be a severe but focal stenosis with a relatively normal distal ICA such that endarterectomy can be performed. Conversely, there may be such diffuse narrowing and thickening of the distal ICA ("string sign") that endarterectomy is not feasible, so that ICA ligation, combined with external carotid endarterectomy if indicated, should be performed.[17] In this event, postoperative anticoagulation therapy may be helpful to prevent distal propagation of the resultant ICA thrombus.

(S) In a patient with persistent carotid symptoms and an arteriographically confirmed ICA occlusion, the ECA may be a conduit for carotid bulb atheroemboli if the normal ECA-ICA collaterals are intact. These collaterals can usually be demonstrated on selective carotid arteriography, with eventual filling of the carotid siphon after common carotid artery (CCA) contrast injection. When such symptoms do not respond to medical therapy, external carotid endarterectomy is indicated together with flush ligation of the ICA origin to eliminate any nidus for thrombus formation.[18]

(T) Following ICA occlusion, patients who have inadequate cerebral collateral circulation may experience ongoing symptoms caused by hypoperfusion. These may manifest as TIAs, often provoked by rising from a lying or sitting position, or as retinal ischemia, manifested as bright light amaurosis. In such patients, it may be possible to improve collateral blood flow through contralateral carotid endarterectomy, vertebral artery intervention, or ipsilateral external carotid endarterectomy; in very selected cases, extracranial-intracranial bypass may be beneficial. It is possible to better characterize cerebral hypoperfusion using acetazolamide-stimulated blood flow studies.[19]

(U) It is theoretically possible for patients with an occluded ICA to experience embolization from a distal ICA thrombus. The diagnosis of such a scenario is confirmed when no other cause for ongoing symptoms can be identified and when symptoms persist despite aggressive antiplatelet management. Warfarin anticoagulation therapy for a period of 3 to 6 months is indicated while the thrombus matures.

REFERENCES

1. Dawson DL, Zierler RE, Strandness DE Jr, et al: The role of duplex scanning and arteriography before carotid endarterectomy: A prospective study. J Vasc Surg 1993;18(4):673.
2. Barnett HJ, Taylor DW, Eliasziw M, et al,: Benefit of carotid endarterectomy in patients with symptomatic moderate or severe stenosis. North American Symptomatic Carotid Endarterectomy Trial Collaborators. N Engl J Med 1998;339(20):1415.
3. Dyken ML: Antiplatelet agents and stroke prevention. Semin Neurol 1998;18(4):441.
4. Marks MP, Marcellus M, Norbash AM, et al: Outcome of angioplasty for atherosclerotic intracranial stenosis. Stroke 1999;30(5):1065.
5. Mattos MA, van Bemmelen PS, Hodgson KJ, et al: The influence of carotid siphon stenosis on short- and long-term outcome after carotid endarterectomy. J Vasc Surg 1993;17(5):902.
6. Kappelle LJ, Eliasziw M, Fox AJ, et al: Importance of intracranial atherosclerotic disease in patients with symptomatic stenosis of the internal carotid artery: The North American Symptomatic Carotid Endarterectomy Trial. Stroke 1999;30(2):282.
7. Streifler JY, Eliasziw M, Fox AJ, et al: Angiographic detection of carotid plaque ulceration: Comparison with surgical observations in a multicenter study. North American Symptomatic Carotid Endarterectomy Trial. Stroke 1994;25(6):1130.
8. Beneficial effect of carotid endarterectomy in symptomatic patients with high-grade carotid stenosis. North American Symptomatic Carotid Endarterectomy Trial Collaborators. N Engl J Med 1991;325(7):445.
9. Randomised trial of endarterectomy for recently symptomatic carotid stenosis: Final results of the MRC European Carotid Surgery Trial (ECST). Lancet 1998;351 (9113):1379.
10. Eliasziw M, Streifler JY, Fox AJ, et al: Significance of plaque ulceration in symptomatic patients with high-grade carotid stenosis. North American Symptomatic Carotid Endarterectomy Trial. Stroke 1994;25(2):304.
11. Rothwell PM, Warlow CP: Prediction of benefit from carotid endarterectomy in individual patients: A risk-modelling study. European Carotid Surgery Trialists' Collaborative Group. Lancet 1999;353(9170):2105.
12. Goldstein LB, McCrory DC, Landsman PB, et al: Multicenter review of preoperative risk factors for carotid endarterectomy in patients with ipsilateral symptoms. Stroke 1994;25(6):1116.
13. Pearce WH, Parker MA, Feinglass J, et al: The importance of surgeon volume and training in outcomes for vascular surgical procedures. J Vasc Surg 1999;29 (5):768.
14. Gomez CR: The role of carotid angioplasty and stenting. Semin Neurol 1998;18(4):501.
15. Gasecki AP, Ferguson GG, Eliasziw M, et al: Early endarterectomy for severe carotid artery stenosis after a nondisabling stroke: Results from the North American Symptomatic Carotid Endarterectomy Trial. J Vasc Surg 1994; 20(2):288.
16. Nicholls SC, Bergelin R, Strandness DE: Neurologic sequelae of unilateral carotid artery occlusion: Immediate and late. J Vasc Surg 1989;10(5):542.
17. Archie JP Jr: Carotid endarterectomy when the distal internal carotid artery is small or poorly visualized. J Vasc Surg 1994;19(1):23.
18. Gertler JP, Cambria RP. The role of external carotid endarterectomy in the treatment of ipsilateral internal carotid occlusion: Collective review. J Vasc Surg 1987;6(2): 158.
19. Webster MW, Makaroun MS, Steed DL, et al: Compromised cerebral blood flow reactivity is a predictor of stroke in patients with symptomatic carotid artery occlusive disease. J Vasc Surg 1995;21(2):338.

SYMPTOMATIC CAROTID ARTERY STENOSIS

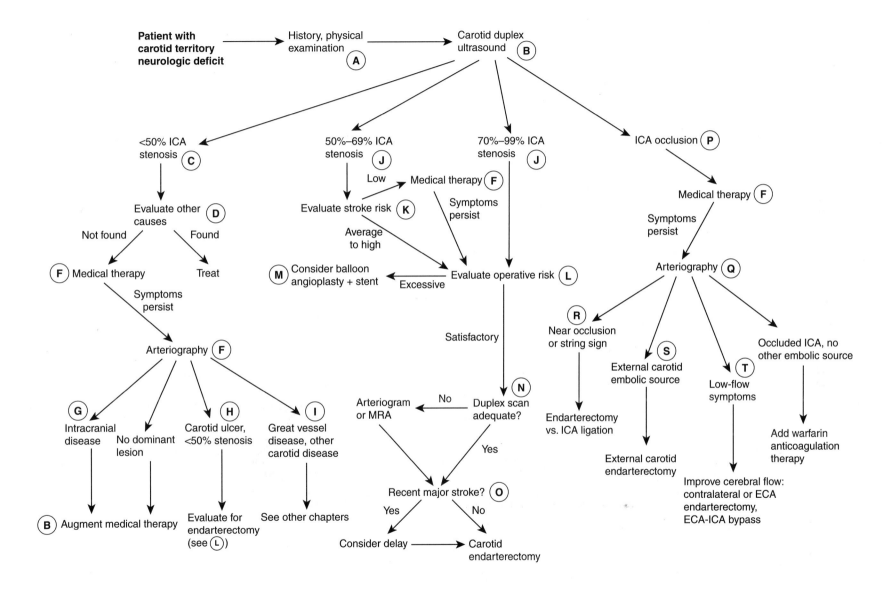

Chapter 8 Asymptomatic Carotid Artery Stenosis

ALIK FARBER, MD • JACK L. CRONENWETT, MD

A Patients at increased risk for carotid artery stenosis are often evaluated with duplex ultrasound surveillance, which is an accurate, noninvasive method of determining stenosis severity. Factors that increase the prevalence of carotid stenosis include (1) a carotid bruit, (2) increasing age, (3) cigarette smoking, and (4) claudication, especially with a low ankle-brachial index (ABI).[1,2] The cost-effectiveness of routine screening for asymptomatic carotid stenosis has been debated, but this is likely beneficial in patients with a predicted high prevalence. Most patients with symptomatic peripheral vascular disease have a sufficiently high prevalence to justify screening.[3]

B Initial evaluation of a patient with an apparently asymptomatic carotid artery stenosis should include a careful history and neurologic examination to confirm the absence of occult neurologic symptoms or signs.

C Patients with asymptomatic internal carotid artery (ICA) stenosis of less than 60% diameter diameter reduction (compared with the normal ICA beyond the stenosis) are at low risk for transient ischemic attack (TIA) or stroke related to the carotid artery. If such stenoses do not progress, the risk of stroke is less than 0.5% per year.[4]

D In asymptomatic patients, less than 60% ICA stenosis can progress to a more severe stenosis that may benefit from carotid endarterectomy. Therefore, duplex ultrasound surveillance is usually recommended for these patients, who would otherwise be candidates for surgery. Stenosis progression is more likely in patients with initially more severe disease. Of patients with mild ICA stenosis (duplex peak systolic velocity [PSV] <175 cm/sec), only 6% progressed to more than 60% stenosis in 4 years, compared with progression in 84% of patients with more severe but still less than 60% initial ICA stenosis.[5]

We recommend a follow-up duplex scan 6 months after the initial evaluation of patients with less than 60% stenosis of the ICA. Subsequent duplex scanning is performed at 2- to 3-year intervals if the stenosis is minimal (peak systolic velocity < 175 cm/sec) and stable. For more severe or progressing stenosis, more frequent follow-up at 6- to 12-month intervals is appropriate.

E Medical therapy for patients with asymptomatic ICA stenosis includes smoking cessation and control of atherosclerotic risk factors such as hyperlipidemia, hypertension, and diabetes. Aspirin has been shown to reduce the stroke rate following TIAs or stroke, but not in asymptomatic patients.[6] However, because aspirin does reduce the risk of vascular death, myocardial infarction, and stroke as a combined endpoint, it is often recommended for asymptomatic patients with known carotid stenosis.[7] Clopidogrel, a new antiplatelet agent, has some additional benefit over aspirin.[8] Because of its higher cost, however, we do not use clopidogrel in asymptomatic patients unless they have a high risk profile or cannot tolerate aspirin.

F The Asymptomatic Carotid Atherosclerosis Study (ACAS), a randomized trial of carotid endarterectomy versus medical management of patients with asymptomatic ICA stenosis of less than 60%, found a significant risk reduction of 53% for ipsilateral stroke in patients undergoing surgery.[9] However, the absolute stroke reduction at 5 years was relatively small, decreasing from 11% in the medically treated group to 5% in the surgical group. A previous Veterans Affairs study yielded nearly identical results.[10] Neither study found that the severity of ICA stenosis within the range of 60% to 99% affected the risk of future stroke; however, neither study determined stenosis severity at the time of subsequent stroke when disease progression is likely to have occurred.

Because ICA stenosis progression is an important predictor of ipsilateral hemispheric stroke, it is intuitive that greater stenosis severity increases stroke risk. In fact, prior to the ACAS, most surgeons reserved endarterectomy for asymptomatic patients with the most severe (>80%) ICA stenosis. One study evaluating 425 patients with stable, asymptomatic 50% to 79% stenosis found that the estimated cumulative 5-year risk of ipsilateral stroke was only 5.4%, which is a rate comparable to that for the surgical patients in the ACAS.[11] Therefore, despite ACAS results, we recommend a more conservative approach for patients with 60% to 79% ICA stenosis compared to those with more than 80% ICA stenosis.

G Progression of carotid stenosis in the asymptomatic patient is a marker of more aggressive atherosclerosis and increases the risk of further progression and symptoms.[11,12] Patients with asymptomatic 50% to 79% carotid stenosis have a 5% annual rate of progression to stenosis greater than 80%.[11] Progression to severe (>80%) ICA stenosis is associated with a 11% annual risk of stroke, whereas absence of progression has an annual risk of stroke lower than 1%.[12] Unfortunately, risk factors that predict stenosis progression in this patient cohort have not been found, and therefore, duplex scan follow-up is important in identifying progressing stenoses.

H For asymptomatic patients with nonprogressing, 60% to 79% ICA stenoses, other risk factors for stroke should be evaluated to identify a higher-risk group that would more certainly benefit from endarterectomy. Because women had both a lower stroke risk under medical therapy and a higher perioperative morbidity rate in the ACAS, we usually do not perform endarterectomy in women until the stenosis reaches 80% unless other additional risk factors are present for stroke.[9] Although it is logical that carotid plaque characteristics should influence stroke risk, this has been difficult to prove. Large, complex ulcers observed at arteriography probably increase stroke risk, but few patients currently undergo arteriogra-

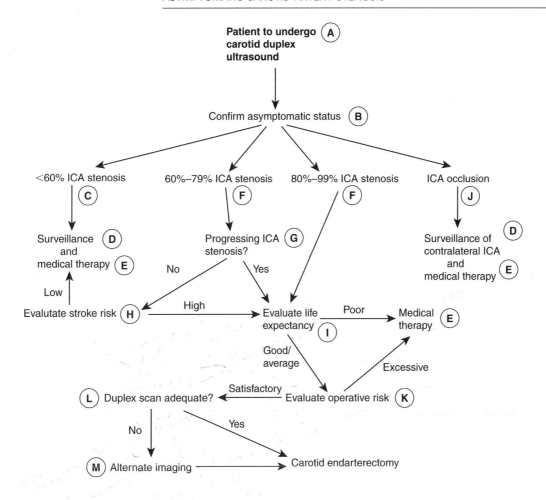

phy. Increasing evidence suggests that echolucent, soft plaque detected by duplex ultrasound scans increases stroke risk compared with the finding of echogenic, calcified plaque.[13] Other factors also appear to increase stroke risk:

- Contralateral ICA occlusion[14]
- Silent ipsilateral infarction on CT scan or silent embolization detected by transcranial Doppler ultrasound surveillance[15]
- Multiple atherosclerotic risk factors

(I) Life expectancy is very important in the decision of whether a patient would benefit from a prophylactic procedure, such as carotid endarterectomy for asymptomatic stenosis. In the ACAS, the late benefit of endarterectomy did not overcome the initial morbidity and mortality until 3 years after surgery.[9] In one cost-effectiveness analysis, we have shown that carotid endarterectomy does not appear cost-effective in the average asymptomatic patient older than 80 years, recognizing that life expectancy depends on many factors other than chronologic age.[16] Patients with an asymptomatic carotid stenosis must choose between the up-front risk of stroke and death versus the gradual reduction of stroke over the ensuing 5 years. In this regard, individual patient preferences and risk aversion are quite variable and must be incorporated into decision making.

(J) Asymptomatic patients with an occluded ICA have a relatively low risk of ipsilateral stroke that may be increased by contralateral ICA stenosis.[14] Endarterectomy is not indicated for ICA occlusion because of the high risk of stroke. These patients are treated medically and are followed up with duplex ultrasound surveillance of the contralateral carotid artery.

(K) At 5 years, the 6% absolute stroke rate reduction afforded by carotid endarterectomy in the ACAS was critically dependent on a low perioperative stroke and death rate, which was only 2.6%.[9] Individual patients must be carefully evaluated in this regard, since a higher perioperative complication rate may eliminate the benefit of endarterectomy. In the ACAS,[17] the following factors increased the perioperative risk of TIA, stroke, or death:

- History of previous stroke
- Contralateral carotid stenosis >60%
- Contralateral siphon stenosis
- Hypertension
- Diabetes mellitus

Another review[18] of carotid endarterectomy performed for asymptomatic stenosis revealed that perioperative stroke and death rates were significantly increased by (1) female gender, (2) age older than 75 years, (3) congestive heart failure, and (4) combined carotid-coronary artery surgery. Operative risk due to coronary artery disease needs to be determined (see Chapters 1 and 20). Individual surgeon and hospital experience are also important determinants of operative outcome. Surgeons who performed fewer than six carotid endarterectomies per year had a significantly higher perioperative stroke and death rates than surgeons who performed more than 12 operations per year.[19] In light of these factors, patients at high perioperative risk can be selected for medical, rather than surgical, therapy.

(L) Duplex ultrasound surveillance has been found to be very accurate in the diagnosis of carotid stenosis. In an effort to avoid the stroke risk and cost of cerebral arteriography, it is used at an increasing number of centers as the sole preoperative study before carotid endarterectomy.[20] This is especially relevant for patients with asymptomatic stenosis, in whom small increases in perioperative risk can nullify the long-term benefit of endarterectomy. This is significant, since 1.2% of the total 2.3% perioperative stroke and death rate in the ACAS was attributable to preoperative arteriography.[17] Even with highly accurate vascular laboratories, however, sometimes preoperative duplex evaluation alone is not adequate. The most important example is evidence of disease in the proximal common carotid or in the distalmost visualized portion of the ICA, since this may significantly alter the conduct of the operation. In addition, severe calcification may obscure duplex insonation, and a loop or kink in the ICA may be difficult to interpret. In these circumstances, selective carotid arteriography or magnetic resonance angiography (MRA) is often beneficial.

(M) Carotid arteriography is the study most often used to evaluate carotid disease when the preoperative carotid duplex study is inadequate. Recently, MRA and CT scans have been used in an effort to avoid complications of arteriography that would eliminate the benefit of endarterectomy in asymptomatic patients. Centers experienced with these techniques have demonstrated their accuracy and utility.[21, 22]

REFERENCES

1. Cheng SW, Wu LL, Ting AC, et al: Screening for asymptomatic carotid stenosis in patients with peripheral vascular disease: A prospective study and risk factor analysis. Cardiovasc Surg 1999;7(3):303.
2. Marek J, Mills JL, Harvich J, et al: Utility of routine carotid duplex screening in patients who have claudication. J Vasc Surg 1996;24(4):572.
3. Ascher E, DePippo P, Salles-Cunha S, et al: Carotid screening with duplex ultrasound in elderly asymptomatic patients referred to a vascular surgeon: Is it worthwhile? Ann Vasc Surg 1999;13(2):164.
4. Johnson BF, Verlato F, Bergelin RO, et al: Clinical outcome in patients with mild and moderate carotid artery stenosis. J Vasc Surg 1995;21(1):120.
5. Nehler MR, Moneta GL, Lee RW, et al: Improving selection of patients with less than 60% asymptomatic internal carotid artery stenosis for follow-up carotid artery duplex scanning. J Vasc Surg 1996;24(4):580.
6. Dyken ML: Antiplatelet agents and stroke prevention. Semin Neurol 1998;18(4):441.
7. Antiplatelet Trialists' Collaboration: Collaborative overview of randomised trials of antiplatelet therapy: I. Prevention of death, myocardial infarction, and stroke by prolonged antiplatelet therapy in various categories of patients [see comments]. BMJ 1994;308(6921):81; erratum, BMJ 1994;308(6943):1540.
8. CAPRIE Steering Committee: A randomised, blinded, trial of Clopidogrel versus Aspirin in Patients at Risk of Ischaemic Events (CAPRIE). Lancet 1996;348(9038):1329.
9. Executive Committee for the Asymptomatic Carotid Atherosclerosis Study: Endarterectomy for asymptomatic carotid artery stenosis. [see comments]. JAMA 1995;273(18):1421.
10. Hobson RW 2nd, Weiss DG, Fields WS, et al: Efficacy of carotid endarterectomy for asymptomatic carotid stenosis. The Veterans Affairs Cooperative Study Group [see comments]. N Engl J Med 1993;328(4):221.
11. Rockman CB, Riles TS, Lamparello PJ, et al: Natural history and management of the asymptomatic, moderately stenotic internal carotid artery. J Vasc Surg 1997;25(3):423.
12. Mansour MA, Mattos MA, Faught WE, et al: The natural history of moderate (50% to 79%) internal carotid artery stenosis in symptomatic, nonhemispheric, and asymptomatic patients. J Vasc Surg 1995;21(2):346.
13. Biasi GM, Sampaolo A, Mingazzini P, et al: Computer analysis of ultrasonic plaque echolucency in identifying high risk carotid bifurcation lesions. Eur J Vasc Endovasc Surg 1999;17(6):476.
14. Faught WE, van Bemmelen PS, Mattos MA, et al: Presentation and natural history of internal carotid artery occlusion. J Vasc Surg 1993;18(3):512.
15. Molloy J, Markus HS: Asymptomatic embolization predicts stroke and TIA risk in patients with carotid artery stenosis. Stroke 1999;30(7):1440.
16. Cronenwett JL, Birkmeyer JD, Nackman GB, et al: Cost-effectiveness of carotid endarterectomy in asymptomatic patients. J Vasc Surg 1997;25(2):298.
17. Young B, Moore WS, Robertson JT, et al: An analysis of perioperative surgical mortality and morbidity in the asymptomatic carotid atherosclerosis study: ACAS Investigators. Asymptomatic Carotid Artheriosclerosis Study [see comments]. Stroke 1996;27(12):2216.
18. Goldstein LB, McCrory DC, Landsman PB, et al: Multicenter review of preoperative risk factors for carotid endarterectomy in patients with ipsilateral symptoms [see comments]. Stroke 1994;25(6):1116.
19. Kucey DS, Bowyer B, Iron K, et al: Determinants of outcome after carotid endarterectomy. J Vasc Surg 1998;28(6):1051.

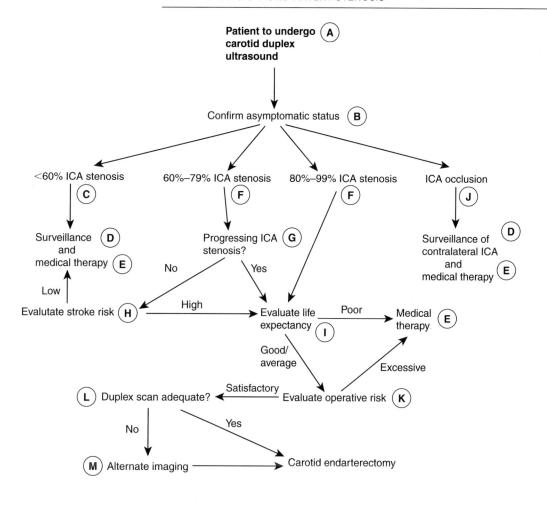

20. Dawson DL, Zierler RE, Strandness DE Jr, et al: The role of duplex scanning and arteriography before carotid endarterectomy: A prospective study. J Vasc Surg 1993;18(4):673.

21. Patel MR, Kuntz KM, Klufas RA, et al: Preoperative assessment of the carotid bifurcation: Can magnetic resonance angiography and duplex ultrasonography replace contrast arteriography? Stroke 1995;26(10):1753.

22. Cinat M, Lane CT, Pham H, et al: Helical CT angiography in the preoperative evaluation of carotid artery stenosis. J Vasc Surg 1998;28(2):290.

Chapter 9 Carotid Endarterectomy

JOSEPH P. ARCHIE, PhD, MD • R. DAVID EDRINGTON, MD

A The choice of general anesthesia versus cervical-regional block anesthesia for carotid endarterectomy (CEA) continues to be controversial. There are no prospective randomized trials to answer the question as to which method may be preferable. Many surgeons prefer one method and are hesitant to change, although surgeons who do so usually go from general to regional block anesthesia.[1-3] We routinely use general anesthesia except in the occasional patient with severe chronic obstructive pulmonary disease or severe left ventricular dysfunction. Other surgeons prefer regional block anesthesia, using it to determine when to selectively shunt, or they believe that it poses a similar[2] or lower[3] incidence of cardiac and pulmonary complications and a lower incidence of perioperative hypertension requiring care in the intensive care unit (ICU). In the past decade, we have observed a striking decrease in the incidence of both perioperative myocardial infarction and hypertension with general anesthesia. The exact reasons for this are undetermined but are probably related to more expert anesthetic management and the increasing number of patients who have had prior coronary artery angioplasty, stenting, or bypass.

B Carotid shunting has a long history of controversy. The choices are obligatory use, selective use based on a monitoring method, and nonuse. Some surgeons, particularly those involved with residency and fellowship training programs, prefer obligatory shunting with general anesthesia. This not only provides instruction in shunt use but alleviates the anxiety associated with prolonged carotid occlusion times. Obligatory shunting as well as all methods of determining when to selectively shunt are deliberately overprotective in terms of identifying the 1% to 2% of patients who need a shunt to prevent cerebral infarction due to inadequate collateral flow during carotid clamping.[4, 5] However, use of a shunt is not without a few drawbacks:

- The danger of embolization or dissection
- The need for a longer arteriotomy
- The tendency to get in the way of the actual endarterectomy

Although only approximately 1% to 2% of intraoperative strokes are attributable to not using a shunt, 7% to 19% of patients experience a transient neurologic deficit after carotid occlusion under regional block or local anesthesia and are accordingly selectively shunted using this technique.[1-3] Frequently used methods of determining when to use a shunt under general anesthesia include electroencephalography, evoked potential, and carotid stump back-pressure. Each of these techniques has its proponents, opponents, and criteria. It is not important which method is used, but it is essential to protect those few patients with inadequate collateral flow. We use a shunt when the mean *internal carotid artery* (ICA) stump back-pressure is below 25 mmHg or when the cerebral perfusion pressure (mean back-pressure − mean jugular venous pressure) is less than 18 mmHg. Over the past two decades and after approximately 2500 carotid endarterectomies, this approach to selective shunting has resulted in an 11% shunt rate and an intraoperative stroke rate *not attributable directly to other causes* of approximately 0.2%.

C When the length of carotid plaque is extensive, when the endarterectomized segment is severely damaged, or when a feathered ICA endpoint cannot be obtained because of a long tongue of plaque, interposition bypass grafting is an appropriate technique. This method has been used in approximately 1% of our carotid endarterectomies.[6] Although we prefer and use saphenous vein grafts, polyester (Dacron) and polytetrafluoroethylene (PTFE) bypass grafts have also produced acceptable outcomes in small series.

D Although eversion endarterectomy has had a long history, it has recently experienced a renewed advocacy. In a prospective, randomized trial comparing standard to eversion carotid endarterectomy, there were no statistically significant differences in outcomes.[7] In this study, however, 60% of the standard or conventional endarterectomies were primarily closed, and of the 40% undergoing patch angioplasty reconstruction, the majority (85%) were performed with synthetic materials.

There is a growing body of evidence that patch angioplasty has a highly significant, threefold to fourfold advantage over primary closure, as measured by perioperative ICA thrombosis, perioperative stroke, and more than 50% restenosis at 1 year.[8, 9] Furthermore, carotid endarterectomies utilizing autologous vein patches have resulted in statistically significantly lower rates of perioperative stroke and restenosis than procedures utilizing Dacron and PTFE patches.[9, 10] Accordingly, we believe that this trial did not compare eversion endarterectomy with the best alternative technique (i.e., standard endarterectomy combined with saphenous vein patch angioplasty reconstruction). Therefore, we see no reason to deviate from the latter procedure. We patch when the arteriotomy necessary to obtain a complete ICA endpoint extends beyond the bulb segment into the uniform diameter artery.[6] This occurs in approximately 96% of our carotid endarterectomies.

E Shortening of redundant endarterectomized ICA segments is becoming a more frequent practice. Although we have used eversion plication at or just distal to the bifurcation, a recent analysis of our experience indicates a significantly *higher* incidence of recurrent stenosis, ≥50% diameter, for the *shortened carotid endarterectomies* in the first 3 years after the procedure when compared to *nonshortened* arteries.[11] Riles and colleagues[12] frequently use eversion plication shortening but perform the procedure more distally near the ICA endpoint of the carotid endarterectomy. Patch angioplasty reconstruction is almost imperative after shortening in order to produce a gradu-

CAROTID ENDARTERECTOMY

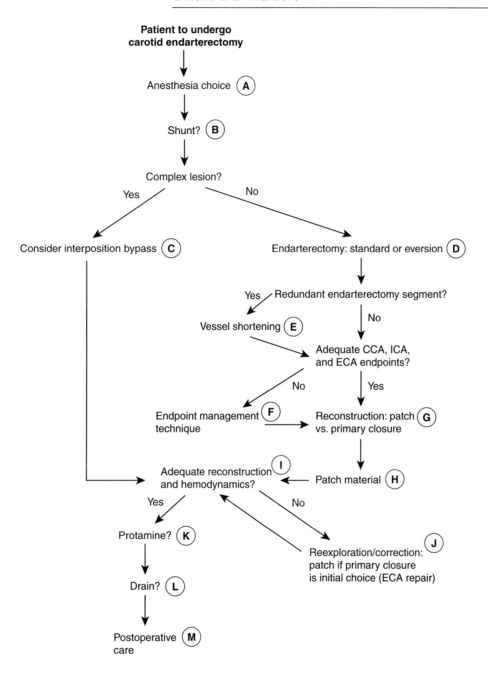

ally tapered transition from the ICA origin to the distal end of the arteriotomy.

(F) Management of incomplete endarterectomy endpoints is uniquely different for each of the three carotid arteries. A completely feathered endpoint of the *common carotid artery* (CCA) is rarely obtainable. Partial or complete circumferential endarterectomy produces a CCA step transition that can be an embolic source and a harbinger of late restenosis.[13] Steps greater than 1 mm in depth can be quickly and easily reconstructed by inversion plication.[13] Beveling the step is an alternative to plication but leaves the thrombogenic diseased media and intima exposed to the blood flow surface, whereas inversion plication does not.

The adequacy of external carotid endarterectomy endpoints is often difficult to determine immediately because they are usually completed blindly with partial eversion. Inspection of the external carotid endarterectomy specimen can be helpful in estimating the adequacy of the endpoint. Continuous wave Doppler ultrasound interrogation after restoring flow can identify major obstructions or occlusions of the *external carotid artery* (ECA). However, even with repair of major defects, the rate of residual and recurrent ECA stenosis is high.[14] The *ICA endpoint* is by far the most important. When a completely feathered endpoint cannot be obtained tacking sutures are required. While these have been necessary in approximately 3% of our operations, the presence of tacking sutures and residual plaque is less than hemodynamically optimal and are harbingers of recurrent stenosis and emboli.

Another way to manage a long tongue of plaque that cannot be completely removed is to use interpositional bypass grafting with a beveled distal anastomosis that tacks over the tongue.[6] The use of additional techniques to manage difficult endpoints usually obligates one to close with a patch angioplasty.

(G) Obligatory patch angioplasty reconstruction, compared with obligatory primary closure, has a statistically significant and powerful (three to four times lower) rate of postoperative ICA thrombosis and perioperative stroke, and a 1-year restenosis rate equal to or more than 50%.[7, 8] The more frequently patch reconstruction is utilized, the lower the incidence of these three outcome endpoints.[7] We use patch angioplasty reconstruction (or occasionally interposition bypass grafting) in the 96% of endarterectomies in which the arteriotomy necessary to obtain a complete ICA endarterectomy endpoint extends beyond the carotid bulb into the uniform diameter distal artery. We limit primary closure to the 4% of cases in which the arteriotomy required to obtain a complete endpoint is limited to the ICA bulb segment.

(H) Controversy over the optimal patch material continues. Meta-analysis of studies in which two or more patch materials were used indicates that greater saphenous vein–patched carotid endarterectomies are associated with statistically significantly and powerfully better outcomes regarding perioperative stroke and restenosis compared with both Dacron and PTFE patches and carry slightly better outcomes than an endarterectomy performed with everted cervical vein patches.[9, 10]

We have found that carotid endarterectomies performed with saphenous vein patches are associated with significantly less restenosis (1.1%) in the first 3 years than when a collagen-impregnated, knitted Dacron patch is used (12.6%).[11] Although saphenous vein is the patch material of choice, vein patches smaller than 3.5 mm in distended diameter carry an increased risk for patch rupture and should not be used.[15] We routinely harvest saphenous veins from the groin in women because many women have small-diameter lower leg veins. Most men have adequate distal veins.

A frequently voiced concern for harvesting greater saphenous veins for a carotid patch is the need for a subsequent autologous bypass. Because only 5 to 6 cm is required for a patch, ankle harvest is rarely a problem. Several investigations have shown that harvest of the first few centimeters of the proximal saphenous vein leaves a patent, adequate, and normal distal vein for possible later use.

(I) Intraoperative confirmation of the adequacy of endarterectomy and reconstruction is highly advisable. Retained plaque and reconstruction technical errors produce hemodynamically disturbed flow, a harbinger of restenosis and thrombosis.[13, 16] For more than two decades, we have used continuous wave bidirectional Doppler interrogation during all carotid endarterectomies. This inexpensive and readily available technology allows qualitative confirmation of normality of blood flow and velocity waveforms in the three carotid arteries as well as the reconstruction zone in most cases. The exception is the difficulty of detecting flow through synthetic patches because of acoustic interference caused by thousands of trapped air pockets. Doppler interrogation plus visual inspection usually identifies major defects, including kinks at the distal end of a patch, dissections, and hemodynamically significant retained atheroma proximally or distally.

Intraoperative arteriography is a commonly used alternative technique, but it is invasive and expensive and frequently adds significant time to the operation. Intraoperative duplex scanning is a more recent technique and is used to confirm the technical adequacy of the surgical result. With advances in imaging and Doppler spectral analysis, there is little doubt that intraoperative duplex scanning is the method of choice for interrogation of the carotid artery after endarterectomy, although this is dependent on operator experience.

(J) Repair or reconstruction of major operative defects in the ICA is mandatory. If residual disease or stenosis in or distal to the endarterectomized segment is identified, the arteriotomy should be extended and patch angioplasty reconstruction performed after the surgeon deals with the defects.

The most common major defect we have identified, although unusual after the learning curve, is

CAROTID ENDARTERECTOMY

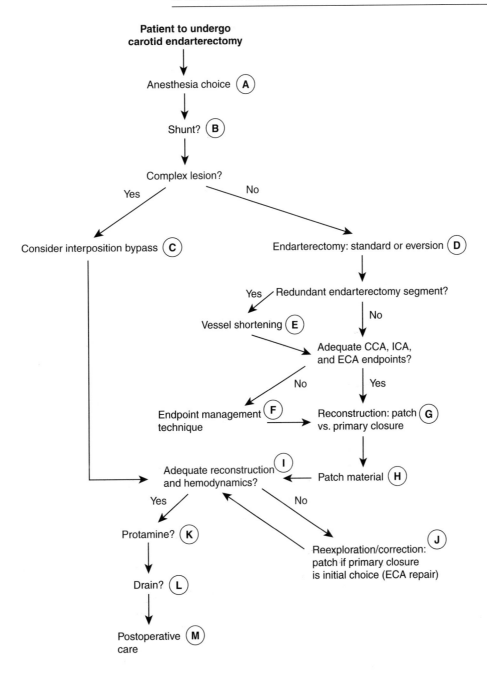

a kink at the distal end of a patch. This is due to failure to taper the patch and artery properly, usually because of too wide a distal patch (toe). This produces an elliptical cross-section or kink in the posterior wall of the native artery and is not visually obvious to the surgeon unless the artery is rotated. The surgeon can best manage repair of an occluded or highly obstructed ECA by excluding it with a clamp across the orifice, elastic loops on the branches, and a completion endarterectomy performed under direct vision. These defects are usually dissection flaps. However, intraoperative repair of these defects has not proved to be highly successful or durable.[14] Although large endarterectomy-produced CCA steps (with or without flaps) can be identified by intraoperative duplex scanning, these are clearly present during endarterectomy and are best managed before reconstruction (see F).

(K) Reversal of heparin with protamine is not advisable unless excessive intraoperative bleeding from suture lines (or the wound in general) or significant postoperative hemorrhage is present. Protamine administration is associated with an increased risk of perioperative stroke.[17,18] It has been suggested that routine use of 3000 units of heparin does not require reversal with protamine.[19] Protamine should be avoided in patients with insulin-dependent diabetes because of the increased risk of hypersensitivity.

The protamine problem is coupled with the controversy over heparin dose. Some surgeons titrate heparin based on body weight and chemical tests, others give a standard dose, such as 5000 units, and others give more when a shunt is used. We normally administer 5000 units of heparin prior to carotid occlusion whether or not a shunt is used, and we do not give protamine unless absolutely necessary to control hemorrhage after other intraoperative methods of hemostasis and blood pressure control have been employed. Most of the approximately 10% of patients to whom we give protamine have been taking warfarin or one of the newer antiplatelet drugs preoperatively.

(L) Routine use of a drain overnight is controversial. Many patients who have satisfactory hemostasis at the time of closure do not need a drain. Unfortunately, we have not been able to determine which patients will need a drain based on the findings at surgery. Therefore, for *all* patients we use a fully perforated, 8-mm wide soft drain with bulb suction. Such drains are beneficial in reducing and evacuating hematomas in the recovery room or later. Obligatory drainage of all endarterectomy incisions is one key reason why our incidence of returning patients to the operating room is less than 2%. Whereas both operative hemostasis and perioperative blood pressure control are the mainstay of hemorrhage and hematoma prevention, a drain provides added protection against unnecessary reexploration. We prefer to bring the drain out of the lower end of the incision and to place a simple suture to be tied when it is removed, prior to early discharge.

(M) After leaving the recovery room, patients are hospitalized overnight, with electrocardiographic and arterial pressure monitoring in a non-ICU bed managed by experienced nursing personnel. Blood pressure control and neurologic monitoring are important. Most patients can be discharged the next day.

REFERENCES

1. Allen BT, Anderson CB, Rubin BG, et al: The influence of anesthetic technique on perioperative complications after carotid endarterectomy. J Vasc Surg 1994;19:834–843.
2. Shah DM, Darling C III, Chang BB, et al: Carotid endarterectomy in awake patients: Its safety, acceptability, and outcome. J Vasc Surg 1994;19:1015–1020.
3. Hartsell PA, Calligaro KD, Syrek JR, et al: Postoperative blood pressure changes associated with cervical block versus general anesthesia following carotid endarterectomy. Ann Vasc Surg 1999;13:104–108.
4. Baker WH, Littooy FN, Hayes AC, et al: Carotid endarterectomy without a shunt: The control series. J Vasc Surg 1984;1:50–56.
5. Ferguson GG: Intra-operative monitoring and internal shunts: Are they necessary in carotid endarterectomy? Stroke 1982;13:387–389.
6. Archie JP: Carotid endarterectomy with reconstruction techniques tailored to operative findings. J Vasc Surg 1993;17:141–151.
7. Cao P, Giordano G, DeRango P, et al: A randomized study on eversion versus standard carotid endarterectomy: Study design and preliminary results. The Everest Trial. J Vasc Surg 1998;27:595–605.
8. Archie JP: Patching with carotid endarterectomy: When to do it and what to use. Semin Vasc Surg 1998;2:24–29.
9. Archie JP: Carotid endarterectomy outcomes: Trials, regional and statewide studies, individual surgeons variance and the influence of patch reconstruction and patch materials. In Whittemore AD (ed): Advances in Vascular Surgery, vol 7. St. Louis, Mosby, 1999, pp 1–22.
10. Archie JP: Carotid patching: What is the optimal patch material. In Goldstone J (ed): Perspectives in Vascular Surgery, vol 10. New York, Thieme, 1999, pp 111–118.
11. Archie JP: Carotid endarterectomy outcome with vein or Dacron graft patch angioplasty and internal carotid artery shortening. J Vasc Surg 1999;29:654–664.
12. Goldman KA, Su WT, Riles TS, et al: A comparative study of saphenous vein, internal jugular vein, and knitted Dacron patches for carotid endarterectomy. Ann Vasc Surg 1995;9:71–79.
13. Archie JP: The endarterectomy-produced common carotid artery step: A harbinger of early emboli and late restenosis. J Vasc Surg 1996;23:932–939.
14. Archie JP: The outcome of external carotid endarterectomy during routine carotid endarterectomy. J Vasc Surg 1998;28:585–590.
15. Archie JP: Carotid endarterectomy saphenous vein patch rupture revisited: Selective utilization based on vein diameter. J Vasc Surg 1996;24:346–352.
16. Bandyk DR, Kaebnick NW, Adams MD, et al: Turbulence occurring after carotid bifurcation endarterectomy: A harbinger of residual and recurrent stenosis. J Vasc Surg 1988;7:261–274.
17. Mauney MC, Buchanan SA, Lawrence WA, et al: Stroke rate is markedly reduced after carotid endarterectomy by avoidance of protamine. J Vasc Surg 1995;22:264–270.
18. Levison JA, Faust GR, Halpern VJ, et al: Relationship of protamine dosing with postoperative complications of carotid endarterectomy. Ann Vasc Surg 1999;13:67–72.
19. Paty PSK, Darling C III, Kreienberg PB, et al: The use of low-dose heparin is safe in carotid endarterectomy and avoids the use of protamine sulfate. Cardiovasc Surg 1999;7:39–43.

CAROTID ENDARTERECTOMY

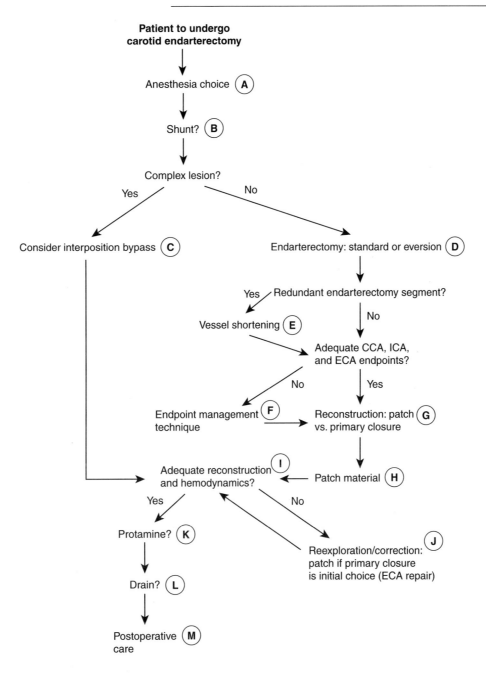

Chapter 10 Recurrent Carotid Stenosis

CARON ROCKMAN, MD • THOMAS S. RILES, MD

(A) The occurrence of new neurologic symptoms at any time in a patient who has undergone carotid endarterectomy should prompt an immediate duplex scan to evaluate both carotid arteries. In particular, hemispheric symptoms ipsilateral to the repaired artery should elicit an urgent evaluation to look specifically for the development of recurrent stenosis or other abnormalities of the surgical site.

(B) Considerable differences persist among experts in this field regarding the clinical significance and natural history of asymptomatic carotid restenosis as well as the role of surgical management and the results and efficacy of carotid reoperations. There is great variation in the reported incidence of recurrent carotid stenosis after prior carotid endarterectomy.

Most large series report less than ideal follow-up of patients after carotid endarterctomy.[1] Perhaps the most accurate incidence of recurrent stenosis is reported by the Asymptomatic Carotid Atherosclerosis Study (ACAS).[2] Early restenosis (>60% reduction in diameter) was found in 7.6% to 11.4% of cases. Late restenosis occurred in 1.9% to 4.9% of cases. Only 5.9% of the patients judged to have recurrent stenosis underwent reoperation, and only one was symptomatic. No correlation was found between the development of late stroke and recurrent disease. Some authors believe that follow-up with serial duplex ultrasound surveillance of the operated carotid artery is not cost-effective, considering the low incidence of recurrent disease.[3-7] Other authors advocate duplex scans early in the postoperative period to document *residual*, as opposed to *recurrent*, stenoses.[3-7]

Certainly, the issue of appropriate postoperative surveillance for carotid endarterectomy patients is an unsettled one at the present time. Our practice has been to perform yearly duplex scans of both carotid arteries following carotid endarterectomy in patients who are asymptomatic after surgery. The optimal interval may increase with stable lesions but decreases with progressing lesions.

(C) Recurrent stenosis of less than 50% in an asymptomatic patient does not necessitate any specific treatment. Yearly scanning should be continued, decreasing in frequency if stability is demonstrated on follow-up studies.

(D) Recurrent moderate stenosis (50% to 79%) in an asymptomatic patient should prompt more frequent surveillance with duplex scans, approximately every 6 months. Alternatively, a magnetic resonance angiogram (MRA) might be performed to gather more anatomic information about a borderline restenotic lesion. However, we do not treat moderate, asymptomatic restenoses surgically.[1]

(E) Severe recurrent stenosis (80% to 99%) in an asymptomatic patient should be confirmed by MRA or conventional cerebral angiography. If a severe recurrent stenosis is not present, the patient should continue with follow-up duplex scans every 6 months.

(F) It is unusual for an asymptomatic patient to develop sudden occlusion of the operated artery during regular duplex follow-up, but this problem does not benefit from surgical treatment. Conservative management, including antiplatelet therapy and continued surveillance of the contralateral carotid artery, is indicated.

(G) If recurrent stenosis of more than 80% is confirmed, our practice has been to treat the lesion, even in the asymptomatic patient. Not all surgeons agree with this aggressive approach.[3, 8] The arguments for nonoperative management of recurrent carotid stenoses are based on possible increased risk of perioperative complications with "redo" surgery. An additional rationale for nonoperative management of recurrent stenoses within 2 years of initial operation is that these most likely represent intimal hyperplasia with less embolic potential than that of atherosclerotic lesions. In our practice, however, we believe that similar surgical indications should be used for secondary carotid surgery as for primary carotid endarterectomy. In part, this is because we have seen patients with early recurrent stenoses caused by intimal hyperplasia who were symptomatic.

In one series reviewing our results with reoperative carotid surgery, 28% of patients who were found to have intimal hyperplasia at reoperative surgery reported preoperative symptoms. Late recurrent stenoses due to atherosclerotic disease carry the same characteristics of primary carotid lesions that predispose them toward embolization and stroke.

At present, we have no accurate way of differentiating which highly stenotic lesions would cause a stroke and which lesions would not. Therefore, we have chosen to treat asymptomatic restenoses that are preocclusive (>80%). With a low perioperative complication rate, the risk-benefit ratio with this approach should remain appropriate.[1]

(H) Recurrent stenoses that develop within 2 years of initial endarterectomy are presumed to be caused by intimal hyperplasia. If anatomic features are appropriate, we have chosen to treat selected asymptomatic, early, severe recurrent lesions with carotid angioplasty and stenting. Our initial experience with seven cases has revealed good technical results and no periprocedural neurologic complications. However, reoperative carotid surgery is still considered if the anatomic features of the recurrent stenosis do not make the lesion a favorable one for percutaneous treatment.

A review by Hobson and coworkers reported the results of carotid angioplasty and stenting in 17 cases of recurrent stenosis caused by neointimal hyperplasia.[9] There were no periprocedural neurologic events and no evidence of secondary recurrent stenoses to date. As with primary treatment of carotid disease, however, the role of ca-

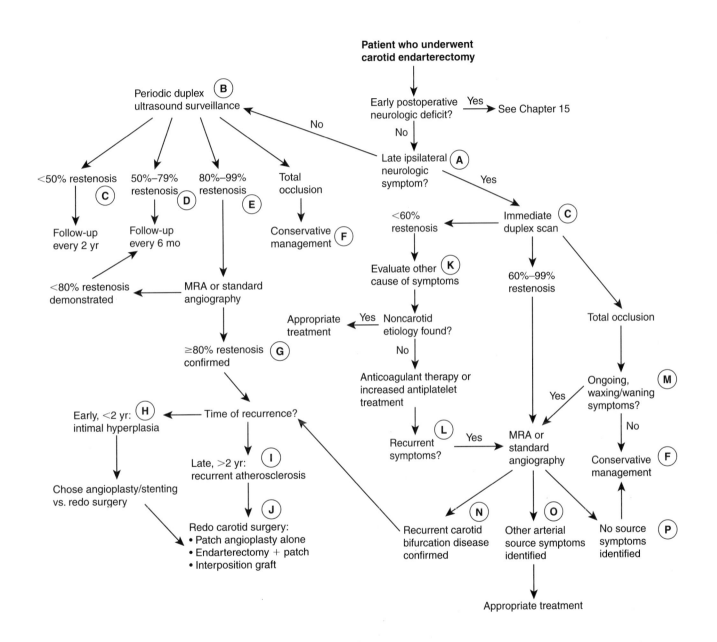

rotid angioplasty and stenting for recurrent stenosis remains to be defined by larger, long-term studies.

(I) Recurrent stenoses occurring later than 2 years after carotid endarterectomy are presumed to be caused by atherosclerosis. Although angioplasty and stenting might be considered in individual patients, reoperative carotid surgery remains the standard approach to these lesions.

(J) Many excellent series concerning reoperations have been published.[10–13] Most of these reports have found only minimally increased perioperative morbidity rates associated with reoperative carotid surgery.[1] In our recent review of 82 carotid reoperations, the perioperative neurologic complication rate was 3.7%; all strokes occurred in patients with unusually complex disease.[1] There was one clinically significant but transient cranial nerve injury. However, the long-term durability of reoperative carotid surgery has not been examined extensively; follow-up of patients with serial duplex surveillance is often lacking.

The ideal surgical technique is also unknown. In nearly all the reported surgically treated cases of recurrent carotid stenosis, patch angioplasty with or without reoperative endarterectomy was used. An earlier review of operations for recurrent stenosis at our institution revealed an important concern.[14] The incidence of late treatment failure after redo surgery was 19.5% (8 of 41 patients), consisting of one stroke, three transient ischemic attacks (TIAs), and four asymptomatic occlusions. We were concerned about these data, which revealed that perhaps surgery for carotid restenosis was less durable than that for primary carotid endarterectomy. Most of the reoperations in this series consisted of redo endarterectomy with vein patch angioplasty. After these results were published, we speculated that perhaps interposition grafting would be a more suitable operation for recurrent carotid artery disease. The goal of our study of 82 carotid reoperations was to determine whether a change in surgical technique influenced the rate of perioperative stroke, late stroke, or secondary restenosis in patients undergoing reoperative carotid surgery.[1]

The choice of which technical procedure to perform during this procedure must be based somewhat on the particular pathologic and anatomic features of the patient's recurrent disease. If typical intimal hyperplasia is found and if the luminal surface is smooth and free of irregularities, patch angioplasty alone of the stenotic lesion can be considered. If the recurrent lesion is found to be recurrent atherosclerotic disease, there are two main options: (1) reoperative endarterectomy and patch angioplasty and (2) replacement of the artery with interposition grafting. These options can be further subdivided into patch angioplasty or interposition grafting with either prosthetic material or autologous vein.

Reoperative endarterectomy can be performed only if it is technically feasible. In cases of recurrent carotid disease, it is often difficult, if not impossible, to establish an appropriate endarterectomy plane or to perform the endarterectomy satisfactorily. This difficulty may be due to the nature of the recurrent lesion or may be secondary to scar tissue in the reoperative area. In this instance, interposition grafting must be considered or it may be the only technical option for reconstruction of the artery. Occasionally, aneurysmal dilatation of a previous vein patch angioplasty is encountered. In this situation, reconstruction with interposition grafting is almost always necessary.

We have reviewed our experience with different materials and configurations used in carotid reoperation. There was a trend toward a higher perioperative neurologic complication rate with interposition grafting than with patch angioplasty (8.6% versus 2.9%; P = not significant). There was also a trend toward higher perioperative neurologic complication rate with prosthetic material than with autologous material (6.4% versus 2.9%; P = not significant). Long-term follow-up (mean, 35 months) also revealed a trend for more late failures (secondary recurrent stenosis, stroke, or occlusion) with patch angioplasty than with interposition grafting (14.6% versus 9.4%; P = not significant). Most notably, there was a statistically significant higher rate of late failures when reconstruction was performed with vein than with any prosthetic material (26.7% versus 2.3%, P = .002).

The reason for the apparent superiority of prosthetic material over autologous material is unclear. However, synthetic grafts appear to be superior to vein grafts in the carotid-subclavian bypass as well.[15, 16]

In summary, the operation performed for recurrent stenosis needs to be individualized and based on the particular operative findings in each patient and on the operating surgeon's judgment. At this point, however, we favor the use of prosthetic material, either polytetrafluoroethylene (PTFE) or polyester (Dacron), for both patch angioplasty and interposition grafting. Our results suggest that interposition grafting may produce a better long-term outcome than reoperative endarterectomy and patch angioplasty. However, a longer period of follow-up is required to confirm this result.

(K) In the case of ipsilateral hemispheric symptoms and recurrent carotid stenosis less than 60%, further evaluation to assess other etiologic factors should be performed. This may include cardiac, neurologic, and ophthalmologic examinations, depending on the specific symptoms. If a noncarotid cause is found, it should be specifically treated. If only a single TIA or ocular symptom has occurred or if the symptom is not well defined, enhanced antiplatelet treatment (increased aspirin, clopidogrel) or warfarin anticoagulation therapy is usually recommended. If the symptom is more compelling, arteriography may be recommended (see L).

(L) If a patient with less than 60% recurrent carotid stenosis manifests multiple hemispheric symptoms despite antiplatelet therapy, further evaluation with either MRA or conventional cerebral angiography is recommended. Occasionally, an extremely ulcerated lesion that is not

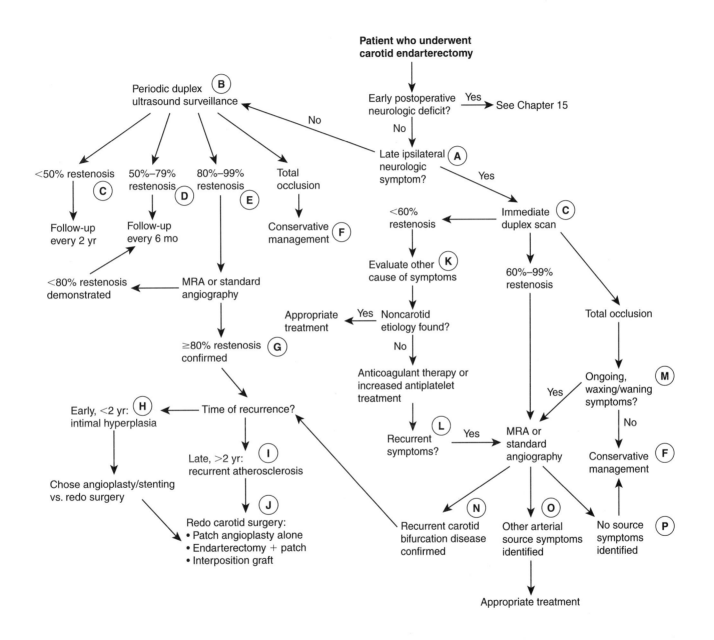

highly stenotic is visualized and found to be the cause of symptoms. Alternatively, the duplex scan may have missed a more stenotic lesion for technical reasons. Finally, more proximal or distal carotid disease may be detected.

(M) In rare instances, a duplex scan performed for the development of ipsilateral hemispheric symptoms may reveal total occlusion of the previously operated artery. If the symptom has been a singular event, conservative management with continued surveillance of the contralateral artery is recommended. However, if the patient experiences ongoing or waxing and waning hemispheric or ocular symptoms, MRA or cerebral angiography is recommended to ensure that the artery is occluded. Reoperative carotid surgery is usually recommended if the artery is found not to be totally occluded, or it would be occasionally recommended if the patient appears to be suffering crescendo embolic events related to an acute occlusion.

(N) If high-quality MRA or conventional cerebral angiography confirms recurrent stenosis of the carotid artery that is most likely the cause of symptoms, redo carotid surgery is recommended. Although the possible role of carotid angioplasty and stenting in this situation is not well defined, we have been reluctant to perform percutaneous treatment of these lesions when the lesion is actively embolizing. If nonembolic, low-flow symptoms are present in an early recurrence from intimal hyperplasia, this option could be considered.

(O) In some cases, emboli may originate from disease proximal or distal to the previous endarterectomy site. Such disease should be treated when possible (see other chapters).

(P) If no convincing source for hemispheric or ocular symptoms is found on angiography, continued conservative treatment with antiplatelet or anticoagulant medication is recommended.

REFERENCES

1. Rockman CB, Riles TS, Landis R, et al: Redo carotid surgery: An analysis of materials and configurations used in carotid reoperations and their influence on perioperative stroke and subsequent recurrent stenosis. J Vasc Surg 1999;29:72–81.
2. Moore WS, Kempczinski RF, Nelson JJ, Toole JF, for the ACAS Investigators: Recurrent carotid stenosis: Results of the Asymptomatic Carotid Atherosclerosis Study. Stroke 1998;29:2018–2025.
3. Ricotta JJ, O'Brien MS, DeWeese JA: Natural history of recurrent and residual stenosis after carotid endarterectomy: Implications for postoperative surveillance and surgical management. Surgery 1992;112:656–663.
4. Roth SM, Bandyk DF, Avino AJ, et al: A rational algorithm for duplex scan surveillance after carotid endarterectomy. J Vasc Surg 1999;30:453–460.
5. Patel ST, Kuntz KM, Kent KC: Is routine duplex ultrasound surveillance after carotid endarterectomy cost-effective? Surgery 1998;124:343–351.
6. Iafrati MD, Salamipour H, Young C, et al: Who needs surveillance of the contralateral carotid artery? Am J Surg 1996;172:136–139.
7. Ricotta JJ, DeWeese JA: Is routine carotid ultrasound surveillance after carotid endarterectomy worthwhile? Am J Surg 1996;172:140–142.
8. Healy DA, Zierler RE, Nicholls SC, et al: Long-term follow-up and clinical outcome of carotid restenosis. J Vasc Surg 1989;10:662–669.
9. Hobson RW II, Goldstein JE, Jamil Z, et al: Carotid restenosis: Operative and endovascular management. J Vasc Surg 1999;29:228–235.
10. Das MB, Hertzer NR, Ratliff NB, et al: Recurrent carotid stenosis: A five-year series of sixty-five reoperations. Ann Surg 1985;202:28–35.
11. Coyle KA, Smith RB, Gray BC, et al: Treatment of recurrent cerebrovascular disease: Review of a 10-year experience. Ann Surg 1995;221:517–524.
12. Mansour MA, Kang SS, Baker WH, et al: Carotid endarterectomy for recurrent stenosis. J Vasc Surg 1997;25:877–883.
13. Meyer FB, Piepgras DG, Fode NC: Surgical treatment of recurrent carotid artery stenosis. J Neurosurg 1994;80:781–787.
14. Gagne PJ, Riles TS, Jacobowitz GR, et al: Long-term follow-up of patients undergoing reoperation for recurrent carotid artery disease. J Vasc Surg 1993;18:991–1001.
15. Ziomek S, Quinones-Baldrich WJ, Busuttil RW, et al: The superiority of synthetic arterial grafts over autologous veins in carotid-subclavian bypass. J Vasc Surg 1986;3:140–145.
16. Law MM, Colburn MD, Moore WS, et al: Carotid subclavian bypass for brachiocephalic occlusive disease: Choice of conduit and long-term follow-up. Stroke 1995;26:1565–1571.

RECURRENT CAROTID STENOSIS

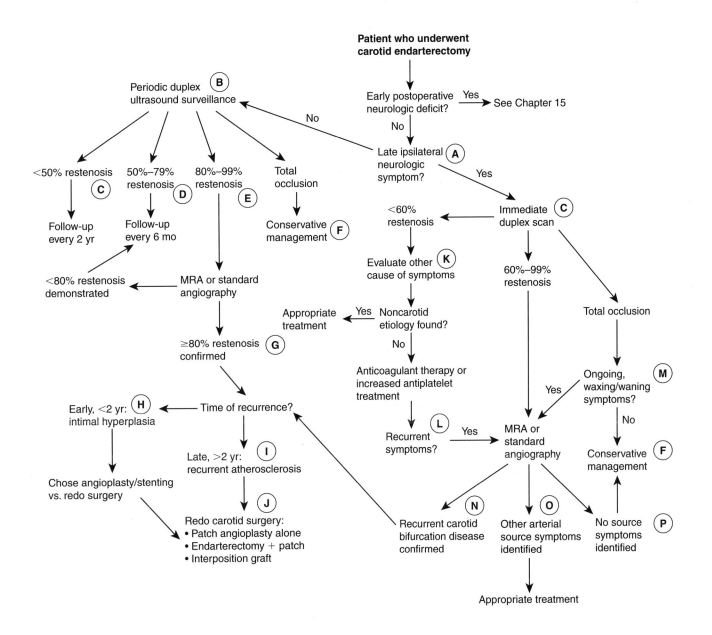

Chapter 11 Acute Stroke

SEAN P. RODDY, MD • WILLIAM C. MACKEY, MD

(A) In 1996, acute stroke was estimated to affect approximately 731,000 Americans, resulting in more than 143,000 deaths with an annual economic cost from health care and lost productivity of nearly $20 billion.[1]

(B) A rapid general history is necessary, with emphasis on risk factors for stroke as well as for prior similar events and the duration and extent of current symptoms. The physical examination includes a general overview to assess hemodynamic stability and airway patency and to exclude cardiac and other etiologic mechanisms. A detailed neurologic examination provides insight into the ischemic territory and the potential for hemorrhage. Routine blood work, electrocardiogram, and chest x-ray should be ordered in the emergency department. The cardiac rhythm should be interpreted. Supplemental oxygen is provided and isotonic volume is administered judiciously, avoiding any hypotension leading to cerebral hypoperfusion. If neurologic symptoms resolve within the first 24 hours, the event is called a transient ischemic attack (TIA). Most TIAs resolve within 1 hour but are considered a harbinger of impending stroke.[2]

(C) An emergent noncontrast head computed tomography (CT) scan is mandatory in all patients. If available on an emergent basis, a magnetic resonance imaging (MRI) scan of the head is an acceptable alternative in suitable patients. MRI may be more sensitive in detecting infarction very early after a neurologic event, but it has limitations in identifying acute subarachnoid hemorrhage. Both CT and MRI allow evaluation for intracranial hemorrhage or early signs of cerebral ischemia.

(D) The decision tree begins with an attempt to exclude patients from potential vascular surgical options who require intense medical or neurosurgical therapies. The criteria used here are essentially all poor prognostic signs for any stroke. These include:

- Intracranial hemorrhage
- A massive infarct
- Cerebral edema
- A mass effect on brain imaging

A depressed level of consciousness is usually indicative of these grave signs and therefore mitigates against aggressive surgical intervention. Seizures must be treated with anticonvulsant agents, and malignant hypertension must be controlled judiciously.

(E) The CT scan may be normal or may show only subtle signs of early infarction. Patients who also possess a preserved level of consciousness and reasonable neurologic findings may be considered candidates for aggressive early intervention with thrombolytic therapy, surgery, or both.

(F) The use of heparin, aspirin, or both remains controversial in acute stroke. Anticoagulants such as heparin are widely used as initial therapeutic agents on the basis of the belief that acute stroke is most likely secondary to thromboembolic occlusion of cerebral vessels. Some data are emerging that contradict this belief. The International Stroke Trial Collaborative Group found that patients given heparin experienced a significant reduction in recurrent ischemic strokes within 14 days (2.9% versus 3.8%), but this effect was offset by an equal increase in hemorrhagic strokes (1.2% versus 0.4%). The difference in death or nonfatal recurrent stroke was not significantly different (11.7% versus 12%), and there was a higher incidence of bleeding with the heparin group, leading the authors to recommend aspirin but not heparin as initial therapy.[3]

(G) A significant neurologic deficit less than 3 hours in duration with no contraindications to thrombolysis is an indication for intravenous thrombolytic therapy in a center with appropriate capabilities. Many formalized exclusion criteria need to be surveyed before these agents are administered. Once a thrombolytic agent is used, the patient either worsens with bleeding and is placed back into medical management or improves or remains unchanged. Patients in the latter category should continue on with carotid duplex evaluation.

The National Institute of Neurologic Disorders and Stroke r-TPA Stroke Study (NINDS study) demonstrated a highly significant benefit in clinical outcome at 3 months for patients given thrombolytic therapy both in global statistics and in each of the four individual components of its analysis. The odds ratio for a favorable outcome was 1.7 ($P = .008$); the absolute increase in the number of patients with minimal or no deficit was 11% (relative benefit, 55%) by the National Institute of Health Stroke Score (NIHSS) and 13% (relative benefit, 50%) by the Rankin score. A significantly higher incidence of intracranial hemorrhage was seen with stroke patients given r-TPA versus control (6.4% versus 0.6%; $P < .001$), but there was no difference in mortality at 3 months (17% versus 21%; $P = $ not significant).[2,4,5]

(H) Once carotid and vertebral imaging are performed, their findings should be interpreted in the context of the clinical presentation, the cardiac rhythm, and the CT scan findings. The rationale for acute intervention in symptomatic patients with critical carotid artery stenoses include the following:

1. Prevention of reinfarction, which can occur up to 20% of the time by 6 weeks.
2. Preservation of ischemic but not infarcted brain tissue (the so-called "ischemic penumbra").
3. Optimal long-term preservation of function.

We define a *significant* internal carotid artery stenosis as greater than 50% and a *critical* stenosis as 80% to 99%.

At this point in the decision tree, the cardiac rhythm is also important. The rate of ischemic stroke among patients with atrial fibrillation averages 5% per year, which is nearly six times the rate of patients without atrial fibrillation.[6] Ischemic strokes associated with atrial fibrillation are probably secondary to embolism of a stasis-induced thrombus that developed in the left atrium. However, 25% of strokes in patients with atrial fibrillation are due to aortic arch atherosclerotic plaque, cerebrovascular atherosclerotic disease, or other cardiac sources of embolism. Data from several recent clinical trials have shown that in patients with atrial fibrillation the use of oral warfarin produces a mean reduction in ischemic stroke of nearly 70% versus a reduction with aspirin of 25%. A patient experiencing this arrhythmia who has not been given anticoagulation therapy with warfarin must undergo echocardiography (see next) regardless of the carotid duplex results.

(I) Patients with noncritical carotid stenoses usually require echocardiographic evaluation, usually by the more sensitive transesophageal route to assess for atherosclerotic disease of the aortic arch, left atrial or ventricular clot, patent foramen ovale, and other conditions. Aortic arch atherosclerosis is an underappreciated source of stroke and may be the second most common cause. Much debate exists in the literature as to the treatment of arch disease.[7] Additionally, if no other etiologic factor is identified, stenoses between 50% and 79% may indicate a carotid source of the event and, therefore, may call for carotid endarterectomy.

(J) Critical stenoses in the carotid territory warrant consideration of early carotid endarterectomy. The North American Symptomatic Carotid Endarterectomy Trial (NASCET) is not directly applicable to patients with acute stroke. We infer, however, that management of these patients is similar and timing is the only unresolved factor. If the findings are fluctuating or if intraarterial thrombus is identified, emergent exploration on the same day is indicated. If the examination reveals neurologic improvement or stability, the patient should be given anticoagulants and be stabilized medically before urgent carotid endarterectomy within that hospital admission. Early intervention is preferred whenever possible, although

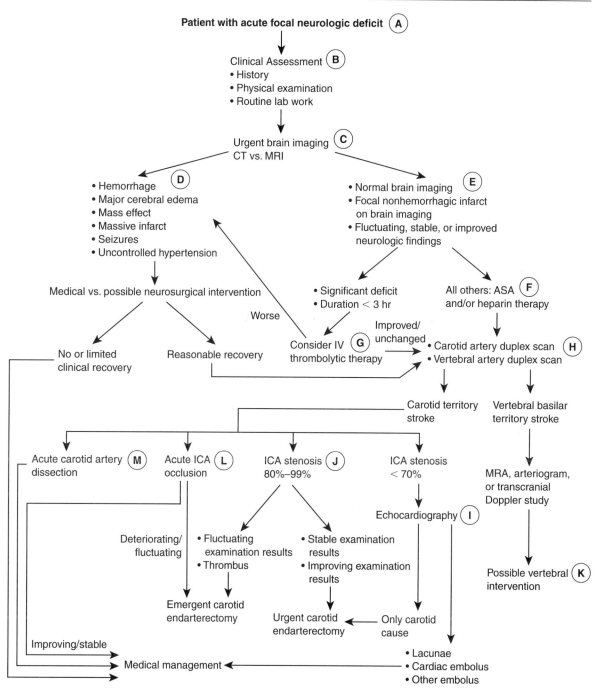

some authors recommend 6 weeks of observation before performing carotid endarterectomy.

Absolute contraindications to early post-stroke carotid endarterectomy[8-10] (see D) include:

- Intracranial hemorrhage
- A massive infarct
- Cerebral edema
- A mass effect on brain imaging
- A depressed level of consciousness

In the setting of two possible etiologic mechanisms, both should be addressed whenever possible. For example, if a patient has both a critical carotid stenosis and atrial fibrillation, an echocardiogram should be performed. If no clot is seen, the patient requires carotid endarterectomy and warfarin therapy should be considered. If a clot is identified, the patient should be first stabilized with anticoagulants and carotid endarterectomy should be considered within 6 weeks.

(K) Infarction within vertebral artery territory mandates more detailed imaging. Magnetic resonance angiography (MRA) or contrast arteriography is required. Transcranial Doppler (TCD) evaluation may help identify the hemodynamic significance of a stenosis in assessment of both intracranial and extracranial disease.

The management of isolated vertebral artery disease is controversial. When vertebral artery disease appears to be the source of the neurologic event, surgical therapy should be directed toward that lesion. In the setting of both carotid and vertebral pathology, the choice of intervention is based on brain imaging and the clinical examination as well as the severity and extent of arterial disease (see Chapter 17).

(L) An extremely controversial topic is the acute carotid occlusion presenting as stroke. If the patient is clinically improving, observation is probably the best course of action. If the patient is deteriorating or has waxing and waning examination results with no evidence of hemorrhage, emergent carotid endarterectomy may be indicated.

The surgeon begins the procedure with no distal clamp prior to arteriotomy in an attempt to prevent distal embolization and then follows with removal of all thrombus by gentle passage of an embolectomy catheter proximal to the cavernous sinus (usually <10 cm), mandatory shunting once back-bleeding is restored, and endarterectomy as indicated. When either poor or no back-bleeding is identified, an on-table arteriogram is performed to establish the patency of the vessel to the circle of Willis. If residual clot cannot be removed or if occlusion is demonstrated at an inaccessible level, ligation of the internal carotid artery is recommended.

(M) Spontaneous or idiopathic acute carotid dissections, when visualized by duplex ultrasound surveillance, require further radiologic confirmation. MRI is recommended because it provides cross-sectional imaging of the carotid artery and the area of the brain affected as well as images of the extracranial and intracranial circulation. Treatment is most often anticoagulation therapy, and the prognosis overall is good. Close monitoring with follow-up duplex scanning is recommended to assess recanalization and the potential need for future endarterectomy.

REFERENCES

1. Broderick J, Brott T, Kothari R, et al: The greater Cincinnati/northern Kentucky stroke study: Preliminary first-ever and total incidence rates of stroke among blacks. Stroke 1998;29:415–421.
2. Kasner SE, Grotta, JC: Ischemic stroke. Neurol Clin 1998;16:355–372.
3. International Stroke Trial Collaborative Group, for the International Stroke Trial (IST): A randomised trial of aspirin, subcutaneous heparin, both, and neither among 19,435 patients with acute ischaemic stroke. Lancet 1997;349:1569–81.
4. National Institute of Neurological Disorders and Stroke rt-PA Stroke Study Group: Tissue plasminogen activator for acute ischemic stroke. N Engl J Med 1995;333:1581–1587.
5. Adams HP Jr, Brott TG, Furlan AJ, et al: Guidelines for thrombolytic therapy for acute stroke–a supplement to the guidelines for the management of patients with acute ischemic stroke: A statement for health care professionals from a special writing group of the Stroke Council, American Heart Association. Circulation 1996;94:1167–1174.
6. Prystowsky EN, Benson DW Jr, Fuster V, et al: Management of patients with atrial fibrillation: A statement for Association. Circulation 1996;93:1262–1277.
5. Adams HP Jr, Brott TG, Furlan AJ, et al: Guidelines for of the aortic arch and the risk of ischemic stroke. N Engl J Med 1994;331:1474–1479.
8. Moore WS, Barnett HJM, Beebe HG, et al: Guidelines for carotid endarterectomy: A multidisciplinary consensus statement from the Ad Hoc Committee, American Heart Association. Stroke 1995;26:188–201.
9. North American Symptomatic Carotid Endarterectomy Trial Collaborators: Beneficial effect of carotid endarterectomy in symptomatic patients with high-grade carotid stenosis. N Engl J Med 1991;325:445–453.
10. Adams HP Jr, Brott TG, Crowell RM, et al: Guidelines for the management of patients with acute ischemic stroke: A statement for health care professionals from a special writing group of the Stroke Council, American Heart Association. Stroke 1994;25:1901–1914.

ACUTE STROKE

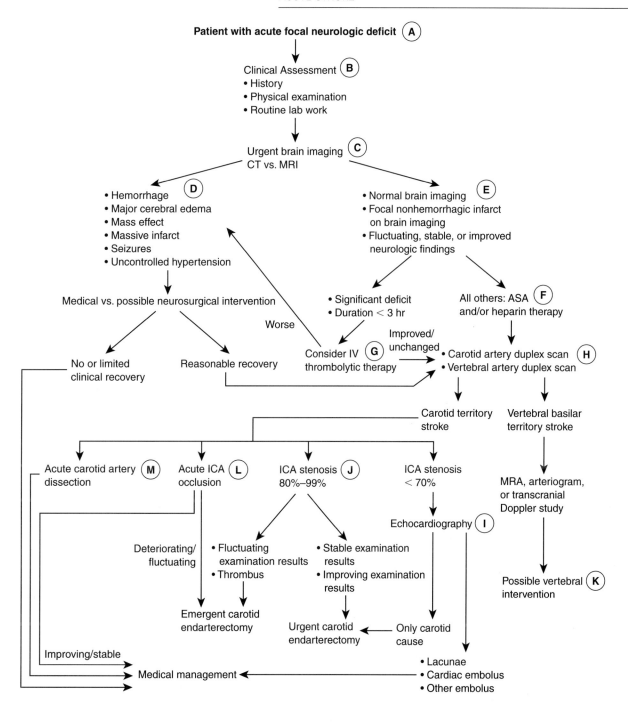

Chapter 12 Carotid Artery Aneurysm

JAMES H. ROTHSTEIN, MD • JERRY GOLDSTONE, MD

(A) Extracranial carotid artery aneurysms are extremely uncommon, with an incidence compared to all extracranial arterial aneurysms of 0.34% to 3.7% and 0.1% to 2% of all carotid operations.[1–7] The largest reported series from a single institution is 67 cases.[3] The initial presentation that prompts further investigation is usually a pulsatile neck mass or neurologic event. In one study of 26 patients, 96% presented with a pulsatile neck mass, 42% had accompanying transient ischemic attacks (TIAs), and 7% presented with rupture. In another study, 92% presented with neurologic symptoms and only 58% had a pulsatile mass.

The type and severity of neurologic deficit can vary from stroke to hemispheric TIA or amaurosis fugax. These are due to either embolic phenomena or thrombosis. Other less common symptoms are secondary to direct compression on contiguous structures and include dysphagia; dyspnea with inspiratory stridor; hoarseness (secondary to recurrent laryngeal nerve involvement); palsies of cranial nerves IX, X, XI, XII; and Horner's syndrome (due to compression of the cervical sympathetic chain). Pain involving the face, eye, and cervical regions can also be a presenting manifestation. Local signs and symptoms of infection may be prominent when an infected aneurysm is present. Rupture into the oropharynx, once common, is now a rare event.[8] Any of these symptoms in the presence of significant cervical trauma should raise the question of the presence of a traumatic carotid pseudoaneurysm.

The differential diagnosis includes peritonsillar or parapharyngeal abscess, cervical lymphadenopathy, tortuosity of the carotid or subclavian arteries, and carotid body tumors.

(B) A pulsatile neck mass is an indication for duplex ultrasound surveillance, which can often establish the correct diagnosis of carotid aneurysm. However, some carotid aneurysms are in the distal extracranial internal carotid artery (ICA) and therefore are not seen by routine duplex scan protocols. Computed tomography (CT) or magnetic resonance imaging (MRI) scans should reveal the size and nature of aneurysms in this location. The evaluation of a stroke or TIA should include a carotid duplex scan and often a diagnostic imaging study of the brain, either with CT or MRI.[6] These studies can usually identify which of the following types of carotid aneurysm is present:

- Degenerative (saccular or fusiform) aneurysm
- Post-dissection aneurysm
- Mycotic aneurysm
- Pseudoaneurysm

(C) Most extracranial carotid aneurysms, like other arterial aneurysms, are degenerative and are associated with atherosclerosis.[3, 7, 8] Trauma is now the next most common cause. Fibromuscular dysplasia and dissection are also well-documented etiologic factors. In multiple studies, severe hypertension, with blood pressure ranging from 170 to 180/105 to 117 mmHg, was present in more than 90% of the patients with the degenerative type of carotid aneurysm. Mycotic aneurysms are rare nowadays. Aneurysms following carotid dissection are discussed in Chapter 13.

(D) Most degenerative carotid aneurysms are fusiform in shape. These are associated with atherosclerosis and can be bilateral. Saccular aneurysms, on the other hand, may be associated with atherosclerosis but are also seen with traumatic injuries and are almost always unilateral. Saccular aneurysms are less likely than fusiform aneurysms to be associated with neurologic symptoms because of their narrow neck; however, this is not true if there is accompanying carotid stenosis. Like other atherosclerotic changes affecting the carotid artery, aneurysmal degeneration is most often located at the common carotid bifurcation with variable extension into the ICA. Distal extension can be significant and may involve the entire extracranial ICA.

(E) More distally located, isolated ICA aneurysms are caused by traumatic injury. Although uncommon, occurring in only 1.7% of penetrating neck injuries, it is an important consideration in these patients with unexplained neurologic symptoms. Blunt trauma to the cervical region more commonly results in intimal disruption and thrombosis of the ICA rather than aneurysm formation. However, disruption of the outer layers of the arterial wall can result in the formation of a pseudoaneurysm. The proposed mechanism is that of hyperextension and rotation of the neck, with impingement of the ICA on the transverse process of the atlas. Of course, disruption of the arterial wall by bone fragments from fractures can also lead to false aneurysm formation. In addition to trauma, pseudoaneurysms of the ICA have also been reported after carotid endarterectomy. This occurrence is a result of patch rupture (vein) or suture line disruption secondary to either technical error or infection. Although rare, infection must be considered as an etiologic possibility in any aneurysm involving a carotid bifurcation that has previously been closed with a synthetic patch.[9] When the diagnosis of infection is confirmed, gram-positive cocci are the most commonly cultured organisms, *Staphylococcus aureus* being the most frequent. Other rare causes of carotid artery pseudoaneurysm formation include connective tissue disorders such as vasculo-Behçet disease and Marfan's syndrome.[10]

(F) Mycotic aneurysms of the carotid artery are also rare; only 50 cases have been reported in the English literature.[11] In the past, syphilitic infection and peritonsillar abscess were most commonly implicated as causes; however, more recent etiologic processes have included intravenous drug abuse, penetrating trauma, dental extractions, and angiographic procedures. Inoculation of the artery can occur either by septic emboli or by direct extension from an adjacent site of infection. The most frequently cultured organism has been *S. aureus*; other reported species include *Streptococcus, Salmonella, Klebsiella, Escherichia coli, Proteus mirabilis, Yersinia,* and *Corynebacterium.*

The initial presentation of a patient with a mycotic carotid aneurysm is usually not subtle and includes fever, chills, and a tender expanding neck mass. This may be associated with Horner's syndrome or even a clinical picture of generalized sepsis. Once the diagnosis is made, the patient should be given broad-spectrum antibiotics and expeditious surgical intervention. Postoperatively, antibiotic coverage specific for the cultured organisms should be continued for 6 weeks.

G After a carotid aneurysm has been identified, the acquisition of additional anatomic information is crucial to planning further management. This information is best obtained by transfemoral selective arteriography, which should include assessment of bilateral carotid and vertebral arteries. This study serves several important purposes; it:

1. Defines the extent of the aneurysm and its relationship to bony structures, particularly the skull base.
2. Delineates the other extracranial and intracranial arteries.
3. Provides anatomic data that will usually establish an etiologic mechanism.
4. Permits both direct measurement of carotid artery back-pressure and a period of temporary carotid occlusion.[12] This is accomplished through the use of an end-hole, balloon-tipped catheter in an awake, anticoagulated patient with blood pressure at baseline values. Occlusion is typically performed for 30 minutes, during which time back-pressure is measured electronically while the patient is clinically observed for development of any neurologic changes.

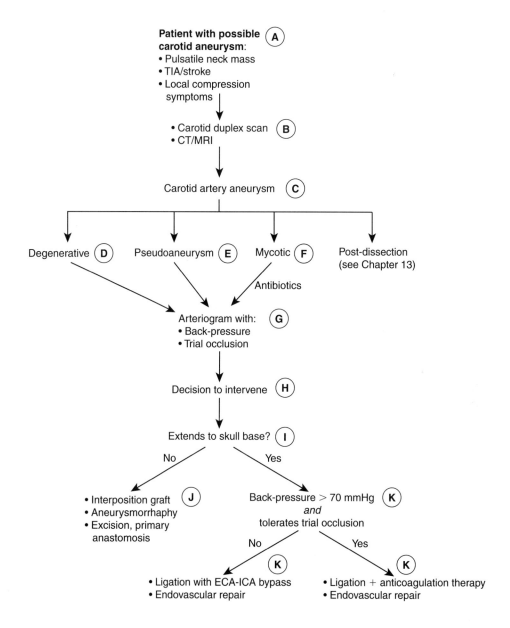

Carotid Artery Aneurysm (continued)

(H) Most extracranial carotid artery aneurysms require treatment to relieve local symptoms, to prevent recurrent or new neurologic events, and to prevent the rare case of rupture.[1,2,3,5,7] Exceptions to this general principle are some small, stable, asymptomatic aneurysms or pseudoaneurysms at or near the base of the skull. Several reports that include serial imaging evaluations have demonstrated that these lesions can remain asymptomatic and anatomically stable over long periods of follow-up. In these special situations, the risks of repair seem to outweigh the risk of untoward lesion-related events.

(I) The relationship of the distal extent of the aneurysm to the base of the skull has a profound influence on the treatment of these lesions. Aneurysms near the skull base reside in an area that is narrow, tapering, unyielding (secondary to bony structures), and congested with critical neurovascular structures. Distal control and adequate exposure to ensure safe and technically accurate distal anastomosis are the challenges that must be overcome.

(J) Fortunately, because most aneurysms occur at or near the carotid bifurcation, proximal and distal control of the vessels can be obtained using standard carotid endarterectomy approaches. The specific surgical procedure required depends largely on the nature and extent of the aneurysm itself. The majority will require resection and interposition grafting. In the presence of infection—either mycotic aneurysms or infected pseudoaneurysms—all infected tissue should be excised including the native artery.

In these cases, reconstructive options are limited to interposition autologous grafting and, less frequently, resection and primary end-to-end anastomosis. The greater saphenous vein is the most commonly used conduit, with other options being sized matched arteries from other locations. In the absence of infection, either autologous or prosthetic reconstruction is appropriate. Occasionally, short defects can be bridged by transposing the transected distal external carotid artery onto the proximal vessel. Some small aneurysms that involve only a partial circumference of the wall can be treated with aneurysmorrhaphy (primary suture or patch). This is most likely to be possible in the rare saccular aneurysm with a small neck.

(K) For aneurysms that extend up to or near the skull base, various techniques are useful to facilitate surgical exposure.[7] These include (1) mandibular subluxation, (2) excision of the styloid process, and (3) use of a nasotracheal rather than an endotracheal tube. Drilling away the temporal bone is another method occasionally used to obtain more working room. As previously mentioned, dissection in this area is difficult and is associated with increased morbidity. If there is room for distal control, treatment options are the same as those described for more proximal lesions, with interposition grafting being the most frequently used.

Other options when distal control is inadequate to perform a safe anastomosis are ligation of the ICA with or without intracranial-extracranial bypass and utilization of an endovascular approach. The decision on whether or not patients can tolerate ICA ligation is based on their response to temporary balloon occlusion as well as the carotid artery back-pressure, which should have been determined during arteriography. The older literature on carotid ligation has reported an incidence of major stroke of 30% to 50%; however, more recent data have shown that the risk has been reduced to 10% when patients are properly selected. This is comparable to the overall risk of surgical repair. A systolic back (stump) pressure of greater than 70 mmHg or half the normal systolic blood pressure, along with an unremarkable period of temporary balloon occlusion, indicates adequate collateral cerebral blood flow to allow safe ligation of the carotid artery.[12] If either of these conditions does not exist, ligation should not be attempted without the addition of an extracranial-intracranial bypass.

There have been reports of delayed cerebral ischemic events of up to 6 weeks following carotid ligation. These events are considered to be secondary to either a low-flow state during an episode of hypotension or an embolic phenomenon from a column of thrombus distal to the point of ligation. These potential high-risk settings can be avoided by maintenance of a normal baseline blood pressure that has been previously recorded and by administration of anticoagulation therapy for a minimum of 6 weeks.

If the aneurysm is not thought to be amenable to open surgical repair and the requirements for ligation are not met, an endovascular approach should be considered.[13] In the case of either a true or false aneurysm, a covered stent may be used to reinforce the vascular wall, thus reducing the risk of rupture.[14–17] During treatment of pseudoaneurysms, a bare stent placed across the neck may cause alteration of flow dynamics within the pseudoaneurysm and result in thrombosis.[18] When stents are used, the patient should receive anticoIf the aneurysm is not thought to be amenable allow endothelialization of the new endoluminal surface.

Other reported endovascular treatments of carotid pseudoaneurysms involve direct occlusion utilizing either detachable coils or liquid polymerizing material, which solidifies within the aneurysm sac; however, long-term follow-up for the complications of stent migration, stenosis, or thrombosis of the artery is not yet available.

REFERENCES

1. Welling RE, Taha A, Goel T, et al: Extracranial carotid artery aneurysms. Surgery 1983;93:319–323.
2. deJong KP, Zondervan PE, van Urk H: Extracranial carotid artery aneurysms. Eur J Vasc Surg 1989;3:557–562.
3. El-Sabrout R, Cooley DA: Extracranial carotid artery aneurysms: Texas Heart Institute Experience. J Vasc Surg 2000;31:702–712.
4. Ito M, Nitta T, Sato K, et al: Cervical carotid aneurysm presenting as transient ischemia and recurrent laryngeal nerve palsy. Surg Neurol 1986;25:346–350.
5. Rittenhouse EA, Radke HM, Sumner DS: Carotid artery aneurysm. Arch Surg 1972;105:786–789.
6. Duvall ER, Gupta KL, Vitek JJ, et al: CT demonstration

of extracranial carotid artery aneurysms. J Comput Assist Tomogr 1986;10(3):404–408.
7. Rosset E, Albertini J-N, Magnan PE, et al: Surgical treatment of extracranial internal carotid artery aneurysms. J Vasc Surg 2000;31:713–723.
8. Liapis CD, Gugulakis A, Misiakos E, et al: Surgical treatment of extracranial carotid aneurysms. Int Angiol 1994;13:290–295.
9. El-Sabrout R, Reul G, Cooley DA: Infected postcarotid endarterectomy pseudoaneurysms: Retrospective review of a series. Ann Vasc Surg 2000;14:239–247.
10. Sasaki S, Yasuda K, Takigami K, et al: Surgical experiences with peripheral arterial aneurysms due to vasculo-Behçet's disease. J Cardiovasc Surg 1998;39:147–150.
11. Grossi RJ, Onofrey D, Tvetenstrand C, et al: Mycotic carotid aneurysm. J Vasc Surg 1987;6:81–83.
12. Ehrenfeld WK, Stoney RJ, Wylie EJ: Relation of carotid stump pressure to safety of carotid artery ligation. Surgery 1983;93:299–305.
13. Ruebben A, Merlo M, Verri A, et al: Exclusion of an internal carotid aneurysm by a covered stent. J Cardiovasc Surg 1997;38:301–303.
14. Perez-Cruet MJ, Patwardhan RV, Mawad ME, et al: Treatment of dissecting pseudoaneurysm of the cervical internal carotid artery using a wall stent and detachable coils: Case report. Neurosurgery 1997;40:622–626.
15. Bernstein SM, Coldwell DM, Prall JA, et al: Treatment of traumatic carotid pseudoaneurysm with endovascular stent placement. J Vasc Interv Radiol 1997;8:1065–1068.
16. Marotta TR, Buller C, Taylor D, et al: Autologous vein-covered stent repair of a cervical internal carotid artery pseudoaneurysm: Technical case report. Neurosurgery 1998;42:408–413.
17. Horowitz MB, Miller G, Meyer Y, et al: Use of intravascular stents in the treatment of internal carotid and extracranial vertebral artery pseudoaneurysms. AJNR Am J Neuroradiol 1996;17:693–696.
18. Higashida RT, Halbach VV, Dowd C, et al: Endovascular detachable balloon embolization therapy of cavernous carotid artery aneurysms: Results in 87 cases. J Neurosurg 1990;72:857–863.

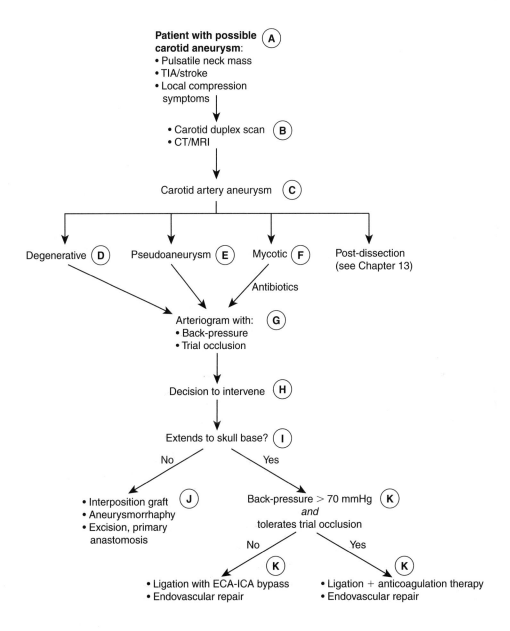

Chapter 13 Carotid Dissection

LAURA K. PAK, MD • LOUIS M. MESSINA, MD

(A) Carotid artery dissections are classified as *traumatic* or *spontaneous*. Traumatic dissections can follow motor vehicle accidents (whiplash injury) or assault, but more often they ensue from "minor trauma" involving rapid rotation or extension of the head, such as coughing, vomiting, wrestling, martial arts, or chiropractic manipulation.[1] The traumatic event may precede initial symptoms by months.

Most (60% to 70%) of all carotid dissections are spontaneous, either idiopathic or presumed secondary to an underlying arterial abnormality. Fibromuscular dysplasia (FMD), Ehlers-Danlos syndrome and Marfan's syndrome are associated with dissection. Electron microscopy of skin biopsy specimens has shown subtle collagen and elastin abnormalities in 68% of patients with internal carotid artery (ICA) dissection, compared with entirely normal connective tissue ultrastructural morphology exhibited in all biopsy specimens from a comparison group of age-matched volunteers.[2] Other possible risk factors for dissection include hypertension, family history of dissection, tobacco, and oral contraceptive use. Of patients with dissection, 30% to 40% report a history of migraine.

(B) Patients can present with symptoms of focal cerebral ischemia, such as hemiparesis, aphasia, and amaurosis fugax. Hemicranial or retro-orbital headache is present in 40% to 80% of patients. When studied prospectively, 52% of patients have ophthalmologic symptoms or signs on initial evaluation, usually manifest as an incomplete Horner's syndrome.[3] Oculosympathetic paresis (miosis and ptosis without anhidrosis) is caused by disruption of sympathetic fibers running along the ICA adventitia, sparing those which control sweating, as these fibers diverge to follow the external carotid artery (ECA) at the bifurcation. Nonembolic ischemic optical neuropathy and ocular motor nerve palsies are less common presenting signs. Dissection must be considered in any patient with the combination of craniocervical pain and either Horner's syndrome or transient monocular blindness. Patients may report pulsatile tinnitus, a bruit that increases in intensity with each heart beat.[4]

(C) Computed tomography (CT) of the head is performed to rule out hemorrhagic cerebral infarct or cerebral edema, which would preclude systemic anticoagulation therapy.

(D) Duplex ultrasonography may identify an extracranial carotid artery dissection. In spontaneous dissections, the flap or thrombus can often be seen just distal to the carotid bulb on B-mode imaging. Traumatic dissections, however, are most frequently located at the skull base, presumably because the injury involves stretching or shearing of the artery against the transverse processes of the cervical vertebrae and the angle of the mandible. The most sensitive ultrasound finding in these cases is a high-resistance Doppler signal with low-flow velocity due to distal stenosis. Intracranial dissections, which constitute 5% to 20% of all carotid dissections, have been identified by transcranial ultrasonography, but findings are not specific enough to guide treatment.[5]

(E) Arteriography remains the "gold standard" in the diagnosis of dissection. The classic but infrequent finding is a double lumen. More commonly, arteriography demonstrates luminal tapering known as the "flame sign," occlusion, or intimal flap. Fibromuscular dysplasia is characterized by intermittent abrupt stricturing, creating a "string of beads." If the diagnosis of fibromuscular dysplasia is confirmed, aortography should be considered to exclude involvement of the renal or external iliac arteries.

Magnetic resonance imaging and angiography (MRI, MRA) have the advantage of being fast, noninvasive, and capable of producing multiplane images without the use of intravenous contrast material. T1-weighted, fat-saturated sagittal images reveal the "eyes of dissection," dark flow voids surrounded by high-intensity thrombus.

Gadolinium-enhanced images may offer greater definition of morphology and composition of the dissected artery as well as a visual representation of flow dynamics across the lesion. Sensitivity and specificity are reported to be 95% to 100%, compared with conventional angiography (i.e., using angiography as the gold standard, the sensitivity and specificity are calculated as 95% and 100%).[6]

(F) Anticoagulants, if not contraindicated, remain the mainstay of treatment, as most cerebral infarcts (84% to 92%) related to dissection are presumed to be embolic rather than hemodynamic in origin.[7] Hemispheric ischemic symptoms related to hypoperfusion can be elicited by clinical history (e.g., arm weakness after a dose of antihypertensive medication) and confirmed by transcranial Doppler or positron emission tomography (PET) or single photon emission computed tomography (SPECT). The use of low-molecular-weight heparin for the treatment of dissection has not been studied. Initial heparin anticoagulation is followed by warfarin for 6 to 12 months, followed by lifelong aspirin therapy.

(G) Radiographic evaluation at 6 months should be done by whichever imaging modality (ultrasound, MRI/MRA, conventional angiography) has best been able to image the dissection at time of diagnosis. In patients who have survived the initial event and who have received anticoagulation therapy, 60% to 85% of dissections recanalize over 2 to 6 months, accompanied by complete or near-complete neurologic recovery. No improvement in luminal diameter is expected after 6 months of anticoagulation therapy. The neurologic prognosis is worse with traumatic dissections than spontaneous dissections and with intracranial than extracranial dissections. There is no correlation, however, between the degree of stenosis and the occurrence of neurologic events.[8–10] Recur-

CAROTID DISSECTION

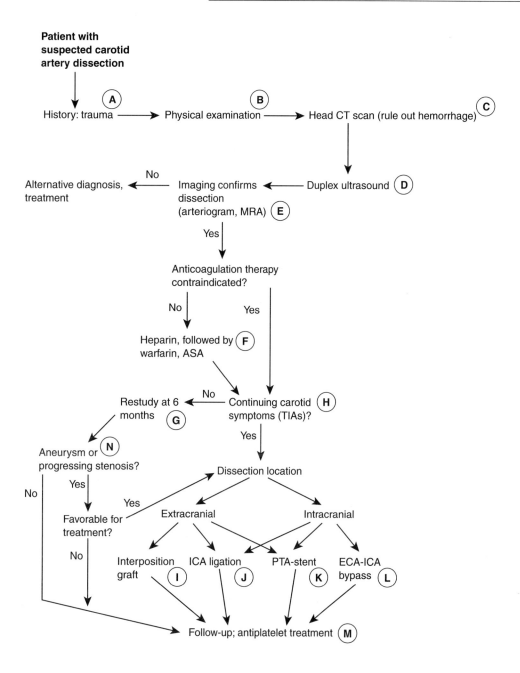

Carotid Dissection (continued)

rence of dissection is estimated at 3% at 3 years and 12% at 10 years and most often involves a different cervical vessel, which justifies the use of long-term aspirin.[11]

(H) Surgery or stenting is indicated for any patient who has progressive or persistent transient ischemic attacks indicating ongoing embolization or low flow or in any symptomatic patient for whom anticoagulation therapy is contraindicated.

(I) Resection of the diseased extracranial ICA with interposition graft using prosthetic material, autologous reversed saphenous vein, or the ECA is the favored operation if distal control is possible.[12]

(J) Ligation of the ICA is considered for treatment of embolization from skull base ICA dissections. If stump pressure is adequate (>70), ICA ligation can be performed with low risk of cerebrovascular accident.[13]

(K) Balloon-expandable and self-expanding endovascular stents have been used for treatment of extracranial dissections. Stroke risk is acceptable and short-term follow-up (3 to 12 months) shows continued ICA patency in greater than 90% in small patient series.[14, 15] Intracranial ICA stenting using flexible coronary stents is performed in few centers, but in case reports it has been successfully applied to symptomatic stenoses and aneurysms of the intrapetrous and intracavernous ICA with minimal morbidity.[16] Stenting precludes the use of follow-up MRI and MRA.

(L) Extracranial to intracranial bypass with ICA ligation is indicated for high cervical and intracranial ICA dissections with impaired cerebral perfusion. The supraclinoid portion of the ICA is the most common location for intracranial dissection. Less often, the intrapetrous or intracavernous ICA is affected.[17] Reversed saphenous vein bypass to the distal ICA or middle cerebral artery is achieved after mastoidectomy or temporal craniotomy and is associated with a 94% 2-year patency rate.[18, 19, 20]

(M) All postoperative patients are maintained on aspirin indefinitely. Patients treated with endovascular stents receive ticlopidine and aspirin for 6 weeks, then aspirin alone.

(N) Treatment of asymptomatic patients with stable moderate-to-severe ICA stenosis, pseudoaneurysm, or progressive stenosis related to dissection is controversial and must be individualized according to patient age, co-morbidities, and surgical risk. Asymptomatic patients with progressive stenosis on reevaluation should continue warfarin therapy and should be reevaluated in 3 months. As many as 25% of patients with extracranial ICA dissection develop an aneurysm. Most of these persist on long-term follow-up but do not appear to enlarge and are associated with negligible risk of rupture or symptomatic thromboembolism in patients maintained on an aspirin regimen alone.[21] Endovascular stenting or resection with arterial reconstruction may be considered for persistent high-grade stenosis and large aneurysms.

REFERENCES

1. Hamann G: Cervicocephalic artery dissections due to chiropractic manipulation. Lancet 1993;341:764–765.
2. Brandt T, Hausser I, Oberk E, et al: Ultrastructural connective tissue abnormalities in patients with spontaneous cervicocerebral artery dissections. Ann Neurol 1998;44:281–285.
3. Biousse V, Touboul PJ, D'Anglejan-Chatillon J, et al: Ophthalmologic manifestations of internal carotid artery dissection. Am J Ophthalmol 1998;126:565–577.
4. Waldvogel D, Mattle HP, Sturzenegger M, Schroth G: Pulsatile tinnitus: Review of 84 patients. J Neurol 1998;245:137–142.
5. Sturzenegger M, Mattle HP, Rivoir A, Baumgartner RW: Ultrasound findings in carotid artery dissection: Analysis of 43 patients. Neurology 1995;45:691–698.
6. Guillon B, Levy C, Bousser MG: Internal carotid artery dissection: An update. J Neurol Sci 1998;153:146–158.
7. Lucas C, Moulin T, Deplanque D, et al: Stroke patterns of internal carotid artery dissection in 40 patients. Stroke 1998;29:2646–2648.
8. Steinke W, Rautenberg W, Schwartz A, Hennerici M: Noninvasive monitoring of internal carotid artery dissection. Stroke 1994;25:998–1005.
9. Kasner SE, Hankins LL, Bratina P, Morganstern LB: Magnetic resonance angiography demonstrates vascular healing of carotid and vertebral artery dissection. Stroke 1997;28:1993–1997.
10. Sturzenegger M: Spontaneous internal carotid artery dissection: Early diagnosis and management in 44 patients. J Neurol 1995;242:231–238.
11. Schievink WI, Mokri B, O'Fallon WM: Recurrent spontaneous cervical artery dissection. N Engl J Med 1994;330:393–397.
12. Balas, P, Ioannou N, Milas P, Klonaris C: Surgical treatment of spontaneous internal carotid dissection. Int Angiol 1998;17:125–127.
13. Schievink WI, Piepgras DG, McCaffrey TV, Mokri B: Surgical treatment of extracranial internal carotid artery dissecting aneurysms. Neurosurgery 1994;35:809–816.
14. Bejjani GK, Monsein LH, Laird JR, et al: Treatment of symptomatic cervical carotid dissections with endovascular stents. Neurosurgery 1999;44:755–761.
15. Hong MK, Satler LF, Gallino R, Leon MB: Intravascular stenting as a definitive treatment of spontaneous carotid artery dissection. Am J Cardiol 1997;79:538.
16. Mericle RA, Lanzino G, Wakhloo AK, et al: Stenting and secondary coiling of an intracranial internal carotid artery aneurysm: Technical case report. Neurosurgery 1998;43:1229–1234.
17. Pelkonen O, Tikkakoski T, Leinonen S, et al: Intracranial arterial dissection. Neuroradiology 1998;40:442–447.
18. Alimi YS, Di Mauro P, Fiacre E, et al: Blunt injury to the internal carotid artery at the base of the skull: Six cases of venous graft restoration. J Vasc Surg 1996;24:249–257.
19. Morgan MK, Sekhon LH: Extracranial-intracranial saphenous vein bypass for carotid or vertebral artery dissections: A report of six cases. J Neurosurg 1994;80:237–246.
20. Vishteh AG, Marciano FF, David CA, et al: Long-term graft patency rates and clinical outcome after revascularization for symptomatic traumatic internal carotid artery dissection. Neurosurgery 1998;43:761–768.
21. Guillon B, Brunereau L, Biosse V, et al: Long-term follow-up of aneurysms developed during extracranial internal carotid artery dissection. Neurology 1999;53:117–122.

CAROTID DISSECTION

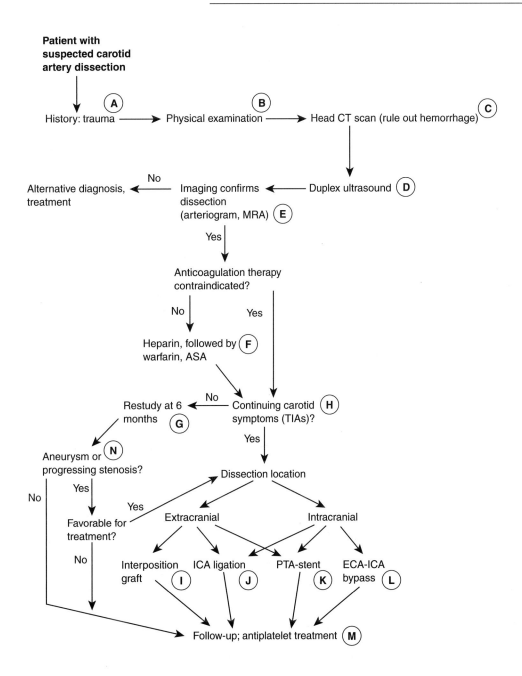

Chapter 14 Fibromuscular Disease of the Carotid Artery

PETER A. SCHNEIDER, MD

(A) Carotid fibromuscular disease (FMD) may present as an asymptomatic bruit, as an incidental finding during a radiologic study, or with cerebrovascular symptoms. Surgical series are heavily weighted with patients presenting with cerebrovascular symptoms. Carotid FMD was found in about 0.5% of consecutive cerebral arteriograms and was the cause of disease in 3.4% of cases in a series of 2000 patients with carotid artery pathology.[1-3] Medial fibroplasia causes 80% to 95% of the cases and produces a "string of beads" appearance on arteriography.[1, 3-5] The disease process tends to involve a more distal segment of the extracranial carotid artery than atherosclerosis and may therefore be difficult to characterize by duplex. Carotid FMD, which is identified by duplex, magnetic resonance angiography (MRA), computed tomography angiography (CTA), or magnetic resonance imaging (MRI) requires standard contrast arteriography if any further evaluation of the lesion is warranted.

(B) Several large series have shown the capacity of carotid FMD to cause transient ischemic attacks (TIAs) or stroke. Hemispheric stroke was the presenting symptom in 12% to 23% of patients, hemispheric TIA in 31% to 42%, and amaurosis fugax in 22% to 28% in three large series.[5-7] Approximately 10% of patients present with significant permanent disability resulting from stroke.[8] Symptomatic patients with carotid FMD require the same level of vigilance and judicious management as patients with carotid atherosclerosis who present in a similar manner.

(C) Among patients with carotid FMD, renal artery FMD occurs in 8% to 40%.[3, 7, 9] The renovascular hypertension that results may be uncontrollable and may complicate the management of carotid disease and any associated intracranial aneurysm disease. If hypertension is present, arteriography is warranted. Percutaneous transluminal balloon angioplasty (PTA) in patients with renal FMD produces excellent and durable results. (see Chapter 51).

(D) Asymptomatic patients with carotid FMD should undergo clinical follow-up, which includes monitoring for hypertension, cerebrovascular symptoms, and other vascular problems. FMD may also involve the external iliac, splenic, hepatic, and axillary arteries. Aspirin or other antiplatelet drugs may be considered as empirical treatment to reduce cerebral emboli. A baseline carotid duplex scan is obtained, and if the study results are adequate, follow-up duplex surveillance is performed. Because of the distal location of FMD in the extracranial vasculature, it may be difficult to fully characterize the disease process or visualize a distal endpoint with duplex scanning. Nevertheless, a positive study can serve as a valuable baseline for detection of future progression or for evaluation of symptoms.

(E) The natural history of asymptomatic carotid FMD is not precisely documented. When small groups of asymptomatic patients have been closely observed, new cerebrovascular symptoms develop in fewer than 10%.[9-11] When serial arteriography has been done, about one third of patients demonstrate significant progression of carotid stenosis over time.[9, 12] Unfortunately, no study has yet prospectively followed a substantial number of asymptomatic patients with significant carotid stenoses due to FMD over an extended period of time.

(F) Arteriography is the best method for evaluation of carotid FMD and is indicated when cerebrovascular symptoms or hypertension is present. This study should include the aortic arch, the extracranial carotid and vertebral arteries, and the intracranial vessels. Because the diseased segment of the internal carotid artery (ICA) may extend over many centimeters with multiple foci of critical stenosis, selective injections of the common carotid arteries with contrast material are usually required to fully delineate the extent of disease. A perpendicular lateral view of the neck with bone landmarking during ipsilateral, selective carotid injection is helpful in determining the extent of distal disease. At the time of arteriography, evaluation should include the renal arteries and any other areas that are symptomatic or are abnormal on physical examination or noninvasive testing. Patients with neurologic symptoms should also undergo CT or MRI of the brain.

(G) Diagnostic imaging may identify associated findings that may potentially influence the management of carotid FMD (see M). If there are no associated findings, treatment of symptomatic carotid FMD is planned.

(H) Medical co-morbidities may pose contraindications to surgery. Fortunately, most patients with symptomatic carotid FMD do not suffer from the systemic complications of atherosclerosis typical of the vast majority of patients with carotid atheromatous disease, and the procedure itself is simpler, making a surgical approach safer in this setting. Occasionally, patients may be poor candidates for surgery because of previous radiation or neck operations.

(I) If there are no contraindications to surgery, the location and accessibility of the lesion determine the approach. The normal carotid artery distal to the diseased segment must be surgically accessible to perform the standard operation of open dilatation with graduated rigid dilators (see J). In patients with FMD, the ICA is often elongated and the bifurcation frequently low. If the disease extends very near or into the skull, however, or if the patient lacks adequate neck flexibility, the lesion may not be accessible to surgical dilatation under direct vision. The advantages of a surgically accessible endpoint are that (1) the rigid dilator can be manually controlled and (2) if perforation, dissection, or occlusion should result, the artery may be replaced.

(J) Dilatation of the ICA with graduated, rigid dilators is the most successful approach with the best long-term follow-up. The origin of the ICA is retracted proximally by placing a sling around it at the carotid bifurcation. Traction on the sling straightens the artery. After exposure of the FMD endpoint is ensured, heparin is administered and the common carotid and external carotid arteries are cross-clamped. Through a small arteriotomy at the base of the bulb, rigid dilators, from 1.5 to 3.5 or 4.0 mm, are introduced and passed through the involved segment. The distal normal ICA is controlled so that the dilator can be properly and safely directed. After each dilator passage, the ICA is back-bled through the arteriotomy.

Large contemporary series with this method show a perioperative stroke rate of 1.4 to 2.6%.[3,6,7] Perforation occurs in fewer than 1% of patients. Cranial nerve injuries may result from distal dissection but are usually transient. They may occur in 5% to 15% of cases.[3,6] Late stroke occurred in 1.8% to 3.2% of patients.[3,6,7] Primary patency was 94% at 5 and 10 years with duplex follow-up surveillance.[6]

(K) When the distal extent of the ICA lesion is not surgically accessible, open balloon angioplasty has been advocated. In this approach, the artery is exposed and balloon dilatation is performed through an arteriotomy with the inflow common carotid artery clamped. Balloon angioplasty is performed under fluoroscopic guidance and the artery is back-bled of debris after dilatation is performed. This approach permits open, controlled dilatation with back-bleeding, which helps to prevent embolization. This technique has been reported in only a small number of patients but appears to produce acceptable results.[13-16] Percutaneous angioplasty of surgically inaccessible lesions may become appropriate if cerebral protection devices can be used, but this awaits further development.

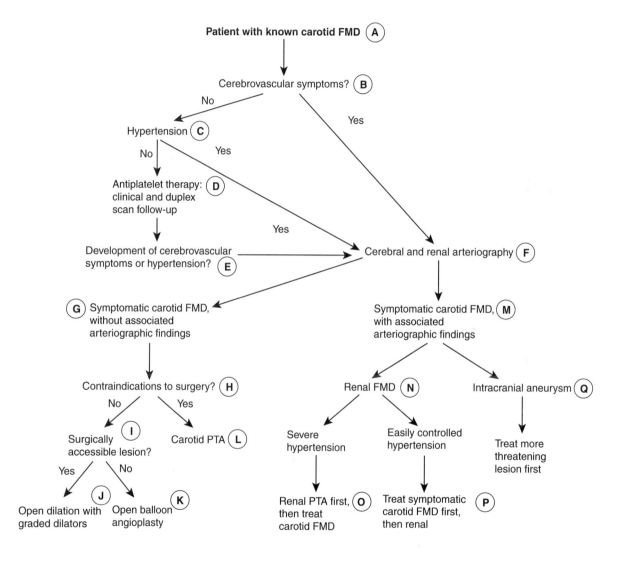

Fibromuscular Disease of the Carotid Artery
(continued)

(L) PTA is an alternative approach for patients with significant contraindications to surgery. PTA has become the treatment of choice for most patients with FMD of the renal artery. Unfortunately, there is little information available to document either the safety or efficacy of PTA for patients with carotid FMD.[17-21] Several cases have been reported, usually as part of a larger group of patients who have undergone angioplasty and specific complication and follow-up data are lacking. There is no substantial information available on percutaneous stent placement for lesions caused by FMD.

Considerations that may influence the future role of percutaneous transluminal angioplasty in the treatment of carotid FMD include the following.

1. Most patients with carotid FMD who are considered for treatment are symptomatic and presumably have had cerebral emboli. Embolization may occur again with percutaneous catheter passage, but is unlikely when an open technique with back-bleeding is used.
2. Surgical dilatation of carotid FMD has been a relatively safe, simple, and durable solution in the typical patient with few co-morbidities.
3. Percutaneous cerebral protection devices are being developed that may reduce embolic risk and that may make this approach more attractive in the future.

(M) A number of associated pathologic processes may be found on arteriography or other imaging studies and must be taken into consideration during the treatment of carotid FMD, including renal artery FMD (see N), intracranial aneurysms (see Q), extracranial aneurysms, vertebral artery FMD, and carotid atherosclerosis.

Extracranial carotid artery aneurysms are uncommon, and those caused by FMD are rare (~2% in one series).[22] These are managed with replacement grafting. Vertebral artery FMD may occur in up to 38% of patients with carotid lesions.[3,6,12] Because vertebral artery FMD only rarely causes symptoms, it does not generally warrant treatment or complicate the management of carotid FMD. Carotid atherosclerosis occurs in up to 20% of patients with carotid FMD.[3,23] The disease process is usually mild, in comparison to the juxtaposed FMD, but on occasion it may not be possible to assign blame to one pathologic process or the other in a symptomatic artery. When FMD and atherosclerosis present simultaneously, they are usually treated together.

(N) Renal FMD may complicate management to a great degree.[3,7,9] Presenting neurologic symptoms may be related to hypertension in some patients (or the postural hypotension associated with aggressive pharmacotherapy) and carotid FMD may be a secondary problem. Patients with intracranial aneurysms are at risk for hemorrhage due to hypertension. Symptomatic carotid FMD that requires surgery is made more risky by uncontrolled hypertension. Either way, proper control of hypertension is mandatory.

(O) Severe or even uncontrollable hypertension may occur as a result of renal artery disease. When this is the case, the best approach is to proceed with renal artery balloon angioplasty, followed soon thereafter with surgery for carotid FMD.

(P) When hypertension is mild or when it can be reasonably controlled, the best approach is to proceed with surgery for symptomatic carotid FMD. The renal artery disease may be treated later if warranted by the clinical situation.

(Q) Intracranial aneurysms are found in 10% to 50% of patients with carotid FMD.[10,12] These lesions pose an independent neurologic risk. In series of patients with carotid FMD, intracranial aneurysms have been responsible for up to half of the symptomatic presentations.[9,10,24] Intracranial aneurysms should be treated on the basis of their own merits, including individual consideration of size, presenting symptoms, and evidence of hemorrhage. When compared with FMD of the carotid artery, the most threatening or symptomatic lesion should be treated first.

REFERENCES

1. Osborn AG, Anderson RE: Angiographic spectrum of cervical and intracranial fibromuscular dysplasia. Stroke Intracranial aneurysms should be treated on the
2. Houser OW, Baker HL: Fibrovascular dysplasia and other uncommon diseases of the cervical carotid artery. Am J Radiol 1968;104:201.
3. Moreau P, Albat B, Thevenet A: Fibromuscular dysplasia of the internal carotid artery: Long-term results. J Cardiovasc Surg 1993;34:465–472.
4. Fisicaro M, Tonizzo M, Mucelli RP, et al: Fibromuscular dysplasia: A case report of multivessel vascular involvement. Int Angiol 1994;13:347–350.
5. Furie DM, Tien RD: Fibromuscular dysplasia of the arteries of the head and neck: Imaging findings. AJR Am J Radiol 1994;162:1205–1209.
6. Chiche L, Bahnini A, Koskas F, et al: Occlusive fibromuscular disease of the arteries supplying the brain: Results of surgical treatment. Ann Vasc Surg 1997;11:496–504.
7. Schneider PA, Cunningham CG, Ehrenfeld WK, et al: Fibromuscular dysplasia of the carotid artery. In Veith FJ, Hobson RW, Williams RA, Wilson SE (eds): Vascular Surgery Principles and Practice. New York, McGraw-Hill, 1994, pp 711–717.
8. Effeney DJ: Surgery for fibromuscular dysplasia of the carotid artery: Indications, technique and results. In Moore WS (ed): Surgery for Cerebrovascular Disease. New York, Churchill Livingstone, 1987, pp 525–533.
9. Stanley JC, Wakefield TW: Arterial fibrodysplasia. In Rutherford RB (ed): Vascular Surgery, 5th ed. Philadelphia, WB Saunders, 2000, pp 387–407.
10. Mettinger KL, Ericson K: Fibrodysplasia and the brain: I. Observations on angiographic, clinical and genetic characteristics. Stroke 1982;13:46.
11. Corrin LS, Sandok BA, Houser OW: Cerebral ischemic events in patients with carotid artery fibromuscular dysplasia. Arch Neurol 1981;38:616.
12. So EL, Toole JF, Dalal P, et al: Cephalic fibromuscular dysplasia in 32 patients: Clinical findings and radiologic features. Arch Neurol 1981;38:619.
13. Smith LL, Smith DC, Killeen JD, et al: Operative balloon angioplasty in the treatment of internal carotid artery fibromuscular dysplasia. J Vasc Surg 1987;6:482–487.

14. de Smul G, Bostoen H: Operative balloon dilatation of fibromuscular dysplasia of the internal carotid artery: Two case reports. Acta Chir Belg 1995;95:139–143.
15. Ballard JL, Guinn JE, Killeen D, et al: Open operative balloon angioplasty of the internal carotid artery: A technique in evolution. Ann Vasc Surg 1995;9:390–393.
16. Lord RSA, Graham AR, Benn IV: Radiologic control of operative carotid dilatation. Cardiovasc Surg 1986; 27:158–161.
17. Jooma R, Bradshaw JR, Griffith HB: Intimal dissection following percutaneous transluminal carotid angioplasty for fibromuscular hyperplasia. Neuroradiology 1985; 27:181–182.
18. Motarjeme A: Percutaneous transluminal angioplasty of the supra-aortic vessels. J Endovasc Surg 1996;3:171–181.
19. Hasso AN, Bird CR, Zinke DE, et al: Fibromuscular dysplasia of the internal carotid artery. Am J Neuroradiol 1981;2:175–180.
20. Tsai FY, Matovich V, Hiesheima G, et al: Percutaneous transluminal angioplasty of the carotid artery. Am J Neuroradiol 1986;7:349–358.
21. Theron JG, Payelle GG, Coskun O, et al: Carotid artery stenosis: Treatment with protected balloon angioplasty and stent placement. Radiology 1996;201:627–636.
22. Miyauchi M, Shionoya S: Aneurysm of the extracranial internal carotid artery caused by fibromuscular dysplasia. Eur J Vasc Surg 1991;5:587–591.
23. Effeney DJ, Ehrenfeld WK: Extracranial fibromuscular disease. In Rutherford RB (ed): Vascular Surgery, 3rd ed. Philadelphia, WB Saunders, 1990, pp 1412–1417.
24. Stewart MT, Moritz MW, Smith RB, et al: The natural history of carotid fibromuscular dysplasia. J Vasc Surg 1986;3:305.

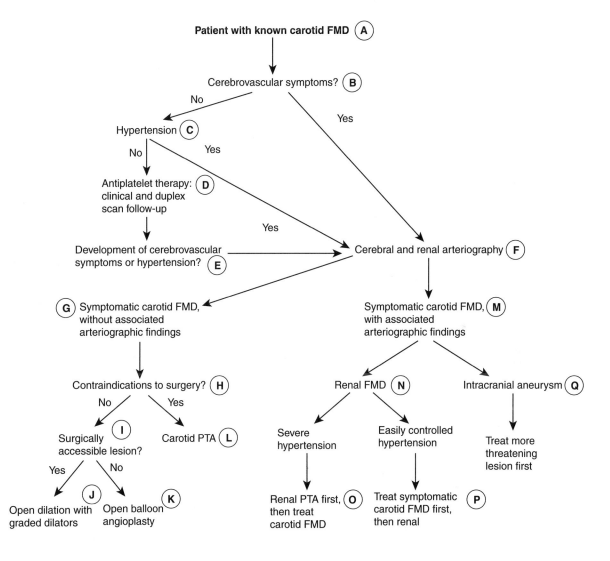

Chapter 15 Carotid Body Tumors

GLENN M. LA MURAGLIA, MD • FARZIN ADILI, MD

(A) Unless they are large, carotid body tumors are generally asymptomatic. Most often, a carotid body tumor presents as a painless, palpable mass deep and lateral in the neck below the angle of the mandible. It is commonly misdiagnosed as an enlarged lymph node.[1] There is a 5% incidence of bilateral tumors and a 10% familial pattern with autosomal dominant transmission.[2,3] Common presentations include swelling below the angle of the mandible or a mass (incidentally discovered) on routine physical examination. A specific risk factor for carotid body tumor is exposure to chronic hypoxia because of significant lung disease or living at a high altitude (3000 to 4000 meters).[4]

(B) Although the patient is commonly asymptomatic, nonspecific symptoms such as dizziness, headache, and local discomfort are sometimes described. Depending on the size of the tumor, there may be some pressure on associated structures, which may induce symptoms from the space-occupying lesion such as hoarseness and dysphagia. Hypertension is found in approximately 6% of patients and can be associated with catecholamine secretion from the tumor.[5]

On examination, the carotid body tumor is an isolated mass that can be pulsatile but not expansive, occasionally accompanied by a bruit. In contrast, carotid aneurysms appear both expansive and pulsatile. Manipulation of the tumor may result in a decrease of heart rate and in dizziness. Carotid body tumors usually demonstrate a characteristic anterior and posterior mobility but are relatively fixed in the vertical axis. When a large medial component to the tumor is present, a large mass can be identified on transoral examination. However, most tumors have approximately equal medial and lateral components from the carotid bifurcation.

(C) When the characteristic findings are highly suggestive of a carotid body tumor, color flow duplex ultrasound imaging is the best screening study.[6] It can suggest the diagnosis by delineating a hypervascular mass nestled in the carotid bifurcation. Typical features include the presence of the solid hypoechoic vascular mass directly in the carotid bifurcation, with wide splaying of the external and internal carotid arteries. Triplex color flow analysis may demonstrate low-resistance arterial flow pattern in the mass but excludes the high turbulent flow patterns characteristic of a carotid aneurysm.[7] This imaging modality may exclude a carotid body tumor or other vascular entities that might be mistaken for a malignant head and neck tumor, thereby avoiding the performance of an ill-advised biopsy procedure, which can result in significant hemorrhage.[8]

Color flow duplex sonography should be performed on both sides of the neck because of the bilateral nature of carotid body tumors. It is also a useful screening test both in sporadic and familial cases for early detection, diagnostic confirmation, and follow-up of nonoperatively managed or postoperative resection of carotid body tumors.

(D) If the patient findings are not characteristic of a carotid body tumor or if color flow duplex ultrasonography does not suggest the diagnosis, patients should be referred for a comprehensive ear-nose-throat evaluation, including oral and nasopharyngeal evaluation. Other causes of neck masses can be confused with carotid body tumors, such as metastatic cancer to the cervical lymph nodes, glomus tumor, brachial cleft cyst, and low parotid tumors. If these findings demonstrate the evidence of a head and neck tumor, staging of the patient and then biopsy are performed. However, if the evaluation does not demonstrate evidence of a head and neck tumor, further diagnostic studies, such as magnetic resonance imaging, computed tomography (CT), or catheter-based angiography should be undertaken, depending on findings of the individual patient.

(E) The characteristics of the carotid bifurcation mass in color flow duplex ultrasonography are important. If the results suggest turbulent flow, as in a true or pseudoaneurysm of the carotid artery, or if there is evidence of an unusual vascular abnormality, diagnostic arteriography should be undertaken. If the mass appears to be solid, however, a carotid body tumor is suggested. Small flow channels can often be detected by duplex ultrasonography in these hypervascular tumors.

(F) When an apparent carotid body tumor is identified by color flow duplex ultrasonography or arteriography, further evaluation is undertaken. Large carotid body tumors may occasionally produce symptoms by pressure on adjacent structures, and there may be hoarseness, dysphagia, stridor, or tongue weakness. The rate of cranial nerve involvement with the tumor has been estimated at 20%, most often the vagus and the hypoglossal nerves.[9] Careful preoperative assessment includes indirect laryngoscopy documentation of vocal cord function and a careful neurologic examination of the other nerves. Although neuroendocrine hypersecretory activity is present in only 5% of patients, they generally have other paragangliomas at other locations, which can be identified with an octreotide scan.[10,11] These patients often complain of headaches, palpitations, hypertension, photophobia, diaphoresis, and cardiac dysrhythmias. Neuroendocrine secretory screening is recommended for all patients, especially those with symptoms or patients with familial, bilateral, or extracervical paragangliomas.

(G) Historically, surgery for these highly vascular and densely adherent tumors to the carotid bifurcation has resulted in high morbidity and mortality,[5] but current series have shown little morbidity and mortality.[1] These factors need to be assessed in the decision to operate on these patients, considering their individual risk factors, tumor size, tumor involvement of adjacent structures, and the slow-growing nature of the tumor.

CAROTID BODY TUMORS

H With the decision not to treat the patient surgically, the tumor size and symptoms of compression on adjacent structures must be considered. If some form of palliative therapy is appropriate, radiation can be considered.

I Radiation therapy has been used but is of only anecdotal benefit, since carotid body tumors are thought to be radioresistant.[12] This concept has been challenged in one study in which there was complete response in 23%, partial response in 54%, and no response in the other 23% of patients treated with radiotherapy.[13] Adjuvant radiotherapy after partial resection, likewise, is of questionable benefit because most of the tumors continue to demonstrate progressive enlargement.

J Medical follow-up is necessary either for patients excluded from surgical consideration without symptoms or for patients who have undergone surgical resection of the carotid body tumor. In patients excluded from surgical consideration, periodic (every 6 months) clinical evaluation of tumor growth and evidence of compression symptoms of adjacent structures should be undertaken. Depending on the findings and the individual patient, appropriate decisions can be made for either surgery or radiation therapy.

For patients who have undergone complete carotid body tumor resection, medical follow-up is dictated on two principles. In patients who have undergone a carotid body tumor resection, it is advisable to obtain a postoperative CT scan with contrast as a baseline study. If there is no evidence of the contralateral or residual tumor on the follow-up study, the patient should be monitored clinically for evidence of a new contralateral or a recurrent carotid body tumor.

For patients who have also undergone a carotid artery reconstruction, such as bypass, additional follow-up should be undertaken for this reconstruction. For a 2-year period, these patients should be evaluated with carotid noninvasive studies starting 6 weeks postoperatively and every 6 months thereafter if there are no significant abnormalities.

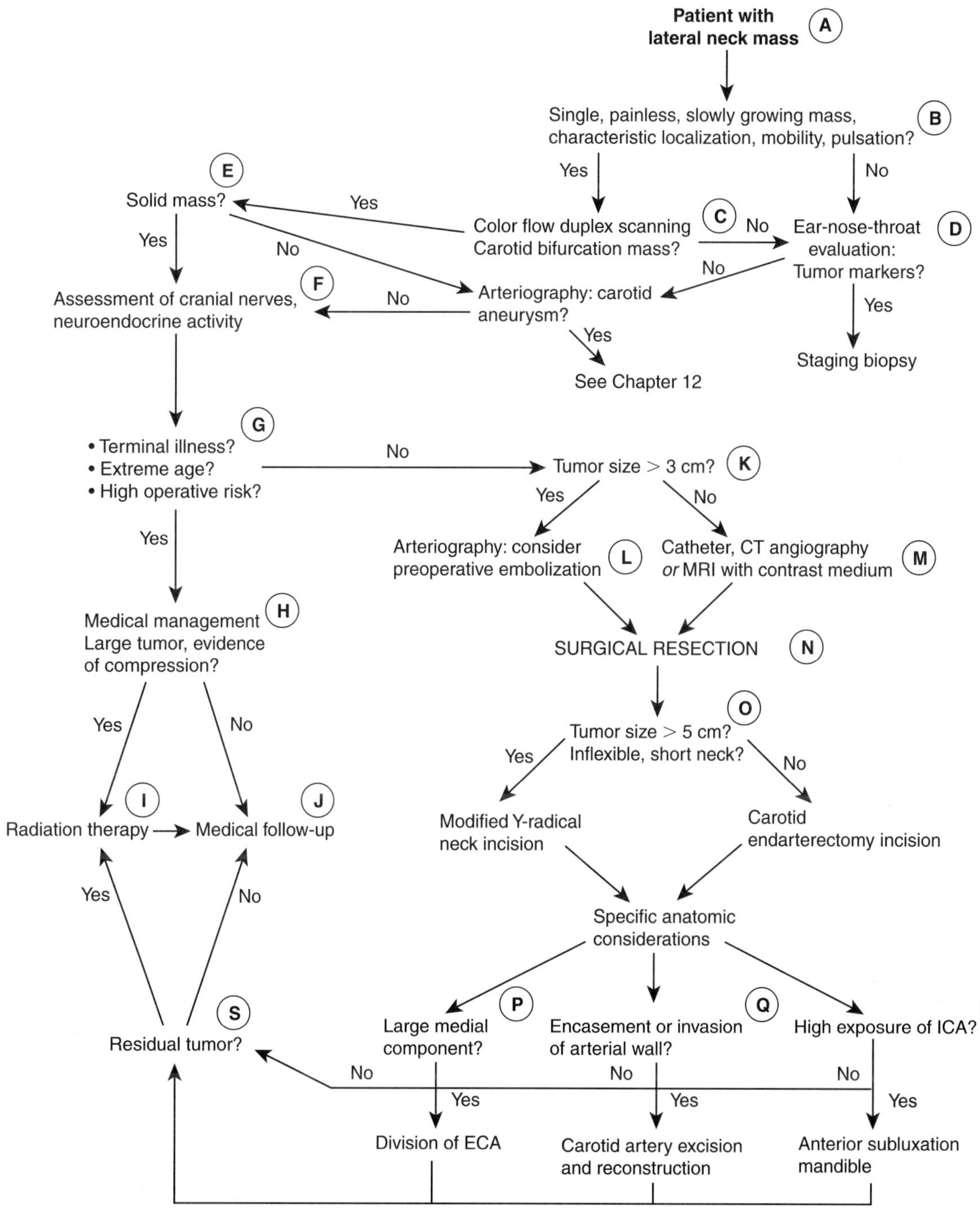

Carotid Body Tumors (continued)

(K) Patients with carotid body tumors larger than 3 cm may benefit from preoperative embolization to decrease the otherwise large intraoperative blood loss, facilitate the operation, and potentially diminish morbidity.[1] However, because this technique has potential hazards (see L), it is not practiced uniformly.

(L) Carotid body tumor embolization is potentially useful to decrease the vascularity of large tumors, but it is a difficult and potentially hazardous procedure that should be undertaken only by highly qualified personnel. Performed before surgical resection, the arteriogram confirms the diagnosis, and the embolization diminishes the highly vascular nature of the tumor and facilitates its surgical removal.

Embolization involves the use of highly selective catheter cannulation of the arteries feeding the tumor. This includes many ascending cervical and external carotid artery branches with occasional branches of the common carotid artery itself. Before injecting the embolic material, the surgeon must first visualize each branch with arteriography for "dangerous anastomoses" to the vertebral or internal carotid artery circulation. Inadvertent embolization of blood vessels that perfuse cranial nerves is also avoided by initial injection of opacified lidocaine into the arteries while neurologic examination is performed to elicit nerve dysfunction.

Vessel embolization is performed by slow injection of polyvinyl alcohol beads (Ivalon, 150 to 300 μm) into the microvasculature of the tumor. Once blood flow in the feeder vessel is negligible, absorbable gelatin sponge (Gelfoam) or a coil is deployed at the vessel origin to induce thrombosis. To avoid tissue edema and reaction around the tumor at the time of surgery, preoperative embolization should be performed on the preoperative day.[1]

(M) If the tumor is smaller than 3 cm, tumor embolization is not worth the risk, because the blood loss and difficulty of dissection are less.[1]

However, the diagnosis needs to be confirmed by an additional imaging modality, such as CT with intravenous contrast material. With reconstruction and the administration of contrast medium, the splaying of the carotid arteries and the presence of a homogenous, highly vascularized mass between the carotid arteries defines the lesion. CT alone cannot distinguish a carotid aneurysm in this area from a carotid body tumor; however, in conjunction with duplex color flow evaluation, a carotid aneurysm can be excluded. MRI may also provide the information similar to that provided by CT, but at a higher cost and without additional useful information.

(N) Despite the surgical challenge of carotid body tumors, surgical excision is the only curative therapy. Nearly 95% of carotid body tumors can be completely resected with a rare mortality (2%).[10] Perioperative stroke affects only 2% to 3% of patients. Careful attention to the anatomy and proximity of the cranial nerves in these tumors is imperative to minimize their injury, which remains, in some series, the highest morbidity (40%) associated with this operation.[10] The team approach of vascular and head and neck surgeons has been advocated, especially for the large tumors, to diminish complications and to facilitate the handling of nerve and artery problems.

(O) The incision used for carotid body tumor resection is determined by tumor size and location. The standard incision should be the oblique incision used for carotid endarterectomy. For larger tumors (>5 cm), high lesions, or a short, inflexible neck needing higher cephalad exposure, a T-shaped incision can be used to center on the inferior aspect of the tumor. Elevation of the superior flap with this incision provides additional exposure.

(P) Division of the external carotid artery can be useful when the tumor is large or when there is a large medial component to the dumbbell-shaped tumor. Division facilitates the medial and posterior dissection of the internal carotid artery and provides valuable exposure of the posterior aspect of the carotid bifurcation, where the tumors are usually very adherent. The artery should be divided in a convenient location, and after removal of the specimen it should be oversewn to avoid dead space.

(Q) Before dissecting the carotid body tumor off the artery, the surgeon should obtain proximal control of the common carotid artery. Careful periadventitial carotid dissection is important to avoid injury to the arterial wall. Bleeding from arterial injury can be repaired by a stitch or patch reconstruction. In large carotid body tumors that significantly splay and stretch the carotid bifurcation, the adventitial surface of the arteries may be attenuated. This principle is in contrast to the situation of a patient with arteriosclerotic disease or metastatic disease in the neck when the carotid artery may be fibrotic. Therefore, the surgeon must take extra care in retracting the artery from the carotid body tumor.

With carotid body tumor encasement or invasion into the artery wall, carotid resection and vascular reconstruction can be indicated. Because this cannot always be predicted before surgery, it is recommended that (1) cerebral perfusion monitoring be used routinely, since it can identify occult thrombosis,[1] and (2) there should be access to the greater saphenous vein if a bypass is required.

(R) High exposure to further improve access to the tumor can be achieved by nasal tracheal intubation and anterior subluxation of the mandible. Fixed mechanical retractors always improve exposure, and with proper positioning, cranial nerve injury can be minimized.

At the most cephalad and posterior point of dissection, the hypoglossal nerve, superior laryngeal nerve, vagus nerve, or mandibular branch of the facial nerve can be injured. If cranial nerves are involved in the capsule and adherent to the tumor, but not frankly invaded, it is important to identify the nerves near the tumor and to dissect them free. However, should the nerves be encased in the tumor and be nonfunctional preoperatively, there is no evidence that freeing them from the tumor can restore their function.

(S) Surgical resection should be complete tumor removal. If extenuating circumstances force residual tumor to be left at the time of surgery, radiation therapy should be considered. All patients should have medical follow-up (see J).

REFERENCES

1. LaMuraglia GM, Fabian RL, Brewster DC, et al: The current surgical management of carotid body paragangliomas. J Vasc Surg 1992;15:1038–1045.
2. Ridge BA, Brewster DC, Darling RC, et al: Familial carotid body tumors: Incidence and implications. J Vasc Surg 1993;7:190–194.
3. Grufferman S, Gillman MW, Pasternak LR, et al: Familial carotid body tumors: Case report and epidemiologic review. Cancer 1980;46:2116–2122.
4. Farr HW: Carotid body tumors: A 40-year study. CA Cancer J Clin 1980;30:260–265.
5. Shamblin WR, ReMine WH, Sheps SG, Harrison EGJ: Carotid body tumor (chemodectoma): Clinicopathologic analysis of ninety cases. Am J Surg 1971;122:732–739.
6. Steinke W, Hennerici M, Aulich A: Doppler color flow imaging of carotid body tumors. Stroke 1989;20:1574–1577.
7. Muhm M, Polterauer P, Gstottner W, et al: Diagnostic and therapeutic approaches to carotid body tumors: Review of 24 patients. Arch Surg 1997;132:279–284.
8. Williams MD, Phillips MJ, Rainer WG: Carotid body tumor. Arch Surg 1992;127:963–968.
9. Davidge-Pitts KJ, Pantanowitz D: Carotid body tumors. Surg Annu 1984;16:203–227.
10. Hallett JWJ, Nora JD, Hollier LH, et al: Trends in neurovascular complications of surgical management for carotid body and cervical paragangliomas: A fifty-year experience with 153 tumors. J Vasc Surg 1988;7:284–291.
11. Lamberts SW, Bakker WH, Reubi JC, Krenning EP: Somatostatin-receptor imaging in the localization of endocrine tumors. N Engl J Med 1990;323:1246–1249.
12. Mitchell DC, Clyne CAC: Chemodectomas of the neck: The response to radiotherapy. Br J Surg 1985;72:903–905.
13. Evenson LJ, Mendenhall WM, Parsons JT, Cassisi NJ: Radiotherapy in the management of chemodectomas of the carotid body and glomus vagale. Head Neck 1998;20:609–613.

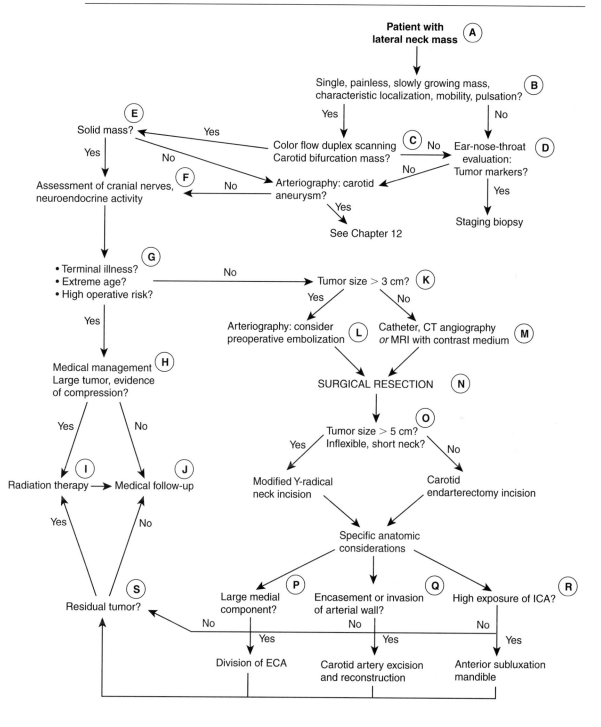

Chapter 16 Stroke Following Carotid Endarterectomy

GREGORY T. SIMONIAN, MD • ROBERT W. HOBSON II, MD

(A) Surgeons have succeeded in reducing the rate of stroke after carotid endarterectomy during the last two decades. Better operative technique and case selection have resulted in declining perioperative stroke and death rates.[1,2] Many centers have reported combined 30-day stroke-death rates of less than 3% in all cases.[3–6] Nevertheless, the management of postoperative stroke is important and deserves a preplanned approach. Properly timed, selective intervention is the key to successful management.

The etiology of stroke after carotid endarterectomy has been documented by several authors.[7,8] The risk of particularly disabling postoperative stroke has been documented through cooperative studies conducted during the 1980s and early 1990s. The Veterans Affairs Cooperative Study on Asymptomatic Carotid Stenosis reported a stroke rate of 2.4%; however, the disabling stroke rate was only 1.0%.[9] The North American Symptomatic Carotid Endarterectomy Trial (NASCET) study reported a 5.8% stroke and death rate; however, the major stroke and death rate was only 2.5%.[10] The Asymptomatic Carotid Atherosclerosis Study (ACAS) on asymptomatic carotid stenosis reported a perioperative stroke and death rate of 2.3%, which included a 1.2% stroke rate after angiography.[11]

Mechanisms responsible for postoperative stroke have been classified in great detail by Riles and colleagues.[7] Most of these events could be assigned to three broad etiologic categories:

1. Stroke resulting from inadequate cerebral perfusion or embolization during the carotid endarterectomy.
2. Stroke due to embolization or fresh thrombus or thrombotic occlusion after restoration of flow in the carotid artery.
3. Stroke from intracerebral hemorrhage probably associated with reperfusion injury.

More than 50% of the postendarterectomy neurologic events are related to the first two of these three categories. On careful review of the VA Study, four of five postoperative strokes were associated with technical errors at the endarterectomy site.[2] The mechanism of stroke will obviously influence postoperative management, but at the outset, the cause may be suspected but is unknown. Therefore, clinical decisions are best keyed initially to the time of stroke discovery and to the findings of appropriate imaging studies.

(B) If general anesthesia is used, patients should be awakened in the operating room so that neurologic status can be assessed. If it is apparent that the patient has experienced a postoperative stroke, we recommend reintubation and exploration of the wound. If there is no carotid artery pulse or if the Doppler signal is abnormal, the arteriotomy is reopened and appropriate corrective measures are carried out (see D). If the pulse and Doppler interrogation are normal, an intraoperative arteriogram is performed including intracranial views. The management of specific findings is discussed below (see D and F). If the arteriogram is normal, the arteriotomy and neck incision are closed and a computed tomography (CT) scan of the brain is obtained later. If ambiguity exists concerning the presence or absence of lateralizing signs or symptoms, the patient is transferred to the recovery room.

(C) If a stroke occurs or is discovered during the first 1 to 3 hours postoperatively, a duplex ultrasound scan is obtained expeditiously. If the scan reveals occlusion, stenosis, or low flow, reexploration is performed (see D). If the scan is negative, a CT scan is performed to evaluate the presence or absence of intracerebral hemorrhage, which, if present, would indicate medical management. If the CT scan is negative, percutaneous (transfemoral) arteriography is recommended to direct further therapy.

(D) The details of immediate or early reexploration for a thrombosed or technically defective carotid endarterectomy are beyond the scope of these comments, but briefly they involve (1) gentle removal of any thrombus present, (2) correction of technical defects, and (3) closure with vein patch angioplasty. A completion arteriogram is indicated to confirm a good result and to exclude distal emboli.

(E) For delayed strokes, a CT scan is obtained to evaluate the presence or absence of intracerebral hemorrhage, which for delayed stroke is generally a part of the reperfusion injury syndrome.[12,13] If no hemorrhage is found, a duplex scan is performed to direct further therapy. If a technical defect or significant thrombus is found, it can be dealt with by reoperation if the evaluation has been expeditious, as it may be for an early in-hospital event. If the delay exceeds 3 hours after the occurrence of stroke, however, observation becomes appropriate. If the CT and duplex scans are normal, transfemoral arteriography is recommended to exclude an intimal flap, intracranial embolism, or other cause.

(F) Arteriographic evidence of an intracranial carotid branch occlusion should stimulate consideration for selective thrombolytic therapy delivered to the area of thrombus distal to the endarterectomy via microcatheter.[14] With the decision to proceed with thrombolytic therapy, it should be recognized that its value in the postoperative patient versus its associated complications has not been rigorously evaluated and its use is based on anecdotal case experience.[15,17] However, in institutions with rapid response evaluation of stroke victims within 3 hours of the event, this option can be considered.[16–18]

(G) Most agree that operating in the presence of a dense neurologic deficit may be associated with higher risk. The area between a mild and severe deficit will continue to be unclear in the absence of better early markers of ischemic damage to the cerebral microcirculation and definitive

STROKE FOLLOWING CAROTID ENDARTERECTOMY

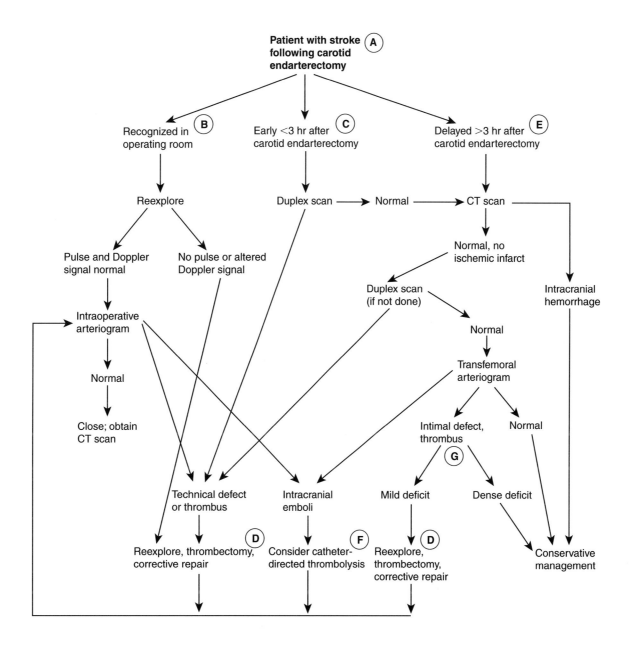

comparative studies. Elapsed time after a stroke may also influence the choice of operative or conservative therapy. Beyond a certain short interval (~3 hours), the risk of operating on acute strokes and exacerbating the ischemic injury or risking intracranial hemorrhage escalates. Considerable time may be required to take control of the patient and to obtain the necessary studies, especially if CT scanning and arteriography are required. Both a dense deficit and a long time delay argue for conservative management.

REFERENCES

1. Till JS, Toole JF, Howard VJ, et al: Declining morbidity and mortality of carotid endarterectomy. Stroke 1987;18:823–829.
2. Towne JB, Weiss DG, Hobson RW: First phase report of cooperative Veterans Administration Asymptomatic Carotid Stenosis Study: Operative morbidity and mortality. J Vasc Surg 1990;11:252–259.
3. Lees CD, Hertzer NR: Postoperative stroke and late neurologic complications after carotid endarterectomy. Arch Surg 1981;116:1561–1568.
4. Thompson JE: Complications associated with carotid endarterectomy and their prevention. World J Surg 3:155, 1979.
5. Kirshner DL, O'Brien MS, Ricotta JJ: Risk factors in a community experience with carotid endarterectomy. J Vasc Surg 1989;10:178–186.
6. Hobson RW, Goldstein J, Jamil Z, et al: Carotid restenosis: Operative and endovascular management. J Vasc Surg 1999;29:228–238.
7. Riles TS, Imparato AM, Jacobowitz GR, et al: The cause of perioperative stroke after carotid endarterectomy. J Vasc Surg 1994;19:206–216.
8. Perdue GD: Management of postendarterectomy neurologic deficits. Arch Surg 1982;117:1079–1081.
9. Hobson RW, Weiss DG, Fields WS, et al: Efficacy of carotid endarterectomy for asymptomatic carotid stenosis. N Engl J Med 1993;328:221–227.
10. North American Symptomatic Carotid Endarterectomy Trial Collaborators: Beneficial effect of carotid endarterectomy in symptomatic patients with high-grade carotid stenosis. N Engl J Med 1991;325:445–453.
11. Executive Committee for the Asymptomatic Carotid Atherosclerosis Study: Endarterectomy for asymptomatic carotid artery stenosis. JAMA 1995;273:1421–1428.
12. Reigel MM, Hollier LH, Sundt TM Jr, et al: Cerebral hyperperfusion syndrome: A cause of neurologic dysfunction after carotid endarterectomy. J Vasc Surg 1987;5:628–634.
13. Piepgras DG, Morgan MK Sundt TM Jr, et al: Intracerebral hemorrhage after carotid endarterectomy. J Neurosurg 1988;68:532–536.
14. Barr JD, Horowitz MB, Mathis JM, et al: Intraoperative urokinase infusion for embolic stroke during carotid endarterectomy. Neurosurgery 1995;36:606–611.
15. Comerota AJ, Eze AR: Intraoperative high-dose regional urokinase infusion for cerebrovascular occlusion after carotid endarterectomy. J Vasc Surg 1996;24:1008–1016.
16. The National Institute of Neurological Disorders and Stroke (NINDS) rt-PA Stroke Study Group: A systems approach to immediate evaluation and management of hyperacute stroke: Experience at eight centers and implications for community proactive and patient care. Stroke 1997;28:1530–1540.
17. The National Institute of Neurological Disorders and Stroke re-PA Stroke Study Group. Tissue plasminogen activator for acute ischemic stroke. N Engl J Med 1995;333(24):1581–1587.
18. Zweifler RM, Drinkard R, Cunningham S, et al: Implementation of a stroke code system in Mobile, Alabama: Diagnostic and therapeutic yield. Stroke 1997;28:981–983.

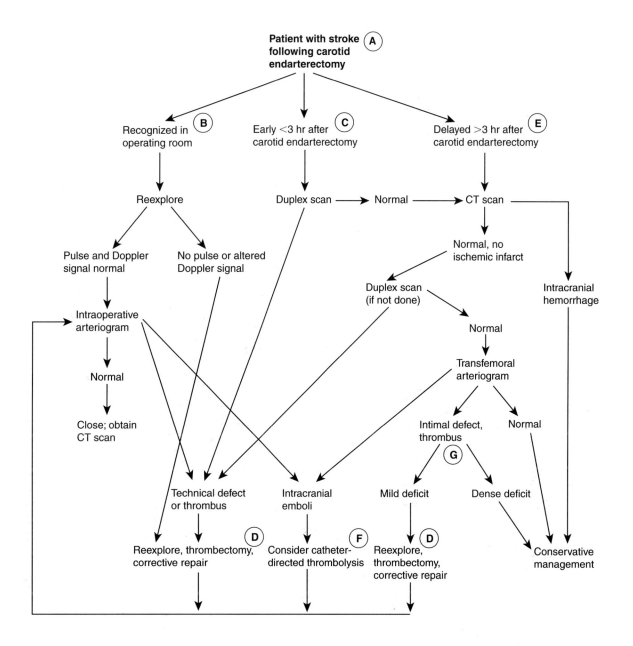

Chapter 17 Vertebral Artery Disease

LISA FLYNN, MD • RAMON BERGUER, MD

(A) The diagnosis of vertebral artery disease may be confirmed by duplex scanning, arteriography, computed tomography, or magnetic resonance imaging (MRI). Vertebral artery disease may be secondary to low-flow (hemodynamic) or to embolic mechanisms. Symptoms may occur spontaneously, may appear during orthostatic maneuvers, or may be related to neck rotation (dynamic).[1] The most common site of atherosclerotic disease of the vertebral artery is at its origin from the subclavian artery. The second most common site for disease is in its second segment (stenosis or occlusion).

(B) Asymptomatic vertebral artery disease is usually noted in studies done for occlusive disease of the carotid bifurcation or supra-aortic trunks. Patients requiring coronary bypass often undergo preoperative carotid duplex ultrasound examination, which may also identify vertebral artery disease.

(C) Symptomatic patients usually present with one or several of the following: ataxia and disequilibrium, orthostatic dizziness, drop attacks, vertigo, blurred vision, hemianopsia, diplopia, cortical blindness, dysarthria, and distal paresthesias.

(D) A dominant but asymptomatic vertebral artery that has more than 75% stenosis at its origin should be corrected in a patient who has bilateral internal carotid artery (ICA) occlusion and who requires coronary bypass.

(E) *Low-flow* (hemodynamic) symptoms of a transient ischemic attack (TIA) may result from severe stenosis, occlusion, or extrinsic compression on the vertebral artery and are usually iterative in nature. MRI findings in these patients are usually negative, and the risk of posterior circulation stroke is low. In contrast, *embolic* TIAs are varied in distribution and are rarely repetitive. The risk of severe stroke in this group is high. In these patients MRI often demonstrates small infarcts in the cerebellum and brain stem.

(F) Stenotic proximal lesions of the vertebral artery are most commonly treated by transposition of this artery to the common carotid artery. A bypass from either the carotid artery or the subclavian artery to the vertebral artery, or reimplantation of the vertebral artery to a new subclavian site are other options.[2] Distal stenotic lesions are often caused by extrinsic compression and are usually corrected with a saphenous vein bypass from the common carotid artery to the distal vertebral artery at the level of C1-C2.[3]

In some cases of extrinsic compression of the vertebral artery at the C0-C1 level, a laminectomy alone may suffice.[4]

If an embolic source is identified as the cause of vertebrobasilar symptoms, surgical intervention is warranted regardless of the degree of ipsilateral stenosis or the condition of the contralateral vertebral artery. When the lesion is bypassed, the proximal embolic source is excluded from the circulation.

(G) Anticoagulation therapy is initially begun with full systemic heparinization aiming at a partial thromboplastin time of 1.5 to 2 times the patient's normal value. Patients are then switched to warfarin, with a goal International Normalized Ratio of 2 to 3. Warfarin therapy is continued for approximately 6 weeks, when another imaging procedure is performed to reevaluate the dissected vertebral artery.

(H) Subsequent imaging is performed after 6 weeks to assess the vertebral artery for healing of the dissection. If the artery is completely healed, anticoagulation therapy may be discontinued. If the dissection persists, there is a potential threat of embolization without anticoagulation. In this scenario, the risks of continued anticoagulation must be weighed against that of either operative intervention (bypass with ligation of the dissected vertebral) or possible embolic posterior circulation stroke.

REFERENCES

1. Ruotolo C, Hazan H, Rancurel G, Kieffer E: Dynamic arteriography. In Berguer R, Caplan L (eds): Vertebrobasilar Arterial Disease. St. Louis, Quality Medical Publishing, 1992.
2. Berguer R, Flynn L, Kline RA, Caplan L: Surgical reconstruction of the vertebral artery: Management and outcome. J Vasc Surg 2000;31:9–18.
3. Berguer R, Morasch MD, Kline RA: A review of 100 consecutive reconstructions of the distal vertebral artery for embolic and hemodynamic disease. J Vasc Surg 1998;27:852–859.
4. Berguer R: Suboccipital approach to the distal vertebral artery. J Vasc Surg 1999;30:344–349.

VERTEBRAL ARTERY DISEASE

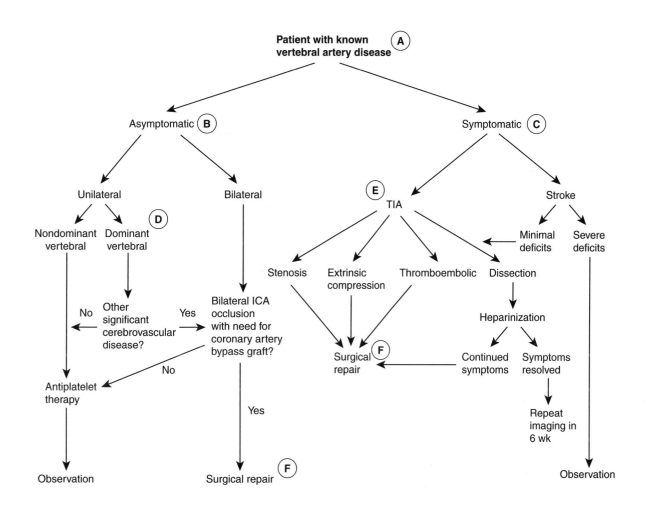

Chapter 18 Subclavian Artery Occlusive Disease

BRUCE A. PERLER, MD • YARON STERNBACH, MD

(A) Unequal arm pressures most commonly are a manifestation of subclavian arterial occlusive disease. The natural history of subclavian stenosis appears relatively benign even when angiographic criteria for subclavian steal are met. One study documented progression to vertebrobasilar symptoms in only 4 of 55 such patients with no strokes reported in a 4-year period.[1] Another report was unable to identify new symptoms in a group of 32 similar patients followed over 2 years.[2] Sonographic follow-up has noted progression of subclavian artery stenoses in only 17% of 67 patients over 2 years.[3] In view of this, asymptomatic patients should be treated conservatively (i.e., observed, with risk factor modification). However, affected patients are susceptible to atherosclerotic disease elsewhere and should therefore undergo broader clinical evaluation.

(B) This clinical scenario represents the "coronary steal syndrome" (CSS), which may develop in patients who have undergone coronary revascularization with an internal mammary artery (IMA). In a Cleveland Clinic series of 66 patients undergoing angioplasty and primary stenting of a subclavian artery, 27 patients (41%) were treated for steal by an IMA bypass and three patients (4.5%) underwent intervention in anticipation of coronary bypass with an IMA.[4] In light of the increasing use of the IMA for coronary revascularization, bilateral arm blood pressure measurements and consideration of CSS is essential in evaluating angina and other manifestations of coronary insufficiency in patients having previously undergone coronary bypass surgery.

(C) Symptoms associated with vertebrobasilar insufficiency (VBI) include drop attacks, ataxia, or other postural disturbances, alternating or bilateral sensory deficits, and homonymous visual changes. The clinical diagnosis of subclavian steal is made when symptoms are identified in the setting of occlusive disease of the ipsilateral subclavian artery or if exercising the ipsilateral arm precipitates them. A wider variety of symptoms may be consistent with the diagnosis of VBI. Among them are dizziness, vertigo, blurred vision, alternating hemiparesis, dysphasia, dysarthria, confusion and loss of consciousness. However, none individually or in combination is pathognomonic. Indeed, numerous other conditions such as vestibular dysfunction, cardiac arrhythmias, and intracerebral small vessel disease may mimic this vascular disorder. For instance, Perler and Williams noted new or recurrent symptoms in 4 of 31 patients who had undergone successful carotid-subclavian bypass despite patent grafts.[5] It is therefore vitally important that patients with unequal arm pressures be comprehensively evaluated to rule out confounding diagnoses before these symptoms are ascribed to VBI.

(D) Upper extremity ischemia alone or in association with VBI is seen in at least 20% of patients with symptomatic subclavian arterial occlusive disease.[5] Most of these patients present with chronic symptoms unless acute distal embolization has occurred from proximal, subclavian disease. Ischemic arm symptoms are usually mild with isolated subclavian disease, causing pain on exertion. Subclavian stenosis affects the left (usually the non-dominant) arm more frequently, and minor symptoms can often be managed conservatively. For more severe symptoms, investigation is required. Synchronous distal arm lesions or distal emboli combined with subclavian disease can cause rest pain or even tissue loss in severe cases.

(E) The vascular laboratory is used to initially assess patients with suspected VBI and arm ischemia. Although the proximal location of subclavian occlusive lesions makes duplex ultrasonography a challenge, this modality can be used to assess patients with arterial disease. Duplex scanning is of particular value in differentiating subclavian stenosis from occlusion, in determining the direction of vertebral artery flow, and in screening for concurrent carotid artery stenosis. An objective assessment of the carotid circulation is mandatory when carotid-subclavian bypass is being considered. Subclavian steal may be present in the absence of retrograde or bidirectional vertebral artery flow at rest. Exercising the limb in question may elicit symptoms and changes in the flow direction. Duplex scans can also be used to assess possibly synchronous arm occlusive disease or emboli. Arm pressure measurement should be obtained in all cases.

(F) Arteriography represents the "gold standard" diagnostic modality. A complete study is indicated in patients who are candidates for interventional treatment. Imaging studies should visualize flow in the arch, the supra-aortic trunks, and the carotid and vertebral systems. Options for immediate endovascular therapeutic intervention exist for lesions with a favorable prognosis.

(G) Patients with distal embolism and severe subclavian stenoses or occlusions are best managed with surgical embolectomy from the proximal artery reconstruction point (subclavian or axillary). If the embolus cannot be extracted from this proximal site, a more distal exposure (e.g., brachial) can be performed. Intraoperative, catheter-directed thrombolytic treatment can be considered for distal emboli. If arm emboli are found with only mild subclavian disease, cardiac sources must be excluded and different treatment strategies considered if treatment is not required for the subclavian lesion. If distal emboli are present but urgent treatment is not required and if the subclavian lesion is amenable to endovascular treatment, percutaneous catheter-directed thrombolysis can be considered.

(H) In view of the variety of surgical options available, their documented low operative mortality and morbidity, and their excellent patency rates, patients with symptomatic subclavian artery occlusions and most patients with symptomatic subclavian stenoses are probably best served by conventional surgical revascularization.

(I) In recent years, experience with the endovascular treatment of subclavian artery occlusive disease has grown. Initial technical success rates exceed 80% and have increased to 100% with the deployment of stents.[4, 6] Comparable results have been achieved in patients with aortoarteritis and arteriosclerosis.[7] Percutaneous transluminal balloon angioplasty (PTA) of complete subclavian occlusion has been associated with greater variability in outcome, generally lower initial and long-term vessel patency, and higher complication rates. Assessment of long-term patency following subclavian PTA or stent placement is confounded by (1) differences in patient selection, (2) a commingling of lesions treated, (3) inconsistency in stent use, and (4) indirect measures of long-term vessel patency. A 3-year patency rate of 84% reported in the Cleveland Clinic experience for primary stenting indicates no benefit over selective stent placement for a suboptimal angioplasty result.[4] The same report noted that complication rates may approach 20% when all technical and local access site complications are tabulated.

(J) Carotid stenosis and indications for carotid endarterectomy are discussed in Chapters 6 to 9). On occasion, significant internal carotid artery disease may be identified in the patient presenting with unequal arm pressures. In the patient requiring operative intervention for symptomatic subclavian arterial occlusive disease, a conventional carotid endarterectomy may be performed synchronously with carotid-subclavian bypass.

Typically, we prefer to originate the graft from the carotid endarterectomy arteriotomy so that the graft also serves as a patch on the endarterectomized vessel. This approach does not appear to increase the inherent morbidity of either procedure.[5] Others have performed simultaneous carotid endarterectomy with axilloaxillary artery bypass with similarly good results.[8] We generally reserve this combined approach for patients with very-high-grade (>70%) asymptomatic carotid stenosis and concurrent symptoms of subclavian arterial occlusive disease.

For patients with VBI from subclavian steal combined with severe ipsilateral carotid disease, we generally perform a combined carotid and subclavian procedure. However, carotid endarterectomy alone may relieve subclavian steal symptoms in many patients with severe carotid disease plus subclavian stenosis or, more commonly, occlusion. Therefore, decision making must be individualized, depending on the apparently dominant lesion, the presence of concomitant arm symptoms, and the experience of the surgeon.

(K) Extra-anatomic carotid-subclavian bypass has emerged as the operative treatment of choice. This procedure has been performed at multiple centers without perioperative mortality. Primary patency rates are superior when synthetic grafts are employed, exceeding 90% at 5 years.[9]

(L) Subclavian artery transposition may be accomplished if an adequate length of the vessel can be mobilized to allow for a single anastomosis to the ipsilateral common carotid artery. The largest reported experience, from Vanderbilt University, was without mortality.[10] Advantages include the avoidance of a synthetic conduit and only a single anastomosis between two native arteries. Durability may even exceed that of carotid-subclavian bypass.

(M) Axilloaxillary artery bypass represents another potential extra-anatomic approach. Multiple series have documented negligible perioperative morbidity. Despite concerns about external compression of this subcutaneously placed graft, 7- to 10-year patency rates between 80% and 90% have been reported.[8, 11-13] This option may be particularly useful for emergent revascularization in the patient with acute upper extremity ischemia if adequate preoperative carotid imaging has not been performed. Alternatively, a subclavian-subclavian bypass can be performed.

(N) Direct reconstruction via a transthoracic approach is generally reserved for patients with multiple-vessel aortic arch disease (including aortoarteritis), which may preclude an extra-anatomic repair (see Chapter 19). Similarly, it may be suitable in patients undergoing simultaneous coronary artery bypass. This anatomic approach was performed prior to the introduction of the extra-anatomic procedures but fell out of favor because of significant rates of perioperative morbidity and mortality. In recent years, however, this approach has become much safer, with mortality rates less than 3% in some centers.[14-16]

REFERENCES

1. Moran KT, Zide RS, Persson AV, et al: Natural history of subclavian steal syndrome. Am Surg 1988;54:643–644.
2. Bornstein NM, Norris JW: Subclavian steal—a harmless hemodynamic phenomenon. Lancet 1986;2:303–305.
3. Ackerman H, Diener HC, Seboldt H, et al: Ultrasonographic follow-up of subclavian stenosis and occlusion: Natural history and surgical treatment. Stroke 1988;19: 431–435.
4. Sullivan TM, Gray BH, Bacharach JM, et al: Angioplasty and primary stenting of the subclavian, innominate and common carotid arteries in 83 patients. J Vasc Surg 1998;28:1059–1065.
5. Perler BA, Williams GM: Carotid subclavian bypass—a decade of experience. J Vasc Surg 1990;12:716–720.
6. Mortajeme A: Percutaneous transluminal angioplasty of supra-aortic vessels. J Endovasc Surg 1996;3:171–181.
7. Tyagi S, Verma PK, Gambhir DS, et al: Early and long-term results of subclavian angioplasty in aortoarteritis (Takayasu's disease): Comparison with atherosclerosis. Cardiovasc Intervent Radiol 1998;21(3):219–224.
8. Chang JB, Stein TA, Liu JP, et al: Long term results with axillo-axillary bypass grafts for symptomatic subclavian artery insufficiency. J Vasc Surg 1997:25:173–178.
9. Ziomek S, Quinones-Baldrich WJ, Busuttil RW, et al: The superiority of synthetic arterial grafts over autogenous veins in carotid subclavian bypass. J Vasc Surg 1986;3: 140–145.
10. Edwards WH, Tapper SS, Edwards WH, et al: Subclavian revascularization: A quarter century experience. Ann Surg 1994;219:673–678.
11. Weiner RI, Deterling RA, Sentissi J, et al: Subclavian artery insufficiency: Treatment with axillo-axillary bypass. Arch Surg 1987;122:876–880.
12. Mingoli A, Feldhaus RJ, Farina C, et al: Comparative results of carotid subclavian bypass and axilloaxillary bypass in patients with symptomatic subclavian disease. Eur J Vasc Surg 1992;6:26–30.
13. Rosenthal D, Ellison RG, Clark MD, et al: Axilloaxillary bypass: Is it worthwhile? J Cardiovasc Surg 1988;29: 191–195.
14. DeBakey ME, Crawford ES, Cooley DA, et al: Cerebral arterial insufficiency: Results following arterial reconstructive operation. Ann Surg 1965;161:921–945.
15. Brewster DC, Moncure AR, Darling RC, et al: Innominate artery lesions: Problems encountered and lessons learned. J Vasc Surg 1985;2:99–112.
16. Kieffer E, Sabatier J, Keskas F, et al: Atherosclerotic innominate artery occlusive disease: Early and long-term results of surgical reconstruction. J Vasc Surg 1995; 21:326–337.

SUBCLAVIAN ARTERY OCCLUSIVE DISEASE

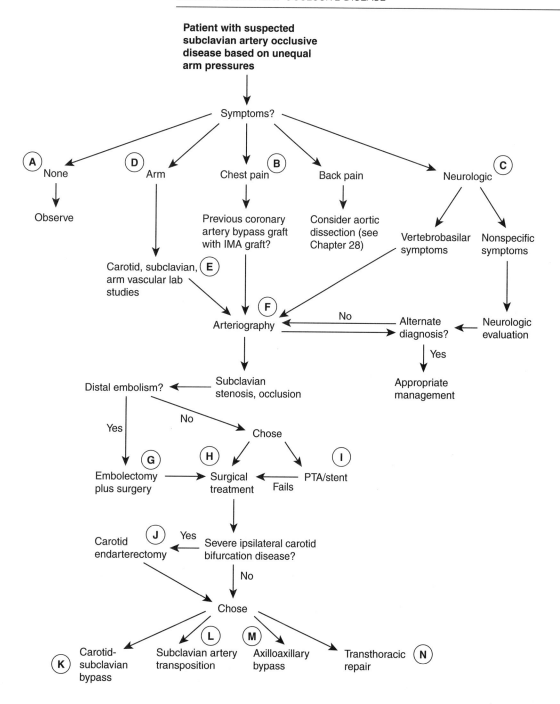

Chapter 19 Brachiocephalic Arterial Occlusive Disease

AUDRA A. NOEL, MD • KENNETH J. CHERRY, JR., MD

(A) Occlusive lesions of the innominate artery and proximal common carotid artery (CCA) are rare, and data on the natural history and surgical outcomes are based primarily on large retrospective series. The Joint Study of Extracranial Arterial Occlusion of 6534 patients found only 17% with more than 30% stenosis of the subclavian or innominate artery.[1] The series of 1961 patients, from Wylie and Effeney at University of California, San Francisco, reviewing operations for carotid bifurcation, vertebral artery, and great vessel disease, documented 7.5% of procedures performed for lesions of the innominate artery, the CCA, or the subclavian artery.[2] Several series report nearly equal gender distribution, and atherosclerosis remains the predominant etiologic factor.[3-6]

Takayasu's arteritis is less common overall and occurs more frequently in women and younger patients. Rarely, radiation may cause great vessel occlusive disease. Mean patient age ranges from 50 to 56 years but is generally younger than the mean age reported for other atherosclerotic lesions. Risk factors are similar to those for lower extremity atherosclerosis, with smoking reported in up to 100% of patients.[4] Diagnosis is based primarily on history and physical examination findings and subsequent confirmation with arteriography or magnetic resonance angiography (see Chapter 6).

(B) Symptoms of innominate artery lesions include right upper extremity, carotid artery (anterior cerebral circulation), or vertebral artery (posterior circulation) transient ischemic symptoms or stroke, or both right arm and neurologic symptoms. In a series from the Mayo Clinic, no patients presented with stroke; however, 77% had neurologic symptoms and 54% had upper extremity complaints (19% with microemboli, 35% with claudication).[3] Berguer's series of 100 consecutive patients reported neurologic symptoms in 83%, stroke in 30% of those patients, and upper extremity symptoms in 4%.[7] Chronic upper extremity symptoms from proximal subclavian lesions are discussed in Chapter 49.

(C) Prophylactic transthoracic repair of asymptomatic stenoses of the innominate artery or CCA to prevent stroke is controversial. In Berguer's series, 13% of patients were asymptomatic, but the authors concluded that operative risk may negate the potential benefit of stroke prevention.[7] In Kieffer's series, 22% of patients were asymptomatic. The authors recommended intervention for asymptomatic disease, especially in the patients with silent cerebral ischemia on cerebral imaging, reduced cerebral flow, or concomitant with coronary artery bypass grafting (CABG).[8]

Because of the small number of asymptomatic patients in all series, it is difficult to derive definitive recommendations. However, simultaneous CABG, particularly with internal mammary artery grafts, is a reasonable indication for intervention for asymptomatic innominate artery or CCA stenoses with a greater than 75% diameter reduction. Further documentation of the safety and efficacy of percutaneous transluminal angioplasty (PTA) may allow for treatment of localized asymptomatic lesions, especially prior to carotid bulb endarterectomy.

(D) Direct repair of innominate lesions is ideal for patients who can tolerate a median sternotomy. Over the past 30 years, median sternotomy has proved to be a safe procedure with limited postoperative pain or respiratory compromise. Direct repair is indicated for reasonably good-risk symptomatic patients with atheroembolic lesions involving the innominate artery and particularly in patients with multiple arch vessel lesions (see I). Mortality rates of direct reconstruction range from 0% to 6.1%, and patency varies from 87% to 98% at 5- to 10-year follow-up.[3-5, 7-9]

(E) In general, direct brachiocephalic reconstruction is preferred over extra-anatomic bypass because of a somewhat higher patency rate. However, these methods have not been rigorously compared, since patients selected for the two approaches are usually not comparable. For patients who are suboptimal candidates for direct reconstruction, either extra-anatomic or endovascular treatment is possible. This includes patients who would require higher-risk reoperative sternotomy, older high-risk patients, and patients with a severely calcified ascending aorta.[4, 5, 7, 8] For patients who are poor candidates for any surgical procedure, balloon angioplasty with and without stenting can be used for brachiocephalic lesions. The choice of cervical bypass versus PTA/stenting depends on institutional experience and continued follow-up of endovascular results.

(F) Small series of patients undergoing PTA of the innominate artery or CCA have been reported.[10-12] Queral and Criado placed 26 primary Palmaz stents in 22 symptomatic patients with an initial success rate of 92%, a patency rate of 85% after a mean of 27 months, and no periprocedure strokes or deaths.[12] In all cases, the procedure was performed in the operating room with open control of the CCA or brachial artery to prevent atheroembolism. Others have reported retrograde balloon angioplasty at the time of carotid endarterectomy.[11] These early reports are sufficiently encouraging that percutaneous endovascular treatment may be considered in patients unable to tolerate direct reconstruction through a median sternotomy. If future reports confirm its efficacy, endovascular treatment may become more widely indicated. For atheroembolic lesions, however, distal control of the artery with a retrograde open approach, or some type of cerebral protection device, is important to prevent intraprocedural emboli.

(G) Innominate endarterectomy is a technically demanding operation that provides excellent results when performed in properly selected pa-

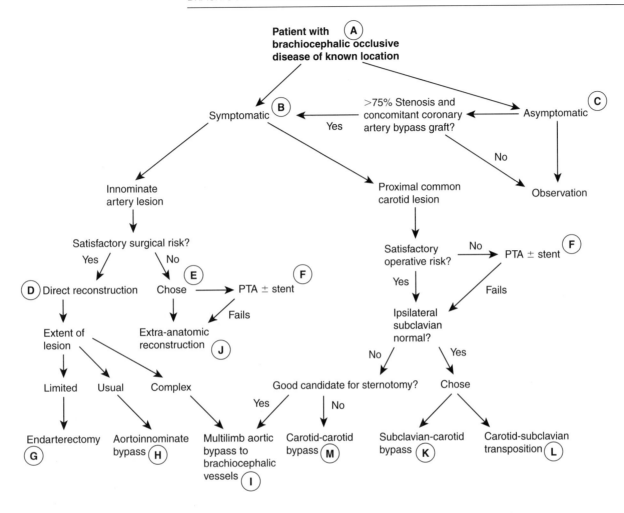

tients. In a series from the Mayo Clinic, there was no difference in recurrence of symptoms for patients undergoing bypass (14.3%) versus endarterectomy (11%).[3] Carlson identified only 3 of 37 patients as not suitable for endarterectomy; however, most centers favor bypass grafting as an easier and more universal procedure.[13] Endarterectomy avoids the use of prosthetic material in young patients and may be performed if the aorta is not severely calcified and if the origin of the left CCA is more than 1.5 cm from the origin of the innominate artery. Contraindications to endarterectomy include arteritis, radiation therapy, recurrent innominate disease, and a common brachiocephalic trunk.

H As stated in G, aorta–innominate artery bypass is preferred in most atherosclerotic patients and in all patients with Takayasu's arteritis, recurrent disease, and previous radiation. The surgeon places a single graft limb from the ascending aorta to the distal innominate artery using an 8- to 10-mm polyester (Dacron) prosthesis.

Several controversies exist regarding specific technical aspects, such as innominate vein division. Although Kieffer reported no complications with vein division and the Mayo Clinic series had only one patient (of four) with transient edema following vein division, Berguer and colleagues reported six patients with upper extremity swelling.[7] Our approach is to leave this vein intact unless it is interfering with adequate visualization, in which case it can be ligated. Neurologic monitoring with electroencephalography may be used for these bypasses, but shunting is rarely required.

(I) If both the right CCA and the right subclavian artery must be bypassed or if bypass of lesions in the left CCA or subclavian artery is desired, we prefer a single-limb graft from the aorta, with side-arms attached as needed, rather than a bifurcated graft. This method reduces the bulk of graft within the mediastinum. Others have successfully used bifurcated grafts, originating from the right side of the ascending aorta, in order to avoid compression by the sternum.[5] However, bifurcated grafts may kink or stenose. When more than two arch branches are reconstructed, such as in the case of Takayasu's disease, side-arms attached to a single graft stem are required.

The results of direct innominate artery reconstructions are excellent, with early relief of symptoms (95%) and good long-term results (87% to 90% of patients symptom-free).[3,5,13,14] Neurologic morbidity ranges from 0% to 8%, and surgical mortality rates range from 0% to 6.1%.[3-5,7-9]

(J) Multiple configurations of extra-anatomic bypass grafts have been used to treat innominate artery lesions. One of the first described was axilloaxillary bypass, but poor patency (50% failure) was observed in several series.[4,15] However, the most recent report by Mingoli and coworkers documented 5- and 10-year symptom-free interval rates of 98% and 94% with 63 crossover axilloaxillary grafts.[16] As expected, overall morbidity (16.1%) and mortality (1.6%) were low with this cervical approach. Other possible origins for crossover bypass include the left carotid or subclavian artery in addition to the left axillary artery. Such grafts may be anastomosed distally to the right axillary or to the subclavian artery. If there is an embolic site in the innominate artery, the right CCA must be divided and revascularized, either with a separate graft, or by implantation into the crossover graft. In such cases, the right subclavian artery (proximal to the vertebral origin) should also be ligated to prevent embolization.[15-17]

In the rare case of a high-risk patient with multiple great vessel disease, femoral to axillary bypass has been reported, with additional crossover grafting as necessary. Our practice has been to use extra-anatomic reconstruction only in patients who are at high risk for median sternotomy. We await the long-term results of endovascular treatment, which we recognize might become the preferred approach in higher-risk patients.

(K) The safest and most effective origin of bypass for a proximal lesion of the CCA is a normal, ipsilateral subclavian artery. Adequacy as a donor artery must be established with imaging and objective noninvasive testing, because subtle degrees of subclavian stenosis are easily missed. The results of this bypass are excellent.[17,18] Saphenous vein graft or prosthetic graft may be used, but several series have reported an apparent advantage of prosthetic grafts in this location.[17,18] If synchronous carotid bifurcation disease is present, it may be managed with concomitant endarterectomy.

(L) Transposition of the CCA onto a patent ipsilateral subclavian artery is appropriate if the CCA is not diseased distal to the planned level of anastomosis. Although this procedure may require more extensive dissection of the CCA, the results are excellent. A series from Berguer and colleagues reported 100% patency of transposition grafts, with a mean follow-up of 53 months.[18]

(M) Carotid-carotid bypass may be considered in poor-risk patients with proximal CCA disease when disease of the ipsilateral subclavian artery precludes its use as an origin for bypass. Good-risk patients, especially those with other arch lesions, have better results with direct arch reconstruction. Retropharyngeal tunneling of a prosthetic graft provides a more direct route than the anterior approach. Although this is an uncommon procedure that is often compiled with other cervical reconstructions, patency results appear good. However, the morbidity of even cervical reconstructions is as high as 9% in symptomatic high-risk patients who are unable to tolerate median sternotomy.[18]

REFERENCES

1. Fields WS, Lemak NA: Joint Study of Extracranial Arterial Occlusion: VII. Subclavian steal—a review of 168 cases. JAMA 1972;222:1139–1143.
2. Wylie EJ, Effeney DJ: Surgery of the aortic arch branches and vertebral arteries. Surg Clin North Am 1979;59:669–680.
3. Cherry KJJ, McCullough JL, Hallett JWJ, et al: Technical principles of direct innominate artery revascularization: A comparison of endarterectomy and bypass grafts. J Vasc Surg 1989;9:718–723.
4. Brewster DC, Moncure AC, Darling RC, et al: Innominate artery lesions: Problems encountered and lessons learned. J Vasc Surg 1985;2:99–112.
5. Reul GJ, Jacobs MJ, Gregoric ID, et al: Innominate artery occlusive disease: Surgical approach and long-term results. J Vasc Surg 1991;14:405–412.
6. Crawford ES, De Bakey ME, Morris GCJ, Howell JF: Surgical treatment of occlusion of the innominate, common carotid, and subclavian arteries: A 10-year experience. Surgery 1969;65:17–31.
7. Berguer R, Morasch MD, Kline RA: Transthoracic repair of innominate and common carotid artery disease: Immediate and long-term outcome for 100 consecutive surgical reconstructions. J Vasc Surg 1998;27:34–41.
8. Kieffer E, Sabatier J, Koskas F, Bahnini A: Atherosclerotic innominate artery occlusive disease: Early and long-term results of surgical reconstruction. J Vasc Surg 1995;21:326–336.
9. Azakie A, McElhinney DB, Messina LM, Stoney RJ: Common brachiocephalic trunk: Strategies for revascularization. Ann Thorac Surg 1999;67:657–660.
10. Ligush JJ, Criado E, Keagy BA: Innominate artery occlusive disease: Management with central reconstructive techniques. Surgery 1997;121:556–62.

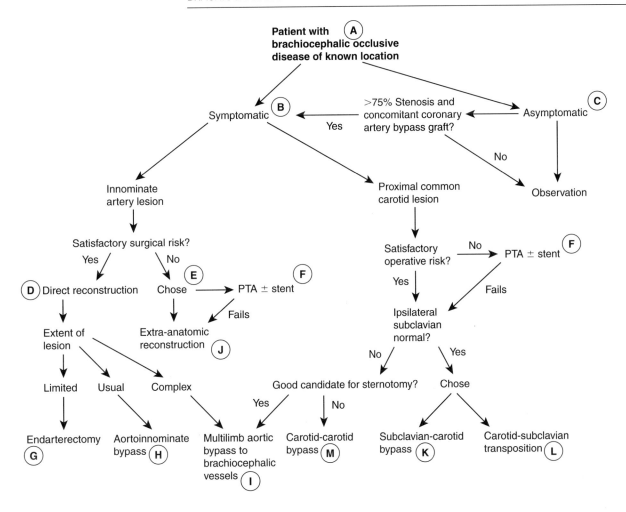

11. Levien LJ, Benn CA, Veller MG, Fritz VU: Retrograde balloon angioplasty of brachiocephalic or common carotid artery stenoses at the time of carotid endarterectomy. Eur J Vasc Endovasc Surg 1998;15:521–527.
12. Queral LA, Criado FJ: Endovascular treatment of aortic arch occlusive disease. Semin Vasc Surg 1996;9:156–163.
13. Carlson RE, Ehrenfeld WK, Stoney RJ, Wylie EJ: Innominate artery endarterectomy: A 16-year experience. Arch Surg 1977;112:1389–1393.
14. Crawford ES, Stowe CL, Powers RW Jr: Occlusion of the innominate, common carotid, and subclavian arteries: Long-term results of surgical treatment. Surgery 1983;94:781–791.
15. Criado FJ: Extrathoracic management of aortic arch syndrome. Br J Surg 1982;69(Suppl):S45–S51.
16. Mingoli A, Sapienza P, Feldhaus RJ, et al: Long-term results and outcomes of crossover axilloaxillary bypass grafting: A 24-year experience. J Vasc Surg 1999;29:894–901.
17. Mingoli A, Feldhaus RJ, Farina C, et al: Comparative results of carotid-subclavian bypass and axillo-axillary bypass in patients with symptomatic subclavian disease. Eur J Vasc Surg 1992;6:26–30.
18. Berguer R, Morasch MD, Kline RA, et al: Cervical reconstruction of the supra-aortic trunks: A 16-year experience. J Vasc Surg 1999;29:239–246.

Chapter 20 Carotid Plus Coronary Disease

JOHN J. RICOTTA, MD • THOMAS BILFINGER, MD, ScD • YARA GORSKI, MD

(A) Stroke remains a major noncardiac complication after coronary artery bypass grafting (CABG), whereas myocardial infarction (MI) is the major non-neurologic cause of *both early and late* morbidity after carotid endarterectomy (CEA). As a result of a better understanding of the multifactorial nature of atherosclerotic disease, there is a trend toward performing routine carotid duplex screening in patients with coronary artery disease (CAD) as well as routine cardiac evaluation prior to carotid endarterectomy. The incidence of severe (>70%) carotid stenosis detected by routine screening after CABG has ranged from 4% to 7.7%[1] and is associated with advanced age, peripheral vascular disease, and smoking. Bilateral severe carotid stenoses increase both perioperative and long-term neurologic events in CABG patients. The incidence of significant CAD in patients with carotid stenosis varies from 30% to 50%. Cardiac screening of patients with markers for CAD can identify patients at risk for both perioperative and late coronary events.

(B) Stroke in evolution or crescendo transient ischemic attacks (TIAs) are rare, but this presentation usually precludes coronary evaluation. Carotid endarterectomy should be performed, but morbidity is increased in this group.

(C) Markers for CAD include age over 70 years, angina pectoris, myocardial infarction, congestive heart failure, diabetes mellitus, and ventricular arrhythmias. Patients with no clinical markers and a reasonable activity level are considered as *low risk* and can undergo carotid endarterectomy without further evaluation of CAD. The number of CAD markers stratifies patients as either *intermediate* or *high risk* (see Chapter 1) and is an indication for further CAD evaluation.[2]

(D) Stress testing is performed to identify patients with evidence of subclinical, inducible myocardial ischemia. Dipyridamole thallium scintigraphy (DTS) and stress echocardiography are the usual options selected (see Chapter 1).

(E) Patients with marked to severe thallium redistribution or marked wall motion abnormalities carry a 30% risk of cardiac complications after carotid endarterectomy and may benefit from coronary revascularization.

(F) Patients with mild thallium redistribution or fixed defects or mild wall motion abnormalities do not benefit from preoperative coronary revascularization. Their cardiac risk associated with carotid endarterectomy is not greatly increased over that in patients without these findings.

(G) Arteriographic confirmation of significant left main or multivessel CAD correlates with both early and late survival, as established in the Coronary Artery Surgery Study (CASS).[3] Some patients are amenable to percutaneous transluminal coronary angioplasty (PTCA); other patients might be considered for CABG based on anatomic findings. Patients with nonreconstructible CAD include those whose disease is not amenable to PTCA or CABG. These patients are at high risk for cardiac events after carotid endarterectomy.

(H) *High neurologic risk* refers to symptomatic unilateral stenosis greater than 70% and asymptomatic bilateral stenosis greater than 80%. Data from the North American Symptomatic Carotid Endarterectomy Trial (NASCET) and the European Carotid Surgery Trial (ECST) indicates a benefit from surgery in patients with symptomatic carotid stenosis greater than 50%.[4] The benefits of surgery increase proportionately to the degree of stenosis. In patients with *high cardiac risk*, the benefit of surgery for a symptomatic stenosis 50% to 69% remains a matter of clinical judgment. The high-risk subgroup of patients, who are not candidates for cardiac revascularization, must be managed individually. Antiplatelet therapy should be maximized. If this measure is not sufficient or if carotid stenosis is severe, carotid endarterectomy can be performed preferentially with regional anesthesia. Carotid stenting may prove useful for these patients in the future.

(I) According to the ACAS, patients with stenosis greater than 60% would benefit from prophylactic carotid endarterectomy.[5] However, this benefit is predicated on a 5-year survival. No data on patients with asymptomatic stenosis and severe nonreconstructible CAD exist. In most cases, the carotid endarterectomy should be deferred until symptoms develop.

(J) Indications for CABG versus PTCA have been developed by a task force of the American Heart Association/American College of Cardiology.[6, 7] Some patients present with carotid stenosis and can be identified by screening for CAD using the preceding sections (C–G) of this algorithm. Others may present with coronary ischemic syndromes and undergo a primary cardiac evaluation. The incidence of significant carotid stenosis in candidates for CABG patients varies from 5% to 15% but is highest in patients with one or more of the following[8, 9]:

- Age older than 60 years
- Peripheral vascular disease
- Earlier neurologic event
- Carotid bruit

Patients with one or more of these characteristics should be screened with carotid duplex ultrasound surveillance before CABG, since the estimated yield in these groups is 8%. Duplex findings may be confirmed by other diagnostic methods such as magnetic resonance angiography or conventional angiography if necessary, depending on the accuracy of the vascular laboratory.

(K) *Low cardiac risk* is difficult to quantify, but the term implies the following:

- A stable anginal pattern (or a pattern that is stabilized with medical therapy)
- Adequate ventricular function
- Absence of severe left main coronary artery stenosis, without a large left ventricular mass at risk

CAROTID PLUS CORONARY DISEASE

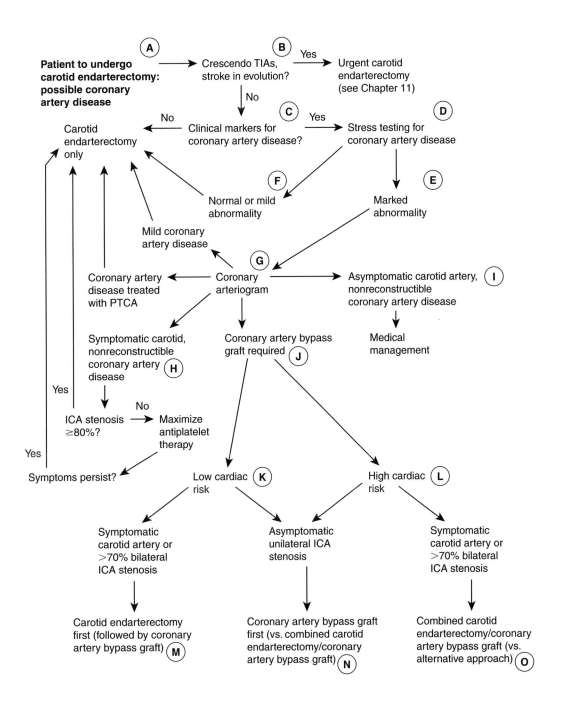

Carotid Plus Coronary Disease (continued)

(L) Patients in the *high cardiac risk* category include those with the following:
- Left main stenosis or severe triple-vessel disease (left main equivalent)
- Unstable angina unresponsive to medical therapy
- Malignant ventricular arrhythmia
- Uncompensated congestive heart failure
- Ejection fraction less than 30%
- Hemodynamic instability requiring inotropic or balloon pump support

Between 40% and 60% of patients who are candidates for CABG probably fall into the high-risk category.[6]

(M) Patients with bilateral carotid stenosis greater than 70% or with unilateral symptomatic carotid stenosis have an increased risk of stroke after CABG alone. In these patients, carotid endarterectomy should be performed prior to or synchronous with CABG.

In patients with *high neurologic risk* and *low cardiac risk*, we prefer carotid endarterectomy first, followed by coronary revascularization. In some centers, with good results, combined procedures are performed. However, the incidence of postoperative stroke in this group is almost double the stroke rate of low-risk carotid stenosis.[7] In patients with bilateral disease, the most severe lesion should be addressed first. This may be done as (1) carotid endarterectomy followed by combined carotid endarterectomy/CABG or as (2) carotid endarterectomy/CABG followed by deferred carotid endarterectomy. When the second carotid endarterectomy is delayed, this period should be for at least 4 to 6 weeks. Data are limited regarding combined CABG and bilateral carotid endarterectomy, but this procedure is not commonly performed.[8]

(N) Patients with unilateral asymptomatic significant carotid stenosis are at the lowest risk of stroke after CABG alone (6.7% in Hertzer's randomized series).[9] Therefore, these patients may be considered for CABG first with delayed carotid endarterectomy. Patients with *low neurologic risk* (asymptomatic and less than 70% internal carotid artery stenosis bilaterally) and *low cardiac risk* should be managed in accord with institutional results. Excellent results have been associated with carotid endarterectomy before (staged) or with CABG (combined). The morbidity and mortality rates in this case vary from 4% to 6%. In centers without good experience with a combined approach, carotid endarterectomy should be delayed, although the risk of stroke is probably increased. In centers with good combined results, this approach is appropriate.

(O) Patients with *low neurologic risk* and *high cardiac risk* can be treated by either combined carotid endarterectomy/CABG or by CABG first with deferred carotid endarterectomy. This decision should be made according to institutional and personal experience. If the overall complication rate (death and stroke) is less than or equal to 8%, combined surgery should be considered. In staged cases, one should defer carotid endarterectomy for 4 to 6 weeks.[10]

(P) As a general rule, patients with *high neurologic risk* and *high cardiac risk* should undergo a combined procedure by an experienced team.[11] A threshold complication rate of 15% to 17% is acceptable, depending on the severity of disease. Carotid endarterectomy with local anesthesia, followed by CABG within 48 hours, has been used in this group; some authors have combined this with prophylactic balloon pump insertion prior to carotid endarterectomy.[12] Others advocate carotid angioplasty prior to CABG, although its efficacy is still unproven. Management of these patients is particularly challenging, and they should be cared for in centers with extensive experience and good results.

REFERENCES

1. Petersen MJ, McBee CM, Bilfinger T, et al: Determinants of morbidity and mortality after combined carotid endarterectomy and open heart surgery. Stroke 1998;29:269.
2. Eagle KA, Coley CM, Newell JB, et al: Combining clinical and thallium data optimizes preoperative assessment of cardiac risk before major vascular surgery. Ann Intern Med 1989;l00:859–866.
3. Myers WO, Gersh BJ, Fisher LD, et al: Medical versus early vessel disease and mild angina pectoris: A CASS Registry study of survival. Ann Thoracic Surg 1987;44:471.
4. Ricotta JJ, Faggioli GL, Castilone A, et al: Risk factors for stroke after cardiac surgery: Buffalo Cardiac Cerebral Study Group. J Vasc Surg 1995;21:359–364.
5. Executive Committee for the Asymptomatic Carotid Atherosclerosis Study: Endarterectomy for asymptomatic carotid artery stenosis. JAMA 1995;273:1421–1428.
6. ACC/AHA Guidelines for Coronary Artery Bypass Surgery: A report of the ACC/AHA Task Force on Assessment of Diagnostic and Therapeutic Cardiovascular Procedures. Circulation 1991;83:1123–1173.
7. Guidelines for Percutaneous Coronary Angioplasty: Report of the ACC/AHA Task Force on Assessment of Diagnostic and Therapeutic Cardiovascular Procedures. J Am Coll Cardiol 1992;22:2033–2054.
8. Ricotta JJ: Carotid endarterectomy and coronary bypass. In Yao J, Pearce WH (eds): Progress in Vascular Surgery. Stamford, Conn, Appleton & Lange, 1997.
9. Hertzer NR, Loop FD, Beven EG, et al: Surgical staging for simultaneous coronary and carotid disease: A study including prospective randomization. J Vasc Surg 1989;9:455-463.
10. Chang BB, Darling RC III, Shah DM, et al: Carotid endarterectomy can be safely performed with acceptable mortality and morbidity in patients requiring coronary artery bypass grafts. Am J Surg 1994;168:94–96.
11. Bilfinger T, Petersen M, Ricotta JJ: In Yao J, Pearce WH (eds): Practical Vascular Surgery. Stamford, Conn, Appleton & Lange, 1999.
12. Allie DE, Lirtzman M, Malik AP, et al: Rapid-staged strategy for concomitant critical carotid and left main coronary disease with left ventricular dysfunction: IABP use. Ann Thoracic Surg 1998;66:1230–1235.

CAROTID PLUS CORONARY DISEASE

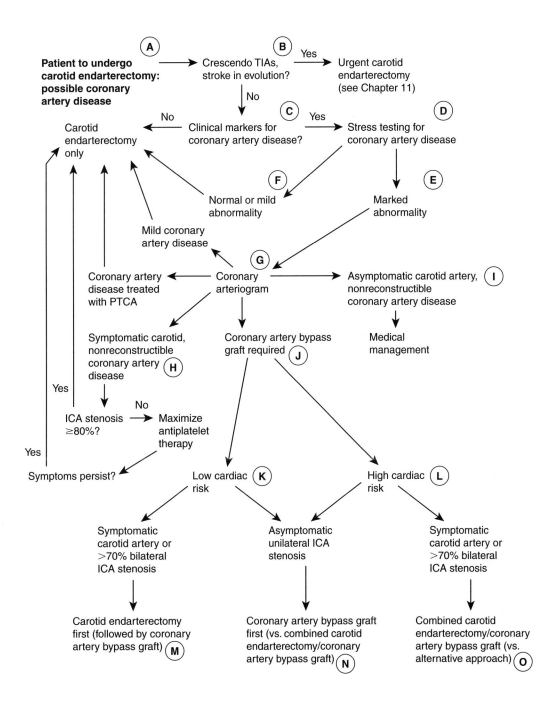

ANEURYSMS

Chapter 21 Abdominal Aortic Aneurysm

MARC L. SCHERMERHORN, MD • JACK L. CRONENWETT, MD

(A) An aneurysm is defined as a focal dilation more than 50% larger than the normal artery diameter, which means that an abdominal aortic aneurysm (AAA) must be larger than 3 cm in diameter. The prevalence of AAAs is 3% to 10% for patients over 50 years of age. Prevalence is increased by a positive family history, older age, male gender, and smoking.[1] Routine physical examination has a low sensitivity to detect an AAA unless the AAA is large: 29% for 3 to 3.9 cm, 50% for 4 to 4.9 cm, and 76% for AAAs larger than 5 cm.[2] Most asymptomatic AAAs are discovered incidentally during imaging studies of the abdomen performed for other reasons.

(B) Patients with a known or suspected AAA should undergo a careful history and physical examination. Factors that increase rupture risk (e.g., hypertension, chronic pulmonary disease, smoking history, positive family history) should be identified. Factors that increase operative risk (e.g., cardiac, pulmonary, and renal diseases) should be quantitated. Life expectancy and quality of life should be evaluated. Physical examination should carefully exclude other aneurysms, especially femoral and popliteal aneurysms, which are often associated. Other factors that might affect the conduct of AAA repair should be identified, such as renovascular hypertension, mesenteric ischemia, and aortoiliac occlusive disease.

(C) Most AAAs are asymptomatic until they rupture (see Chapter 23). Occasionally, they may cause distal embolization, which is more often seen with small AAAs that have an irregular, stellate configuration of the contained thrombus. Rarely, they may thrombose, causing acute, severe ischemia. Pain and tenderness associated with AAAs are difficult to assess, and other causes should be sought before impending rupture is presumed; however, inflammatory AAAs can present this way. All of these symptomatic presentations are usually indications for urgent or emergent surgical repair.

(D) Ultrasound scanning is a noninvasive, accurate, and relatively inexpensive method for determining the diameter of the abdominal aorta.[3] It is more difficult to image the suprarenal aorta with ultrasound scanning, but most aortic aneurysms confined to the abdominal segment are largest in the infrarenal location, so that they can still be detected and measured with this modality. Ultrasound should be the initial study to confirm a suspected AAA and to measure its diameter. Ultrasound is also appropriate for screening patients at increased risk for an aneurysm, such as relatives (>50 years of age) of patients with known AAAs.

Computed tomography (CT) is sometimes used instead of ultrasound as the first diagnostic step if surgery is anticipated, such as in patients with obviously large AAAs on physical examination. Although CT diameter measurements are more accurate, measurements obtained by ultrasound are usually sufficient for initial decision making and should be within 3 mm of the true diameter using modern equipment.

(E) In a patient with an asymptomatic AAA, the first step in decision making is to estimate the risk of aneurysm rupture. Of the factors known to increase rupture risk, diameter is the most important and the most useful in decision making. Current best estimates of rupture risk as a function of diameter are shown in Table 21-1.

The wide range of these estimates reflects both imprecise data and variation between patients. Because most known AAAs are repaired before rupture, the risk of rupture can seldom be determined from observational studies. Furthermore, other factors influence rupture risk, which explains why not all AAAs rupture at the same size threshold. In addition to larger diameter, rapid expansion, smoking and chronic obstructive pulmonary disease (COPD), a strongly positive family history, hypertension, and eccentric aneurysm shape, all appear to increase rupture risk.[4-9]

Unfortunately, there is no precise formula that incorporates these risk factors to calculate rupture risk. However, we can use these risk factors in combination to estimate AAA rupture risk as low, average, or high (Table 21-2). Patients with low risk of rupture are best managed conservatively with careful ultrasound surveillance unless they are very young with long life expectancy, such that the eventual AAA repair, because of expansion, is almost certain. In this case, early surgical repair may be recommended if the patient understands the risk tradeoffs and prefers more aggressive management.

(F) If AAA rupture risk is average or high, the next step in decision making is to estimate a patient's life expectancy to determine whether prophylactic repair would yield long-term benefit. Obviously, patients with a short life expectancy because of co-morbid disease are less likely to die of AAA rupture and are less likely to benefit from AAA repair.

Unfortunately, there is no precise formula to determine a recommendation for management based solely on life expectancy. Because of commonly associated co-morbid disease, such as hypertension and coronary artery disease (CAD), the late survival rate of patients after elective AAA repair is significantly less than age-matched and sex-matched patients without AAAs (60% versus

TABLE 21-1
Estimated Risk of Aneurysm Rupture Related to Diameter

Diameter (cm)	Rupture Risk (%/year)
<4	0
4–5	0.5–5
5–6	3–15
6–7	10–20
7–8	20–40
>8	30–50

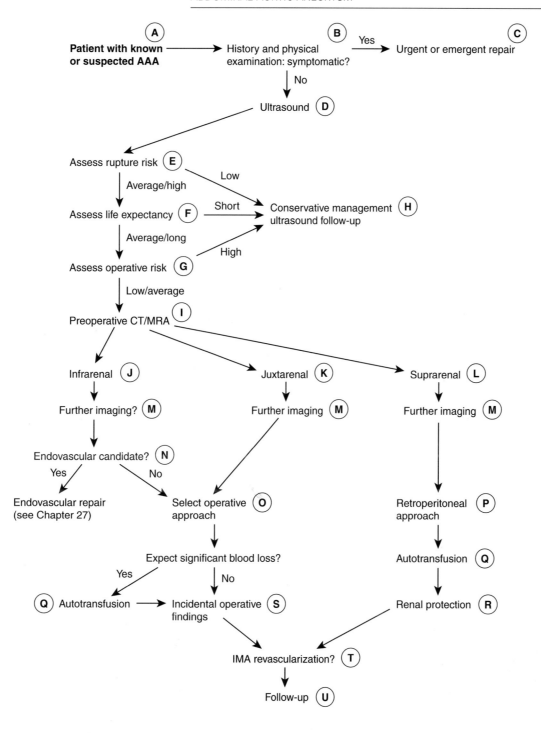

Abdominal Aortic Aneurysm (continued)

TABLE 21-2
Factors Influencing Risk of Aneurysm Rupture

	Low Risk	Average Risk	High Risk
Diameter	<5 cm	5-6 cm	>6 cm
Expansion	<0.3 cm/year	0.3-0.6 cm/year	>0.6 cm/year
Smoking/COPD	None, mild	Moderate	Severe/steroids
Family history	No relatives	One relative	Numerous relatives
Hypertension	Normal blood pressure	Controlled	Poorly controlled
Shape	Fusiform	Saccular	Very eccentric

COPD, chronic obstructive pulmonary disease.

79% at 6 years).[10] Table 21-3 estimates life expectancy by age, sex, and race for patients with AAA.[11] Estimates for individual patients must be refined by a careful assessment of their overall health, especially other factors that might drastically affect survival, such as malignancy. In general, the lower the rupture risk, the longer life expectancy should be for surgical repair to be recommended. Patients with a short life expectancy are best managed conservatively unless the risk of AAA rupture is very high.

(G) The final step in decision making for potential AAA repair is to assess operative risk. Operative mortality is dependent on major organ dysfunction as well as surgeon and hospital volume. A meta-analysis by Steyerberg and colleagues provides a useful, quantitative estimate for operative mortality in patients undergoing open AAA repair (Table 21-4).[12] Increased operative risk should increase the threshold for surgical repair and should be balanced against rupture risk and life expectancy. For borderline decisions, more precise determination of cardiac risk with echocardiography or stress imaging may be useful (see Chapter 1). In some cases, better medical management, including perioperative β blockade, can modify high operative risk.[13] Coronary artery bypass graft (CABG) or interventional treatment before AAA repair is probably beneficial *if* the patient with CAD would otherwise benefit from this treatment.

In patients with high operative risk, conservative management of an AAA is usually recommended unless the risk of rupture is very high or if the AAA diameter increases during follow-up. The most difficult decision making often involves patients with small (4 to 5.5 cm) AAAs. The United Kingdom Small Aneurysm Trial showed no improvement in life expectancy after early AAA repair in these patients, but in this study 61% of patients undergoing ultrasound surveillance underwent AAA repair after a median time of only 2.9 years, usually because of increased size.[14] Furthermore, even during very rigorous follow-up, 1% of patients experienced rupture each year in the United Kingdom Trial. There was a trend for surgical benefit in younger patients (<72 years of age) and in patients with larger AAAs (>4.5 cm). Decision analysis suggests that early surgery can be beneficial and cost-effective if operative risk is low.[15]

Thus, surgical repair can be recommended for small AAAs but only if the operative risk is known to be low and the life expectancy long. Patient preferences have an important role in these decisions, especially when the relative risks and benefits of immediate surgery versus conservative management are borderline.

TABLE 21-3
Life Expectancy (Years) for Patients with Abdominal Aortic Aneurysms Related to Age, Sex, and Race

		Male		Female	
Age (yr)	Total	White	Black	White	Black
60	13	12	11	14	13
65	11	11	10	12	11
70	10	9	8	10	10
75	8	8	7	9	8
80	6	6	6	7	6
85+ over	5	4	4	5	5

From U.S. Bureau of the Census: Statistical Abstract of the United States, 118th ed. Washington, DC, Government Printing Office, 1998.[11]

TABLE 21-4
Operative Risk: Independent Risk Factors for Operative Mortality After Elective Aneurysm Repair

Risk Factor	Odds Ratio*	95% CI
Creatinine > 1.8 mg/dL	3.3	1.5-7.5
Congestive heart failure	2.3	1.1-5.2
ECG ischemia	2.2	1.0-5.1
Pulmonary dysfunction	1.9	1.0-3.8
Older age (per decade)	1.5	1.2-1.8
Female gender	1.5	0.7-3.0

*Odds ratio indicates relative risk compared to patients without that risk factor.
CI, confidence interval; ECG, electrocardiographic.
From Steyerberg EW, Kievit J, de Mol Van Otterloo JC, et al: Perioperative mortality of elective abdominal aortic aneurysm surgery: A clinical prediction rule based on literature and individual patient data. Arch Intern Med 1995;155:1998-2004.[12]

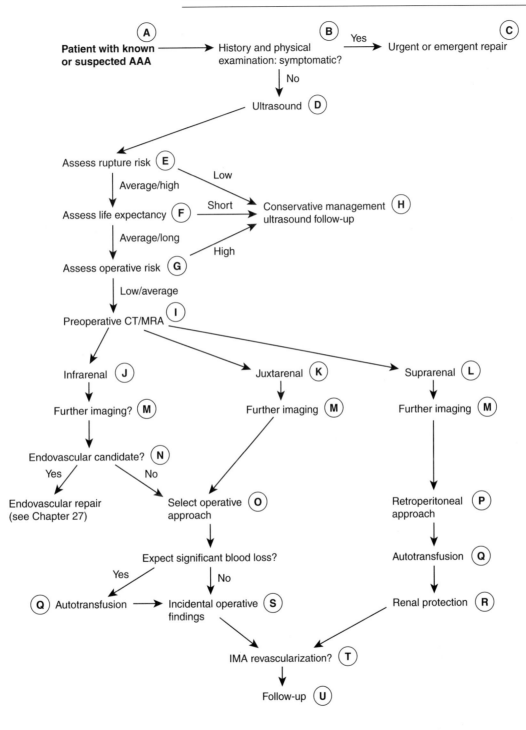

Abdominal Aortic Aneurysm (continued)

(H) Medical management of AAAs is designed to reduce expansion and rupture rate and to detect expansion that might warrant surgical repair. Smoking cessation and hypertension control are paramount. Increasing evidence suggests that low-dose propranolol reduces expansion rate independent of hemodynamic effects and is appropriate for patients without contraindications.[16] Because steroid treatment of patients with COPD has been implicated in AAA expansion, steroid therapy should be discontinued if possible.[8] Ultrasound surveillance to detect expansion should be performed at 6-month intervals in patients who could be candidates for surgical repair. Expansion rate is a function of size and averages an increase in diameter of 10% per year.[17] Rapid expansion (>1 cm/year) is generally an indication for surgical repair of even small AAAs.[6]

(I) CT scanning with intravenous (IV) contrast medium is most commonly used preoperatively to obtain anatomic information necessary to plan surgical repair. Most important is to define the proximal and distal extent of the AAA. Important anatomic variants are easily detected with CT scanning, such as a circumaortic or retroaortic left renal vein, left-sided inferior vena cava, and horseshoe or pelvic kidney. Spiral CT with three-dimensional (3-D) reconstruction provides information about mesenteric, renal, and iliac arterial disease. Specialized 3-D software can provide detailed information concerning the location of soft and calcified plaque, which can help identify an optimal site for aortic clamping, particularly when this involves the suprarenal aorta. Spiral CT with 3-D reconstruction also provides important information in guiding endograft repair of AAAs.

Magnetic resonance angiography (MRA) is an alternative that avoids IV contrast and radiation exposure and provides better images of major aortic branches. However, MRA is more expensive and time-consuming than CT scanning and is not as readily available.

(J) Most AAAs are infrarenal (i.e., those that can be managed with an aortic clamp placed below both renal arteries). Pararenal AAAs account for 2% to 20% of AAAs (depending on referral patterns) and include both suprarenal and juxtarenal AAAs. Concurrent iliac aneurysms occur in 10% to 25%.

(K) Juxtarenal AAAs extend to the inferior margin of the renal arteries such that they require aortic clamp placement above at least one renal artery but do not require renal artery reimplantation. Operative risk is similar to that of infrarenal AAAs, since renal ischemic time is minimal and often involves only one kidney.

(L) Suprarenal AAAs extend above the renal arteries but not above the diaphragm. Typically, supraceliac clamp placement with attendant renal and mesenteric ischemia is required. Operative risk is increased relative to infrarenal AAAs.[18] Therefore, detection of a suprarenal AAA requires reevaluation of the appropriateness of surgery. Because the risk of surgery is increased, the optimal diameter threshold for elective repair is usually higher, by approximately 1 cm.

(M) After high-quality CT scanning, catheter-based arteriography is not usually necessary for preoperative evaluation of infrarenal AAAs for surgical repair; it is helpful, however, for patients with occlusive disease of the renal, mesenteric, or iliac-femoral arteries who might benefit from simultaneous repair.[19] Furthermore, it is required to delineate aberrant renal arteries associated with horseshoe or ectopic kidney, or to clarify questionable details on the CT scan. As noted, MRA is increasingly used for this purpose when available, especially in patients with renal insufficiency, to avoid the nephrotoxicity of radiographic contrast agents. Juxtarenal and suprarenal AAAs are usually evaluated with preoperative arteriography to define relevant anatomy and pathology of the mesenteric and renal arteries unless 3-D CT scanning or MRA has clearly shown these details.

(N) Selection of patients with infrarenal AAAs for endovascular repair (see Chapter 27) is currently under investigation, although long-term follow-up is not yet available. However, experience to date suggests that endovascular repair will become appropriate for many patients with infrarenal AAAs because of lower morbidity and mortality.

(O) Infrarenal AAAs can be approached with either a transperitoneal or retroperitoneal incision. The *transperitoneal* approach allows exploration of the abdomen if other pathologic processes must be evaluated and provides easier access to the right and left iliac and renal arteries simultaneously. Either a midline or transverse incision can be used, although we prefer the latter because of easier pain control postoperatively with less respiratory splinting.

The *retroperitoneal* approach, usually from the left side, also minimizes pulmonary complications as a result of easier postoperative pain control and is probably associated with less ileus than transperitoneal operations. It is optimal if multiple previous operations have created intraperitoneal adhesions. The retroperitoneal approach is also useful for inflammatory AAAs in which visceral organs may be densely adherent to the anterior aorta, and it is beneficial for patients with horseshoe kidney because extensive mobilization or division of the kidney can be avoided. A right-sided retroperitoneal approach can be used when specific anatomic situations favor this, such as a larger right iliac aneurysm or prior left retroperitoneal surgery.

(P) Although suprarenal AAAs can be approached with a transperitoneal midline incision, this method requires medial visceral rotation and is associated with an increased risk of iatrogenic splenic trauma. Thus, the left retroperitoneal approach is generally preferred. Similarly, although juxtarenal AAAs can be approached transperitoneally, the left retroperitoneal approach provides more flexibility if the AAA extends more proximally than appreciated. Usually, careful mobilization allows adequate exposure of the proxi-

ABDOMINAL AORTIC ANEURYSM

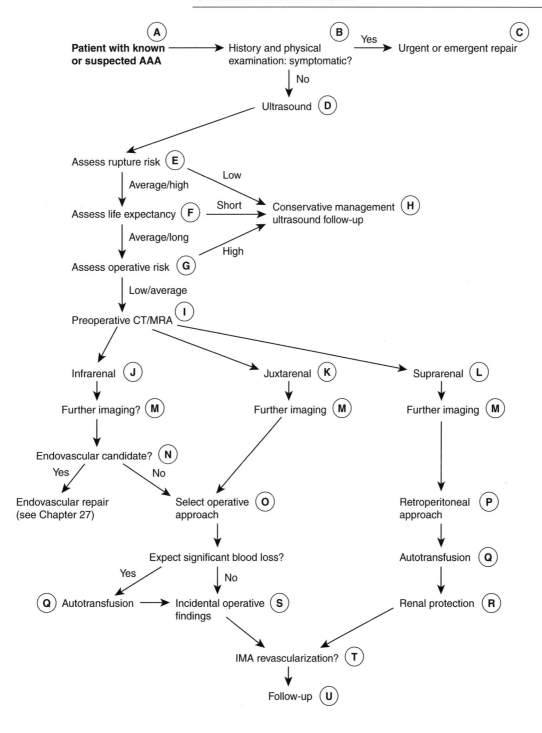

mal right renal artery and right common iliac artery through this approach, although occasionally a separate pelvic counter-incision may be needed for complete right iliac exposure.

(Q) Autotransfusion has not been cost-effective for routine infrarenal AAAs, since transfusion is frequently unnecessary.[20] It is cost-effective, however, when larger blood loss is anticipated, such as in suprarenal or juxtarenal AAA repair or in complicated infrarenal repair. If blood loss cannot be accurately predicted, costs can be minimized by initial use of only the reservoir of such devices, withholding the more expensive, disposable components until shed blood processing and autotransfusion are deemed necessary.

(R) Postoperative renal dysfunction after infrarenal AAA repair can result from renal artery atheroemboli during aortic clamping or from inadequate volume replacement. With suprarenal clamping, renal dysfunction is more likely related to renal ischemia. Prior to suprarenal clamping, we ensure adequate volume status and give IV mannitol as an oxygen free radical scavenger. If we anticipate renal ischemia longer than 15 minutes, we use iced saline solution as cold perfusion for the renal arteries.

(S) Occasionally, unexpected operative findings, such as metastatic cancer, might preclude elective AAA repair. However, preoperative CT scanning has markedly reduced the likelihood of unexpected intra-abdominal pathology. A nonobstructing colon cancer might be encountered but should generally be treated in a later procedure and should not preclude AAA repair. This is generally true for other unexpected, nonemergent intra-abdominal disease that might result in aortic graft infection if treated simultaneously with AAA repair. The simultaneous treatment of asymptomatic cholelithiasis during AAA repair is more controversial because of the smaller potential risk of graft infection compared with intestinal operations.

In general, our approach has been to avoid simultaneous cholecystectomy. Aortocaval fistula, if not diagnosed preoperatively, will be apparent by profuse venous bleeding after opening the aneurysm. The fistula should be controlled by direct pressure and repaired from within the aneurysm, with care taken not to embolize thrombotic debris or air into the venous system.

(T) Revascularization of the inferior mesenteric artery (IMA) is generally not necessary after AAA repair because of collateral flow from superior mesenteric and internal iliac artery branches. If the IMA is patent, it is initially controlled with a vascular clamp or vessel loop until aortoiliac revascularization is completed. The IMA occlusion is then released, and back-bleeding is assessed. In the presence of pulsatile back-bleeding and a normal-appearing sigmoid colon, the IMA is ligated at its orifice, with care taken to preserve collateral branches near its origin. In the presence of minimal back-bleeding and a dusky-appearing sigmoid colon without Doppler flow signals, the IMA orifice is reimplanted onto the side of the aortic graft and a localized orificial endarterectomy is performed if necessary.

Although IMA back-pressure can be measured to assess collateral flow, we have found this method cumbersome and use the scheme described earlier. IMA revascularization is more likely required if:

- The internal iliac arteries are diseased
- The internal iliac arteries are partially excluded by the aneurysm repair
- Prior colon surgery has interrupted the mesenteric collateral arteries
- Known superior mesenteric artery occlusive disease is present

(U) Long-term follow-up of patients after AAA repair is warranted to detect new aneurysms that may develop in the remaining aorta, the anastomoses, or the iliac arteries. Aneurysms large enough to warrant surgery have been seen in 14% of patients on follow-up CT scanning after 8 to 9 years.[21] Routine CT follow-up at 5 years is therefore recommended in younger patients who are more likely to survive long enough for the potential development of an additional aneurysm that would benefit from surgical repair.

REFERENCES

1. Lederle F, Johnson G, Wilson S, et al: Prevalence and associations of abdominal aortic aneurysm detected through screening. Ann Intern Med 1997;126:441–449.
2. Lederle F, Simel D: Does this patient have abdominal aortic aneurysm? (The rational clinical examination). JAMA 1999;281:77–82.
3. Jaakkola P, Hippelainen M, Farin P, et al: Interobserver variability in measuring the dimensions of the abdominal aorta: Comparison of ultrasound and computed tomography. Eur J Vasc Endovasc Surg 1996;12:230–237.
4. Cronenwett JL, Murphy TF, Zelenock GB, et al: Actuarial analysis of variables associated with rupture of small abdominal aortic aneurysms. Surgery 1985;98:472–483.
5. Reed WL, Hallett JW Jr, Damiano MA, et al: Learning from the last ultrasound: A population-based study of patients with addominal aortic aneurysm. Arch Intern Med 1997;157:2064–2068.
6. Limet R, Sakalihassan N, Albert A: Determination of the expansion rate and incidence of rupture of abdominal aortic aneurysms. J Vasc Surg 1991;14:540–548.
7. Verloes A, Sakalihasan N, Koulischer L, Limet R: Aneurysms of the abdominal aorta: Familial and genetic aspects in three hundred thirteen pedigrees. J Vasc Surg 1995;21:646–655.
8. Lindholt J, Heickendorff L, Antonsen S, et al: Natural history of abdominal aortic aneurysm with and without coexisting chronic obstructive pulmonary disease. J Vasc Surg 1998;28:226–233.
9. Vorp DA, Raghavan ML, Webster MW: Mechanical wall stress in abdominal aortic aneurysm: Influence of diameter and asymmetry. J Vasc Surg 1998;27:632–639.
10. Johnston KW: Nonruptured abdominal aortic aneurysm: Six-year follow-up results from the multicenter prospective Canadian aneurysm study. J Vasc Surg 1994;20:163–170.
11. U.S. Bureau of the Census: Statistical Abstract of the United States, 118th ed. Washington, DC, Government Printing Office, 1998.
12. Steyerberg EW, Kievit J, de Mol Van Otterloo JC, et al: Perioperative mortality of elective abdominal aortic aneurysm surgery: A clinical prediction rule based on literature and individual patient data. Arch Intern Med 1995;155:1998–2004.
13. Mangano D, Layug E, Wallace A, Tateo I: Effect of atenolol on mortality and cardiovascular morbidity after noncardiac surgery: Multicenter Study of Perioperative Ischemia Research Group [erratum appears in N Engl J Med

1997;336:1039]. N Engl J Med 1996;335:1713–1720.
14. The U.K. Small Aneurysm Trial Participants: Mortality results for randomised controlled trial of early elective surgery or ultrasonographic surveillance for small abdominal aortic aneurysms. Lancet 1998;352(9141):1649–1655.
15. Schermerhorn M, Birkmeyer J, Gould D, Cronenwett J: Cost-effectiveness of surgery for small abdominal aortic aneurysms based on data from the U.K. small aneurysm trial. J Vasc Surg 2000;31:217–226.
16. Englund R, Hudson P, Hanel K, et al: Expansion rates of small abdominal aortic aneurysms. Aust N Z J Surg 1998;68:21–24.
17. Cronenwett JL, Sargent SK, Wall MH, et al: Variables that affect the expansion rate and outcome of small abdominal aortic aneurysms. J Vasc Surg 1990;11:260–269.
18. Jean-Claude J, Reilly L, Stoney R, Messina L: Pararenal aortic aneurysms: The future of open aortic aneurysm repair. J Vasc Surg 1999; 29:902–912.
19. Campbell JJ, Bell DD, Gaspar MR: Selective use of arteriography in the assessment of aortic aneurysm repair. Ann Vasc Surg 1990;4:419–423.
20. Clagett G, Valentine R, Jackson M, et al: A randomized trial of intraoperative autotransfusion during aortic surgery. J Vasc Surg 1999;29:22–31.
21. Kalman P, Rappaport D, Merchant N, et al: The value of late computed tomographic scanning in identification of vascular abnormalities after abdominal aortic aneurysm repair. J Vasc Surg 1999;29:442–450.

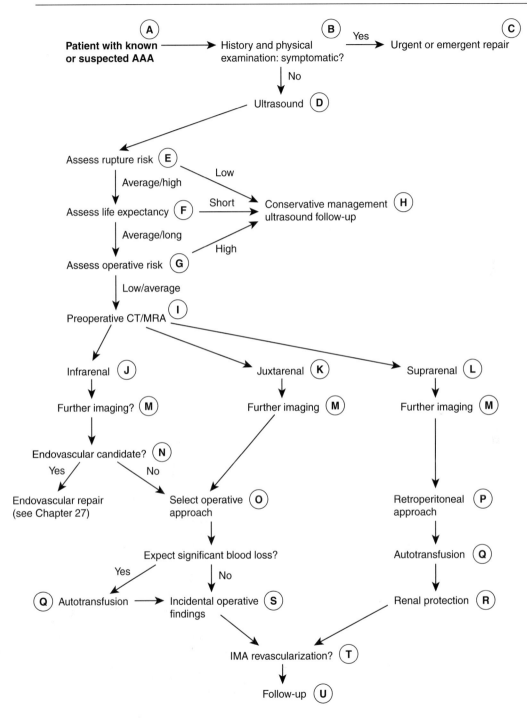

Chapter 22 Thoracoabdominal Aortic Aneurysm

RICHARD P. CAMBRIA, MD

(A) Thoracoabdominal aortic aneurysms (TAAs) involve contiguous segments of the thoracic and abdominal aorta and/or the visceral aortic segment. They are relatively uncommon, constituting 2% to 5% of the spectrum of degenerative aneurysms, and are classified according to extent of aortic involvement (Crawford classification). Features distinguishing TAAs from abdominal aortic aneurysms (AAAs) include:

1. The cause; 20% of TAAs are sequelae of chronic dissection.
2. The clinical presentation; 20% of TAAs are treated in urgent or ruptured circumstances.
3. The demographic profile; in our experience, the male-to-female sex ratio is 1:1 for TAAs but 4:1 for AAAs.
4. The scope and potential complications of surgical treatment.

In contemporary clinical series from centers of excellence, overall operative mortality ranges from 5% to 10% with similar figures for postoperative spinal cord ischemic complications.[1–6] Our experience has been that these figures are approximately halved when only elective operations are taken into account.[2]

(B) Although seemingly self-evident, accurate assessment of the size and extent of TAA—with fine-cut, contrast-enhanced computed tomography (CT) scan the primary diagnostic tool—is vital to clinical decision making. Frequent errors, usually in the direction of overestimating TAA diameter, are related to tangential (rather than perpendicular) measurements in regions of buckling or angulated aortic segments. Requirements are as follows:

1. Crawford *type I* and *II* TAAs call for resection of the entire descending thoracic aorta. *Type II* also calls for resection of the entire abdominal aorta.
2. *Type III* TAAs typically involve the lower half of the descending thoracic aorta and variable extents of the abdominal aorta.
3. *Type IV* (total abdominal aneurysm) is distinguished from a suprarenal AAA by virtue of the need to extend the proximal suture line cephalad to the celiac axis.

(C) Natural history data indicate that 6 cm is the appropriate size threshold to consider intervention for type I to III TAAs.[7, 8] Since type IV is a total abdominal aneurysm, a 5-cm threshold comparable to that for AAA is maintained for these lesions. Other mitigating factors, such as the presence of Marfan's syndrome and chronic dissection, and young age (as might be observed in a patient with aortitis as an etiologic mechanism of aneurysm), should lower the size threshold for intervention.

Similar to observations on AAA natural history, the presence of significant chronic obstructive pulmonary disease (COPD) increases the risk of TAA expansion and rupture[7]; alternatively, such antecedent pulmonary dysfunction clearly increases perioperative risk. Accordingly, the decision to recommend operation considers the variables related to the risk of TAA rupture and risk of operative repair. The latter is predicated upon knowledge of surgical detail and a thorough assessment of co-morbid conditions.

(D) Assessment of operative risk involves cardiopulmonary profiling and evaluation of renal function and overall functional capacity. We routinely perform dipyridamole-thallium scanning or an equivalent test to assess myocardial ischemic potential when surgery would entail supraceliac clamping. In addition, patients with symptoms or a history indicative of left ventricular dysfunction undergo echocardiography. Patients with an ejection fraction below 30% are poor candidates for elective operation, in view of the limitations on life expectancy and clearly increased operative mortality.

Although history alone can usually discern major pulmonary limitations, routine pulmonary function tests are performed. We have found that 24% of our patients undergoing operation had significant impairment of pulmonary reserve (FEV_1 < 50% predicted); this in turn correlates with postoperative pulmonary complications—the most frequent source of perioperative morbidity. While optimization of respiratory status preoperatively (most importantly, cessation of smoking) is desirable, this should not include introduction of corticosteroid therapy, which may precipitate TAA rupture in our experience.

Assessment of renal function and renovascular anatomy is crucial in patients being considered for TAA resection; occlusive lesions of the mesenteric and renal arteries occur in about 30% of TAA patients.[2, 3] At least partly related to macroscopic renovascular disease, we noted significant impairment of renal excretory function (creatinine ≥ 1.8 mg/day) in 15% of operated TAA patients, with such renal dysfunction correlated with operative mortality.[2, 9] We reported a relative risk of early postoperative mortality of 6.5 for patients who sustain clinically significant perioperative renal failure, and antecedent renal dysfunction is the most powerful correlate of postoperative renal failure.[2, 9]

In my view, the presence of major excretory dysfunction (creatinine ≥ 2.5 mg/dl) *without* the potential favorable impact of concomitant renovascular repair constitutes a relative contraindication to operation. Alternatively, when clinical and anatomic findings dictate the necessity for renovascular repair, the surgical imperative is thereby strengthened.

(E) In patients with prohibitive operative risk, a small TAA, advanced age, or fragility, operation should be deferred, risk factors predictive of rupture controlled, and sequential observation initiated. Three interventions—cessation of cigarette smoking, rigid control of hypertension, and institu-

THORACOABDOMINAL AORTIC ANEURYSM

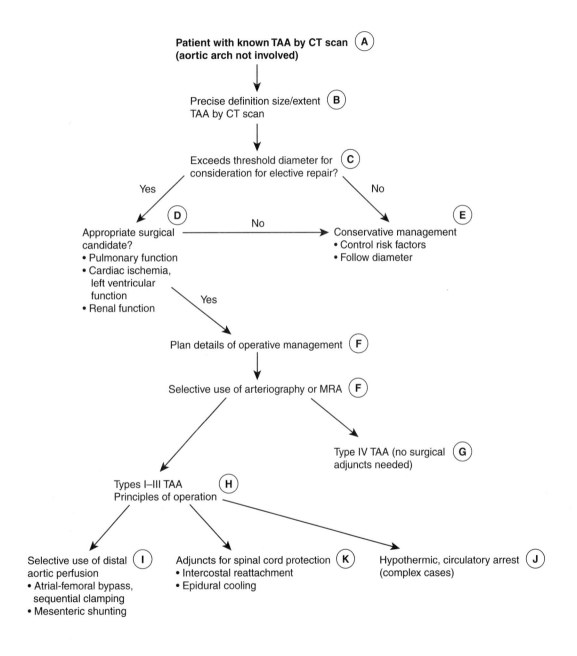

Thoracoabdominal Aortic Aneurysm (continued)

tion of β blockade irrespective of blood pressure—are mandatory in patients selected for nonoperative therapy according to the contribution of these variables to TAA expansion and rupture. Sequential observation with serial CT scanning is indicated for potential surgical candidates, as TAA expansion rate (as intuitively expected) has been implicated in the risk of rupture in contemporary natural history studies.[7, 10] Finally, if the TAA anatomy is amenable to a combined open or endovascular approach (for the thoracic component), we have applied this method for TAA repair in patients who would otherwise not be operative candidates.

(F) The next issue in planning operative management is the desirability of further imaging studies. As stated in B, the primary imaging modality for accurate assessment of TAA size and extent is the fine-cut, contrast-enhanced CT scan. Such a study also permits assessment of the following variables important to surgical planning:

1. Arch involvement.
2. Presence of dissection.
3. Presence and topography of mural thrombus in the critical (T_9-L_1) intercostal segment (i.e., prediction of patent intercostal arteries therein).
4. Patency and topographic relationships of mesenteric and renal arteries (but only inferences about origin of stenoses).
5. Kidney size and nephrograms.
6. Distal extent of the TAA and possible major iliac aneurysms.

It is, therefore, clear that the CT scan is the principal test for deciding where proximal and distal suture lines are placed.

Angiography is used selectively; it is preferred in the following circumstances:

1. Chronic dissection.
2. Patients with Marfan's syndrome.
3. Evidence of hemodynamically significant iliac disease.
4. Remaining questions about proximal extent or arch involvement.
5. Complexities of mesenteric circulation (e.g., earlier colon resection) or symptoms of mesenteric vascular insufficiency or superior mesenteric artery (SMA) compromise on other imaging studies.
6. Prior proximal or distal aortic graft placement (seen in 30% of TAA patients).[2, 3]

Magnetic resonance angiography or imaging (MRA/MRI) can often be substituted for arteriography, and we prefer this modality in patients with any degree of renal insufficiency. Furthermore, the gadolinium-enhanced nephrograms can give important information about the prospects for renal function retrieval with renovascular repair (see D). We prefer to specifically avoid contrast arteriography when:

1. The patient has significant azotemia.
2. There is a patient history or clinical evidence of atheroembolism.
3. Shaggy aortic mural thrombus is demonstrated on the CT scan in the visceral aortic segment.

(G) Separate consideration of type IV TAA is appropriate because many of the technical nuances used in types I to III TAA repair are unnecessary in the repair of type IV TAA. The overall scope of operation and attendant morbidity and mortality associated with type IV TAA repair should approach that of routine AAA repair. Type IV TAAs can be repaired with an eighth interspace thoracoabdominal incision, with limited lateral diaphragmatic incision, and with surgical dissection confined almost exclusively to below the diaphragm. Our experience indicates that at least 50% of these lesions can be repaired with a simplified beveled proximal anastomosis wherein the proximal aorta, celiac artery, SMA, and right renal arteries are reconstructed with a single suture line. Accordingly, visceral and renal cross-clamp times can typically be kept under 30 minutes and the variety of adjuncts directed against spinal cord and mesenteric ischemia (see I and K) are generally not required.

(H) On the basis of an enormous experience in more than 1500 patients, Crawford's colleagues concluded that a simplified operative approach emphasizing an expeditious operation with brief cross-clamp intervals and avoidance of perioperative hemorrhage produced the best results. Despite admirable overall results, particularly considering the long time interval over which the experience was accumulated, these investigators expressed frustration with a 16% incidence of spinal cord ischemic complications and an 18% rate of perioperative renal failure.[6] Accordingly, the evolution of the technical conduct of operation has largely been driven by efforts to minimize the major complications, in particular, spinal cord ischemia.

Controversy persists over the two fundamental approaches to operation, namely, a clamp-and-sew technique (usually with adjuncts directed toward the principal complications) versus a partial left heart bypass method (most often, left atriofemoral bypass [AFBP]) to provide distal aortic perfusion and, at least in theory, to minimize intercostal and visceral and renal ischemia.

Despite different approaches, we have documented that overall results from centers of excellence were actually quite similar (and favorable) with either technique.[2, 11] Our principal objections to the routine use of AFBP is that it (1) adds complexity, (2) necessitates heparin, (3) increases blood turnover,[3] and (4) contributes to systemic hypothermia and "saves" only the cross-clamp time required to complete the proximal anastomosis.

Because of topographic proximity of the critical (T_9-L_1) intercostal segment and the visceral aortic segment, it is generally not possible to perform separate reconstruction of these segments with a sequential clamping technique. Our technique is more properly referred to as "clamp and sew with adjuncts"—in that we utilize specific maneuvers intended to minimize the principal complications.

THORACOABDOMINAL AORTIC ANEURYSM

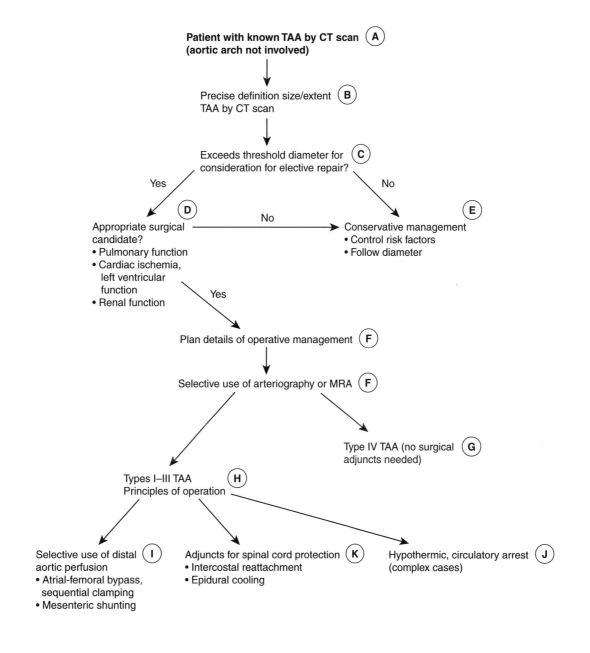

These include (1) epidural cooling for spinal cord protection,[12] (2) regional renal hypothermia,[9] and (3) in-line mesenteric shunting[13] to minimize visceral ischemia and its potential contribution to metabolic derangements and coagulopathy.

Important technical components of operation include (1) maintaining adequate exposure, (2) managing the diaphragm, (3) weighing the advisability of intercostal artery reconstruction (see J) and (4) deciding the mode of renal artery reconstruction. Although radial division of the diaphragm affords rapid and complete exposure, it results in irrevocable paralysis of the left hemidiaphragm that contributes to postoperative respiratory compromise. We agree with Engle and colleagues[14] that a phrenic nerve–sparing method of managing the diaphragm decreases respiratory morbidity. Potential loss of the right renal artery by orificial compromise in the visceral inclusion button can be prevented by interrogation of the renal artery orifice with a 12 French catheter to appreciate its orientation. A side-arm bypass has been our preferred mode of left renal artery reconstruction.

(I) Whereas some surgeons use left atriofemoral bypass or distal aortic perfusion as the preferred technique for most TAA repairs, others use this method only for type I and II TAAs. Since the principal advantage of this method is the application of a sequential clamp technique during the proximal anastomosis, we use AFBP only in circumstances of undue technical complexity in the region of the proximal aortic anastomosis. This is principally in patients with chronic dissection as the cause of TAA wherein the aorta may be dissected at the point where the proximal anastomosis is being constructed. In such cases, circumferential division and reapproximation of the aortic layers in the anastomosis are often required, resulting in the need for substantially more time than with the typical degenerative aneurysm. AFBP should be considered in certain other situations:

1. Patients with significant azotemia (in order to absolutely minimize renal ischemia).
2. The demonstration on preoperative studies of multiple patent intercostal vessels (as often seen with chronic dissection).
3. Substantial baseline cardiac disease in which the mechanical "unloading" of the left ventricle during cross-clamping may be advantageous.

(J) Occasionally, when the proximal extent of type I and II TAAs involve the transverse portion of the aortic arch, proximal clamp placement may be hazardous or impossible. Hypothermic circulatory arrest, as employed in ascending/arch reconstruction, may be necessary to achieve repair. At least one group has advocated this approach for routine repair of extensive TAAs, with the rationale that it affords maximum spinal cord protection.[15] However, the results achieved have not compared favorably with those achieved by other methods. We adhere to the majority opinion that the attendant morbidity of circulatory arrest (fluid shifts, coagulopathy) in the setting of extensive TAA resection is such that this method should be applied only when no other technical option exists. In fact, I have used this technique in only a single instance of TAA repair.

(K) Most surgeons employ spinal cord protective maneuver as a component of their overall operative approach. Such maneuvers fall into two general categories[11]:

1. Surgical or nonsurgical methods to preserve spinal cord blood supply, including widely applied techniques such as intercostal artery reconstruction[16] and cerebrospinal fluid pressure monitoring and drainage.[1,5,17]
2. So-called neuroprotective adjuncts, either some variation of hypothermic protection or a pharmacologic therapy such as endorphin-receptor blockade with naloxone.[1]

Our operative approach has been consistent with the "majority opinion" that reconstruction of intercostal arteries (when technically feasible) in the critical T_9-L_1 intercostal segment is an important adjunct to prevent cord ischemia. Our experience is consistent with that of other reports implicating the sacrifice of such arteries as correlated with cord injury.[4,12,16] Intercostal reconstruction is typically a "blind" maneuver and is probably unnecessary in many patients. However, failing some *reliable* intraoperative monitoring technique, the anatomic variables relevant to the potential for cord ischemia (size and continuity of the anterior spinal artery, potential medullary contributions of individual intercostal arteries) are generally unknown to the surgeon. Recent work with motor-evoked potential monitoring suggests that it may provide such intraoperative information.[18] Hypothermia for cord protection is firmly based on experimental data and can be a component of a variety of operative strategies.

Our preference has been to maintain systemic normothermia and to exploit the *regional* hypothermia achievable with epidural cooling for spinal cord protection. This technique has now been used in more than 200 patients over a 5-year interval. It has been most effective in reducing the immediate, devastating paraplegia from intraoperative cord ischemia, but the variables contributing to delayed deficit remain problematic and may not be influenced by operative conduct. With this technique, overall cord ischemic complications in truly elective operations have been reduced to the 3% range.[12]

REFERENCES

1. Acher CW, Wynn MM, Hoch JR, Kranner PW: Cardiac function is a risk factor for paralysis in thoracoabdominal aortic replacement. J Vasc Surg 1998;27:821–830.
2. Cambria R, Davison JK, Zannetti S, et al: Thoracoabdominal aneurysm repair: Perspectives over a decade with the clamp-and-sew technique. Ann Surg 1997;226:294–305.
3. Coselli JS, LeMaitre SA, Poli de Figueiredo L, Kirby RP: Paraplegia after thoracoabdominal aortic aneurysm repair: Is dissection a risk factor? Ann Thorac Surg 1997;63:28–36.
4. Grabitz K, Sandmann W, Stuhmeirer K, et al: The risk of ischemic spinal cord injury in patients undergoing graft replacement for thoracoabdominal aortic aneurysms. J Vasc Surg 1996;23230–240.

5. Safi H, Hess KR, Randel M, et al: Cerebrospinal fluid drainage and distal aortic perfusion: Reducing neurologic complications in repair of thoracoabdominal aortic aneurysms, type I and type II. J Vasc Surg 1996;23:223–228.
6. Svensson LG, Crawford ES, Hess KR, et al: Experience with 1509 patients undergoing thoracoabdominal aortic operations. J Vasc Surg 1993;17:357–370.
7. Juvonen T, Ergin MA, Galla JD, et al: Prospective study of the natural history of thoracic aortic aneurysms. Ann Thorac Surg 1997;63:1533–1545.
8. Perko MJ, Norgaard M, Herzog TM, et al: Unoperated aortic aneurysm: A survey of 170 patients. Ann Thorac Surg 1995;59:1204–1209.
9. Kashyap VS, Cambria RP, Davison JK, L'Italien GJ: Renal failure after thoracoabdominal aortic surgery. J Vasc Surg 1997;26:949–957.
10. Lobato AC, Puech-Leao P: Predictive factors for rupture of thoracoabdominal aortic aneurysm. J Vasc Surg 1998;27:446–453.
11. Cambria RP, Giglia J: Prevention of spinal cord ischaemic complications after thoracoabdominal aortic surgery. Eur J Vasc Endovasc Surg 1998;15:96–109.
12. Cambria RP, Davison JK, Carter C, et al: Epidural cooling for spinal cord protection during thoracoabdominal aneurysm repair: A five-year experience. J Vasc Surg 2000;31:1093–1102.
13. Cambria RP, Davison JK, Giglia JS, Gertler JP: Mesenteric shunting decreases visceral ischemic time during thoracoabdominal aneurysm repair. J Vasc Surg 1998;27:745–749.
14. Engle J, Safi HJ, Muller CC, et al: The impact of diaphragm management on prolonged ventilator support following thoracoabdominal aortic repair. J Vasc Surg 1999;29:150–156.
15. Kouchoukos N, Daily BB, Rokkas CK, et al: Hypothermic bypass and circulatory arrest for operations on the descending thoracic and thoracoabdominal aorta. Ann Thorac Surg 1995;60:67–77.
16. Safi HJ, Miller CC III, Carr C, et al: Importance of intercostal artery reattachment during thoracoabdominal aortic aneurysm repair. J Vasc Surg 1998;27:58–68.
17. Coselli JS, LeMaire SA, Koksay C, et al: Cerebrospinal fluid drainage reduces paraplegia following thoracoabdominal aortic aneurysm repair: Results of a prospective randomized trial. J Vasc Surg (in press).
18. Jacobs MJ, Meylaerts SA, de Haan P, et al: Strategies to prevent neurologic deficit based on motor-evoked potentials in types I + II thoracoabdominal aortic aneurysm repair. J Vasc Surg 1999;29:48–59.

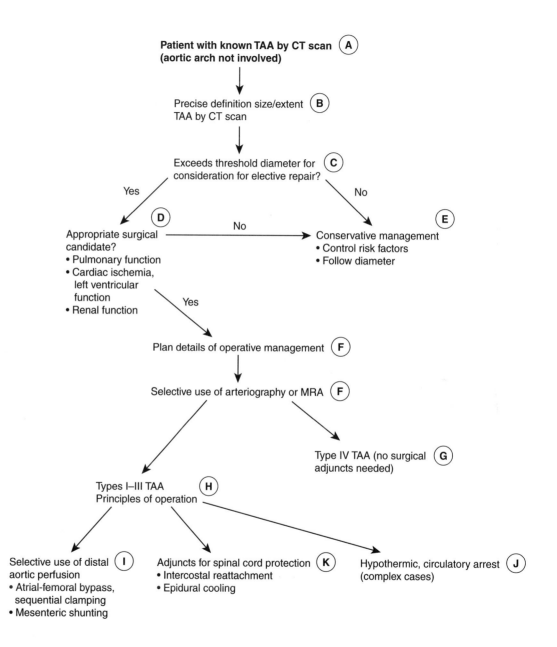

Chapter 23 Ruptured Abdominal Aortic Aneurysm

JOHN W. HALLETT, JR., MD • TODD E. RASMUSSEN, MD

(A) Nearly all patients with ruptured abdominal aortic aneurysms (AAAs) present with acute abdominal or back pain.[1-3] The pain is generally sudden in onset and is often associated with light-headedness or collapse as a result of sudden hypovolemia. If an AAA ruptures into the retroperitoneum against a ureter, pain can be referred to the ipsilateral testicle. Rarely, an AAA may rupture into the vena cava, producing an acute arteriovenous fistula manifested by acute shortness of breath, pulmonary edema, and lower limb congestion and swelling.

(B) If the patient's history and physical findings suggest a ruptured AAA, one must ascertain rapidly the presence or absence of an aortic aneurysm. This can usually be accomplished by asking the patient or family, as most patients with known AAAs are aware of their diagnosis and are undergoing periodic surveillance. Occasionally, a patient may even know the size of the AAA. Approximately 50% of patients with ruptured AAAs are unaware that they have an aneurysm until the day of rupture.[3] When possible, one should also ascertain whether there is a family history of AAA with or without rupture.

(C) If the patient is hemodynamically stable, an immediate abdominal computed tomography (CT) scan is appropriate to establish the presence or absence of an AAA and to identify any signs of rupture. Generally, such a CT scan is performed with intravenous (IV) contrast medium with or without oral contrast. Many emergency departments have the ability to perform bedside abdominal ultrasonography to determine the presence or absence of an aneurysm. Although an ultrasound study is fast, it is not accurate for delineating evidence of rupture.

(D) If the patient is hemodynamically unstable or has had a documented episode of hypotension or syncope, one must establish quickly the presence or absence of an AAA either by history, physical examination, or ultrasound scan. Once the presence of an aneurysm is established, the unstable patient should be moved expeditiously to an operating room.

(E) During the initial evaluation, one should obtain an emergent electrocardiogram (ECG) unless a patient is hemodynamically unstable with a known AAA. Sometimes acute myocardial infarction presents with epigastric pain and hypotension, suggesting a ruptured AAA. If the ECG suggests myocardial infarction, medical stabilization should be initiated. It should be kept in mind that any myocardial ischemia may be due to anemia or shock. This is an extremely difficult branch in the algorithm because an unnecessary, emergent laparotomy in a patient with an acute myocardial infarction is potentially lethal. Alternatively, delay in repair of a ruptured AAA is also lethal.

If the ECG is unremarkable and if the patient is hemodynamically stable or becomes stable after fluid resuscitation is begun, it must be decided whether an abdominal CT scan should be performed. One must weigh the risk of taking the time to obtain an abdominal CT scan when a possible ruptured AAA exists against the benefit of the additional information it offers.

(F) When an abdominal CT scan demonstrates a ruptured AAA, the patient must be moved quickly to the operating room. Delays in radiology may result in continued hemorrhage, progressive shock, and cardiac arrest.

(G) When the AAA is not ruptured but tender, the aneurysm should be considered symptomatic and should be repaired as soon as the patient is optimized medically. In such a patient, this treatment should be carried out in the intensive care unit (ICU). Inflammatory AAAs can present this way but should be detected by CT scan. If a ruptured or symptomatic AAA has been excluded, other causes for the patient's symptoms must be considered.[4-8] Common examples that may be associated with abdominal or back pain and hypotension include a perforated ulcer, acute pancreatitis, and perforated diverticulitis. Some of these conditions may require laparotomy and surgical treatment.

(H) Resuscitation should be initiated with Ringer's lactate while blood and blood products are being typed and cross-matched. If a delay of more than 15 to 20 minutes is encountered in obtaining cross-matched blood, one should initiate emergency release (type O⁻) blood transfusion in the hemodynamically unstable patient.

Generally, one should prepare 6 units of packed red blood cells (pRBCs) with a communication that more may be required. An autotransfusion system should be used if available. In addition, one should anticipate the need for fresh frozen plasma (FFP) and platelets. A general guideline is to transfuse 2 to 4 units of FFP and 6 packs of platelets for every 6 to 8 units of pRBCs required.

(I) Most would advocate proceeding directly to the operating room for resuscitation if the patient has typical pain, a pulsatile abdominal mass, and *hypotension*. If there is a lingering question, an ultrasound study of the abdomen to assess the abdominal aorta, and even a transesophageal echocardiogram to further assess cardiac function or wall motion abnormality, can be performed in the operating room.

(J) Whenever possible, the operating team should include an experienced vascular surgeon and vascular anesthesiologist. Studies have demonstrated lower operative morbidity and mortality when such an experienced team can be assembled.[9]

It is important for the operating surgeon to identify the circulating nurse in charge, the chief scrub nurse, and the anesthesia team leader and to communicate his or her operative strategy with each. In the setting of a ruptured AAA, the operating room may be hectic. The surgeon in charge must organize a coordinated effort with as much calm leadership as possible. This increases the chances that the sequence of events will proceed in a manner consistent with the surgeon's plan.

When the need for ruptured AAA repair is anticipated, the operating room personnel should be notified and asked to warm the room to 72° to 75°F. Warm ambient air is one of the best methods of minimizing core body heat loss. Hypothermia (core temperature < 35°C or 95°F) has adverse effects on outcome by causing increased levels of circulating catecholamines and by contributing to coagulopathy.[10] Perioperative normothermia is associated with reduced incidence of intraoperative cardiac events such as dysrhythmias. In addition to increasing the temperature of the operating room, one can enhance normothermia by warming IV fluids with a countercurrent warming mechanism. Such a system is especially important during infusion of multiple units of cooled blood products.

The sterile surgical preparation should extend from the patient's mid-chest to knees and to the table on both sides. A Foley catheter with a urinometer should be routine. A nasogastric tube should be placed to minimize gastric distention, vomiting, and aspiration and to facilitate identification of the esophagus if supraceliac aortic cross-clamping is necessary.

(K) The most crucial maneuver in the intraoperative management of a ruptured AAA is expeditious, uncomplicated clamping of the aorta. Extensive retroperitoneal hematoma makes the infrarenal aortic exposure problematic because of increased risk of injury to the duodenum and the left renal vein as one searches for the obscured aorta. In this situation, initial supraceliac aortic cross-clamping is safer.

A series of steps facilitates safe, expeditious exposure and clamping of the supraceliac aorta.[11] One must keep in mind that temporary, manual occlusion of the aorta at the hiatus may be achieved by one's hand, a sponge stick, a Richardson retractor, or a special T-bar aortic compressor. This step may temporarily stabilize a patient and

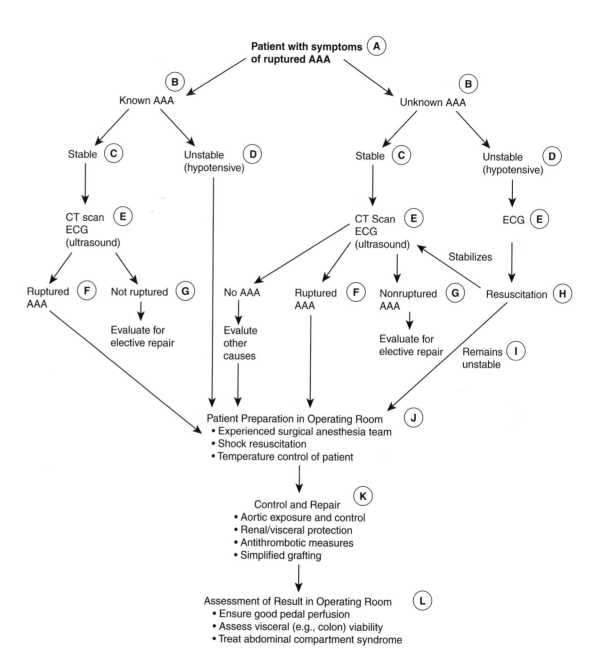

may allow time for the maneuvers to be described. The steps are as follows:

1. Identify the aorta and esophagus at the diaphragmatic hiatus. A nasogastric tube helps to identify the esophagus, which is moved to the left upper quadrant. The left lateral segment of the liver usually must be mobilized and retracted to the right; otherwise, it can be retracted cephalad.
2. Open the gastrohepatic ligament to expose the crus of the diaphragm, and palpate the aortic pulse.
3. With scissors, spread the crus of the diaphragm to expose the supraceliac aorta.
4. Complete periaortic dissection bluntly with the fingers or a suction device.
5. Use the index and middle fingers of the left hand to guide the clamp over the aorta and clamp it above the celiac artery.

After the infrarenal aorta is dissected safely from the duodenum and left renal vein, a second aortic clamp is applied below the renal arteries and the supraceliac clamp is released slowly. The supraceliac clamp is usually in position for 8 to 10 minutes while the infrarenal aortic neck is isolated and clamped. If such dissection is hazardous because of hematoma and unclear landmarks, the aneurysm can be opened and the proximal anastomosis constructed internally, as proposed by Crawford. This may be done with the aid of a balloon (e.g., Foley) catheter inflated in the aorta above the aneurysm neck, with the catheter first passed through the graft. The supraceliac clamp is then moved onto the graft before completion of the distal anastomosis.

The surgeon can achieve distal control externally before opening the aneurysm by clamping the iliac arteries or internally with balloon catheters once the aneurysm is opened.

Visceral organ hypoperfusion, especially renal shock, affects all hypotensive patients and is best minimized by rapid resuscitation and avoidance of prolonged hypotension and supraceliac aortic cross-clamping. IV mannitol (12.5 to 25 g) may be beneficial both to augment diuresis and to act as a scavenger of oxygen free radicals. Although controversial, low-dose IV dopamine infusion (2 to 3 μg/kg per minute) may enhance renal perfusion and diuresis.

The role of systemic anticoagulation with IV heparin is also debatable and should be adjusted for each individual. In patients with massive rupture and hypothermia, systemic coagulopathy may already be under way, and heparin is unlikely to be beneficial. Small doses of heparin (2500 units) may prevent distal iliofemoral arterial thrombosis, which may occur during aortic cross-clamping and can be used on an individual case basis, as can regional heparinization down each iliac artery.

To keep the operative time as brief as possible, one should simplify graft configuration and attempt to employ a tube graft whenever possible. In the setting of ruptured AAA and shock, small (<2 cm) iliac aneurysms should not be repaired. For larger iliac aneurysms, generally a bifurcated aortoiliac or aortofemoral graft is necessary. The graft material is the surgeon's choice. However, it should generally be a graft that does not require preclotting (e.g., collagen-coated or polytetrafluoroethylene).

Investigational trials of new endovascular stent grafts are nearing completion, and the role of these stents for a ruptured AAA is not known. A few successful instances in this setting have been reported. These stents may offer some benefit in the stable patient with a contained rupture, presuming expertise with this technique.

After the graft is placed, it is essential to ensure perfusion to both the feet and the bowel. Pulses may not be palpable in patients with vasoconstriction or in patients with peripheral femoropopliteal diseases. If pulses are absent, perfusion should be confirmed with a continuous wave Doppler or with calf-level pulse volume recordings.

Continuous wave Doppler examination of the colon (especially left and sigmoid) and small bowel can be performed, and sigmoidoscopy can be done in the early postoperative period if colon viability is questionable.

The concept of delayed abdominal closure in the management of ruptured AAAs has been receiving increased attention.[12] Massive retroperitoneal hematoma and edematous bowel from shock and capillary leak syndrome make primary abdominal closure difficult in many patients. A tight primary closure can lead to intra-abdominal hypertension (bladder pressure > 30 mmHg) and intra-abdominal compartment syndrome, which may compromise respiratory, renal, and intestinal recovery. One option is the use of prosthetic mesh, sewn either to the skin or fascia, allowing ample room for swelling of intra-abdominal contents in the immediate 48 to 72 postoperative hours. This closure also allows for a planned second look to examine questionably viable bowel. This approach of late abdominal closure may confer physiologic (pulmonary, renal, and gastrointestinal) and survival benefits in selected patients with ruptured AAAs.

REFERENCES

1. Hallett JW Jr: Abdominal aortic aneurysm: Natural history and treatment. Heart Dis Stroke 1992;1:303–308.
2. Johansen K, Kohler TR, Nicholls SC, et al: Ruptured abdominal aortic aneurysm: The Harborview experience. J Vasc Surg 1991;13:240–247.
3. Gloviczki P, Pairolero PC, Mucha P, et al: Ruptured abdominal aortic aneurysms: Repair should not be denied. J Vasc Surg 1992;15:851–859.
4. Dardik A, Burleyson GP, Bowman H, et al: Surgical repair of ruptured abdominal aortic aneurysms in the state of Maryland: Factors influencing mortality among 527 recent cases. J Vasc Surg 1998;28:413–420.
5. Valentine RJ, Barth MJ, Myers SI, Clagett GP: Nonvascular emergencies presenting as ruptured abdominal aortic aneurysms. Surgery 1993;113:286–289.
6. Melin MM, Gloviczki P, Cherry KJ Jr, et al: Laparotomy for presumed ruptured abdominal aortic aneurysm: Outcome of deceptive emergencies. Vasc Surg 1997;31:523–530.
7. Sullivan CA, Rohrer MJ, Cutler BS: Clinical management of the symptomatic but unruptured abdominal aortic aneurysm. J Vasc Surg 1990;11:799–803.
8. Cambria RA, Gloviczki P, Stanson AW, et al: Symptomatic

nonruptured abdominal aortic aneurysms: Are emergent operations necessary? Ann Vasc Surg 1994;8:121–126.
9. Ouriel K, Geary K, Green RM, et al: Factors determining survival after a ruptured aortic aneurysm: The hospital, the surgeon, and the patient. J Vasc Surg 1990;11:493–496.
10. Frank SM, Fleisher LA, Breslo MJ, et al: Perioperative maintenance of normothermia reduces the incidence of morbid cardiac events: A randomized clinical trial. JAMA 1997;277:1127–1134.
11. Veith FJ, Gupta S, Daly V: Technique for occluding the supraceliac aorta through the abdomen. Surg Gynecol Obstet 1990;151:427–429.
12. Oelschlager BK, Boyle EM, Johansen K, Meissner MH: Delayed abdominal closure in the management of ruptured abdominal aortic aneurysms. Am J Surg 1997; 172: 411–415.

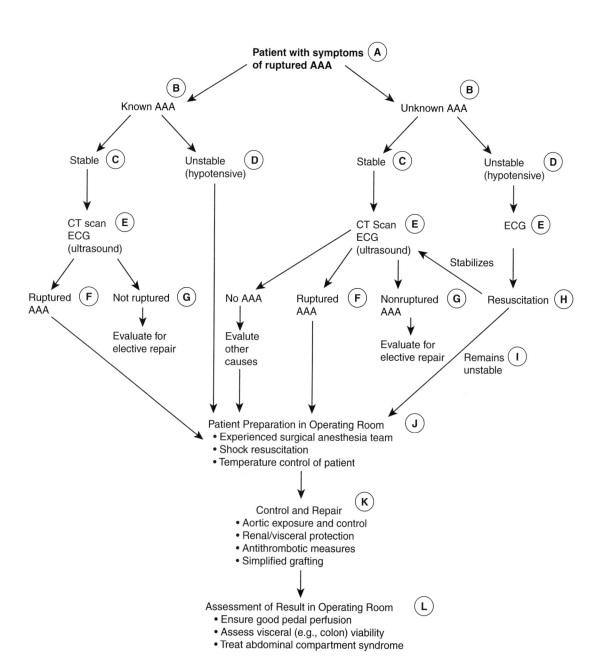

Chapter 24 Aortovenous Fistula

M. ASHRAF MANSOUR, MD

(A) Aortovenous fistulae are encountered infrequently in clinical practice. The etiologic mechanism of this abnormal arteriovenous communication may vary as follows:

Congenital fistulae are rare.[1]

Traumatic fistulae are caused by penetrating abdominal injuries (gunshot or stab wound) or by an iatrogenic injury (e.g., during lumbar laminectomy).

Spontaneous fistulae are the most frequently encountered type and constitute 90%.[2] The fistula results from erosion or rupture of an atherosclerotic infrarenal abdominal aortic aneurysm (AAA) into an adjacent venous structure. In 90% of cases, the erosion occurs at or near the aortic bifurcation, causing an *aortocaval fistula* (ACF).[2] Less commonly, fistulous communication may occur from the aorta to an iliac vein, left renal vein, or mesenteric vein.[3-7] There have been more than 200 published reports of aortocaval fistula.[8] It is estimated that aortocaval fistula is encountered in 2% to 4% of ruptured AAAs but in fewer than 2% of elective AAA repairs.[8-10]

(B) A history of AAA or some form of penetrating trauma (including disc surgery) is usually found in patients presenting with aortocaval fistula. Most AAAs are asymptomatic, but most patients with aortocaval fistula and AAAs present with symptoms.

In a review of aortocaval fistulae associated with AAAs, abdominal pain was a presenting symptom in 51% of patients, back pain in 38%. A pulsatile abdominal mass was detected on physical examination in 88% of patients.[8] Depending on the size of the fistula, symptoms of high cardiac output failure, such as dyspnea, and even lower extremity edema from increased venous pressure may be present. Patients with post-traumatic aortocaval fistula often present with a gradual onset of these symptoms some years after the initial trauma. This may obscure the diagnosis until the symptoms become severe if the significance of the initial traumatic event is not appreciated.

(C) Patients with aortocaval fistula due to AAA may also present with a frankly ruptured aneurysm (see Chapter 23). Since emergent surgery is required in these patients, the aortocaval fistula may not be detected preoperatively. Occasionally, an aortocaval fistula may present with enough pain and hypotension that AAA rupture is presumed, when the only "rupture" has been into the vena cava and not outside the vasculature.

(D) One can detect an unknown aortocaval fistula or other arteriovenous fistula in the operating room by noting a retroperitoneal thrill and pelvic congestion with a prominent, if not pulsatile, venous pattern in the pelvis. In other cases, the diagnosis may not be made until a ruptured or nonruptured AAA is opened. Uncontrolled bleeding, despite proximal and distal control, then raises this possibility. Although this is venous bleeding, the venous blood may not be obviously darker if the patient is breathing 100% oxygen. Compression at the site of bleeding controls this bleeding until the cause can be determined and until repair can proceed (see I).

(E) Physical examination reveals important clues of aortocaval fistula. An epigastric bruit or thrill is detected in 66% of these patients; other signs observed include dyspnea (39%), congestive heart failure (CHF) (38%), lower extremity edema (33%), renal insufficiency (24%), and hematuria (20%).[8] These findings increase with the size of the fistula and with the experience of the examiner.

When the fistula between the aorta and inferior vena cava (IVC) is large enough, a relatively high volume of arterial blood flow can be shunted into the central venous system, causing significant venous hypertension, which in the lower extremity leads to leg swelling. Higher venous return increases the cardiac output significantly, leading to symptoms of CHF, including dyspnea, orthopnea, and ankle swelling.

On physical examination, engorged neck veins and an S_3 gallop can be demonstrated. Microscopic or gross hematuria is reported with aortocaval fistula alone, but it may also be a sign of AAA rupture.[11] In a review of the literature, hematuria was observed in 100% of patients presenting with aorta to left renal vein fistula.[6] Patients with aortocaval fistula may also have impaired renal function that is usually reversed after successful repair of the AAA and fistula closure.[12]

(F) The most expeditious confirmatory noninvasive test is a color flow duplex ultrasound study. The examination can be performed rapidly at bedside avoiding unnecessary delay and transportation of unstable patients to the radiology suite. High-velocity turbulent flow can be detected in the adjacent vein, either the IVC or the left renal vein.[13] The presence and size of an associated AAA can also be established with ultrasound.

Computed tomography (CT) scan of the abdomen and pelvis with intravenous contrast also establishes the diagnosis.[14, 15] Additional valuable information can be gained from this study to help plan the operation. CT can evaluate the proximal and distal extent of the AAA, as well as any congenital venous anomalies that may be present, such as retroaortic left renal vein or left side IVC.

Early opacification of the IVC is a clue to the presence of an arteriovenous fistula. In patients with compromised renal function, MRI would be the test of choice to replace angiography and avoid contrast induced nephrotoxicity.[16] While much information can be gained from a color flow duplex and a CT scan with contrast, the precise location of the aortovenous fistula may not be found. Arteriography can help localize the site of the fistula, although partial venous balloon occlusion may be necessary to find the exact site because of otherwise very high flow rates.

(G) Renal vein anomalies are uncommon; however, in 20 reports of aorta to left renal vein fistula (ALRVF), the left renal vein was retroaortic in 95%.[6, 17, 18] Turbulent flow in the left renal vein suggests the presence of aorta–left renal fistula.[13] No contrast uptake on CT scan in an otherwise normal left kidney is usually seen with aorta–left renal vein fistulae.[6, 17] This less frequent form of aortovenous fistula requires repair, but these patients are usually more stable hemodynamically than those with aortocaval fistula.

The repair is described in *I*. Overall, circumaortic left renal vein is encountered in 6% of patients, whereas a retroaortic left renal vein is seen in 3.3% of patients.[17, 19] It is essential to acquire this information preoperatively in order to alert the surgeon that dissection around the neck of the aneurysm should be done with caution to avoid venous injury.

H Once the diagnosis of aortovenous fistula is confirmed, plans for expeditious repair should be made. An arterial line and pulmonary artery catheter should be placed. The hyperdynamic circulation caused by the larger arteriovenous fistula leads to an increased cardiac output that typically decreases to normal levels after the fistula is closed.[18] Close monitoring during the operation is essential. A cell saver for autotransfusion can be very helpful.[20]

I The conduct of the operation follows a standard sequence. Proximal and distal arterial control is first obtained. It is not necessary to control the IVC circumferentially; in fact, this step should be avoided, since it is difficult because of

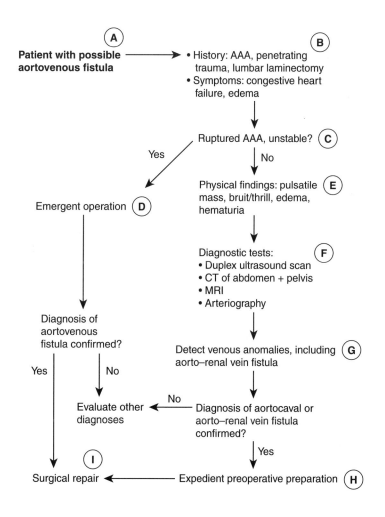

surrounding inflammation and it usually leads to venous injury. However, the surgeon should identify the points at which manual compression can be applied to limit venous bleeding. It is usually possible to palpate a significant thrill on the aorta or AAA during dissection. In several case reports, however, the fistula was found to be occluded by a large amount of thrombus in the AAA and the inferior vena cava was thrombosed.[9,10] Dislodging such a thrombus after the AAA is opened may cause significant venous bleeding or pulmonary embolism.

Alternatively, a large opening into the IVC may lead to air embolism after the AAA is opened.[9] After placing the arterial clamps and being prepared with a method for control of venous backbleeding should this opening be large, the surgeon opens the AAA, controls the venous bleeding as necessary, and identifies the location of the fistula. The anesthesiologist should be warned that if the IVC is temporarily occluded, a marked decrease in venous return will lead to a precipitous drop in blood pressure. Balloon occlusion catheters for venous control through the fistula should be available but are seldom required.[21] Primary fistula closure from within the aneurysm sac, with or without a patch, is preferred. Some authors have elected to exclude the aneurysm and to perform a bypass,[22] but this is rarely necessary. A modest defect can be closed primarily without encroachment on the lumen of the IVC. Larger defects may require patch closure to avoid narrowing the IVC.[10] If an iliac aneurysm has ruptured, it may be necessary to obtain distal control of the femoral artery in the groin.

Repair of an aortic–left renal vein fistula is more straightforward. Because the fistula is smaller, the patient is more stable and the diagnosis should be known preoperatively. The IVC does not need to be controlled. Proximal control of the aorta is important, however, and differs from the usual approach to AAAs. Knowing that there is a retroaortic left renal vein dictates that circumaortic dissection be avoided and that the proximal clamp be placed well above the level of the renal vein so as to not crowd the repair. Once control is obtained and the AAA is opened, the renal vein fistula will be found just at the posterior rim of the aortic neck. It can be repaired by simple suture closure. Even if the renal vein is somewhat narrowed by the repair, the venous drainage of the left kidney will be adequate through undisturbed and well-developed collateral veins.

Although endovascular techniques have been used to treat traumatic arteriovenous fistulae, arterial occlusive disease, and AAAs, no reports have addressed aortovenous fistulae specifically.[23-25] For a traumatic fistula and an aorta of normal size, this will likely be a successful option, since a supported endograft would exclude the venous fistula. However, for aortocaval fistulae caused by AAAs, the endograft might not prevent residual flow from lumbar arteries into the venous fistula. Further assessment is required before an endograft can be recommended.

REFERENCES

1. Kuint J, Bilik R, Heyman Z, et al: Congenital aorto-caval fistula in the newborn: A case report. J Pediatr Surg 1998;33:743–744.
2. Alexander JJ, Imbembo AL: Aorta–vena cava fistula. Surgery 1989;105:1–12.
3. Baker WH, Sharzer LA, Ehrenhaft JL: Aortocaval fistula as a complication of abdominal aortic aneurysms. Surgery 1972;72:933.
4. Brewster DC, Cambria RP, Moncure AC, et al: Aortocaval and iliac arteriovenous fistulas: Recognition and treatment. J Vasc Surg 1991;13:253.
5. Gomes MMR, Bernatz PE: Arteriovenous fistulas: A review and ten-year experience. Mayo Clin Proc 1970;45:81.
6. Mansour MA, Rutherford RB, Metcalf RK, Pearce WH: Spontaneous aorto–left renal vein fistula: The "abdominal pain, hematuria, silent left kidney" syndrome. Surgery 1991;109:101–106.
7. Vammen S, Sandermann J: Aortovenous fistula to the inferior mesenteric vein in a ruptured abdominal aortic aneurysm. Eur J Vasc Endovasc Surg 1998;15:84–85.
8. Bednarkiewicz M, Pretre R, Kalangos A, et al: Aortocaval fistula associated with abdominal aortic aneurysm: A diagnostic challenge. Ann Vasc Surg 1997;11:464–466.
9. Tsolakis JA, Papadoulas S, Kakkos K, et al: Aortocaval fistula in ruptured aneurysms. Eur J Vasc Endovasc Surg 1999;17:390–393.
10. Davis PM, Gloviczki P, Cherry KJ, et al: Aorto-caval and ilio-iliac arteriovenous fistulae: Rare and challenging problems. Am J Surg 1998;176:115–118.
11. Salo JA, Verkkala KA, Ala-Kulju KV, et al: Hematuria is an indication of rupture of an abdominal aortic aneurysm into the vena cava. J Vasc Surg 1990;12:41–44.
12. Brunkwall J, Lanne T, Bergentz SE: Acute renal impairment due to a primary aortocaval fistula is normalised after a successful operation. Eur J Vasc Endovasc Surg 1999;17:191–196.
13. Mansour MA, Russ PD, Subber SW, Pearce WH: Aorto-left renal vein fistula: Diagnosis by duplex sonography. AJR Am J Roentgenol 1989;152:1107–1108.
14. Rosenthal D, Atkins CP, Jerrius HS, et al: Diagnosis of aortocaval fistula by computed tomography. Ann Vasc Surg 1998;12:86–87.
15. Sheward SE, Spencer RR, Hinton RT, et al: Computed tomography of primary aorto-caval fistula. Comput Med Imaging Graph 1992;16:121.
16. Lupetin AR, Dash N, Contractor FM: MRI diagnosis of aortocaval fistula secondary to ruptured infrarenal abdominal aneurysm. Cardiovasc Intervent Radiol 1987;10:24–27.
17. Thompson RW, Yee LF, Natuzzi ES, Stoney RJ: Aorta–left renal vein fistula syndrome caused by rupture of a juxtarenal abdominal aortic aneurysm: Novel pathologic mechanism for a unique clinical entity. J Vasc Surg 1993;18:310–315.
18. Jabbour N, Radulescu OV, Flogiates T, Stahl W: Hemodynamics of an aorta-left renal vein fistula: A case report and a review of the literature. Crit Care Med 1993;21:1092–1095.
19. Bartle EJ, Pearce WH, Sun JH, Rutherford RB: Infrarenal venous anomalies and aortic surgery: Avoiding vascular injury. J Vasc Surg 1987;6:590–593.
20. Doty DB, Wright CB, Lamberth WC, et al: Aortocaval fistula associated with aneurysm of the abdominal aorta: Current management using autotransfusion techniques. Surgery 1978;84:250.
21. Ingoldby CJ, Case WG, Primrose JN: Aortocaval fistulas and the use of transvenous balloon tamponade. Ann R Coll Surg Engl 1990;72(5):335.
22. Woolley DS, Spence RK: Aortocaval fistula treated by aortic exclusion. J Vasc Surg 1995;22:639–642.

23. Scharrer-Pamler R, Gorich J, Orend KH, et al: Emergent endoluminal repair of delayed abdominal aortic rupture after blunt trauma. J Endovasc Surg 1998;5:134–137.
24. Semba CP, Kato N, Kee ST, et al: Acute rupture of the descending thoracic aorta: Repair with use of endovascular stent-grafts. J Vasc Interv Radiol 1997;8:337–342.
25. Desgranges P, Mialhe C, Cavillon A, et al: Endovascular repair of posttraumatic thoracic pseudoaneurysm with stent graft. AJR Am J Roentgenol 1997;169:1743–1745.
26. May J, White GH, Yu W, et al: Application of stent-graft in arteriovenous fistulae or peripheral aneurysms. In Yao JST, Pearce WH (eds): Techniques in Vascular and Endovascular Surgery. Stamford, Conn, Appleton & Lange, 1998.
27. Marin ML, Hollier LH: Endovascular grafts. Semin Vasc Surg 1999;12:64–73.
28. Zajko AB, Little AF, Steed DL, Curtiss EI: Endovascular stent-graft repair of common iliac artery to inferior vena cava fistula. J Vasc Interv Radiol 1995;6:803–806.
29. Miyata T, Ohara N, Shigematsu H, et al: Endovascular stent graft repair of aortopulmonary fistula. J Vasc Surg 1999;29:557–560.

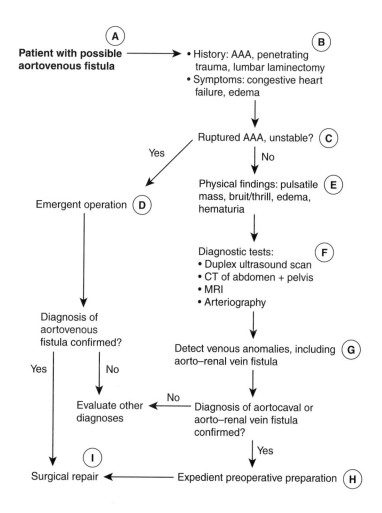

Chapter 25 Aortoenteric Fistula

SEAN P. O'BRIEN, MD • CALVIN B. ERNST, MD

(A) Secondary aortoenteric fistula (AEF) occurs in 0.4% to 2.4% of patients after aortic reconstructive procedures.[1-3] The incidence increases to 40% with primarily infected aortic grafts.[4-6] A careful history and physical examination should be the initial diagnostic step. The classic triad of symptoms includes bleeding, sepsis, and abdominal pain, although all three symptoms together present in fewer than 30% of patients. Gastrointestinal (GI) hemorrhage is the most common initial symptom, occurring in more than 80% of cases of AEF.

Events predisposing to infection, such as repair of ruptured aneurysms, increase the likelihood of fistula formation. The incidence of AEF is 1.7% after repair of ruptured aneurysms, compared with 0.7% with elective aneurysms repair and 0.2% with elective aortic occlusive disease reconstruction.[4] The interval from aortic reconstruction to the onset of hemorrhage averages 2 to 6 years after graft placement.[7-9] Signs of infection occur in 15% of patients, including fever of unknown origin; generalized malaise; purulent, draining groin wounds; or cellulitis and septicemia. Abdominal pain rarely occurs with AEF and is usually associated with aneurysm expansion in primary AEF. Secondary AEF is uniformly fatal with nonoperative treatment.[1,2,10]

(B) There is ample time to pursue a definitive diagnosis in more than 90% of patients, as the majority have an early presentation with a "herald bleed." The hemorrhage may manifest as hematemesis, hematochezia, melena, or chronic anemia.[1,11,12] Massive GI hemorrhage inevitably follows the herald bleed, with variable timing. Usually the patient remains stable after the initial herald bleed, which allows for time to conduct a deliberate but expeditious evaluation.

Any patient with an aortic graft who experiences GI bleeding should be considered to have an AEF until findings prove otherwise.[1,2,13] Although the incidence of AEF in patients with GI bleeding with a history of aortic reconstruction is only 2%, the failure to diagnose this problem is uniformly fatal because of massive exsanguinating hemorrhage. Preoperative diagnostic accuracy is only 50%, but the attempt should be made if the patient is clinically stable.[1,14,15]

(C) Fewer than 5% of initial bleeding episodes present as massive hemorrhage without antecedent bleeding.[12] The patients are unstable and continue to have GI hemorrhage. There is no time for the preoperative diagnostic tests recommended for the early herald bleed presentation, and the patient must be prepared for an immediate operation. The patient will succumb to hemorrhage unless the AEF is operatively controlled very quickly. All patients with a history of aortic surgery and GI bleeding should be considered to have an AEF until findings prove otherwise.[1,2,13]

(D) Upper GI endoscopy with visualization through the third and fourth portions of the duodenum is the first study of choice when the patient is clinically stable. Endoscopic findings suggestive of an AEF include bleeding from the duodenum wall, punctate mucosal ulcerations of the distal duodenum, and visualization of the graft, which may be found in up to one third of patients.[16,17] Other sources of hemorrhage may be identified, such as a bleeding peptic ulcer or gastric varices. Bleeding may originate from several sources, and hemorrhage should not be attributed to another cause until AEF is definitively ruled out. The endoscope may dislodge a tamponading thrombus, and the physician must therefore be prepared to proceed immediately to the operating room.[18,19]

(E) Computed tomography (CT) with contrast medium complements nondefinitive endoscopic studies and should follow a negative or indeterminate endoscopic examination. Findings suggestive of AEF include perigraft fluid or gas bubbles more than 6 weeks after aortic reconstruction, pseudoaneurysm formation around the proximal anastomosis, thickening of adjacent bowel wall, and leakage of oral contrast.[20,21] Perigraft infection and AEF cannot be differentiated with CT, but the presence of either can be detected with a high sensitivity (94%) and specificity (85%).[21] Magnetic resonance imaging (MRI) is very accurate in the diagnosis of perigraft infection and may be very helpful in identifying an AEF, but more experience with this modality is necessary to ensure a definitive diagnosis.

(F) Further diagnostic imaging can assist preoperative preparation in a patient with a known or strongly suspected AEF. Aortography helps in identifying visceral vessel patency and lower extremity circulation, and it serves as a preoperative road map. Aortography also identifies findings consistent with AEF in one third of patients, although actual contrast extravasation through the fistula is uncommon.[22,23] In many cases, spiral CT scanning with three-dimensional reconstruction can also supply this type of preoperative information.

(G) Other potentially helpful tests in AEF diagnosis not apparent with endoscopy or CT scan include indium-labeled leukocyte and red blood cell scanning, and indium-labeled immunoglobulin G. These nuclear imaging techniques have demonstrated a high sensitivity in detecting graft infection, but their role in the diagnosis of AEF remains undefined. GI contrast studies should be deferred until arteriographic procedures have been performed to avoid obscuring radiographic findings. Helpful radiographic findings include the "coiled spring" sign from contrast extravasation outlining the aortic prosthesis and duodenal irregularities from extrinsic duodenal compression or clot in the duodenum.

(H) If all findings are negative and the patient remains stable with no further bleeding, observation is a viable option. If the patient experi-

AORTOENTERIC FISTULA

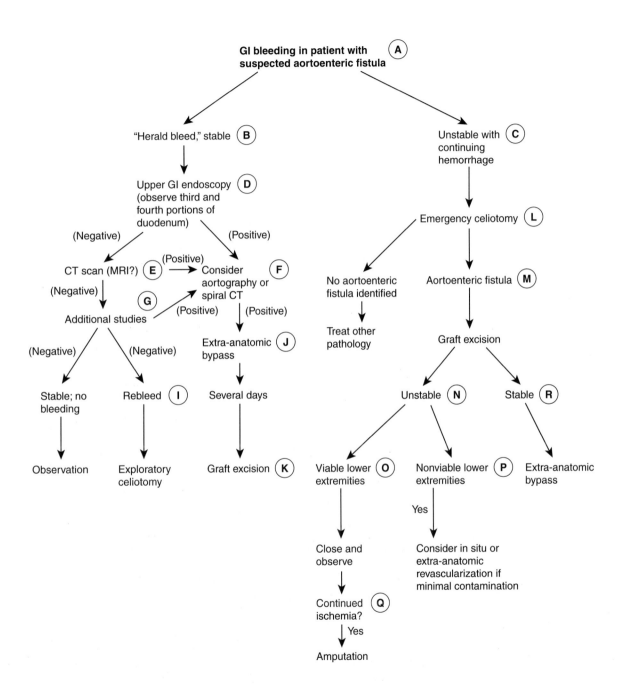

ences no further hemorrhage and the index of suspicion for an AEF is low, the patient can be closely observed in the hospital with serial hemoglobin and hematocrit studies, with a low threshold to proceed to the operating room.

(I) If all diagnostic studies are negative and rebleeding occurs, an urgent exploratory celiotomy is indicated. If left untreated, mortality is certain from either massive exsanguinating hemorrhage or overwhelming sepsis. Preoperative medical stabilization includes fluid resuscitation, blood typing and crossmatching, and broad-spectrum antibiotic coverage.

The preparatory steps for celiotomy require preparing and draping the entire abdomen, thorax, neck, upper arms, groin, and upper thighs. The abdomen is entered through a vertical midline incision, with room left for the extra-anatomic bypass tunnels along the lateral thorax and abdomen. A thorough exploration of the abdomen and retroperitoneum is essential, especially since a preoperative diagnosis has not been made. Control of the supraceliac aorta is obtained, followed by proximal and distal control of the infrarenal aorta. The bowel overlying the aortic prosthesis must be mobilized completely for accurate identification of an AEF.

(J) When the diagnosis of AEF has been established preoperatively with diagnostic testing in a clinically stable patient, a two-stage approach is the most appropriate plan. Axillobifemoral bypass is performed initially, followed by aortic graft excision, bowel repair, and aortic stump closure several days later. Occluding the limbs of the original prosthesis during the initial extra-anatomic revascularization induces graft thrombosis, thereby simplifying excision of the infected graft several days later.[24] The extra-anatomic bypass must be passed through clean tissue planes to distal arterial segments free of infection. Thus, the distal anastomosis may need to extend to the distal superficial femoral, deep femoral, or proximal popliteal arteries, depending on the extent of aortic graft infection.

(K) The staged approach, although usually satisfactory in stable patients, has several potential problems. Possible complications include (1) continued hemorrhage from the AEF before definitive repair and (2) risk of bacterial seeding of the new prosthesis. In one large series, the risk of secondary infection of the extra-anatomic bypass was only 16%.[25] In addition, the actual risk of ongoing hemorrhage from the AEF is small and patient survival is improved by the less stressful two-stage approach.[25]

The most feared complication of graft excision is aortic stump dehiscence, with stump closure in a potentially infected field precipitating this complication. Stump blowout occurs in up to one third of patients, despite varying methods of stump closure with omental flaps, muscle flaps, and serosal patches.[26, 27]

(L) An unstable patient with continuing hemorrhage requires an emergency celiotomy after immediate resuscitation and stabilization. The abdomen should be explored in the manner previously described to rule out an AEF. If the exploratory celiotomy results are negative, further evaluation of the source of GI bleeding should be continued after completion of the operation.

(M) If an AEF is discovered during the exploratory celiotomy, the first step must be control of the hemorrhage with excision of the graft. Graft excision must precede extra-anatomic bypass. The aortic stump must be securely closed with two rows of nonabsorbable suture, applied distal to the renal arteries. All nonviable aortic wall is removed, with only healthy aortic wall used for the closure. The bowel defect is closed transversely. If the extent of bowel involvement obviates primary closure, the third portion of the duodenum is oversewn. A loop of jejunum is brought up for an anastomosis to the proximal duodenum.

(N) If the patient remains clinically unstable after excision of the graft and control of the AEF, selective lower extremity revascularization is employed. The aorta is oversewn, and the abdomen is closed with careful observation of lower extremity viability. The immediate clinical condition of the lower extremities determines the next step of the algorithm.

(O) Viable lower extremities allow for a period of observation and time to stabilize the patient. Graft excision alone is more likely be tolerated if the original operation has been for aortoiliac occlusive disease with the presence of well-developed collateral vessels. The excision alone may be sufficient if an end-to-side aortic anastomosis was performed originally, if the original graft has thrombosed, or if the patient is an amputee.[14]

(P) After all incisions are closed, critical assessment of lower extremity viability is required. If the lower extremities appear nonviable or if Doppler blood flow in the groins cannot be detected, extra-anatomic revascularization becomes necessary. The surgeon constructs the bypass through clean tissue planes to avoid contaminating the new prosthesis. The patient's condition must be stable enough to tolerate the additional procedures so that life is not jeopardized. In situ graft replacement has been suggested in situations of minimal retroperitoneal contamination to obviate aortic stump blowout and to decrease the stress involved with multiple operations.[28–31]

Kieffer and coworkers reported a series of 43 patients with AEFs or infected grafts replaced with in situ cadaveric preserved allografts followed for an average of almost 14 months.[29] They reported 81% operative success and 88% initial survival, with only 25% late graft-related complications. In situ graft placement may be applied as a bridge to delayed prosthetic reconstruction. With a grossly contaminated wound, in situ aortic reconstruction is contraindicated. Aortic replacement with superficial femoropopliteal veins (SFPVs) has proved successful for aortic graft infection.[32] However, patients with graft infection as a result of an AEF constitute a special category, and under such circumstances Clagett and colleagues have not recommended SFPV reconstruction.[32]

AORTOENTERIC FISTULA

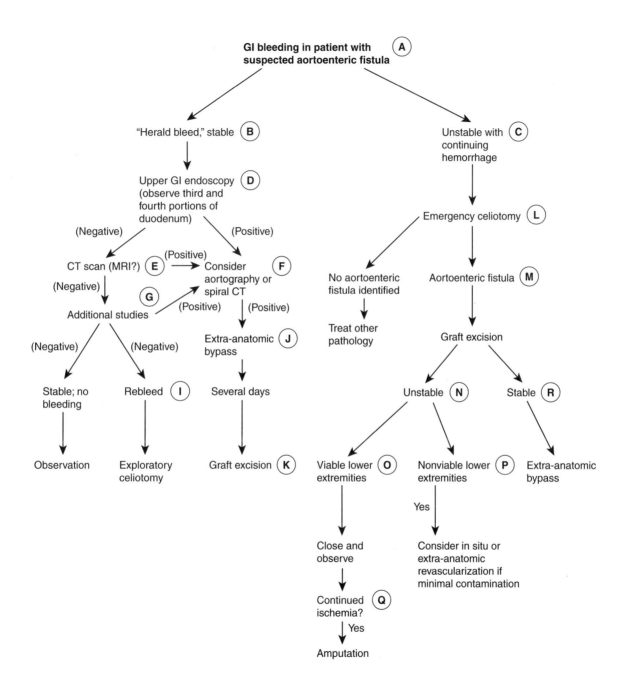

Q If the patient remains clinically unstable after graft excision and closure of the AEF, close observation without extra-anatomic or in situ bypass is indicated. The patient must be able to tolerate the secondary reconstructive procedure. If severe ischemia continues with impending gangrene and the patient's condition remains uncertain, amputation is the only alternative.

R Graft excision should be followed by extra-anatomic bypass in clinically stable patients who require emergency celiotomy upon presentation. Timing of the secondary extra-anatomic bypass depends on the patient's condition and response to celiotomy. Immediate extra-anatomic bypass after graft excision taxes the already stressed patient, reflected by the increased mortality rates among patients undergoing concomitant (37%) versus stages (13%) revascularization.[23] Delaying the axillofemoral bypass may be advisable if the extremities are not too ischemic.

REFERENCES

1. Bunt TJ: Synthetic vascular graft infections: II. Graft-enteric erosions and graft-enteric fistulas. Surgery 1983;94:1.
2. Dossa CD, Ernst CB: Aortoenteric fistula. In Greenhalgh and Hollier (eds): Emergency Vascular Surgery. London, WB Saunders, 1992, pp 18.1–18.15.
3. Schütte HE: Angiographic signs of aortic graft-enteric fistulae. Clin Radiol 1987;38:503.
4. Busuttil RN, Reese W, Baker JD, et al: Pathogenesis of aortoduodenal fistula: Experimental and clinical correlates. Surgery 1979;85:1.
5. DeWeese MS, Fry WJ: Small bowel erosion following aortic resection. JAMA 1962;179:882.
6. O'Mara CS, Williams GM, Ernst CB: Secondary aortoenteric fistula: A 20-year experience. Am J Surg 142:203, 1981.
7. Champion MC, Sullivan SN, Coles JC, et al: Aortoenteric fistula: Incidence, presentation, recognition, and management. Ann Surg 1982;195:314.
8. Ernst CB: Aortoenteric fistulas. In Haimovici H (ed): Vascular Emergencies. New York, Appleton-Century-Crofts, 1982, pp 365–385.
9. Perry MO, Melichar R, Heimbach DM: Duodenal erosion by aorto-renal Dacron graft. J Cardiovasc Surg 1977;18:77.
10. Moulton S, Adams M, Johansen K: Aortoenteric fistula: A 7-year experience. Am J Surg 1986;151:607.
11. Crawford ES, Manning LG, Kelly TF: "Redo" surgery after operations for aneurysm and occlusion of the abdominal aorta. Surgery 1977;81:41.
12. Salo J, Verkkala K, Ketonen P, et al: Graft-enteric fistulas and erosions: Complications of synthetic aortic grafting. Vasc Surg 1986; March/April, 88.
13. Ernst CB: Axillary-femoral bypass graft patency without aortofemoral pressure differential. Ann Surg 1975;181:424.
14. Higgins RSD, Steed DL, Zajko AB, et al: Computed tomographic scan confirmation of paraprosthetic enteric fistula. Am J Surg 1991;162:36.
15. Perdue GD Jr, Smith RB, Ansley JD, et al: Impending aortoenteric hemorrhage: The effect of early recognition on improved outcome. Ann Surg 192:237, 1980.
16. Campbell HC Jr, Ernst CB: Aortoenteric fistula following renal revascularization. Am Surg 1978;44:155.
17. Ng E, Copperman LR: Erosion of the small intestine with hemorrhage following aortic resection: Roentgen findings. Clin Radiol 1970;21:87.
18. O'Donnell TF Jr, Scott G, Shepard A, et al: Improvements in the diagnosis and management of aortoenteric fistulas. Am J Surg 1985;149:481,.
19. Skibba RM, Greenberger NJ, Hardin CA: Paraprosthetic-enteric fistula: Role of preoperative endoscopy. Dig Dis 1975;20:1081.
20. Gordon SL, Nicholas GG, Carter SL, et al: Aortoenteric fistula presenting as multicentric osteomyelitis. Clin Orthop 1978;131:255.
21. King RM, Sterioff S, Engen DE: Renal artery graft-to-duodenum fistula: Unusual presentation of a recurrent flank abscess. J Cardiovasc Surg 1985;26:509.
22. Reckless JPD, McColl I, Taylor GW: Aortoenteric fistulae: An uncommon complication of abdominal aortic aneurysms. Br J Surg 1972;59:458.
23. Sheil AGR, Reeve TS, Little JM, et al: Aortointestinal fistulas following operations on the abdominal aorta and iliac arteries. Br J Surg 1969;56:840.
24. Dossa CD, Pipinos II, Shepard AD, Ernst CB: Primary aortoenteric fistula: Part I. Ann Vasc Surg 1994;8:113.
25. Ott DJ, Kerr RM, Gelfand DW: Aortoduodenal fistula. Gastrointest Endosc 1978;24:296.
26. Lorimer JW, Goobie P, Rasuli P, et al: Primary aortogastric fistula: A complication of ruptured aortic aneurysm. J Cardiovasc Surg 1996;37:363.
27. Morrow C, Safi H, Beall AC Jr: Primary aortoduodenal fistula caused by *Salmonella* aortitis. J Vasc Surg 1987;6:415.
28. Garrett HE, Beall AC Jr, Jordan GL Jr, et al: Surgical considerations of massive gastrointestinal tract hemorrhage caused by aortoduodenal fistula. Am J Surg 1963;105:6.
29. Kieffer E, Bahnini A, Koskas F, et al: In-situ allograft replacement of infected infrarenal aortic prosthetic grafts: Results in forty-three patients. J Vasc Surg 1993;17:349.
30. Thomas WEG, Baird RN: Secondary aorto-enteric fistulae: Towards a more conservative approach. Br J Surg 1986;73:875.
31. Walker WE, Cooley DA, Duncan JM, et al: The management of aortoduodenal fistula by in situ replacement of the infected abdominal aortic graft. Ann Surg 1987;205:727.
32. Clagett GP, Valentine RJ, Hagino RT: Autogenous aortoiliac/femoral reconstruction from superficial femoral-popliteal veins: Feasibility and durability. J Vasc Surg 1997;25:255.

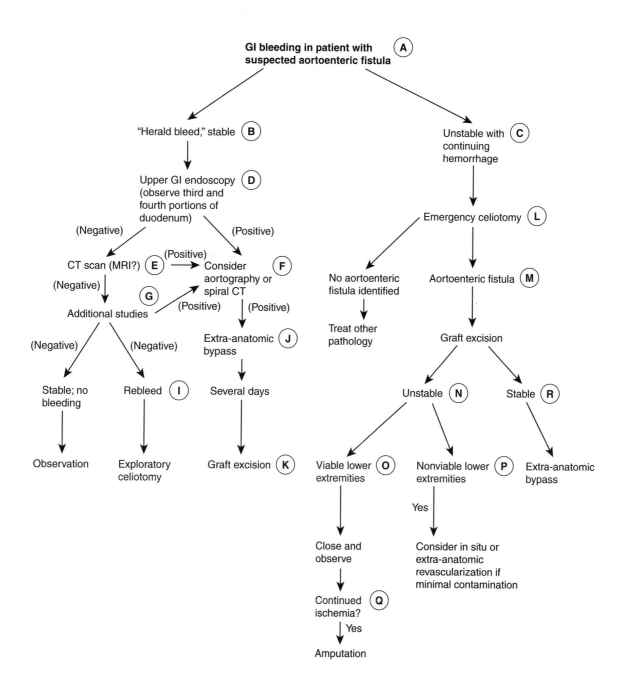

Chapter 26 Sigmoid Ischemia After Aortic Surgery

PETER G. KALMAN, MD • K. WAYNE JOHNSTON, MD

(A) Sigmoid ischemia after aortic surgery is an infrequent but potentially devastating complication. It may present with overt peritonitis, but more often the findings are more subtle and include:

- Abdominal pain (out of proportion with recent surgery)
- Abdominal distention
- Diarrhea with or without blood
- Fever of unknown origin
- Leukocytosis and thrombocytopenia
- Unexplained acidosis
- Increased fluid requirements

Unfortunately, the diagnosis is frequently entertained only after a significant delay; therefore, a high index of suspicion is essential in order to recognize this occurrence at a stage when successful management is feasible.

(B) The complication usually involves the sigmoid colon, although ischemia after abdominal aortic surgery isolated to the rectum[1] or other segments has been reported. Clinically apparent colon ischemia has been reported to occur with an incidence of 1% to 2%[2,3]; however, with routine postoperative colonoscopy, an incidence of 6% was detected.[2] This incidence was significantly reduced when aggressive efforts toward colonic and pelvic revascularization were made.[4] Although these efforts can minimize the occurrence of this complication, early recognition of clinical signs and predisposing factors can maximize the chances of avoiding mortality.

(C) The most common predisposing factor for sigmoid ischemia is ruptured aortic aneurysm repair, with an incidence as high as 35%.[5,6] It has been suggested that patients undergoing repair of an elective abdominal aortic aneurysm (AAA) are at higher risk than patients with occlusive disease because of their previous development of collateral circulation. Ernst and colleagues reported an incidence of 7.4% after aneurysm repair and 4.3% after revascularization in patients with aortoiliac occlusive disease.[2]

Other potential predisposing factors[2-4] may include:

- Mesenteric or internal iliac occlusive disease observed on the preoperative arteriogram
- Ligation of a large patent inferior mesenteric artery (IMA), particularly with coexistent superior mesenteric artery (SMA) disease
- Retrograde filling of SMA from the IMA
- A large, meandering mesenteric artery

Also to be considered are:

- Advanced age
- Interruption of collateral circulation because of prior colectomy
- Previous pelvic radiation[7]
- Failure to maintain perfusion to at least one internal iliac artery
- Perioperative hypotension

The cause is generally multifactorial, and it becomes incumbent upon the surgeon to identify patients at increased risk with clues from the preoperative arteriogram (mesenteric or internal iliac disease) or by using noninvasive intraoperative methods to detect occult colon ischemia, such as measurement of intramural colon pH,[8] photoplethysmography,[9] intravenous fluorescein,[10] and laser Doppler flowmetry.[11] Once potential or occult ischemia is suspected, it is important to emphasize operative strategies to minimize the risk.[12-14]

(D) If the patient with possible sigmoid ischemia clearly has peritonitis, laparotomy is indicated, but most surgeons would perform rigid or flexible sigmoidoscopy first to confirm the diagnosis. Surgical management of peritonitis or transmural involvement on sigmoidoscopy involves a resection of colon of questionable viability and a proximal diverting colostomy or ileostomy. A primary colon anastomosis should be avoided. The abdomen is thoroughly irrigated, and the retroperitoneum is covered with omentum if feasible. Surgical intervention should also be considered when medical management fails or when an indolent, septic course ensues.

(E) Colonoscopy generally provides the definitive diagnosis. Mild mucosal ischemia appears pale with petechial hemorrhage. With severe transmural involvement, the mucosa appears darker with areas of sloughing and ulceration. Brandt and associates[15] performed flexible lower endoscopy in 18 patients (mean, 4.4 days postoperatively) because of bloody stools (67%), hemodynamic instability or sepsis (44%), and acidosis (22%). They concluded that sigmoidoscopy reliably diagnoses colonic ischemia and can differentiate full-thickness ischemia from more superficial mucosal ischemia. They recommended laparotomy when full-thickness involvement was identified (or when peritonitis was present) and follow-up with serial endoscopy when nonconfluent mucosal ischemia was observed.

(F) In the presence of mild colon ischemia on endoscopy, medical management is indicated unless there are signs of systemic toxicity or otherwise unexplained clinical deterioration. Such indications might include peritonitis, shock, acidosis, rapidly rising white blood cell count, and deterioration of mental status.

(G) Medical management consists of maintaining nothing-by-mouth status, broad-spectrum antibiotics to cover aerobes and anaerobes, hydration, and consideration of parenteral nutrition. Additionally, other low-flow states (e.g., those due to low cardiac output) should be identified and treated, and medications known to cause mesenteric arterial vasospasm should be discontinued if possible.

(H) Long-term follow-up should include questioning of colonic function. There is the potential for stricture formation secondary to fibrosis in regions of partial-thickness involvement. A change in bowel habits should prompt investigation by colonoscopy.

REFERENCES

1. MacKay C, Murphy P, Rosenberg IL, Tait NP: Rectal infarction after abdominal aortic surgery. Br J Surg 1994;67:497–498.
2. Ernst CB, Hagihara PF, Daughtery ME, et al: Ischemic colitis incidence following abdominal aortic reconstruction: A prospective study. Surgery 1976;80:417–421.
3. Kalman PG, Johnston KW, Lipton IH: Prevention of severe intestinal ischemia following reconstruction of abdominal aorta. Can J Surg 1981;24:634–637.
4. Zelenock GB, Strodel WE, Knol JA, et al: A prospective study of clinically and endoscopically documented colonic ischemia in 100 patients undergoing aortic reconstructive surgery with aggressive colonic and direct pelvic revascularization, compared with historic controls. Surgery 1989;106:771–780.
5. Piotrowski JJ, Ripepi AJ, Yuhas JP, et al: Colonic ischemia: The Achilles heel of ruptured aortic aneurysm repair. Am Surg 1996;62:557–561.
6. Levison JA, Halpern VJ, Kline RG, et al: Perioperative predictors of colonic ischemia after ruptured abdominal aortic aneurysm. J Vasc Surg 1999;29:40–45; discussion, 45–47.
7. Israeli D, Dardik H, Wolodiger F, et al: Pelvic radiation therapy as a risk factor for ischemic colitis complicating abdominal aortic reconstruction. J Vasc Surg 1996;23:706–709.
8. Fiddian-Green RG, Amelin PM, Herrmann JB, et al: Prediction of the development of sigmoid ischemia on the day of aortic operations: Indirect measurements of intramural pH in the colon. Arch Surg 1986;121:654–660.
9. Ouriel K, Fiore WM, Geary JE: Detection of occult colonic ischemia during aortic procedures: Use of an intraoperative photoplethysmographic technique. J Vasc Surg 1988;7:5–9.
10. Bergman RT, Gloviczki P, Welch TJ, et al: The role of intravenous fluorescein in the detection of colon ischemia during aortic reconstruction. Ann Vasc Surg 1992;6:74–79.
11. Redaelli CA, Schilling MK, Carrel TP: Intraoperative assessment of intestinal viability by laser Doppler flowmetry for surgery of ruptured abdominal aortic aneurysms. World J Surg 1998;22:283–289.
12. Seeger JM, Coe DA, Kaelin LD, Flynn TC: Routine reimplantation of patent inferior mesenteric arteries limits colon infarction after aortic reconstruction. J Vasc Surg 1992;15:635–641.
13. Connolly JE, Ingegno M, Wilson SE: Preservation of the pelvic circulation during infrarenal aortic surgery. Cardiovasc Surg 1996;4:65–70.
14. Hassen-Khodja R, Pittaluga P, Le Bas P, et al: Role of direct revascularization of the internal iliac artery during aortoiliac surgery. Ann Vasc Surg 1998;12:550–556.
15. Brandt CP, Piotrowski JJ, Alexander JJ: Flexible sigmoidoscopy: A reliable determinant of colonic ischemia following ruptured abdominal aortic aneurysm. Surg Endosc 1997;11:113–115.

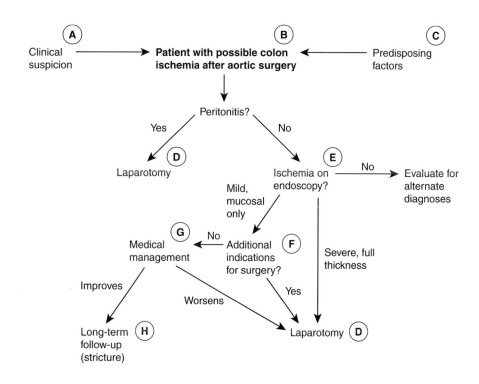

Chapter 27 Endovascular Abdominal Aortic Aneurysm Repair

MARK FILLINGER, MD

(A) Decision making for endovascular abdominal aortic aneurysm (AAA) repair begins by judging whether intervention is appropriate. In general, the indications for endovascular AAA repair are no different than those for open AAA repair. A Markov decision analysis based on quality-adjusted life-years indicates that the option of endovascular repair can alter the threshold for intervention, but the difference is important only in older, sicker patients who have appropriate anatomy for endovascular repair.[1] For younger patients in generally good health, the threshold for intervention based on AAA size is essentially the same for both types of repair.

In the past, "appropriate indications for intervention" would also have included the proviso that symptomatic or ruptured aneurysms are not appropriate for endovascular repair. However, anecdotal reports suggest that experienced surgeons from centers with experience in this intervention can perform endovascular repair in this situation with good results.[2] In the patient with a symptomatic AAA, there is generally time for an urgent computed tomography (CT) scan and adequate measurements to determine whether endovascular repair is worth pursuing. A patient with a ruptured AAA may not be stable enough to tolerate a CT scan, and consequently transfer to the operating room is mandatory. Endovascular repair in an urgent or emergent setting, however, requires a rapid evaluation while excellence in imaging accuracy and patient selection are maintained. Moreover, a large stent-graft inventory is necessary in this setting. Since it is thus expected that endovascular repair for symptomatic or ruptured AAAs would be limited to selected tertiary care centers for the near future, specific deviations for more urgent repair are not discussed further here.

Finally, the algorithm in this chapter assumes referral for consideration of AAA endografting and is geared to the near future, when improved devices, hopefully, will have proven long-term stability. Until this is achieved, this approach must be considered under trial and good-risk patients might be better served by standard open AAA repair.

(B) Most AAAs are discovered incidentally, and initial anatomic information often consists of an ultrasound study or a CT scan performed with a protocol directed toward another disease process. Evaluation of potential endovascular repair requires much more detailed anatomic information, and this is best provided by spiral CT or magnetic resonance angiography (MRA).

CT angiography (CTA) describes a protocol in which data are collected by spiral CT with a small x-ray beam thickness (thin collimation of 3 to 5 mm) over the entire volume of interest during the "arterial phase" of the contrast injection. The CT images are reformatted for view in multiple planes, including axial reformats at 2- to 3-mm intervals (specifying a small reformat interval is not the same as specifying thin collimation).[3-5] This technique provides ample anatomic information for the initial evaluation. Although more detailed image processing is needed to definitively characterize the anatomy, enough information can be provided by conventional CTA to discuss the likely options with the patient.

In general, CTA is preferred to MRA because of its greater availability, lower acquisition time, better resolution, lower technical demands for acquiring adequate images, fewer issues of claustrophobia, and lower cost. In patients with renal insufficiency, however, MRA is an excellent alternative. When MRA is used as a primary study, CT without contrast medium is recommended as an adjunctive study because MRA generally does not display calcifications that may have a significant impact on surgical decision-making.

(C) Preliminary anatomic information that can be obtained from CTA includes the following:
- Aortic neck diameter
- The native common iliac artery and external iliac artery diameter bilaterally
- The extent of aneurysm involvement
- An evaluation (with good imaging) of clinically significant occlusive disease in the visceral vessels and the iliac arteries

Although many CT scanners do not have adequate workstations or software available for accurate length measurements in three-dimensional (3-D) space, an attempt should be made to estimate the potential length for fixation and sealing at the aortic neck and both iliac attachment sites. The quality of the attachment sites can also be evaluated with preliminary imaging (i.e., the extent of calcified and noncalcified plaque at attachment sites). Most of these parameters can also be evaluated with MRA, with the notable exception of calcification (and in some cases noncalcified atheroma or thrombus).

Once adequate preliminary anatomic information is obtained, many patients can be excluded immediately from consideration for endovascular repair without the use of more sophisticated imaging studies. For example, the aortic neck or iliac diameters may require endograft sizes that are unavailable, a small iliac artery diameter may preclude femoral access, or superior mesenteric artery (SMA) occlusive disease with a large patent internal mammary artery (IMA) may make endovascular repair a poor option. In other cases, it may be obvious that the patient is not a candidate for endovascular repair because of an inadequate infrarenal aortic "neck" or the presence of a suprarenal aortic aneurysm. Adequate renal function

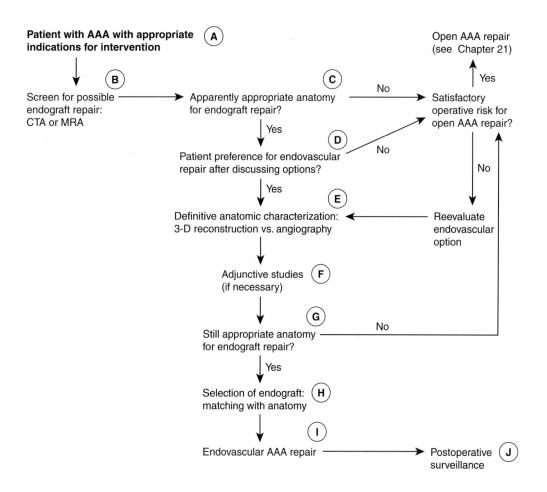

Endovascular Abdominal Aortic Aneurysm Repair
(continued)

to tolerate contrast medium has been a general requirement for endovascular repair, although this study can be performed with minimal or no iodinated contrast with the use of carbon dioxide angiography, gadolinium angiography, or intravascular ultrasound in centers with those capabilities

(D) The surgeon should consider patient preference for open versus endovascular repair before proceeding to definitive anatomic characterization. This discussion must balance the decreased morbidity, shorter hospital stay and shorter recovery time associated with endovascular repair against the lesser durability of endovascular repair, the potential for conversion to open repair, and the increased need for postoperative follow-up imaging after an endograft is placed.

At this point, it is also crucial that a patient undergoing endovascular AAA repair be willing to return for regular postoperative imaging studies because much remains unknown about endograft durability and AAA morphology changes after AAA exclusion (see J). Statistical data to help frame this discussion continue to become more reliable, but these data are extremely device-dependent and constantly changing. This discussion must balance the decreased durability of endovascular repair versus open repair, the possible need for conversion to open repair, and the need for indefinite postoperative follow-up imaging after an endograft is placed against the decreased morbidity, shorter hospital stay and recovery time that endovascular repair offers, and the increased need for postoperative follow-up imaging after an endograft is placed.

After an informed discussion of the various options, the patient may not be willing to consider endovascular repair, and thus further time and expense for definitive anatomic characterization may be avoided.

(E) If preliminary imaging indicates the patient may be a candidate for endovascular repair, it is appropriate to proceed with *definitive* anatomic characterization of the patient's anatomy. Generally, this consists of CT plus at least one other complementary study. The most commonly employed methods are spiral CT plus conventional arteriography with a graduated "marker" catheter, or spiral CT plus evaluation using 3-D reconstruction and specialized measurement software. These studies provide complementary information that must be obtained for appropriate evaluation. Definitive anatomic evaluation includes a more accurate evaluation of occlusive disease and more precise measurements of arterial diameters and lengths.

If the preliminary evaluation used conventional CT or a spiral CT with a suboptimal protocol, the first step would probably be to obtain a spiral CT based on a protocol optimized for AAA imaging. This allows reconstruction or reformatting at very small intervals in multiple planes, providing information that is not available from conventional CT.[4] Information regarding arterial occlusive disease and the extent of aneurysmal disease is also much more accurate with spiral CT.[3] Measurements using calipers and a small hard copy image are not optimal. It is preferable to minimize measurement error by performing electronic measurements on a CT workstation. Spiral CT images using collimation of 3 to 5 mm, reformat intervals of 2 mm, and reformats perpendicular to the vessel are preferable for measurements of diameter, and they also provide more accurate measurements of length.[5]

Evaluation of occlusive disease is crucial for many reasons. The presence of significant SMA occlusive disease and a patent IMA is a relative contraindication to endovascular repair because it would exclude perfusion of the IMA origin. Internal iliac artery occlusive disease may be important because occlusion of one internal iliac artery is generally well tolerated if the other internal iliac artery is relatively free of disease. Occlusion of both internal iliac arteries, however, increases the risk of severe buttock claudication, colon ischemia, and perhaps even the risk of paraplegia.

Conventional CT is not adequate for evaluation of occlusive disease.[3,5] Spiral CT and/or CT angiography is relatively accurate for the evaluation of mesenteric, renal, and iliac occlusive disease but still comes with problems regarding accuracy of length measurements.[5]

Conventional arteriography is excellent for the evaluation of arterial occlusive disease (mesenteric, renal, iliac) and is also reasonably good for length measurements, including estimated graft length. Notably, the marker catheter tends to take a shorter path than the endograft because the catheter has a much smaller diameter. More important, conventional arteriography is relatively poor for evaluating the extent of aneurysmal disease and results can be misleading with regard to the extent of occlusive disease if multiple views are not obtained. Because the adventitia carries the structural load for the stent-graft, endograft diameter sizing should be based on measurements from adventitia to adventitia rather than the luminal diameter, as seen on angiography. Thus, the use of spiral CT and conventional arteriography with a marker catheter are both required to provide all of the information necessary to plan endovascular AAA repair.

Spiral CT plus 3-D reconstruction and specialized measurement software has emerged as an alternative to spiral CT plus arteriography with a marker catheter. This method incorporates the preferred elements of CT angiography, CT reformats perpendicular to the vessel, electronic measurements of highly magnified CT images, and 3-D reconstructions (preferably multiobject reconstructions). Key diameter and length measurement problems are eliminated by combining these preferred techniques, and the cost and morbidity of an invasive test are eliminated.[5-7] In cases of renal insufficiency, one can also perform 3-D reconstruction from MRA using similar software. Creation of multiobject 3-D reconstructions does have two disadvantages:

1. This method is time-consuming, even for experienced technicians.
2. Physician time and training are required in order to provide an accurate and detailed analysis of hundreds of spiral CT reformat images and the 3-D reconstruction itself.

Nonetheless, this method can reveal anatomic abnormalities and potential problems for endovascular repair that may not be revealed by conventional spiral CT and arteriography.[3-7] It appears that CT plus 3-D reconstruction and specialized measurement software will emerge as the method of choice as a result of equal or greater measurement accuracy, elimination of an invasive modality, and better patient selection.

(F) Adjunctive studies regarding patient anatomy are generally not necessary and are avoided following definitive anatomic characterization (see E), but duplex ultrasound surveillance may be useful for evaluation of iliac, renal, or mesenteric occlusive disease. Adjunctive studies with duplex scan, captopril renal scan, or MRA are similar for open or endovascular repair and are not discussed further here.

Therapeutic maneuvers for renal and iliac artery occlusive disease are generally avoided preoperatively. Renal stents often protrude into the aortic lumen and may complicate delivery or precise placement of the aortic stent-graft. Iliac angioplasty creates a dissection as part of the process, and this may cause "snowplowing" of the large endograft delivery device. Iliac stents can become extremely deformed and also complicate passage of these large delivery devices. Thus, iliac disease is treated by avoidance, bypass using iliac-femoral conduits, or the "Dotter" technique at the time of device delivery. Endovascular treatment of renal disease is generally avoided or treated after the aneurysm is excluded by the aortic stent-graft.

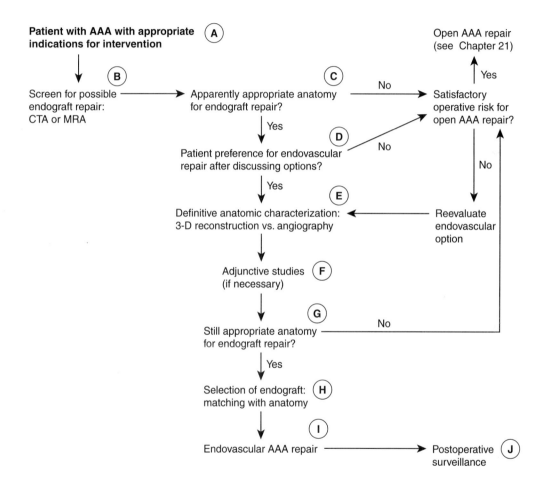

Endovascular Abdominal Aortic Aneurysm Repair
(continued)

G It is important to follow manufacturer specifications regarding appropriate candidates for endovascular AAA repair with each particular device. In general, the following are required:

1. An infrarenal aortic neck length of 15 mm from the lowest renal artery to the aneurysm sac.
2. An aortic neck-body angle that is 60 degrees or less.
3. Aortic bifurcation diameter adequate to accommodate the limbs of a bifurcated endograft without undue compression of the limbs.
4. Iliac seal zones or attachment sites 15 mm or more in length.
5. Absence of significant plaque that might cause problems in the attachment or "seal" zones.
6. An absence of external iliac artery diameter problems that might prevent access of the delivery devices (including absence of severe occlusive disease or tortuosity).
7. Availability of a device of adequate size so that appropriate "oversizing," sealing, and attachment are likely.

Conversion to open repair as a result of failed endovascular repair is associated with a significantly increased mortality rate (11% mortality for acute conversion, 7% for late conversion),[8] which is greater than the mortality for elective open repair in most cases. Thus, attempting endovascular repair under unfavorable anatomic conditions is to be discouraged.

H Each endograft system has differences in stent-graft or delivery device design that predispose the system to certain types of anatomy. Many of the differences have an obvious impact on matching the endograft with a patient's anatomy, such as the range of available aortic stent-graft "trunk" diameters, the range of iliac limb diameters, and the available lengths. The impact of the profile (diameter) of the main delivery device and contralateral limb device is also relatively obvious.

Other important differences in flexibility, pushability, and "torqueability" for the various delivery devices, however, can affect the question of whether device delivery would be possible in a particular patient. Patient selection can also be affected by differences in the necessary degree of endograft oversizing, recommended characteristics of the vessel at the attachment sites, and the required length of the attachment sites. All of these criteria must be reviewed carefully, with specific reference to the endograft manufacturer specifications.

A learning curve is associated with endovascular repair, and the available data suggest a learning curve of approximately 30 endovascular repairs.[9, 10] Once experience is obtained with one device for endovascular AAA repair, learning another device may be easier. Nonetheless, appropriate training regarding device-specific aspects of patient selection, device delivery, and follow-up imaging should be obtained from an experienced user before using any new device.

I A description of specific techniques regarding endovascular AAA repair is beyond the scope of this text, but some generalities apply to endovascular AAA repair with all types of endograft. General, continuous spinal, epidural, or even local anesthesia may be used. Preparing and draping the patient should be performed in anticipation of a possible need for open repair.

Since the need for emergent conversion to open repair is always possible, the environment should be one in which open repair can be safely and quickly performed. Although uncommon, infection of a prosthetic graft in the aortic position is associated with a mortality rate of 20% to 50%. Thus, sterile technique is crucial.

Ideally, the environment includes the same standards of sterility required for an operating room along with excellent imaging capabilities.[11] In general, a preprocedure arteriogram is obtained on the operating room table as a "road map" for delivery of the device. After the procedure is completed, arteriography is obtained with delayed imaging adequate for the detection of late or slow-filling endoleaks, so images must also be excellent. Generally, a state-of-the-art portable C-arm and a carbon fiber table are adequate for this task.[11] The surgeon should correct attachment site endoleaks or modular stent-graft junction endoleaks before leaving the operating room or endovascular suite, if possible. Problems may ultimately be associated with aneurysm growth and rupture if left untreated.

J Because the long-term durability of endovascular repair remains a matter of concern, postoperative follow-up is mandatory. Unfortunately, no single imaging modality is optimal for postoperative surveillance, and a combination of modalities is thus needed.[12]

Current recommendations are for a clinic visit with history and physical examination, ankle-brachial indices, abdominal x-rays (three or four views), and contrast-enhanced CT with or without 3-D reconstruction. Abdominal x-rays are used primarily to evaluate the stent framework for deformation and fractures.

CT is used primarily to evaluate stent-graft migration, fixation, or apposition to the vessel wall, endoleak, branch vessels (renal, mesenteric and internal iliac arteries), and aneurysm size (diameter and possibly volume).

Duplex scanning employing color Doppler ultrasound or power Doppler can also be used to detect aneurysm size and potential endoleak, but accuracy tends to be on the order of 85%.[12, 13] Contrast enhancement may increase accuracy, but duplex scans are highly operator-dependent, are subject to difficulties with bowel gas or obesity, and are less accurate for determining migration and stent-vessel apposition. In addition, ultrasonography is generally less accurate than CT for measurement of diameter.[12, 14]

Contrast-enhanced CT should include the "arterial phase" at a minimum, with the addition of a noncontrast phase if extensive calcifications (and potential artifact) are present.[12] If the aneurysm enlarges at any time point or shows no signs of shrinkage within 1 year, evaluation should be directed toward finding a potential endoleak or attachment site problem. If there is no evidence of endoleak on arterial phase CT, a "venous phase" CT scan (a repeat scan 2 to 5 minutes following contrast injection) is warranted.[12, 15] If no endoleak is detected using the delayed venous phase technique, consideration should be given to transmission of pressure without actual flow of contrast.[15, 16] Three-dimensional reconstruction of CT or MRA data (including special reformats and magnified views) can be useful for detecting the source of an endoleak, for evaluating appropriate fixation, and for detecting changes in shape and volume. At present, aneurysm enlargement seems to be detected more accurately by changes in volume than by changes in diameter.[12, 17]

Follow-up is recommended at 1, 6, and 12 months postoperatively and thereafter at 6-month or 12-month intervals. More frequent monitoring or intervention is generally required when endoleak is detected or when the aneurysm is not clearly shrinking.

Repair is recommended for all type I (attachment site) endoleaks, type III (graft material defects or modular junction separation) endoleaks, all new (secondary) endoleaks, and any endoleak with signs of aneurysm expansion. Intervention is also necessary for cases of stent-graft deformation that lead to occlusions. Correction of endoleak and occlusion may be via endovascular or open repair, but in most cases endovascular repair is possible.[18] Because a number of problems can occur more than 1 year after endovascular AAA repair,[18] the physician should emphasize the importance of indefinite, long-term follow-up even if the endograft is functioning perfectly after 1 year.

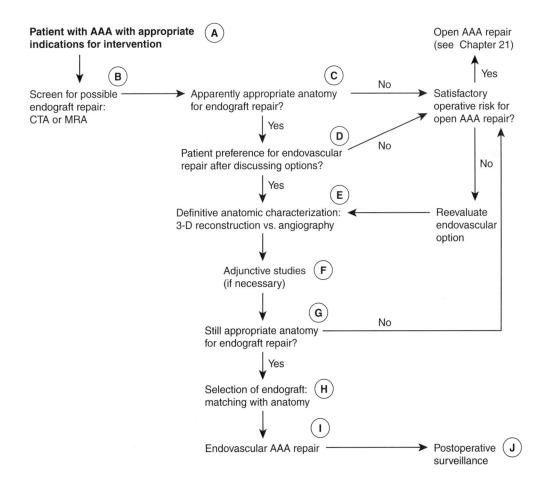

Endovascular Abdominal Aortic Aneurysm Repair
(continued)

REFERENCES

1. Finlayson SR, Birkmeyer JD, Fillinger MF, Cronenwett JL: Should endovascular surgery lower the threshold for repair of abdominal aortic aneurysms? J Vasc Surg 1999;29:973–985.
2. Ohki T, Veith FJ, Sanchez LA, et al: Endovascular graft repair of ruptured aortoiliac aneurysms. J Am Coll Surg 1999;189:102–112; discussion, 112–113.
3. Fillinger MF: Utility of spiral CT in the preoperative evaluation of patients with abdominal aortic aneurysms. In Whittemore AD (ed): Advances In Vascular Surgery. St. Louis, Mosby–Year Book, 1997, pp 115–131.
4. Fillinger MF: Computed tomography and three-dimensional reconstruction in evaluation of vascular disease. In Rutherford RB (ed): Vascular Surgery, 5th ed. Philadelphia, WB Saunders, 2000, pp 230–269.
5. Fillinger MF. New imaging techniques in endovascular surgery. Surg Clin North Am 1999;79:451–475.
6. Broeders I, Blankensteijn J, Olree M, et al: Preoperative sizing of grafts for transfemoral endovascular aneurysm managment: A prospective comparative study of spiral CT angiography, arteriography, and conventional CT imaging. J Endovasc Surg 1997;4:252–261.
7. Beebe HG, Jackson T, Pigott JP: Aortic aneurysm morphology for planning endovascular aortic grafts: Limitations of conventional imaging methods. J Endovasc Surg 1995;2:139–149.
8. Jacobowitz GR, Lee AM, Riles TS: Immediate and late explantation of endovascular aortic grafts: The endovascular technologies experience. J Vasc Surg 1999;29:309–316.
9. Cuypers P, Buth J, Harris PL, et al: Realistic expectations for patients with stent-graft treatment of abdominal aortic aneurysms: Results of a European multicentre registry. Eur J Vasc Endovasc Surg 1999;17:507–516.
10. Harris PL: The highs and lows of endovascular aneurysm repair: The first two years of the Eurostar Registry. Ann R Coll Surg Engl 1999;81:161–165.
11. Fillinger MF, Weaver JB: Imaging equipment and techniques for optimal intraoperative imaging during endovascular interventions. Semin Vasc Surg 1999;12:315–326.
12. Fillinger MF: Postoperative imaging after endovascular AAA repair. Semin Vasc Surg 1999;12:327–338.
13. Sato DT, Goff CD, Gregory RT, et al: Endoleak after aortic stent graft repair: Diagnosis by color duplex ultrasound scan versus computed tomography scan. J Vasc Surg 1998;28:657–663.
14. Thomas PR, Shaw JC, Ashton HA, et al: Accuracy of ultrasound in a screening programme for abdominal aortic aneurysms. J Med Screen 1994;1:3–6.
15. Schurink GW, Aarts NJ, Wilde J, et al: Endoleakage after stent-graft treatment of abdominal aneurysm: Implications on pressure and imaging—an in vitro study. J Vasc Surg 1998;28:234–241.
16. Marty B, Sanchez LA, Ohki T, et al: Endoleak after endovascular graft repair of experimental aortic aneurysms: Does coil embolization with angiographic "seal" lower intraaneurysmal pressure? J Vasc Surg 1998;27:454–461; discussion, 462.
17. Balm R, Kaatee R, Blankensteijn JD, et al: CT-angiography of abdominal aortic aneurysms after transfemoral endovascular aneurysm management. Eur J Vasc Endovasc Surg 1996;12:182–188.
18. Umscheid T, Stelter WJ: Time-related alterations in shape, position, and structure of self-expanding, modular aortic stent-grafts: A 4-year single-center follow-up. J Endovasc Surg 1999;6:17–32.

Chapter 28 begins on the following page

Chapter 28 Aortic Dissection

ANTHONY W. DiSCIPIO, MD • LARS V. SVENSSON, MD

A Aortic dissection is the most common aortic emergency, occurring twice as often as ruptured abdominal aortic aneurysms (AAAs). Descending dissections affect older patients with degenerative, atherosclerotic disease, whereas ascending dissections are more common in younger patients, especially those with Marfan's syndrome. However, any age group can be affected, including women during pregnancy. Mortality of untreated ascending aortic dissection is high, greater than 1% per hour. Unfortunately, this diagnosis is often overlooked, such that the condition remains undiagnosed in 30% to 50% of patients who present with chest pain related to aortic dissection before death.[1-3]

B Approximately 75% of patients with aortic dissection present with sudden-onset, sharp, tearing pain. For ascending aortic dissections, this is usually in the anterior chest, with pain radiating into the neck and arms, followed by interscapular pain with progression down into the back and sometimes into the legs. With descending aortic dissections, the pain more typically begins in the interscapular area, then radiates down the back and down into the legs. Thus, pain from dissections is described by "three Ss": sudden, sharp, and shifting.

The other 25% of patients present with ischemic symptoms from aortic branches obliterated by the dissection, including stroke, anuria, mesenteric ischemia, and extremity ischemia. Patients are frequently hypertensive on presentation. However, shock may result from rupture, tamponade, or acute aortic regurgitation. Physical examination should include a detailed pulse examination, with extremity blood pressure measurements, neurologic evaluation, and assessment of urine output.

C Hypertensive patients with suspected dissection require emergent blood pressure control. Intravenous β blockers should be used to reduce both heart rate and cardiac contractility before sodium nitroprusside is added for blood pressure control to avoid increased contractility associated with nitroprusside alone.

D The diagnosis of aortic dissection can be confirmed by several imaging modalities. The preferred initial technique is either spiral computed tomography (CT) scanning or transesophageal echocardiogram, depending on which is the first available at an institution.[4,5] Spiral CT is accurate and can image the visceral and iliac arteries. Transesophageal echocardiography is also accurate and is useful for evaluation of aortic valve regurgitation or cardiac tamponade but not visceral arteries. These tests accurately delineate ascending from descending aortic dissection, which determines immediate management. Arteriography is also accurate in the diagnosis of dissection but is more time-consuming. It is now generally reserved for situations in which evaluation of aortic branch flow is important. Magnetic resonance imaging (MRI) is generally too time-consuming for the acute setting.

E Aortic dissection can be confused with acute myocardial infarction, pulmonary embolism, acute abdominal processes, peripheral embolism, ruptured abdominal aneurysm, and a variety of other acute illnesses. If imaging does not disclose a dissection, careful evaluation is mandatory. If no cause is found, subsequent imaging with a different modality should be considered to further exclude dissection.

F For ascending aortic dissections, immediate operation is required; hypothermic arrest, an open distal anastomosis, transection of the aorta, and often right subclavian artery perfusion are used.[1,3] When surgical treatment is necessary, descending aortic dissections are approached via a left thoracotomy. The aortic segment containing the origin of the dissection just distal to the left subclavian artery is replaced with a prosthetic graft. The new aortic graft should be as short as possible, without leaving an aneurysm, to reduce risk of spinal cord ischemia. Similarly, whenever feasible, the operation should be conducted with distal perfusion, mild hypothermia, cerebrospinal fluid drainage (with or without intrathecal papaverine), and reperfusion of the true lumen.[1,3,6,7]

G It is important to ascertain whether rupture of descending aortic dissections has occurred; if so, emergent surgery rather than the preferred conservative treatment is necessary.[8] Diagnosis of rupture is made by CT scan showing contrast extravasation or blood in the pleural space. Unfortunately, early surgery for acute descending dissection is associated with a high (10% to 20%) mortality rate.[1,9]

H Patients with a nonruptured descending aortic dissection are managed medically in an intensive care unit with rigorous blood pressure control. In this circumstance, recurrent pain may indicate further expansion or possible rupture. Repeated CT scanning may be helpful, but persistent pain despite hypertension control is generally considered an indication for urgent surgical repair to prevent impending rupture.[6]

I Visceral, renal, or extremity ischemia may be treated nonoperatively with stents or stent grafts or with balloon septostomy.[10] In our experience, this has been a very useful technique to avoid the need for surgery to reverse ischemia. If ischemia is noted before surgery in patients who require proximal ascending/arch repairs for dissection, we have found these endovascular techniques useful before aortic repair.

J If endovascular techniques do not reverse visceral, renal, or leg ischemia, surgical revascularization is indicated if the patient can tolerate such a procedure. The Stanford group has recommended direct repair of the aortic dissection, if not already done, to obliterate the false lumen and to restore true lumen flow.[11]

The alternative approach is infrarenal aortic

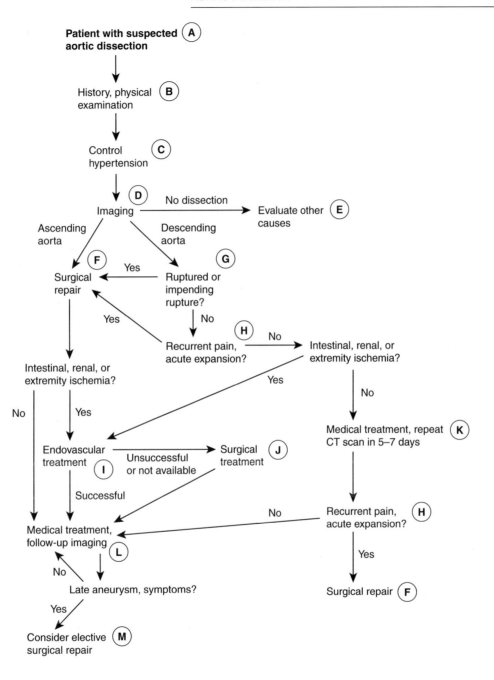

graft placement with surgical septostomy to create a proximal reentry into the false lumen, which may correct renal or visceral ischemia, and allows closure of the distal false lumen to restore lower extremity blood flow. If this attempt is unsuccessful, direct renal or visceral revascularization is possible, as is direct excision of the suprarenal septum with orificial endarterectomy as required.[12,13] Unfortunately, there is a high mortality related to the need for such extensive surgical intervention and the associated visceral and renal ischemic interval. If only the legs are ischemic, femorofemoral or axillobifemoral bypass provides a less invasive option if the ischemia cannot be treated with angioplasty or stent placement.

(K) Blood pressure should be reduced to 100 to 110 mmHg systolic and the heart rate to below 60 beats per minute using β blockers and antihypertensive therapy (see B). With lowering of blood pressure, pain should be reduced, if not abolished. Addition of morphine further helps control pain. Persisting or progressive pain may indicate extension of dissection, rupture, or visceral or extremity ischemia. As aggressive medical therapy is instituted, it is important to watch for the development of ischemia, manifested by low urine output or poor tissue perfusion. Even in stable patients without pain or ischemia, it is important to repeat a CT scan in 5 to 7 days because the descending aortic diameter may increase substantially. If the thoracic aorta expands to more than 6 cm in diameter, surgery should be considered in the subacute setting.

(L) Careful long-term follow-up with repeated CT scan or MRI is important for patients who are treated medically. Generally, if patients initially have an aorta of less than 4 cm in diameter, aortic dilatation does progress rapidly unless the patient has Marfan's syndrome or uncontrolled hypertension. Uncontrolled high blood pressure appears to be the most important risk factor for aneurysm development other than the initial diameter of the aorta. In our patients, late rupture of chronic dissections treated medically occurred in approximately one third.[7] Thus, periodic follow-up, increasing from 6- to 12-month intervals, is appropriate.

(M) Indications for surgical repair of a descending thoracic or a thoracoabdominal aneurysm following dissection include symptoms (pain) of acute expansion or enlargement larger than 6 cm in diameter. Rupture risk must be balanced against operative risk, including paraplegia, in these often high-risk elderly patients. Decision making is often difficult and must be individualized.

When elective aneurysm repair is being planned, it is critical to evaluate the aortic arch to determine the best operative approach. If the aortic arch at the left subclavian artery shows aneurysmal dilatation, calcification, or atheroma, or if the patient is undergoing a reoperation, deep hypothermic circulatory arrest is usually recommended to avoid the necessity of a proximal aortic clamp.

If only the aorta distal to the mid-descending portion needs to be repaired, for example, for a penetrating ulcer with associated dissection, the evidence for the use of distal perfusion for spinal cord protection is not as strong, in contrast to the clamp-and-sew repair technique. In this segment, however, the reattachment of intercostal arteries below T7 to and including L2 is important, particularly for thoracoabdominal aneurysm repairs.

If the proximal descending aorta is involved, distal perfusion with adjunctive measures appear to be useful in preventing spinal cord and visceral organ damage. If such a patient requires a thoracoabdominal aneurysm repair, usually because the aorta is larger than 3.5 cm at the diaphragmatic hiatus, distal perfusion with hypothermia, cerebrospinal fluid drainage, and reattachment of the intercostal arteries between T7 and L2 is important in the prevention of spinal cord neurologic injury (see Chapter 22).

REFERENCES

1. Svensson LG, Crawford ES: Cardiovascular and Vascular Disease of the Aorta. Philadelphia, WB Saunders, 1997.
2. Kouchoukos NT, Dougenis D: Surgery of the thoracic aorta. N Engl J Med 1997;332:1876–1888.
3. Svensson LG, Labib SB: Aortic dissection and aortic aneurysm surgery. Curr Opin Cardiol 1994;9:191–199.
4. Keren A, Kim CB, Hu BS, et al: Accuracy of biplane and multiplane transesophageal echocardiography in diagnosis of typical acute aortic dissection and intramural hematoma. J Am Coll Cardiol 1996;28:627–636.
5. Sommer T, Fehske W, Holzknecht N, et al: Aortic dissection: A comparative study of diagnosis with spiral CT, multiplanar transesophageal echocardiography, and MR imaging. Radiology 1996;199:347–352.
6. Fann JI, Smith JA, Miller DC, et al: Surgical management of aortic dissection during a 30-year period. Circulation 1995;92(Suppl 9):II113-II121.
7. Svensson LG, Crawford ES, Hess KR, et al: Dissection of the aorta and dissecting aortic aneurysms: Improving early and long-term surgical results. Circulation 1990;82(Suppl 5):IV24–IV38.
8. Schor JS, Yerlioglu ME, Galla JD, et al: Selective management of acute type B aortic dissection: Long-term follow-up. Ann Thorac Surg 1996;61:1339–1341.
9. Elefteriades JA, Hartleroad J, Gusberg RJ, et al: Long-term experience with descending aortic dissection: The complication-specific approach. Ann Thorac Surg 1992;53:11–20; discussion, 20–21.
10. Slonim SM, Nyman U, Semba CP, et al: Aortic dissection: Percutaneous management of ischemic complications with endovascular stents and balloon fenestration. J Vasc Surg 23;241–251.
11. Fann JI, Sarris GE, Mitchell RS, et al: Treatment of patients with aortic dissection presenting with peripheral vascular complications. Ann Surg 1990;212:705–713.
12. Cambria RP, Brewster DC, Gertler J, et al: Vascular complications associated with spontaneous aortic dissection. J Vasc Surg 1988;7:199–209.
13. Webb TH, Williams GM: Abdominal aortic tailoring for renal, visceral, and lower extremity malperfusion resulting from acute aortic dissection. J Vasc Surg 1997;26:474–480.

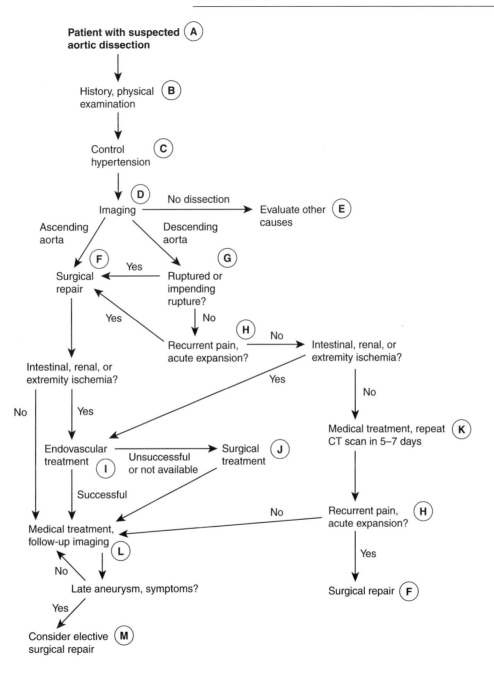

Chapter 29 Iliac Artery Aneurysm

WILLIAM C. KRUPSKI, MD • MARK R. NEHLER, MD

(A) An iliac artery aneurysm (IAA) is defined as a focal dilation more than 1.5 times the normal iliac artery diameter (10 mm in men and 9 mm in women[1]). Patients with coexistent abdominal aortic aneurysms (AAAs) have diffuse iliac artery enlargement, on average about 1.7 cm.[2] Traditional clinical definitions of IAAs have varied between 2 and 2.5 cm diameter. Isolated IAAs not in continuity with aortoiliac aneurysms represent a low percentage of all intra-abdominal aneurysms.[3] In a recent autopsy series, there were seven isolated IAAs in 26,251 postmortem examinations over a 15-year period, for an incidence of 0.03%. However, there were 202 iliac artery aneurysms among 1287 AAAs, for a prevalence of 16%. Others have reported higher occurrences of solitary IAAs, from 2.2% of all intra-abdominal aneurysms in one study to as high as 7% to 11.5% in others.[4–6]

Seventy percent of IAAs involve the common iliac artery, and most others involve the internal iliac artery. Isolated external iliac artery aneurysms are rare. IAAs involve multiple segments in more than one third of patients.[4]

(B) More than 90% of IAAs are combined with an AAA either as a direct extension (fusiform aortoiliac) or as coexistent.[7, 8] Conversely, about 10% to 20% of aortic aneurysms involve the iliac segments.[3]

(C) It is unusual for patients to present with a small AAA and coexistent large IAAs. If IAAs warrant repair because of their size or a patient's symptoms, a bifurcated aortic graft to replace both the iliac aneurysm and aorta should be performed in order to avoid future AAA expansion; this also facilitates the proximal anastomosis.

(D) More commonly, an IAA is discovered during the evaluation of an AAA that does warrant repair. The preoperative abdominal/pelvic computed tomography (CT) scan demonstrates this anatomy. Traditionally, arteriography has been used in patients with IAAs to plan arterial reconstruction that will optimize pelvic blood flow, including maintaining antegrade inflow to at least one internal iliac artery. Spiral CT scanning or magnetic resonance angiography (MRA) can also provide this information in most cases.

(E) Traditionally, a diameter of 2.5 to 3.0 cm has been the size considered for elective IAA repair on the basis of minimal incidence of rupture below 3.5 cm.[4, 9, 10] However, Santilli and coworkers[11] have reported retrospective follow-up of 189 patients with enlarged iliac arteries for a mean of 20 months. This study included a mixture of isolated IAAs and IAAs coexistent with AAAs. No IAAs below 5.0 cm diameter ruptured. These authors concluded that repair of asymptomatic IAAs is indicated only when the diameter is larger than 4.0 cm. However, most iliac arteries entered into this database were small; only 10% were larger than 3.0 cm in diameter. Moreover, the authors suggested a lower threshold for IAA repair in the setting of AAA repair, especially in younger patients.

(F) As stated, IAAs under 2.5 cm in diameter are considered to have a low risk of rupture. As with surgery for aortic aneurysms, indication and extent of operation frequently is influenced by the patient's age and medical condition. Thus, it is reasonable to ignore a relatively small IAA in a high-risk patient who requires AAA repair because the increased morbidity associated with a bifurcation graft outweighs the low rupture risk, especially in an older patient.

(G) In the evaluation of a patient with pelvic artery aneurysms, several basic principles are important:

1. Exposure of bilateral aneurysms is usually easier with a transperitoneal approach. If a retroperitoneal approach is employed, leave the left kidney down to provide optimal access to the pelvis.
2. Maintain antegrade perfusion to one of the internal iliac arteries to avoid colonic or pelvic ischemia and impotence.
3. Minimize unnecessary dissection (include minimal aneurysmal wall resection) to prevent injury to the iliac veins, the ureters, and the parasympathetic nerve plexus, which is responsible for sexual function.
4. Use fixed retractors with multiple special deep blades to facilitate exposure.
5. Because of the depth of the dissection, use a high-intensity fiberoptic headlight; standard overhead operating room lights are usually inadequate.

(H) If the AAA is not a fusiform aneurysm in continuity with the iliac aneurysms, a tube graft is often preferable in patients with IAAs smaller than 2.5 cm or in elderly, high-risk patients because the risk of complications outweighs the risk of rupture. Placement of tube grafts avoids difficult pelvic exposure and dissection, and only one large distal anastomosis is required. Older patients (in their upper 70s and 80s), patients with multiple significant co-morbid risk factors, and patients with prior extensive pelvic surgery or irradiation that would make operative exposure hazardous should be managed in this manner if the IAAs are small, are presumably asymptomatic, and are not associated with other pelvic pathologic processes (e.g., ureteral obstruction, peripheral nerve compression).

(I) Isolated IAAs are rare, constituting 1% to 11% of all IAAs[3, 5, 8, 10] (see A). They occur with equal frequency on the right and left. Up to 80% involve multiple iliac segments; 70% are in the common iliac artery, 20% are in the internal iliac artery, and the remainder are located in the external iliac artery.[4, 8]

(J) A high percentage of patients with isolated IAAs experience symptoms. IAAs are associated with a higher rupture rate than AAAs, although this conclusion may be erroneous; the deep pelvic location of these aneurysms makes them less likely to be detected by physical examination or routine ultrasound study, and they therefore often reach large sizes before discovery.[4, 6, 8, 12, 13]

Compression or erosion of surrounding structures due to expansion in a fixed pelvic space is usually responsible for detection. Ureteral obstruction and subsequent pyelonephritis can lead to urosepsis. Erosion into the ureter or bladder can cause massive hematuria.[14] Compression of femoral, sciatic, or obturator nerves can produce neurologic symptoms.[14] Most commonly, patients complain of vague abdominal pain.[10]

(K) Case reports of infected IAAs describe a wide range of causes. Most infected aneurysms result from the following:

1. Hematogenous seeding from bacteremia (gram-positive endocarditis, fungemia, or salmonellosis).[15, 16]
2. Local spread from adjacent structures (gram-negative urinary tract infections, gram-negative or anaerobic infections from colon obstruction, or perforation).[17, 18]
3. Introduction of infection coincident with intravascular interventions (arteriography, percutaneous transluminal angioplasty (PTA), or stent placement).[19]

(L) The treatment of choice for infected IAAs is aneurysm exclusion with excision of all grossly infected tissue.[15, 18, 20, 21] If consequent ischemia is anticipated, extra-anatomic bypasses or in situ revascularization with autogenous conduits may be required. Occasionally, the iliac arteries are sufficiently redundant to allow aneurysmal resection and primary end-to-end arterial reconstruction after extensive arterial mobilization.[10] Despite this recommendation, however, infected IAAs are extremely difficult to excise completely without potentially life-threatening pelvic venous hemorrhage owing to the proximity of numerous thin-walled veins adjacent to pelvic artery aneurysms.

Successful embolization has been accomplished in selected high-risk patients.[22, 23] The mortality

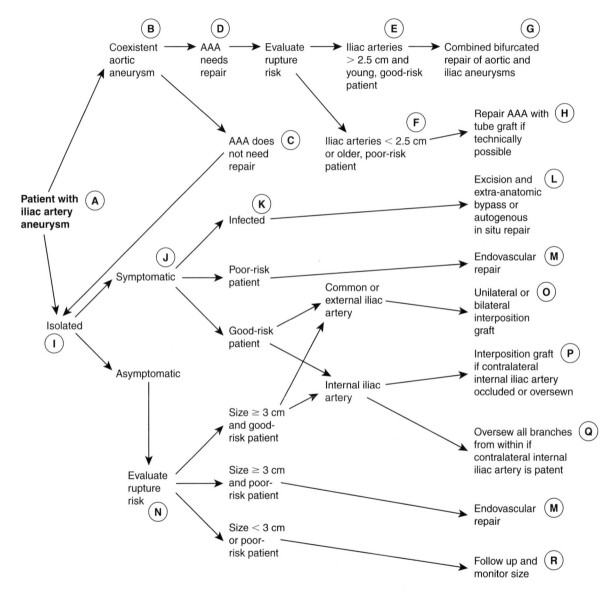

rate for infected IAA repair is similar or greater than the 10% to 15% death rate associated with repair of infected infrarenal aortic aneurysms because the deep pelvic location of iliac aneurysms makes exposure more difficult.[24,25]

(M) Successful endovascular treatment of IAAs in high-risk patients has been reported in small series.[26-28] Endovascular repair is a viable option for both symptomatic high-risk patients with variably sized IAAs (see J) as well as asymptomatic patients with large IAAs (see N). The aneurysms are excluded by means of various types of covered stent grafts via a transfemoral approach. The mean follow-up period in most reported cases is short. Long-term data will determine the general applicability of this approach.

(N) Determination of operative risk versus rupture risk requires recognition of many variables in the repair of isolated IAAs in asymptomatic patients. The smallest IAA that was reported to rupture measured 3.5 cm intraoperatively, but the value may be inaccurate owing to the patient's hemodynamic instability.[10] More recently, Santilli and colleagues reported rupture only in IAAs measuring 4 cm or larger.[11]

We recommend surgical repair of asymptomatic IAAs measuring 3 cm in diameter in relatively younger, good-risk patients. In patients with IAAs measuring more than 3 cm in maximum diameter who are poor operative candidates, endovascular repair may be considered, although long-term results are as yet uncertain.

In patients with IAAs smaller than 3 cm who are poor operative risks, regular observation with serial ultrasound studies or CT examinations is recommended. Although ultrasound is a less expensive technique for serial follow-up, the pelvic location and associated bowel gas often make accurate measurements difficult. Thus, we favor CT scans in most patients for this purpose.

(O) Unilateral, common IAAs should be repaired with unilateral interposition grafts, usually via a retroperitoneal approach. Bilateral aneurysms can be treated with separate bilateral interposition grafts, or with an aortobi-iliac graft. The latter is usually preferred, since one less anastomosis is required and possible future aneurysmal degeneration of the intrarenal aorta is avoided. If technical or other issues preclude this, separate bilateral iliac grafts can be placed.

(P) For treatment of isolated internal IAAs, it is prudent to maintain flow to at least one internal iliac artery whenever technically possible. Overall, the incidence of pelvic ischemia in modern aortoiliac surgery is less than 1%, but most cases involve bilateral internal iliac artery interruption, either from surgery or from emboli.[29,30] Patients with pelvic ischemia suffer buttock symptoms (claudication, rest pain, or necrosis), genital necrosis, spinal cord injury, or colorectal infarction. The mortality rate ranges from 60% to 100%.[31] Some authors have recommended revascularization of the inferior mesenteric artery if the circulation of neither internal iliac artery can be maintained.[32]

(Q) Exclusion of internal IAAs is best managed from within the lumen. All branches are oversewn from within the opened aneurysm to minimize the amount of dissection required in proximity to adjacent veins. Avoiding major venous injury is a critical technical component for this procedure.

(R) Small IAAs should be monitored yearly with computed tomography (see N). Rapid increase in size (>0.5 cm/year), size greater than 3 cm, and development of symptoms should prompt consideration of repair, either by operation for good-risk patients[8] or by endovascular techniques for poor-risk patients.[28]

REFERENCES

1. Pedersen OM, Aslaksen A, Vik-Mo H: Ultrasound measurement of the luminal diameter of the abdominal aorta and iliac arteries in patients without vascular disease. J Vasc Surg 1993;17:596–601.
2. Armon MP, Wenham PW, Whitaker SC, et al: Common iliac artery aneurysms in patients with abdominal aortic aneurysms. Eur J Vasc Endovasc Surg 1998;15:255–257.
3. Brunkwall J, Hauksson H, Bengtsson H, et al: Solitary aneurysms of the iliac arterial system: An estimate of their frequency of occurrence. J Vasc Surg 1989;10:381–384.
4. Richardson JW, Greenfield LJ: Natural history and management of iliac aneurysms. J Vasc Surg 1988;8:165–171.
5. Nachbur BH, Inderbitzi RG, Bar W: Isolated iliac aneurysms. Eur J Vasc Surg 1991;5:375–381.
6. Minato N, Itoh T, Natsuaki M, et al: Isolated iliac artery aneurysm and its management. Cardiovasc Surg 1994;2:489–494.
7. Lawrence PF, Lorenzo-Rivero S, Lyon JL: The incidence of iliac, femoral, and popliteal artery aneurysms in hospitalized patients. J Vasc Surg 1995;22:409–415.
8. Krupski WC, Selzman CH, Floridia R, et al: Contemporary management of isolated iliac aneurysms. J Vasc Surg 1998;28:1–11.
9. McCready RA, Pairolero PC, Gilmore JC, et al: Isolated iliac artery aneurysms. Surgery 1983;93:688–693.
10. Krupski WC: Isolated iliac artery aneurysms, in Current Therapy in Vascular Surgery. St. Louis, Mosby–Year Book, 1994, pp 296–302.
11. Santilli SM, Wernsing SE, Lee ES: Expansion rates and outcomes for iliac artery aneurysms. J Vasc Surg 2000;31:114–121.
12. Desiron Q, Detry O, Sakalihasan N, et al: Isolated atherosclerotic aneurysms of the iliac arteries. Ann Vasc Surg 1995(9 Suppl);S62–S66.
13. Sacks NP, Huddy SP, Wegner T, Giddings AE: Management of solitary iliac aneurysms. J Cardiovasc Surg (Torino) 1992;33:679–683.
14. Krupski WC, Bass A, Rosenberg GD, et al: The elusive isolated hypogastric artery aneurysm: Novel presentations. J Vasc Surg 1989;10:557–562.
15. Tsunezuka Y, Urayama H, Ohtake H, Watanabe Y: A solitary iliac artery aneurysm caused by *Candida* infection: Report of a case. J Cardiovasc Surg (Torino) 1998;39:437–439.
16. Huang PL, Chua S, Guo GB, Fu M: Mycotic aneurysm leading to iliac arteriovenous fistula diagnosed by vascular duplex color scan. J Ultrasound Med 1998;17:513–516.
17. Van DH, Keppenne V, Sakalihasan N, et al: Ureteroarterial fistula: Two observations. Acta Chir Belg 1997;97:133–136.
18. Hassan D, Ulmer BG, McFadden D: Infected internal iliac artery aneurysm: A case report. Can J Surg 1996;39:67–69.
19. Kolvenbach R, el Basha M: Secondary rupture of a common iliac artery aneurysm after endovascular exclusion and stent-graft infection [letter]. J Vasc Surg 1997;26:351–353.

20. Grandmougin D, Warembourg H, Fayad G: Successful treatment of primary pneumococcal multilocular mycotic aneurysms. Eur J Cardiothorac Surg 1997;12:133–137.
21. Tatebe S, Kanazawa H, Yamazaki Y, et al: Mycotic aneurysm of the internal iliac artery caused by Klebsiella pneumoniae. Vasa 1996;25:184–187.
22. Akomea-Agyin C, Reidy JF, Deverall PB: Transcatheter embolization of mycotic iliac aneurysm after aortic valve replacement because of bacterial endocarditis. J Thorac Cardiovasc Surg 1996;112:1671–1672.
23. Hoeffel JC: [Mycotic aneurysm of the iliac artery (letter)]. Arch Pediatr 1994;1:696–697.
24. Moneta GL, Taylor LMJ, Yeager RA, et al: Surgical treatment of infected aortic aneurysm. Am J Surg 1998;175:396–399.
25. Sessa C, Farah I, Voirin L, et al: Infected aneurysms of the infrarenal abdominal aorta: Diagnostic criteria and therapeutic strategy. Ann Vasc Surg 1997;11:453–463.
26. Marin ML, Veith FJ, Lyon RT, et al: Transfemoral endovascular repair of iliac artery aneurysms. Am J Surg 1995;170:179–182.
27. Razavi MK, Dake MD, Semba CP, et al: Percutaneous endoluminal placement of stent-grafts for the treatment of isolated iliac artery aneurysms. Radiology 1995;197:801–804.
28. Parsons RE, Marin ML, Veith FJ, et al: Mid-term results of endovascular stented grafts for the treatment of isolated iliac artery aneurysms. J Vasc Surg 1999;30:915–921.
29. Hassen-Khodja R, Pittaluga P, Le BP, et al: Role of direct revascularization of the internal iliac artery during aorto-iliac surgery. Ann Vasc Surg 1998;12:550–556.
30. Paty PK, Shah DM, Chang BB, et al: Pelvic ischemia following aortoiliac reconstruction. Ann Vasc Surg 1994;8:204–206.
31. Iliopoulos JI, Howanitz PE, Pierce GE, et al: The critical hypogastric circulation. Am J Surg 1987;154:671–675.
32. Byrne JL, Zaman SN, Meade JW, Aronski WP: Operative management of bilateral internal iliac artery aneurysms. J Cardiovasc Surg (Torino) 1989;30:241–243.

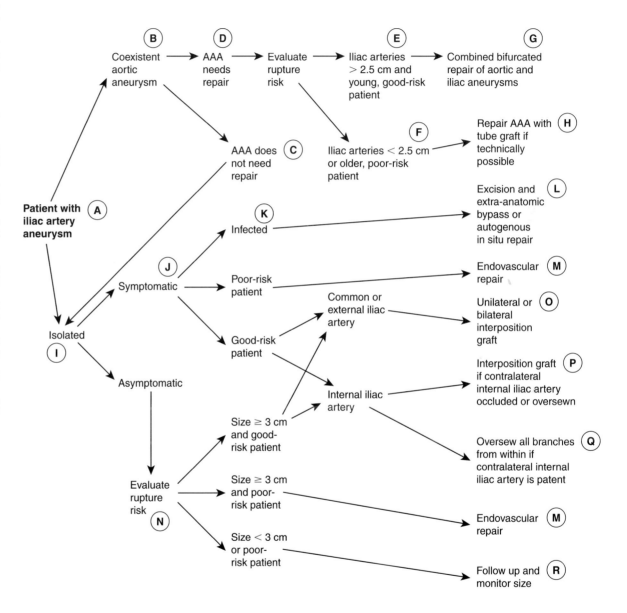

Chapter 30 Femoral Artery Aneurysm

MARK R. NEHLER, MD • WILLIAM C. KRUPSKI, MD

A A *true* femoral aneurysm involves all vessel wall layers. A *false* femoral artery aneurysm *(pseudoaneurysm)* develops from a defect in the arterial wall or from an earlier anastomosis, beginning with extravasation of blood into a contained extravascular space and maturing into an aneurysm-like hematoma. Most femoral aneurysms and pseudoaneurysms are detected as asymptomatic, pulsatile groin masses. Pain associated with rapid expansion or pressure on the adjacent femoral nerve is seen almost exclusively in anastomotic or traumatic pseudoaneurysms.

B The clinical scenario has a major impact on the diagnostic and treatment algorithm because true aneurysms and pseudoaneurysms behave differently. Hemodynamically significant bleeding usually occurs only in association with traumatic pseudoaneurysms *(iatrogenic or noniatrogenic)*. Rarely, this bleeding can be localized to the retroperitoneum, producing hemodynamic and hematocrit changes without obvious local signs in the groin. Therefore, a history of arterial trauma (catheterization, indwelling lines, intravenous drug use) or previous vascular operations (grafts, patches) should be sought. True aneurysms enlarge gradually without a dramatic beginning. In contrast, because true aneurysmal disease is often multifocal, a history of prior aortic or popliteal aneurysms should be sought.

C Added to the history (arterial trauma or operation), ultrasound examination may help to differentiate a true aneurysm (fusiform ultrasonographic appearance) from a pseudoaneurysm (saccular ultrasonographic appearance). Furthermore, management is altered according to aneurysm or pseudoaneurysm size and the presence of intraluminal thrombus. Ultrasound studies are accurate for detecting femoral aneurysms and pseudoaneurysms larger than 2.0 cm.[1,2] Although small amounts of intraluminal thrombus can be missed, ultrasound scanning is also the noninvasive method of choice for detecting clot formation. The additional use of arteriography, computed tomography (CT), or magnetic resonance angiography (MRA) is often recommended for the evaluation of anastomotic pseudoaneurysms for several reasons:

1. Detection of pseudoaneurysms at other anastomotic sites (particularly proximal aortic grafts) changes management.
2. Precise location of the aneurysm with respect to the femoral bifurcation assists in planning the reconstruction.
3. Identification of coexistent occlusive disease may warrant intervention.

D The common femoral artery (CFA), after the iliac and popliteal arteries, is the third most common site of peripheral arterial aneurysms. With true femoral aneurysms, 44% are isolated to the CFA, 56% involve the femoral bifurcation, and fewer than 1% are isolated to the superficial femoral or profunda femoris (deep femoral) arteries.[3-5] Although the definition of an aneurysm has traditionally been a 50% increase in arterial diameter, the clinical application of this definition to femoral aneurysms remains unclear. The CFA mean diameter is 9.8 mm in men and 8.2 mm in women.[6] However, the CFA increases in size throughout life, and diameter correlates with weight, height, and body surface area. For practical purposes, clinical decisions are based on the presence of a femoral aneurysm greater than 2.0 cm. in diameter.

E Approximately 50% of patients with a true aneurysm of the femoral artery have a coexistent abdominal aortic aneurysm (AAA). About one third of patients with a femoral artery true aneurysm have a coexistent popliteal artery aneurysm. The incidence of bilateral femoral artery aneurysms is extremely variable (range, from 20 to 70%).[7,8] These relationships justify screening with ultrasonography for these other aneurysms.

F Most femoral artery aneurysms are asymptomatic. Symptoms associated with femoral aneurysms are usually related to distal ischemia secondary to thromboembolism or to compression of adjacent structures. In rare instances (<5% of cases), these aneurysms may rupture when they are extremely large.[9] Acute ischemia may result from aneurysm thrombosis (usually involving both the superficial femoral and profunda femoris arteries and, therefore, typically profound) or from distal embolization producing the "blue toe syndrome" or more extensive ischemia, depending on the location of embolic debris. Chronic compressive symptoms may involve the femoral nerve (nonspecific groin and anterior-medial thigh pain or numbness) or the femoral vein or lymphatics (unilateral edema). In general, symptomatic aneurysms warrant repair in all but very-high-risk patients.

G The natural history of small (<3 cm in diameter) femoral artery aneurysms is usually benign. Graham and coworkers[9] monitored 105 CFA aneurysms over a mean of 28 months, and only 3 produced limb ischemia. Observation is appropriate with yearly clinical and ultrasound examinations. The management of femoral aneurysms with substantial intraluminal thrombus is uncertain. These aneurysms may pose increased thrombotic and embolic risks; however, because the amount of thrombus also increases with size, the effect of these two is difficult to separate.

H The optimal threshold diameter for elective repair has not been precisely established; it varies with operative risk and life expectancy. However, larger (>3 cm in diameter) femoral aneurysms (with or without intraluminal thrombus) are likelier to cause symptoms from compression and to contain laminated intraluminal thrombus, which presumably increases risk of thrombosis and embolization. Thus, repair is recommended in patients at reasonable risk.

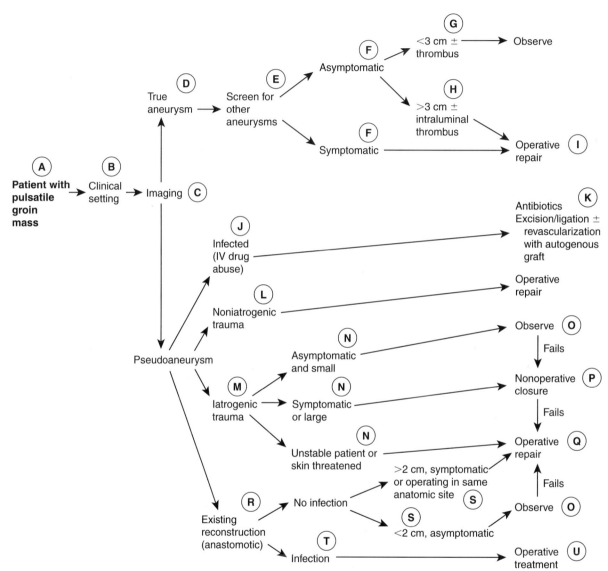

I Repair of true aneurysms of the CFA usually requires interposition grafting to exclude the aneurysmal segment. Leaving some posterior wall intact may help in determining appropriate graft length. The conduit of choice is either polyester (Dacron) or polytetrafluoroethylene (PTFE). If the aneurysm involves the femoral bifurcation, two separate grafts that join the superficial femoral and profunda femoris arteries posteriorly to recreate the bifurcation may be required. As with all prosthetic grafts placed in the groin, meticulous wound closure is important to avoid wound complications and risk of graft infection.

J Intravenous drug abuse (IVDA) is the most common cause of an infected CFA pseudoaneurysm. Patients with infected pseudoaneurysms usually present with gross signs of infection, including erythema, induration, and purulence in the groin area. They may also have signs of systemic sepsis. Infected arteries frequently present initially with intermittent arterial bleeding ("herald bleed"). Urgent evaluation and expeditious surgical exploration are indicated.

K The best management of infected pseudoaneurysm is controversial regarding the choice between autogenous arterial reconstruction and primary excision with ligation. A prudent approach is to proceed with excision and ligation, reserving autogenous bypass for those who would otherwise suffer limb loss, as predicted by absent pedal Doppler signals following excision. When possible, continuity between the superficial and deep femoral arteries should be maintained to increase collateral flow after CFA excision and ligation.

Despite IVDA, most of these patients have saphenous vein in the mid-thigh that is potentially usable for arterial reconstruction. Reddy and colleagues[10] performed reconstruction in patients with infection involving only the femoral bifurcation, with an amputation rate of 12% in 60 patients. When in situ autogenous reconstruction is not feasible or is inappropriate because of local conditions and critical ischemia exists, an extra-anatomic bypass, such as through the obturator foramen, may be considered.

Femoral Artery Aneurysm (continued)

(L) Pseudoaneurysms resulting from noniatrogenic penetrating trauma should always be repaired because the extent of disruption of the wall of the CFA is usually much greater than with iatrogenic injuries. The natural history of these traumatic lesions is uncertain, but continued expansion resulting in increased perioperative surgical morbidity at the time of later repair has been reported.[11] Because of the potential for contamination, autogenous repair is performed when possible.

(M) Two reviews reporting more than 2000 diagnostic cardiac catheterizations have documented a 0.5% incidence of bleeding complications (hemorrhage or pseudoaneurysm).[12, 13] Arterial complications are more common after therapeutic than diagnostic procedures (1.5%), especially when procedures include insertion of intravascular devices, such as stents (up to 15%).[14]

The diameter of the device being inserted is the major risk factor related to arteriographic complications. Patient-related factors (e.g., peripheral vascular disease with calcified arteries, obesity preventing adequate hemostatic compression, and concurrent anticoagulation) are also important. Technique-related factors include (1) introducer size, (2) through-and-through arterial puncture, and (3) puncture or laceration of the circumflex or deep femoral branches that cannot be adequately compressed after the procedure. These observations explain why hemorrhagic complications occur in some patients but not in others.

Despite the increased use of percutaneous closure devices (which themselves can cause a variety of complications), hemorrhagic complication rates have not been dramatically reduced in large series.[15] Hematomas are easily differentiated from early pseudoaneurysms by duplex ultrasound surveillance.

Indications for surgical evacuation of postprocedural hematomas include:

1. Expanding size.
2. Blood loss sufficient to require transfusion.
3. Mass effect producing nerve compression, venous obstruction, or a threat to viability of the overlying skin.

(N) Small (<2 cm), asymptomatic iatrogenic pseudoaneurysms may be followed with ultrasound surveillance, since some may spontaneously thrombose and resolve; however, treatment is usually recommended for symptomatic or larger pseudoaneurysms.[16, 17] Nonoperative treatment is used initially in most cases. For rapidly expanding or very large pseudoaneurysms that cause hemodynamic instability or threaten skin viability from tension, emergent operative repair is indicated.

(O) Observation is an alternate approach to femoral artery pseudoaneurysms, as suggested by Toursarkissian and associates.[18] In this series, lesions with clear indications for surgery (i.e., symptoms, diameter > 4 cm, earlier operation at the same anatomic site) underwent immediate operative repair. Other lesions were observed with serial duplex scanning until closure occurred or one of the aforementioned endpoints mandated surgery. Of the approximately 300 lesions encountered, 50% required immediate operation and 50% were observed. Of those lesions observed, 86% closed spontaneously within a mean of 23 days. If confirmed by other studies, these results indicate that many of the pseudoaneurysms currently being treated by compression or thrombin injection may carry a favorable outcome when simply observed, implying that more selective application of nonoperative closure techniques may be possible.

(P) Ultrasound-guided compression therapy has been used extensively for treatment of many acute iatrogenic femoral artery pseudoaneurysms. Duplex ultrasound scanning is used to localize the communication between artery and pseudoaneurysm cavity. The ultrasound head is then used for concise compression of the pseudoaneurysm (via the B-mode ultrasound image), limiting flow into the pseudoaneurysm without occluding the artery.

A typical protocol prescribes initial compression for 20 to 30 minutes. If flow into the pseudoaneurysm is not eliminated, a subsequent compression for a similar period is often successful. Few pseudoaneurysms are successfully obliterated if these first two compressions are unsuccessful. Initial success rates of 90% have been reported in multiple series,[19, 20] including success rates of 70% even in patients receiving uninterrupted anticoagulation therapy.[21] The best results are achieved with acute lesions smaller than 4 cm in diameter (particularly in patients receiving anticoagulation). Compression of acute pseudoaneurysms, especially those with considerable surrounding hematoma, is painful, and inability of patients to tolerate the compression is a significant limitation of the procedure. Because recurrence affects as many as 10% of patients, subsequent scanning to confirm thrombosis is indicated the next day. Most recurrent pseudoaneurysms can be obliterated by repeated compression.

Kang and coauthors[22] initially reported successful treatment of femoral pseudoaneurysms by percutaneous thrombin injection directly into the pseudoaneurysm cavity, producing immediate thrombosis in 70 of 71 patients. The potential of direct intravascular thrombin injection to produce serious thrombotic complications (one patient in the Kang series) has not been significant in some recent series.[23, 24] Avoidance of painful compression and immediate successful obliteration are attractive features of this technique, which appears to also be somewhat more efficacious than ultrasound compression.[23, 24]

(Q) Operative repair consists of a vertical groin incision, proximal control, and opening the hematoma with suture control of the traumatic arterial opening. Femoral pseudoaneurysm repair is most conveniently performed with the patient under general or regional anesthesia, but local anesthesia can be used if necessary. The cost of operative therapy for this relatively frequent clinical problem, the occasionally precarious medical condition (particularly cardiac) of the patient population, and the potential for significant wound complications are all significant disadvantages of the operative approach.

(R) Anastomotic pseudoaneurysms occur most frequently after prosthetic bypasses. Now that silk sutures are no longer used for arterial anastomoses, important risk factors for development of noninfected anastomotic pseudoaneurysms include:

1. Local wound complications after the initial operation.
2. Female sex.
3. A previous anastomotic pseudoaneurysm.[25]

One review from Denmark demonstrated an incidence of 4.3%, occurring at a mean interval of 9 years after the original bypass procedure.[26]

(S) It is generally safe to follow small (<2 cm), noninfected and asymptomatic femoral anastomotic pseudoaneurysms. In a series of recurrent anastomotic pseudoaneurysms, those smaller than 2 cm were observed without sequelae.[25] The optimal threshold size for elective repair is not clear. In general, we recommend repair of anastomotic femoral pseudoaneurysms in the presence of symptoms, rapid expansion, or a diameter greater than 2 cm. We advocate repair of all femoral anastomotic pseudoaneurysms in patients requiring ipsilateral infrainguinal reconstruction to remove a potential source of embolization that may threaten the graft in the future.[27] In 99 CFA repairs (60% for aneurysmal disease), the perioperative mortality rate was 2%; the 5-year assisted primary patency and limb salvage rates were 77 and 95%, respectively. Resection of the involved portion of the old graft, débridement to healthy native artery, and interposition grafting are more durable than imbrication of the defect.

(T) Graft infection, either obvious or occult, must always be suspected as an etiologic factor in the development of anastomotic pseudoaneurysms. Pseudoaneurysms presenting at multiple anastomotic sites increase suspicion of graft infection. CT scanning (to detect perigraft fluid and soft tissue stranding) and radioisotope-labeled white blood cell scanning have been used to confirm an infected pseudoaneurysm. When

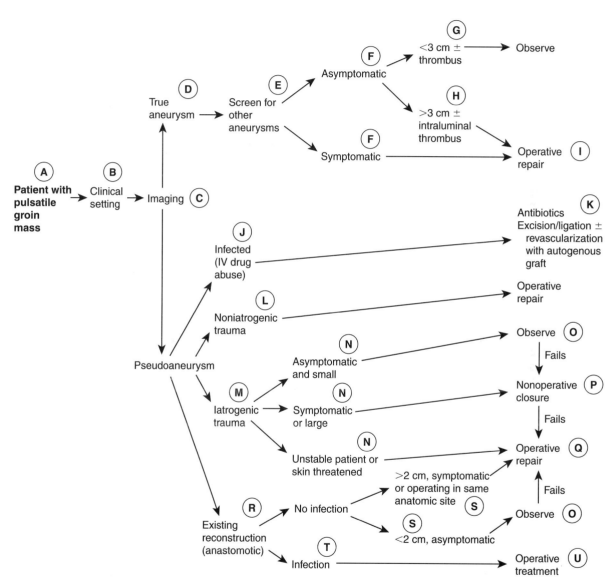

occult infection is not detected, in situ repair usually results in recurrent anastomotic pseudoaneurysms.

Using sonication techniques, Seabrook and colleagues[28] recovered coagulase-negative staphylococcus species in more than 50% of partial graft explants in patients with anastomotic pseudoaneurysms, suggesting that occult infection is more common than generally appreciated. For this reason, sonicated graft culture should always be performed and long-term antibiotic therapy considered if results are positive.

(U) Operative treatment is required for all infected femoral anastomotic pseudoaneurysms. Although some centers have advocated in situ replacement of indolent late-appearing infected grafts when they are demonstrated to be caused by low-virulence organisms, such as *Staphylococcus epidermidis*, these recommendations have generally excluded those with pseudoaneurysms.

Alternative treatment includes extra-anatomic reconstruction using remote sites, followed by graft excision and femoral artery autogenous patching, which is the procedure of choice for grossly infected grafts with suture line disruption. If only a single limb of a bifurcation graft is involved, the limb may be transected via a retroperitoneal approach, which preserves the remainder of the aortofemoral graft. This is followed by obturator or some other extra-anatomic bypass.

Operative mortality rates range from 14% to 50%, with 5-year limb salvage rates averaging 75%.[29, 30] However, 20% of the extra-anatomic reconstructions become infected over time, with a high rate of eventual limb loss (see Chapters 40 and 44).

REFERENCES

1. Gooding GA, Effeney DJ: Ultrasound of femoral artery aneurysms. AJR Am J Roentgenol 1980;134:477–480.
2. Neiman HL, Yao JS, Silver TM: Gray-scale ultrasound diagnosis of peripheral arterial aneurysms. Radiology 1979;130:413–416.
3. Levi N, Schroeder TV: Arteriosclerotic femoral artery aneurysms: A short review. J Cardiovasc Surg (Torino) 1997;38:335–338.
4. Yahel J, Witz M: Isolated true atherosclerotic aneurysms of the deep femoral artery. Case report and literature review. J Cardiovasc Surg (Torino) 1996;37:17–20.
1. Gooding GA, Effeney DJ: Ultrasound of femoral artery artery aneurysm—an uncommon site of aneurysm formation. Eur J Vasc Endovasc Surg 1995;10:502–504.
6. Sandgren T, Sonesson B, Ahlgren R, Lanne T: The diameter of the common femoral artery in healthy human: influence of sex, age, and body size. J Vasc Surg 1999;29:503–510.
7. Adiseshiah M, Bailey DA: Aneurysms of the femoral artery. Br J Surg 1977;64:174–176.
8. Howell JF, Crawford ES, Morris GCJ, et al: Surgical treatment of peripheral arteriosclerotic aneurysm. Surg Clin North Am 1966;46:979–989.
9. Graham LM, Zelenock GB, Whitehouse WMJ, et al: Clinical significance of arteriosclerotic femoral artery aneurysms. Arch Surg 1980;115:502–507.
10. Reddy DJ, Smith RF, Elliot JP, et al: Infected femoral false aneurysms in drug addicts: Evolution of selective vascular reconstruction. J Vasc Surg 1986;3:718–724.
11. Perry MO: Complications of missed arterial injuries. J Vasc Surg 1993;17:399–407.
12. Fruhwirth J, Pascher O, Hauser H, Amann W: [Local vascular complications after iatrogenic femoral artery puncture]. Wien Klin Wochenschr 1996;108:196–200.
13. Ricci MA, Trevisani GT, Pilcher DB: Vascular complications of cardiac catheterization [see comments]. Am J Surg 1994;167:375–378.
14. Lumsden AB, Miller JM, Kosinski AS, et al: A prospective evaluation of surgically treated groin complications following percutaneous cardiac procedures. Am Surg 1994;60:132–137.
15. Gerckens U, Cattelaens N, Muller R, et al: [Percutaneous suture closure of the femoral artery access after diagnostic heart catheter examination or coronary intervention]. Dtsch Med Wochenschr 1996;121:1487–1491.
16. Waller DA, Sivananthan UM, Diament RH, et al: Iatrogenic vascular injury following arterial cannulation: The importance of early surgery. Cardiovasc Surg 1993;1:251–253.
17. Perler BA: Surgical treatment of femoral pseudoaneurysm following cardiac catheterization. Cardiovasc Surg 1993;1:118–121.
18. Toursarkissian B, Allen BT, Petrinec D, et al: Spontaneous closure of selected iatrogenic pseudoaneurysms and arteriovenous fistulae. J Vasc Surg 1997;25:803–808.
19. Cox GS, Young JR, Gray BR, et al: Ultrasound-guided compression repair of postcatheterization pseudoaneurysms: Results of treatment in one hundred cases. J Vasc Surg 1994;19:683–686.
20. Langella RL, Schneider JR, Golan JF: Color duplex-guided compression therapy for postcatheterization pseudoaneurysms in a community hospital. Ann Vasc Surg 1996;10:27–35.
21. Dean SM, Olin JW, Piedmonte M, et al: Ultrasound-guided compression closure of postcatheterization pseudoaneurysms during concurrent anticoagulation: A review of seventy-seven patients. J Vasc Surg 1996;23:28–34.
22. Kang SS, Labropoulos N, Mansour A, et al: Expanded indications for ultrasound guided thrombin injection of pseudoaneurysms. J Vasc Surg 2000;31:289–298.
23. Taylor BS, Rhee RY, Muluk S, et al: Thrombin injection versus compression of femoral artery pseudoaneurysms. J Vasc Surg 1999;30:1052–1059.
24. Paulson EK, Sheafor DH, Kliewer MA, et al: Treatment of iatrogenic femoral arterial pseudoaneurysms: Comparison of US-guided thrombin injection with compression repair. Radiology 2000;215:403–408.
25. Ernst CB, Elliott JPJ, Ryan CJ, et al: Recurrent femoral anastomotic aneurysms: A 30-year experience. Ann Surg 1988;208:401–409.
26. Levi N, Schroeder TV: Anastomotic femoral aneurysms: Is an increase in interval between primary operation and aneurysms formation related to change in incidence? Panminerva Med 1998;40:210–213.
27. Nehler MR, Taylor LMJ, Lee RW, et al: Interposition grafting for reoperation on the common femoral artery. J Vasc Surg 1998;28:37–42.
28. Seabrook GR, Schmitt DD, Bandyk DF, et al: Anastomotic femoral pseudoaneurysm: An investigation of occult infection as an etiologic factor. J Vasc Surg 1990;11:629–634.
29. Yeager RA, Moneta GL, Taylor LMJ, et al: Improving survival and limb salvage in patients with aortic graft infection. Am J Surg 1990;159:466–469.
30. Karner-Hanusch J, Staudacher M, Prager M, et al: [Management of severe infection complicating aortofemoral grafts]. Wien Klin Wochenschr 1998;110:721–724.

FEMORAL ARTERY ANEURYSM

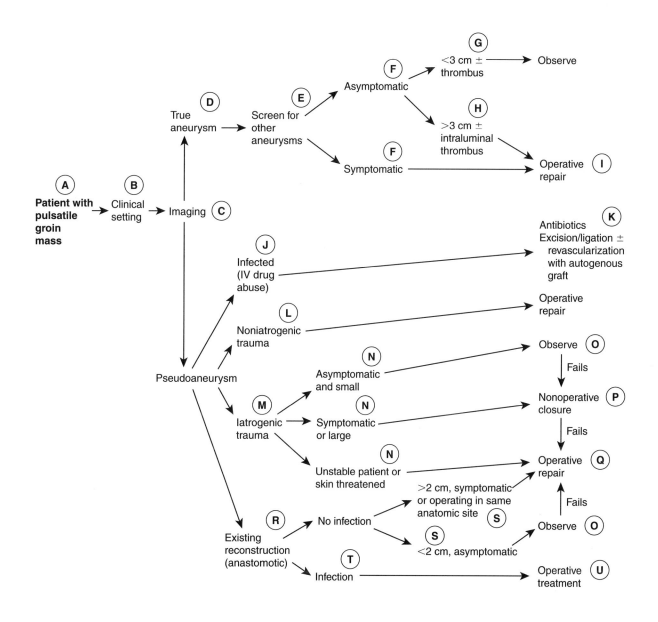

Chapter 31 Femoral Artery Pseudoaneurysm from Trauma

DANIEL J. REDDY, MD

(A) Clinical diagnosis of a traumatic femoral pseudoaneurysm is often difficult, making confirmatory diagnostic testing advisable. The management of a femoral artery pseudoaneurysm resulting from iatrogenic arterial puncture for catheter access, as well as the collateral damage sustained by this artery from chronic use of the adjacent femoral vein for habitual intravenous (IV) drug abuse, is included in the algorithm. Excluded is the management of femoral artery injuries following noniatrogenic vascular trauma (see Chapters 30 and 66).

(B) Hemorrhage sufficient to cause significant hemodynamic instability should prompt the treating surgeon to curtail detailed workup and to proceed with urgent operation in most patients regardless of etiology.

(C) Details of an urgent operation are presented in G, U, and X later.

(D) If clinical signs suggest a femoral pseudoaneurysm and a history of recent percutaneous femoral puncture, a color flow duplex ultrasound examination should be obtained for diagnosis as well as possible compression therapy, as for other traumatic pseudoaneurysms. Although a pseudoaneurysm is approximately 10 times more likely to occur after a therapeutic procedure, compared with a diagnostic procedure alone, other etiologic factors need to be considered. The following factors increase the likelihood of a pseudoaneurysm versus a simple hematoma[1-3]:

- Ongoing anticoagulation therapy
- Altered platelet function
- Long duration of procedure
- Large catheter size
- The need for several catheter exchanges

(E) Color flow imaging, combined with spectral Doppler ultrasound and with the typical use of a 5-MHz linear array transducer, promptly confirms or rules out the diagnosis in most clinical settings. Importantly, other findings influencing management decisions are also readily available with this examination. For example, the presence or absence of an associated deep venous thrombosis (DVT) in the common femoral vein can be determined.[4-6]

(F) When investigations determine that there is an associated arteriovenous (A-V) fistula, femoral nerve deficit, very large hematoma or complex arterial injury, operative repair is ordinarily the best option. Ultrasound guided nonoperative strategies do not effectively eradicate an A-V fistula. Evacuation of a large hematoma promotes soft tissue healing and relieves femoral nerve compression, whereas complex arterial injuries require open repair because there are no reliable nonoperative or minimally invasive options.

(G) Standard vascular surgical repair techniques that emphasize direct suture repair, when possible, and autogenous tissue for angioplasty or bypass are highly effective.

(H) On a duplex scan, a pseudoaneurysm appears as extravascular, swirling blood flow both toward and away from the probe. Bidirectional blood flow is identified in the tract connecting the cavity and the adjacent injured artery.[4-10]

(I) If no pseudoaneurysm or other relevant pathologic process is identified (see B and F) the patient is observed. Although it would not be incorrect to observe a very small pseudoaneurysm, implied in such a decision would be the need for a follow-up scan confirming spontaneous resolution.

(J) Ultrasound-guided compression to treat a pseudoaneurysm is highly successful in most patients, but adequate sedation and analgesics are required so that the patient can tolerate the applied pressure and time involved in this treatment modality. Operator stamina to apply sufficient controlled force to accomplish pseudoaneurysm occlusion while avoiding native artery occlusion is also involved in the decision, as is pseudoaneurysm "neck" size. A larger "neck" favors compression over thrombin injection, while DVT in the adjacent vein argues against employing either of these newer methods. Highly successful, ultrasound-guided thrombin injection is easier on the patient and more readily accomplished.[4-10] Although the potential for errant thrombin injection would raise the risk profile for this modality, its reported safety record to date has been excellent.[11-12]

(K) With the pseudoaneurysm "neck" observed, sufficient pressure is applied by the duplex scan probe to produce cessation of blood flow into the pseudoaneurysm while allowing normal flow in the femoral artery. Pressure is maintained for 10 to 15 minutes before the sac is scanned again to check for any residual inflow from the "neck." Multiple compression sequences totaling 45 to 60 minutes may be needed in one treatment session. Rescanning of the common femoral artery and vein upon completion to determine success in monitoring more distal extremity pulses during compression also prevents excessive compression of the native artery.

(L) Depending on patient tolerance of procedure discomfort, ultrasound-guided compression can be attempted again after a short interval, such as on the following day.

(M) Following successful treatment and several hours of bed rest for the patient, a follow-up duplex scan the next day is performed to verify thrombosis of the pseudoaneurysm sac.

(N) The goal of ultrasound-guided compression is to thrombose the pseudoaneurysm rather than avoid operation. Accordingly, the treatment should be abandoned when repeated attempts have failed.

(O) The technique consists of 0.5 mL of a sterile 1000 U/mL solution of bovine thrombin injected percutaneously directly into the pseudoaneurysm sac (remote from the "neck") under continuous monitoring of the ultrasound image to monitor prompt thrombus formation. In a minority of patients, repeated injections may be required. As experience with this method accumulates, it appears that it may become the primary treatment choice.[11–12]

(P) Post-traumatic pseudoaneurysms occurring in the setting of IV drug abuse are almost always infected and underlie the injection site. This site is a chronic, draining, umbilicated skin and soft tissue lesion or "track." A postphlebitic leg is typical, as is chronic adenopathy, lymphedema, and soft tissue sepsis. Important elements of the history are inadvertent arterial punctures ("hit a pinkie") or postinjection arterial bleeding ("skeeting red blood"). Herald bleeds as well as inadvertent arterial injections ("leg trip") may have occurred, causing severe distal extremity ischemia and closed-space sepsis.[13–16]

(Q) If infection is a possibility, blood specimens should be obtained for culture and screens for hepatitis and human immunodeficiency virus should be performed. Tetanus immunization should be updated (active and passive, if necessary). Bacterial endocarditis should be considered. Gram-negative and methicillin-resistant *Staphylococcus aureus* (MRSA) antibiotic coverage should be started pending culture results.

(R) Owing to the typical presentation of these patients, digital subtraction arteriography is favored over duplex ultrasound because the associated changes in the soft tissue, venous, and lymphatic structures degrade the diagnostic accuracy of noninvasive testing. The groin examination findings, chronically positive in these patients, warrant a low threshold for definitive arteriographic study.[13]

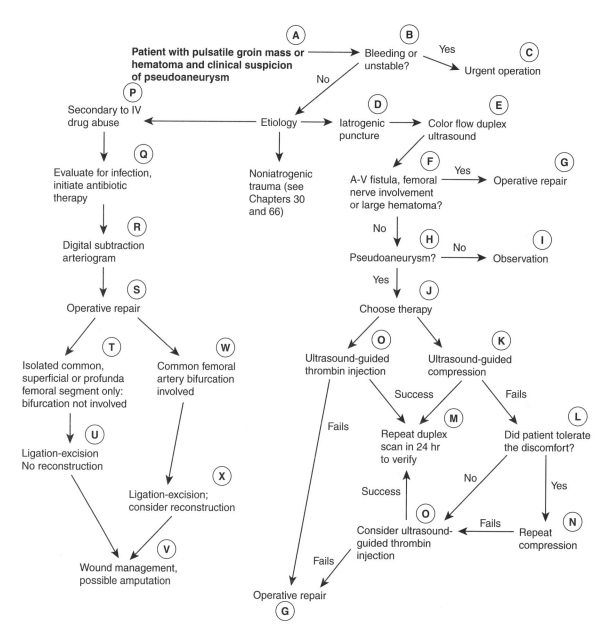

(S) Operative repair for this complex life-threatening lesion employs the following priority sequence:
1. Prevent death from hemorrhage.
2. Achieve control of sepsis.
3. Accomplish wound healing.
4. Preserve the lower extremity, if possible.

(T) The operative plan includes general anesthesia and sterile access in the operative field to the entire extremity and involves proximal control *above* the inguinal ligament when needed. Operative findings and preoperative arteriography facilitate identification, as precisely as possible, of which of the four anatomic subsegments of the femoral artery is involved.

(U) Amputation is unlikely when the femoral artery bifurcation can be maintained for axial flow into the superficial or deep femoral arteries. Moreover, collateral flow through an intact bifurcation below an excised common femoral artery is usually sufficient to avoid critical ischemia in this patient population. Accordingly, reconstruction is not routinely considered in such cases as the risk-benefit profile does not warrant it.[13]

(V) Managing the wound often challenges the surgical team to apply many general, vascular and plastic surgical techniques. Typically, reoperation for wound inspection, débridement, and dressing changes with the patient under general anesthesia is required. In some cases, major amputation is also necessary (see *U* and *W*).

(W) Although most patients with the common femoral artery bifurcation involved can be managed by ligation-excision alone, many come to amputation even at the above-knee level because of resulting ischemia and insufficient collateral flow.

(X) In a minority of cases, sepsis may be limited and easily controlled at the time of triple ligation-excision of the femoral artery bifurcation. In this unusual clinical setting, arterial reconstruction with autogenous tissue may be advisable to lessen the risk of amputation; however, innovation and very careful wound management are necessary. Special attention to graft protection and long-term follow-up is mandatory.[13]

REFERENCES

1. Messina LM, Brothers TE, Wakefield TW, et al: Clinical characteristics and surgical management of vascular complications in patients undergoing cardiac catheterization: Interventional versus diagnostic procedures. J Vasc Surg 1993;13:593–600.
2. Babu SC, Piccorelli GO, Shah PM, et al: Incidence and results of arterial complications among 16,350 patients undergoing cardiac catheterization. J Vasc Surg 1989;10:113–116.
3. Kresovik TF, Khoury MD, Miller BV, et al: A prospective study of the incidence and natural history of femoral vascular complications after percutaneous transluminal coronary angioplasty. J Vasc Surg 1991;13:328–336.
4. Feld R, Patton GM, Carabasi RA, et al: Treatment of iatrogenic femoral artery injuries with ultrasound-guided compression. J Vasc Surg 1992;16:832–840.
5. Hajarizadeh H, LaRosa CR, Cardullo P, et al: Ultrasound-guided compression of iatrogenic femoral pseudoaneurysm failure, recurrence, and long-term results. J Vasc Surg 1995;22:425–430.
6. Hertz SM, Brener BJ: Ultrasound-guided pseudoaneurysm compression: Efficacy after coronary stenting and angioplasty. J Vasc Surg 1997;26:913–918.
7. Dean SM, Olin JW, Piedmonte M, Grubb M, Young JR: Ultrasound-guided compression closure of postcatheterization pseudoaneurysms during concurrent anticoagulation: A review of seventy-seven patients. J Vasc Surg 1996;23:28–34.
8. Hood DB, Mattos MA, Douglas MG, et al: Determinants of success of color-flow duplex-guided compression repair of femoral pseudoaneurysms. Surgery 1996;120:585–588.
9. Kazmers A, Meeker C, Nofz K, et al: Nonoperative therapy for postcatheterization femoral artery pseudoaneurysms. Am Surg 1997;63:199–204.
10. Kumins NH, Landau DS, Montalvo J, et al: Expanded indications for the treatment of postcatheterization femoral pseudoaneurysms with ultrasound-guided compression. Am J Surg 1998;176:131–136.
11. Liau CS, Ho FM, Chen MF, Lee YT: Treatment of iatrogenic femoral artery pseudoaneurysm with percutaneous thrombin injection. J Vasc Surg 1997;26:18–23.
12. Kang SS, Labropoulos N, Mansour MA, Baker WH: Percutaneous ultrasound guided thrombin injection: A new method for treating postcatheterization femoral pseudoaneurysms. J Vasc Surg 1993;27:1032–1038.
13. Reddy, DJ, Smith RF, Elliott JP Jr, et al: Infected femoral artery false aneurysm in drug addicts: Evolution of selective vascular reconstruction. J Vasc Surg 1986;3:718–724.
14. Padberg F Jr, Hobson R 2d, Lee B, et al: Femoral pseudoaneurysm from drugs of abuse: Ligation or reconstruction? J Vasc Surg 1992;15:642–648.
15. Ting AC, Cheng SW: Femoral pseudoaneurysms in drug addicts. World J Surg 1997;21:783–786.
16. Welch GH, Reid DB, Pollock JG: Infected false aneurysm in the groin of intravenous drug abusers. Br J Surg 1990;77:330–333.

FEMORAL ARTERY PSEUDOANEURYSM FROM TRAUMA

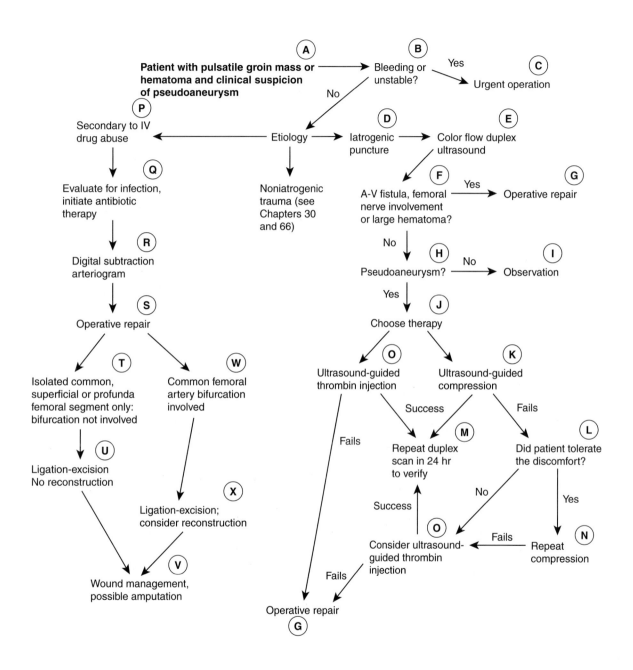

Chapter 32 Popliteal Artery Aneurysm

RICHARD J. POWELL, MD

(A) Popliteal artery aneurysms are the most common peripheral aneurysm. They occur predominantly in men (94% in one series[1]) and are bilateral in two thirds of cases. There is a 30% to 60% incidence of abdominal aortic aneurysms (AAAs) associated with bilateral popliteal artery aneurysms. A popliteal artery is considered aneurysmal when it is 1.5 to 2 times the size of the native artery, which may vary according to the size of the individual. Certainly, popliteal arteries greater than 2 cm in diameter are considered aneurysmal.

Popliteal artery aneurysms can present as an asymptomatic, pulsatile mass found behind the knee on routine physical examination, or they may be identified on ultrasonography as part of an investigation for a contralateral popliteal artery aneurysm. Symptomatic patients can present with either claudication or acute, often limb-threatening ischemia, from thrombosis or distal embolization (see C).

(B) A duplex ultrasound study is performed to confirm the presence and size of a popliteal artery aneurysm and any contained thrombus. This is an accurate study that is not expensive. If a popliteal aneurysm is identified, additional ultrasound studies of the contralateral popliteal artery and abdominal aorta are warranted to detect concomitant aneurysms. If the diagnosis of an AAA is confirmed, that aneurysm should be repaired before the repair of an asymptomatic popliteal artery aneurysm or a chronically symptomatic, but non-limb-threatening popliteal artery aneurysm. A patient with an acutely symptomatic popliteal artery aneurysm with a threat to the limb should undergo repair prior to repair of an asymptomatic AAA.

Other studies that have been used to identify or size popliteal aneurysms include magnetic resonance imaging (MRI) and computed tomography (CT). Both are accurate but are more expensive than ultrasound. Arteriography is not a good technique for aneurysm identification because only the flow lumen is visualized, which can result in an underestimation of the size of a thrombus-containing aneurysm. It is also important to obtain ankle-brachial indices (ABIs) to determine whether significant atheroembolization or atherosclerosis exists in the tibial outflow arteries.

(C) Symptomatic aneurysms can present with chronic or acute thromboembolic complications. Many patients present with chronic calf claudication similar to that caused by atherosclerotic occlusive disease. However, acute thrombosis of the aneurysm can present with limb-threatening ischemia that warrants emergent intervention if limb loss is to be avoided. Although large aneurysms rarely rupture, they can cause a mass effect in the popliteal fossa and result in leg swelling due to compression of the popliteal vein.

Although several studies have suggested that aneurysms pose increased thromboembolic risk as they enlarge, this has not been confirmed in the majority of studies, and small aneurysms may still cause these sequelae, especially if they are found to contain thrombus on an ultrasound study.

Acute symptoms typically result from thrombosis of the aneurysm or sudden embolization, both of which result in distal ischemia. The patient frequently presents with abrupt onset of a cool, pulseless leg from the knee down. The differential diagnosis in this situation usually includes embolic events of cardiac origin and thrombosis of preexisting atherosclerotic disease. The differential diagnosis can often be refined with history and physical examination. The contralateral leg should be carefully examined, since an aneurysm here increases the probability of an ipsilateral aneurysm. In contrast, normal contralateral pulse findings suggest an embolus of cardiac origin, whereas a chronically absent pulse suggests that the patient's symptoms may be due to thrombosis of preexisting atherosclerotic disease.

Chronic symptoms from popliteal aneurysms may also be due to recurrent embolic events with subsequent gradual occlusion of the tibial outflow arteries. This presents as chronic ischemia of the affected limb and is often manifested by calf claudication similar to that of atherosclerotic occlusive disease involving these arteries.

(D) Asymptomatic patients with aneurysms smaller than 2 cm in diameter that contain no thrombus or patients at high surgical risk because of medical co-morbidities should be monitored with serial duplex ultrasonography every 6 to 12 months.

(E) Patients with aneurysms greater than 2 cm in diameter or with smaller-diameter aneurysms that contain thrombus are at increased risk for symptoms and should be considered for surgical therapy. It is expected that symptoms will occur in 36% to 57% of patients who initially present with an asymptomatic popliteal artery aneurysm.[2,3] Michaels and Galland have used a Markov decision analysis model to determine the criteria for treatment of asymptomatic popliteal aneurysms.[4] These investigators have found that asymptomatic patients with a popliteal artery aneurysm should undergo surgical repair. However, the advantages of surgical repair are maintained only if the operative mortality is less than 2% to 3% and if the chance of symptom development is greater than 10% per year. These authors conclude that at present there is a significant difference between nonsurgical and surgical therapy in favor of elective surgical treatment for most patients.

(F) Arteriography is usually performed in patients with a symptomatic popliteal artery aneurysm whether the symptoms are acute or chronic. In addition, arteriography is indicated in patients who are being considered for surgery for asymptomatic aneurysms whose ABI is below 0.9. The purpose of arteriography is not only to assess the extent of the aneurysm but also to identify a potential distal target for bypass. Alternative im-

POPLITEAL ARTERY ANEURYSM

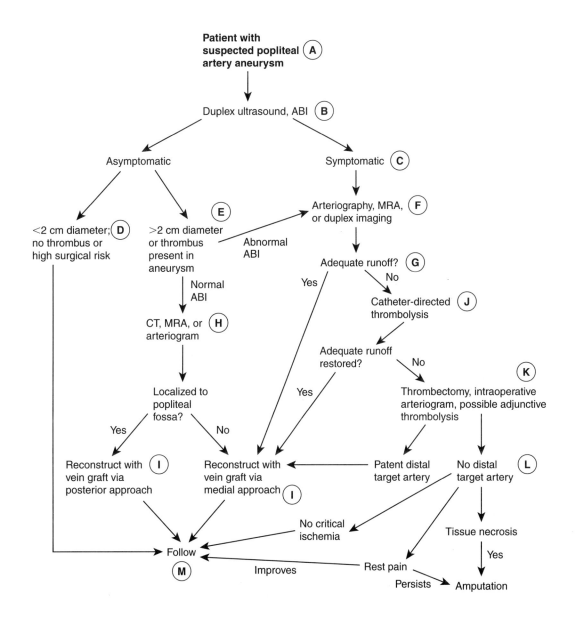

Popliteal Artery Aneurysm (continued)

aging modalities may be needed for patients at risk for renal failure as a result of contrast agents. These include carbon dioxide arteriography, magnetic resonance arteriography (MRA), and duplex arteriography. The choice of modality is commonly based on local expertise and experience.

(G) If adequate runoff is identified on the arteriogram (i.e., either a below-knee popliteal artery or a tibial artery in continuity to the foot), the surgeon can then proceed with reconstruction of the aneurysm with a vein graft. If the arteriogram indicates inadequate runoff with no distal tibial artery suitable for bypass, the surgeon should consider thrombolytic therapy (see J).

(H) In asymptomatic patients with normal ABIs, we have found that a spiral CT scan usually provides sufficient information to plan surgical repair without arteriography. This is often supplemented by duplex scanning. It is important to define the proximal and distal extent of the aneurysm, especially when one is planning to use a posterior approach. However, MRA/MRI or contrast arteriography can also define the extent of the aneurysm and is preferred by many for preoperative evaluation of all popliteal aneurysms.

(I) Aneurysms limited to the popliteal fossa can be considered for reconstruction with the use of the lesser saphenous vein and a posterior approach to the popliteal fossa. Patients with aneurysms that extend either proximally or distally out of the popliteal fossa should be considered for reconstruction using a vein graft and a medial approach. In either instance, the aneurysm needs to be excluded above and below the popliteal fossa or, in the case of the posterior approach, with endoaneurysmorrhaphy. In the absence of adequate greater saphenous vein, other autogenous vein (e.g., the lesser saphenous or an arm vein) may be used. Prosthetic material may be used in the absence of autogenous vein, especially if the required bypass is short.

(J) In acute situations when limb-threatening ischemia exists as a result of a thrombosed popliteal artery aneurysm and no runoff can be identified, preoperative thrombolysis has been suggested by several groups as a technique to lyse thrombus in the infrageniculate vessels to provide outflow for a bypass. The largest series has been reported by Carpenter and coworkers.[5] These investigators treated seven patients with complete thrombosis of both the aneurysm and all runoff arteries with preoperative thrombolytic therapy in an attempt to open a distal tibial artery suitable for bypass grafting. These patients showed significantly improved graft patency and limb salvage when compared with similar patients treated by emergency operation that included tibial artery thrombectomy and attempted bypass.

In the Carpenter study,[5] the mean time to complete thrombolysis was 29 hours; however, the mean time to reperfusion for adequate limb salvage was much shorter than this. One of the additional benefits of thrombolysis appeared to be a more gradual reperfusion of the lower extremity; as a result, no episodes of compartment syndrome occurred in these patients. Other considerations in the future may include the use of various rheolytic thrombectomy catheters in order to open tibial arteries to identify a target vessel in the acute setting.

In patients who present with acute limb ischemia with associated motor and sensory compromise, there may not be sufficient time to revascularize the lower extremity using catheter-directed therapy. In these situations, consideration should be given to operative exploration of the below-knee popliteal artery, tibial thrombectomy, and intraoperative arteriography. Following thrombectomy, bypass to the thrombectomized vessel can be performed.[6]

(K) If thrombolysis is not available or unsuccessful, the below-knee popliteal artery should be explored, with either mechanical thrombectomy of the tibial vessels using a balloon or rheolytic thrombectomy catheter, or intraoperative thrombolysis. Following this measure, intraoperative arteriography may be used to identify a distal tibial target vessel to perform the necessary bypass.

(L) If no distal tibial target artery can be identified after intraoperative thrombectomy, thrombolysis, and arteriography, bypass attempts are unlikely to be successful. Consideration can be given to blind exploration of pedal arteries; in our experience, however, this has not yielded a vessel suitable for bypass if it was not identified on operative arteriography or preoperative duplex examination. Patients with critical leg ischemia may require amputation, whereas patients without signs of critical ischemia may be observed initially.

(M) Follow-up of patients with popliteal artery aneurysms includes serial ultrasound examinations every 6 months with ABIs, since 35% of the patient population experiences claudication symptoms from embolization that reduce the ABI.[3] If symptoms develop or the size of the aneurysm increases significantly, repair should be undertaken.

REFERENCES

1. Whitehouse WM, Wakefield TW, Graham LM, et al: Limb-threatening potential of arteriosclerotic popliteal artery aneurysms. Surgery 1983;93:694–699.
2. Dawson I, van Bockel JH, Brand R, et al: Popliteal artery aneurysms: Long-term follow-up of aneurysmal disease and results of surgical treatment. J Vasc Surg 1991;13:398–407.
3. Szilagyi DE, Schwartz RL, Reddy DJ: Popliteal artery aneurysms: Their natural history and management. Arch Surg 1981;116:724–728.
4. Michaels JA, Galland RB: Management of asymptomatic popliteal aneurysms: The use of a Markov decision tree to determine the criteria for a conservative approach. Eur J Vasc Surg 1993;7:136–143.
5. Carpenter JP, Barker CF, Roberts B, et al: Popliteal artery aneurysms: Current management and outcome. J Vasc Surg 1994;19:65–73.
6. Dormandy JA, Rutherford RB, and the TASC (Trans-Atlantic Intersociety Consensus) Working Group: Management of peripheral arterial disease (PAD). J Vasc Surg 2000;31:S151–158.

POPLITEAL ARTERY ANEURYSM

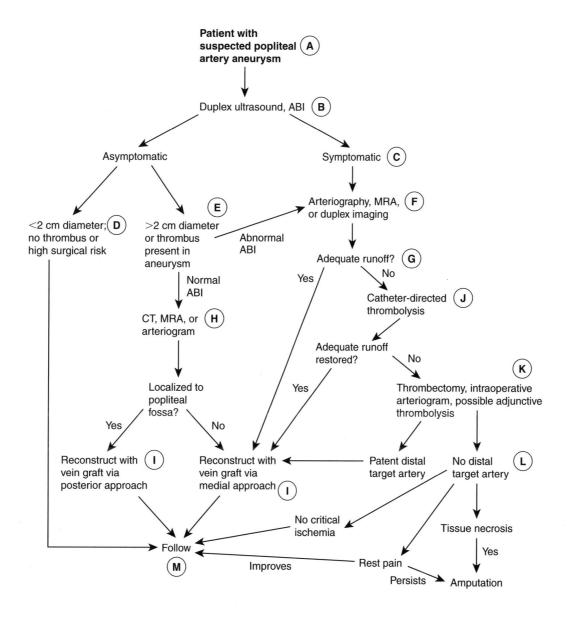

Chapter 33 Hepatic and Renal Artery Aneurysms

GERALD B. ZELENOCK, MD

Hepatic Artery Aneurysm

(A) Hepatic artery aneurysms are the second most common splanchnic aneurysm.[1,2] They account for approximately 20% of aneurysms within the splanchnic circulation and are being recognized more frequently in contemporary experience secondary to the widespread use of advanced imaging techniques, such as computed tomography (CT) and magnetic resonance imaging/angiography (MRI/MRA). The male-to-female ratio is approximately 2:1. Generally, hepatic artery aneurysms occur in older patients but post-traumatic pseudoaneurysms are seen in younger patients.

(B) CT or MRI can be used to confirm the presence of and to determine the size of hepatic artery aneurysms. For preoperative planning, however, the precise location of the aneurysm should be determined with selective hepatic arteriography or MRA. In the case of a ruptured hepatic artery aneurysm, the urgency of the clinical presentation clearly influences the extent of imaging possible. A rapid-sequence spiral CT scan usually establishes the diagnosis sufficient for emergent surgical treatment.

(C) Most hepatic artery aneurysms are asymptomatic and are discovered incidentally at the time of an imaging study. Some hepatic artery aneurysms cause such symptoms as right upper quadrant or epigastric pain. If these aneurysms are large, they may occasionally compress the bile duct and cause obstructive jaundice. Rupture of larger aneurysms can also occur, either into one of the major biliary ducts presenting as hemobilia, or into the peritoneal cavity, causing hypotension and shock. All symptomatic hepatic artery aneurysms should be considered for repair, with rupture demanding emergent treatment.[1-3]

(D) The likelihood of rupture of asymptomatic hepatic artery aneurysm has not been accurately determined. In addition to larger size, rapid expansion and hypertension probably increase rupture risk. In general, elective repair of asymptomatic hepatic artery aneurysms is considered when they exceed 2 cm diameter.[1,2]

(E) Observation of small hepatic artery aneurysms involves (1) periodic assessment of size with an appropriate imaging study, and (2) checking for any relevant symptoms that might stimulate elective repair.[4]

(F) Surgical risk must be assessed and balanced against aneurysm rupture risk, with the context of life expectancy considered for each patient.

(G) A major consideration during planning hepatic artery aneurysm treatment is the location of the aneurysm, especially whether it is intrahepatic or extrahepatic.[1-3] Intrahepatic aneurysms can be ligated with open surgical techniques, but substantial hepatic resection may be required simply to exclude the aneurysm. Because of this, endovascular techniques that also obliterate the aneurysm without requiring hepatic resection are preferred unless the aneurysm involves a very proximal (and more surgically accessible) hepatic artery branch that might benefit from surgical reconstruction to avoid ischemic injury to a large hepatic segment. Given a normal portal circulation, however, such ischemic injury is uncommon; thus, most intrahepatic aneurysms are optimally managed by obliterative endovascular techniques.

(H) Both endovascular and traditional surgical treatments of hepatic artery aneurysms require the operator to keep in mind the relatively common anatomic variants in the hepatic circulation, including replaced right or left hepatic arteries, which may occur in 15% to 20% of patients. Endovascular treatment of hepatic artery aneurysms is usually obliterative and depends on reliable proximal and distal occlusion of the aneurysm and all feeding branches.[5-7] Selective and subselective catheterization of intrahepatic hepatic artery arcades, followed by deployment of coils, absorbable gelatin sponge (Gelfoam), or other obliterative material, is usually successful in the treatment of such aneurysms.

(I) Surgical treatment of extrahepatic artery aneurysm depends on their location and the extent of collateral circulation. Because of the excellent collateral circulation involving the common hepatic artery, aneurysms in this location can usually be simply ligated. Test clamping can be performed and the liver inspected if there is any question about this. If ischemic changes are seen, the surgeon can repair the common hepatic artery aneurysm by inline vascular reconstruction utilizing an autogenous saphenous vein or a prosthetic conduit. Since most common hepatic artery aneurysms can be ligated, they may also be treated by endovascular obliteration if it is possible to localize the obliteration to this segment of the artery.

Proper hepatic artery aneurysms are not as well collateralized and most often require direct arterial reconstruction with an autogenous saphenous vein or prosthetic bypass graft. In general, the more peripheral in the extrahepatic circulation, the more likely that reconstruction will be required. Occasionally, because of the dual blood supply to the liver from both the hepatic arterial circulation and the portal venous circulation, ligation of the proper hepatic artery is acceptable. Simple intraoperative test clamping for a period of 5 to 10 minutes can usually establish the safety of hepatic artery ligation.

REFERENCES

1. Stanley JC, Thompson NW, Fry WJ: Splanchnic artery aneurysms. Arch Surg 1970;101:689.
2. Zelenock GB, Stanley JC: Splanchnic artery aneurysms. In Rutherford RB (ed): Vascular Surgery, 5th ed. Philadelphia, WB Saunders, 2000.
3. Lumsden AB, Mattar SG, Allen RC, Bacha EA: Hepatic artery aneurysms: The management of 22 patients. J Surg Res 1996;60:345–350.
4. Athey PA, Sax SL, Lamki N, Cadavid G: Sonography in the diagnosis of hepatic artery aneurysms. AJR Am J Roentgenol 1986;147:725.
5. Baker JS, Tisnado J, Cho SR, Beachley MC: Splanchnic artery aneurysms and pseudoaneurysms: Transcatheter embolization. Radiology 1987;163:135.
6. Goldblatt M, Goldin AR, Shaff MI: Percutaneous embolization for the management of hepatic artery aneurysms. Gastroenterology 1977;73:1142.
7. Jonsson K, Bjernstad A, Eriksson B: Treatment of a hepatic artery aneurysm by coil occlusion of the hepatic artery. Am J Roentgenol 1980;134:1245.

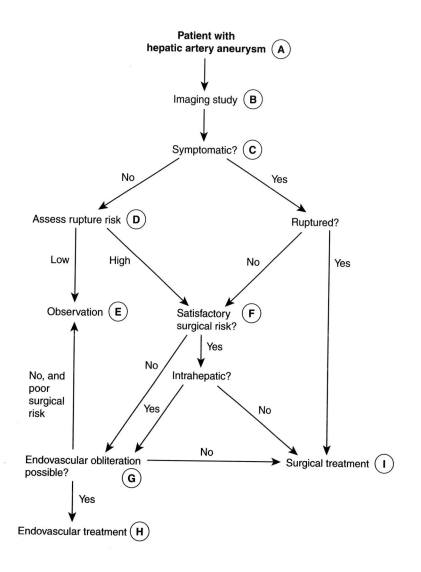

Hepatic and Renal Artery Aneurysms (continued)

Renal Artery Aneurysm

(A) True renal artery aneurysms are uncommon.[1-3] Their incidence in the general population is approximately 0.09%. Their clinical significance is still controversial and may be overestimated by reports that describe operative rather than population-based experience. Similarly, many clinical reports do not make distinctions between true renal artery aneurysms, renal artery dissecting aneurysms, aneurysmal dilations associated with medial fibrodysplastic disease, and arteritis-related and vasculitis-related aneurysms.[3-5] True renal artery aneurysms affect women slightly more than men (1.2:1); however, this probably reflects the inclusion of patients with arterial fibrodysplasia, since there is no obvious gender predilection when such patients are excluded.

Renal artery aneurysms are usually saccular and are located at bifurcations of the renal artery. Approximately 90% are extraparenchymal, with 75% occurring at first-order or second-order renal artery branches.

(B) CT, MRI, or ultrasound studies can be used to confirm the presence and to assess the size of renal artery aneurysms. For preoperative planning, however, the precise location of a renal artery aneurysm should be determined with selective renal arteriography or MRA. With a ruptured renal artery aneurysm, the urgency of the clinical presentation clearly influences the extent of imaging possible. A rapid-sequence spiral CT scan can usually establish the diagnosis sufficient for emergent surgical treatment.

(C) Most renal artery aneurysms are asymptomatic. They may be discovered as a flank calcification on a plain film of the abdomen or may be identified by other imaging studies performed for unrelated reasons. Uncommonly, emboli from renal artery aneurysms can cause enough renal infarction to incite flank pain. However, patients with a ruptured renal artery aneurysm exhibit acute flank and abdominal pain and, eventually, hemodynamic instability. These patients require emergent surgical repair.

Rupture is the most dreaded complication of a renal artery aneurysm. However, the reported cumulative rupture incidence of 3% is probably overstated because of the tendency to cite surgical reports rather than population-based experiences. In surgical series, the mortality rate for rupture is fully 10%; for loss of a kidney, it is nearly 100%.

Renal artery aneurysms discovered during pregnancy are an exception to the generally accepted benign nature of most bland aneurysms. Ruptures in a pregnant woman do not seem to be associated with age, uncontrolled blood pressure, or the number of pregnancies; with rupture, however, they are associated with a 55% maternal mortality rate and an 85% fetal mortality rate.

(D) Whether a renal artery aneurysm itself is the cause of hypertension is debatable. Several mechanisms whereby such aneurysms may cause hypertension have been identified. Embolization of aneurysmal contents, specifically intra-aneurysmal thrombus, or thrombotic occlusion of the adjacent renal artery may cause renal ischemia and renovascular hypertension. Furthermore, compression or kinking of a perianeurysmal renal artery may cause flow reduction and may produce renovascular hypertension, as may a web-like stenosis in the renal artery.

Some believe that small renal artery aneurysms are manifestations of, or exacerbated by, poststenotic dilatation that occurs in conjunction with such web-like stenosis. Whether the renovascular hypertension is secondary to the aneurysm or is simply associated with it, fully 80% of patients with renal artery macroaneurysms are hypertensive.

Poorly controlled hypertension is an indication for repair of renal artery aneurysms because the aneurysm may be contributing to the hypertension and hypertension increases the rupture risk. Not infrequently, small renal artery aneurysms are discovered during evaluation of renovascular hypertension and are treated during the surgical procedure performed to correct the more proximal renal artery stenosis.

(E) An accepted indication for repair of renal artery aneurysms is embolization of thrombus contained within the aneurysm, for this can occlude distal arteries and may reduce renal function.

(F) In the absence of hypertension or renal emboli, the other indication for elective repair of renal artery aneurysms is prevention of rupture. It is important to acknowledge that increased risk of rupture in large aneurysms has not been clearly proven in the clinical literature; as with other aneurysms, however, size is considered the best potential predictor of rupture. There is considerable debate about an appropriate diameter threshold at which to recommend repair, but my colleagues and I begin to consider prophylactic treatment when the diameter exceeds 1.5 cm.

Rupture risk is also increased during pregnancy, such that all but the smallest aneurysms discovered during pregnancy should probably undergo repair at that time. Rapid expansion likely increases rupture risk, but the extent of calcium in the aneurysm wall has not been linked to rupture risk. Rupture risk must also be balanced against surgical risk, in the context of life expectancy, before aneurysm repair can be recommended in an individual patient.

(G) Observation of small renal artery aneurysms entails follow-up of three clinical parameters: (1) size of the aneurysm, (2) the presence or absence of hypertension, and (3) renal function. Increasing size, poorly controlled hypertension, or loss of renal function suggesting embolization should prompt reevaluation of the benefit of surgical repair.

(H) Surgical risk must be assessed and balanced against the risk of aneurysm rupture, taken in the context of life expectancy for each patient.

(I) Aneurysmorrhaphy, saphenous vein patch, and/or aortorenal bypass are preferred techniques for repair of renal artery aneurysms.[2] The saccular nature of the aneurysm and its location at branch points commonly lend themselves to aneurysm excision and aneurysmorrhaphy. Saphenous vein bypass to the level of the first-order or second-order branches is an alternative technique familiar to most vascular surgeons.

Nephrectomy is used as the last resort because the goal of surgical therapy is to eliminate the aneurysm without loss of the kidney or compromise of its function. In the event of massive hemorrhage or with large or functionally important aneurysms, however, nephrectomy may occasionally be required.

Endovascular treatment of renal artery aneurysms has been reported.[6,7] Embolization or occlusion of the aneurysm and covered stent grafts have been employed with apparent good results, although anecdotal initial reports are too few to suggest treatment guidelines at this time.

REFERENCES

1. Stanley JC, Rhodes EL, Gewertz BL, et al: Renal artery aneurysms: Significance of macroaneurysms exclusive of dissections and fibrodysplastic mural dilations. Arch Surg 1975;110:1327.
2. Stanley JC: Natural history of renal artery stenosis and aneurysms. In Calligaro KD, Dougherty MJ, Dean RH (eds): Modern Management of Renovascular Hypertension and Renal Salvage. Baltimore, Williams & Wilkins, 1996, p 15.
3. Lumsden AB, Salam TA, Walton KG: Renal artery aneurysm: A report of 28 cases. Cardiovasc Surg 1996;4:185.
4. Martin RS III, Meacham PW, Ditesheim JA, et al: Renal artery aneurysm: Selective treatment for hypertension and prevention of rupture. J Vasc Surg 1989;9:26.
5. Panayiotopoulos YP, Assadourian R, Taylor PR: Aneurysms of the visceral and renal arteries. Ann R Coll Surg Engl 1996;78:412.
6. Bui BT, Oliva VL, Leclerc G, et al: Renal artery aneurysm: Treatment with percutaneous placement of a stent-graft. Radiology 1995;195:181.
7. Klein GE, Szolar DH, Breinl E, et al: Endovascular treatment of renal artery aneurysm with conventional non-detachable microcoils and Guglielmi detachable coils. Br J Urol 1997;79:852.

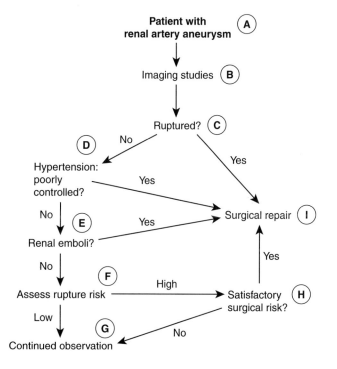

EXTREMITY OCCLUSIVE DISEASE

Chapter 34 Patients with Leg Pain While Walking

MARTHA McDANIEL, MD

A In most cases, arteriogenic claudication as a cause of leg pain while a person is walking can be diagnosed by history alone according to the criteria developed by Geoffrey Rose and adopted by the World Health Organization[1] (see algorithm). Sensitivity of the criteria for identifying patients with arterial occlusive disease is not relevant in this algorithm, since patients enter the algorithm by reporting leg pain while walking. However, the specificity of the Rose criteria is excellent[2] and only about 1% of patients with arteriogenic claudication do not meet the listed criteria. The most common reasons that patients with true arteriogenic claudication do not respond to these questions in the expected manner include (1) irreproducibility of symptoms with exercise and promptness of relief with rest (perhaps both related to other systemic factors such as variation in cardiac output or mood), and (2) having symptoms of fatigue (or "giving out") rather than symptoms of pain.

B Other conditions that lead to leg pain during walking can complicate the differential diagnosis. Most common among these are:

- Neurogenic claudication (secondary to nerve compression, irritation)
- Arthritis of the hip or knee
- Neuropathic pain (due to intrinsic neuropathy)
- Fatigue of muscular deconditioning

Although the sensation of calf cramping experienced by patients with either neurogenic or arteriogenic claudication may be similar, pain stemming from the former cause is frequently present when the patient is standing still or sitting and may be relieved by a change in position (e.g., stooping over). Localized pain in the back is also common in neurogenic claudication. If the objective lower extremity arterial examination of choice (Doppler pressures or pulse volume recording) yields normal findings at rest, treadmill testing may be useful in differentiating neurogenic from arteriogenic claudication.

Patients are usually able to localize the pain of arthritis to the affected joint and not to the calf or buttock. Arthritic pain is often present at rest and may be worse after a period of immobilization (after sleep or prolonged sitting).

Neuropathic pain, most often seen in conjunction with diabetes but also due to chronic alcohol ingestion and other systemic diseases, is frequently present at rest, is associated with diminished tactile sensation, is bilateral, and may be present in the upper extremities. It tends to progress from distal to proximal extremities and is thus likely to be worse in the foot than in the calf. It is not made worse with exercise. Neuropathic pain is more frequently confused with ischemic rest pain (see Chapter 35) than with arteriogenic claudication.

Some patients report fatigue rather than pain as their primary symptom of arterial insufficiency when walking. Objective testing is useful in distinguishing patients who are suffering from muscular deconditioning from patients with true claudication.

Patients may have any of these confusing conditions concomitantly with true arteriogenic claudication. Accurate attribution of the degree to which symptoms are related to one, as opposed to the other, is the mark of a seasoned clinician and can be quite difficult.

C Ischemic ulceration and/or gangrene may develop in a patient with claudication; this causes them to be moved into the chronic critical ischemia category, which is managed differently (see Chapter 35). However, not all skin ulcers are ischemic or fail to heal because of ischemia. Skin ulcers occur when the skin cannot remain intact in its environment, but a difficult environment (i.e., trauma or pressure or both) may contribute to the development of an ulcer. Venous, arterial, neurotrophic, and traumatic ulcers are the most common types. Ulcers due primarily to arterial insufficiency are most frequently found on the distal extremity (toes or forefoot), do not exhibit active granulation, and usually occur in conjunction with ischemic rest pain. Chronic venous insufficiency or diabetic neuropathy may coexist with arterial disease. In this case, minor trauma may precipitate an ulcer that fails to heal because of either arterial or venous insufficiency or because of the absence of protective sensation.

Although many factors contribute to ulcer healing, an adequate oxygen supply by the circulation at the site of ulceration is always a requirement for healing. Spontaneously appearing lesions in the foot can usually be expected to heal if the ankle arterial pressure is above 50 to 80 mmHg or if the toe pressure exceeds 30 mmHg.[3] By extrapolation of data obtained from foot ulcerations,[4] lesions in other parts of the lower extremity can generally be expected to heal if $TcPo_2$ exceeds 30 mmHg.

D At this point in the algorithm, the diagnosis of arteriogenic claudication has been made. The most common cause of this in most Western populations is atherosclerosis, which is a systemic disease. Complications of atherosclerosis in arterial beds outside the lower extremities cause most of the excess deaths in claudicants, who die at a rate of roughly 7% per year.[5] Regardless of the treatment offered for arteriogenic claudication, systemic risk factor control is a primary goal because it may decrease not only the progression of disease in the lower extremities but the risk of death from systemic atherosclerotic complications.

Diabetes, smoking, and hypertension are recognized to be associated with an increased risk of death and of disease progression in the lower extremities. Limited data are available concerning the efficacy and cost-effectiveness of risk factor modification in improving health for claudicants, but a consensus is emerging, by extrapolation from extensive study of patients with coronary artery disease, that these factors as well as hyper-

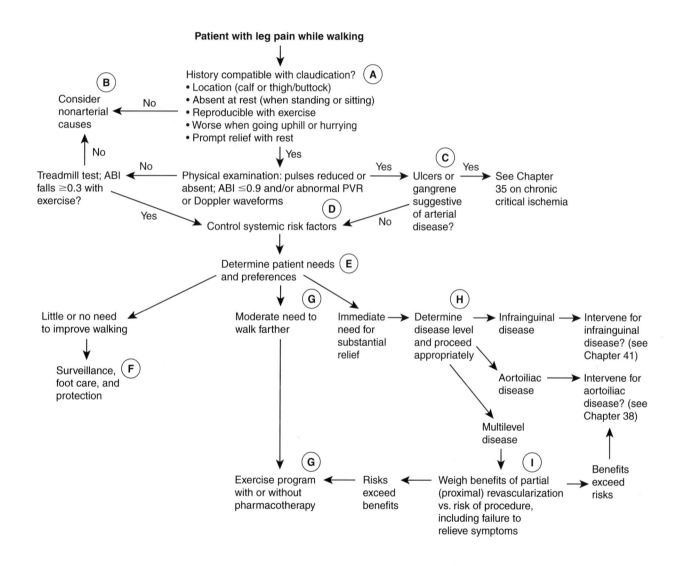

cholesterolemia should be controlled if possible (see Chapter 2, which covers management of hyperlipidemia). Addition of an antiplatelet agent to the medical regimen also reduces the frequency of secondary cardiovascular events.[6] Smoking cessation is most likely to occur in the context of a special program.[7]

There is no clear consensus among physicians as to whether specific treatment should be offered for claudication if a patient continues to smoke. The likelihood that a patient will be successful in quitting smoking, the degree of his or her disability, and local practice patterns all play a role in this decision. Pain-free walking distance may not improve on cessation of smoking,[8] and it is therefore unwise to predict such a benefit with smoking cessation.

(E) Patients' life circumstances and co-morbidities combine to help dictate their needs and preferences concerning specific therapy for claudication. The degree of walking impairment and systemic disability may be determined by questionnaire (e.g., Walking Impairment Questionnaire [WIQ],[9] Short-Form Health Survey [SF-36][10]), interview, or quantitative testing such as on the treadmill. Ultimately, however, the patient's needs can usually be categorized into one of three groups (see algorithm). The time period over which the patient would like to see a change in walking ability, the change in pain-free walking distance that would make a clinical difference, and the amount of time a patient is willing or able to devote to the chosen therapy should all enter into the decision.

(F) Patients who are content with their present pain-free walking distance or those who may not benefit from specific treatment of claudication (such as those who are equally limited in walking by exertional dyspnea) may still benefit from control of systemic risk factors (see D). In addition, they may benefit from receiving reassurance that the natural history of their condition as it affects their lower extremities is relatively benign.[5] Most patients in this category also need to know how they can affect this natural history, including appropriate preventive care of their compromised feet. This knowledge is particularly important for patients with very poor lower extremity perfusion in whom healing of a traumatic lesion would be unlikely if one occurred.

(G) Patients with a moderate walking disability or a moderate need to walk farther are the ideal candidates for a trial of an exercise program or drug therapy. The choice among these alternatives may be influenced by the availability of a structured exercise program in the local community, possible systemic benefits of exercise, the amount of time the individual is willing or able to devote to treatment, concurrent co-morbidities, and drug sensitivities.

In the United States today, only two drugs (pentoxifylline and cilostazol) have been approved by the Food and Drug Administration (FDA) for use in patients with claudication. Of the two, cilostazol appears more likely to yield a clinically significant increase in walking distance in most patients.[11, 12]

Patients who pursue a walking-based exercise program, in general, can expect to double their baseline pain-free walking distance. Success has been greater with supervised exercise than with home-based programs.[13] Full utilization of such programs has been limited by the facts that (1) most major health insurers do not presently reimburse the costs of *supervised* exercise programs for claudication and (2) such programs are not widely available.

(H) Determining the levels (aortoiliac, infrainguinal, multilevel) of arterial occlusive disease is generally straightforward with the aid of segmental limb pressures and Doppler waveforms or segmental pulse volume recording. Situations in which these tests might be misleading or difficult to interpret include (1) iliac artery disease, in which femoral waveforms may fail to reflect hemodynamically significant iliac disease,[14] and (2) definitive detection of a second lesion if a highly hemodynamically significant lesion is present at a more proximal level. A physician's level of suspicion for inaccuracies in these relatively simple tests must be high if the clinical history is incompatible with the objective findings.

Increasingly, physicians rely on noninvasive tests to define the degree and location of occlusive lesions. Experience is accumulating with the use of duplex examination as the sole study prior to anatomic intervention.[15] Nevertheless, most surgeons still employ arteriography once the decision is made to intervene with open or endovascular surgery.

When infrainguinal disease is the cause of claudication, more controversy exists as to the appropriateness of anatomic intervention than for aortoiliac disease. In the case of infrainguinal disease, axial arterial lesions are long and occlusive and percutaneous intervention is unlikely to be durable; aortoiliac disease, in contrast, is often focal and can be well treated with endovascular techniques. Thus, for infrainguinal disease, surgical bypass is usually required, with its attendant risks and complications.[16] In this setting, the possible benefits of drug and/or exercise treatment should be reconsidered.

(I) In the presence of hemodynamically significant multilevel occlusive disease, anatomic intervention is complex. One must consider the relative contributions of each level of occlusive disease to the overall reduction in flow and the likelihood of clinical success after proximal revascularization alone as well as the morbidity and mortality of the contemplated procedures, given the patient's co-morbidities. A risk-benefit analysis must be settled in the patient's interest and with the patient's full understanding. Segmental limb pressures and Doppler waveforms or segmental pulse volume recording usually allow an estimate of the extent to which symptoms can be attributed to aortoiliac disease or to infrainguinal disease. The magnitude of expected improvement from treatment of the inflow (aortoiliac) component can be estimated and compared with the patient's

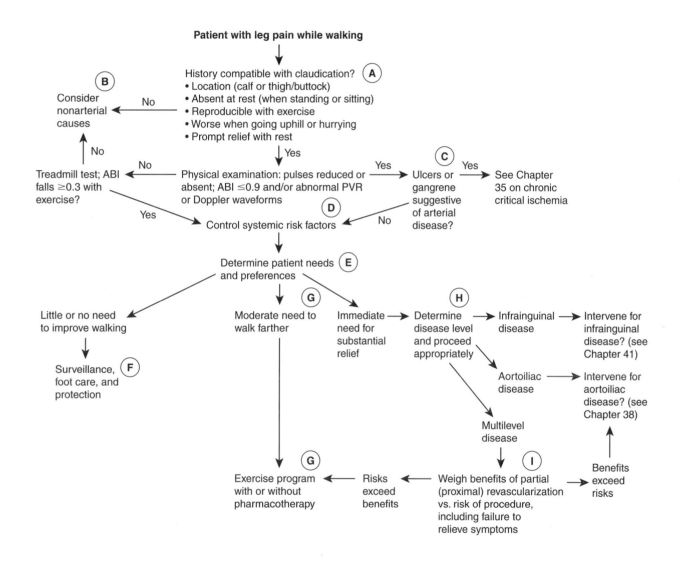

needs and preferences. If complex or open multilevel intervention would be required to achieve the patient's goals, careful consideration is required. In this circumstance, many patients and physicians would opt for a trial of drug and/or exercise therapy.

REFERENCES

1. Rose G: The diagnosis of ischaemic heart pain and intermittent claudication in field surveys. Bull WHO 1962; 27:645–658.
2. Criqui M, Fronek A, Klauber M, et al: The sensitivity, specificity, and predictive value of traditional clinical evaluation of peripheral arterial disease: Results from noninvasive testing in a defined population. Circulation 1985; 71:516–522.
3. Wutschert R, Bounameaux H: Predicting healing of arterial leg ulcers by segmental systolic pressure measurements. Vasa 1998;27:224–228.
4. Ballard J, Eke C, Bunt T, Killeen J: A prospective evaluation of transcutaneous oxygen measurements in the management of diabetic foot problems. J Vasc Surg 1995; 22:485–490.
5. McDaniel M, Cronenwett J: Basic data related to the natural history of intermittent claudication. Ann Vasc Surg 1989;3:273–277.
6. Secondary prevention of vascular disease by prolonged antiplatelet treatment: Antiplatelet Trialists' Collaboration. Br Med J (Clin Res) 1988;296:320–331.
7. Hughes J, Goldstein M, Hurt R, Shiffman S: Recent advances in the pharmacotherapy of smoking. JAMA 1999;281:72–76.
8. Girolami B, Bernardi E, Prins M, et al: Treatment of intermittent claudication with physical training, smoking cessation, pentoxiphylline, or nafronyl: A meta-analysis. Arch Intern Med 1999;159:337–345.
9. Regensteiner J, Steiner J, Panzer R, Hiatt W: Evaluation of walking ability by questionnaire in patients with peripheral arterial disease. J Vasc Med Biol 1990;2:142–152.
10. Ware J, Sherbourne C: The MOS 36-item Short-Form Health Survey (SF-36): I. Conceptual framework and item selection. Med Care 1990;30:473–483.
11. Green R, McNamara J: The effects of pentoxifylline on patients with intermittent claudication. J Vasc Surg 1988;7:356–362.
12. Money S, Herd J, Isaacson J, et al: Effect of cilostazol on walking distances in patient with intermittent claudication caused by peripheral vascular disease. J Vasc Surg 1998;27:267–275.
13. Patterson R, Pinto B, Marcus B, et al: Value of a supervised exercise program for the therapy of intermittent claudication. J Vasc Surg 1997;25:312–319.
14. Currie I, Jones A, Wakely C, et al: Non-invasive aortoiliac assessment. Eur J Vasc Endovasc Surg 1995;9:24–28.
15. Moneta G, Yeager R, Lee R, Porter J: Noninvasive localization of arterial occlusive disease: A comparison of segmental Doppler pressures and arterial duplex mapping. J Vasc Surg 1993;17:578–582.
16. Byrne J, Darling RD III, Chang B, et al: Infrainguinal arterial reconstruction for claudication: Is it worth the risk? An analysis of 409 procedures. J Vasc Surg 1999; 29:259–269.

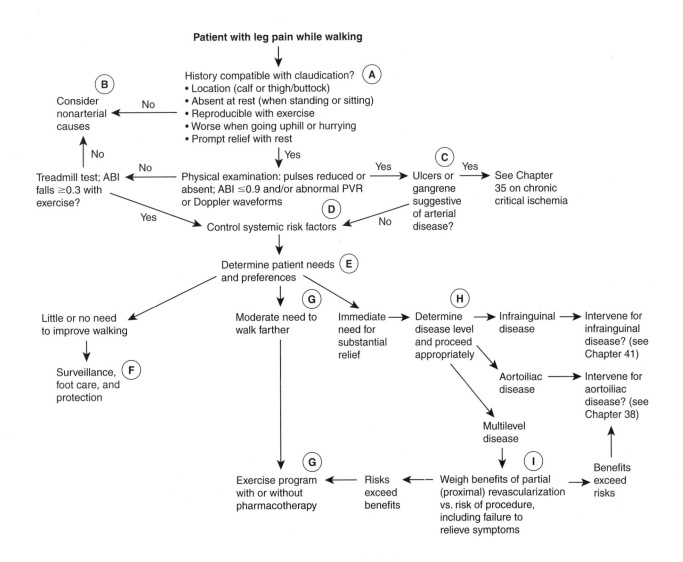

Chapter 35 Chronic Critical Limb Ischemia

JOHN V. WHITE, MD • SCOTT VAN DUZER, MD

A Critical limb ischemia (CLI) results from a reduction in peripheral perfusion to the extent that basal metabolic needs of the tissues are not adequately met. This commonly leads to rest pain, the formation of ischemic ulcers of the toes or forefoot, or ischemic gangrene of these areas. Although the presentation of CLI is frequently obvious, there are causes other than vascular for symptoms of rest pain and leg ulceration that must be considered. Disorders that may cause leg pain include diabetic neuropathy, nerve root compression, and reflex sympathetic dystrophy, whereas ulceration may be induced by venous disease, diabetic neuropathy, and collagen vascular disease.

B There is a subgroup of patients with severely impaired distal perfusion without manifestations of rest pain, ulceration, or ischemic gangrene. Although these patients have an asymptomatic form of chronic CLI, termed *subcritical ischemia*, they are at high risk for rapid deterioration and limb loss after an inciting event, such as minor trauma to the toes or a transient reduction in systemic blood pressure.[1] In a study of 713 patients with CLI who required below-knee amputation, more than half were noted to be without symptoms 6 months or more prior to the required procedure.[2] Although patients with subcritical ischemia do not require interventional therapy, the severity of the distal arterial occlusive disease should be assessed in the noninvasive laboratory and the risk factors for atherosclerosis identified and controlled. These patients should then be placed in surveillance programs.

C After the history is obtained and the physical examination is performed, determination of the ankle pressure and ankle-brachial index (ABI) is the most fundamental diagnostic test for the documentation of chronic CLI. Because heavily calcified distal vessels can yield falsely elevated indices, pulse-volume recordings and/or toe pressures should also be obtained when the clinical suspicion is high. An ankle pressure below 50 mmHg, an index of or below 0.40, or a toe pressure below 30 mm Hg associated with nearly monophasic pulse volume recordings in the foot indicate CLI. The ABI is also the best predictor of mortality from all vascular causes. A patient with an ABI of 0.3 or lower is at increased relative risk for death of 1.8 compared with patients whose ABI is 0.31 or greater.[3]

D Because CLI is associated with severe systemic atherosclerosis, evaluation of risk factors and determination of the presence at other sites of significant occlusive disease are warranted in the patient who has not undergone such an assessment. Risk factor determination with measurement of fasting blood glucose level, cholesterol (total, high-density lipoprotein, and low-density lipoprotein) profile, complete blood count with platelet count, and serum creatinine should be undertaken. Homocysteine levels should be obtained in younger patients with more aggressive forms of arterial occlusive disease.[4] A resting electrocardiogram (ECG) and duplex imaging of the carotid arteries should be performed because of the association of coronary and carotid artery disease in patients with severe peripheral arterial occlusive disease.[5, 6]

E Correction or control of risk factors for arterial occlusive disease is essential for patients with chronic CLI. More than 20% of patients with CLI die within 1 year of presentation and 40% to 70% die within 5 years.[7, 8] Cigarette smoking increases the rate of progression and the severity of peripheral arterial occlusive disease and the amputation rate. Diabetes increases the likelihood of progression of CLI to gangrene.[9] These risk factors should be rigorously addressed.[10]

Although coronary artery disease is likely to be identified in patients with CLI and should warrant the initiation of antiplatelet therapy, intervention *prior to* lower extremity revascularization is often not required.[11] Treatment of ulcers and infection should begin immediately with appropriate therapies, including local wound care, topical antibacterial agents, and systemic antibiotics as needed.

F *Primary* amputation should be considered in patients in whom there is necrosis of significant portions of weight-bearing areas of the foot, a fixed, unremediable flexion contracture of the leg, or other nonvascular condition that makes the limb useless for weight bearing, or a very limited life expectancy due to a terminal illness or comorbid conditions. Even though more aggressive forms of revascularization with myocutaneous reconstruction can be performed, these should be reserved for younger patients and for patients able to withstand the multiple procedures required.[12] The appropriate level and type of amputation is covered in Chapter 46.

G If the limb can be salvaged and can become a useful, weight-bearing extremity and if the patient is an acceptable candidate for intervention, imaging of the inflow and outflow arteries should be undertaken. Because of the diffuse nature of occlusive lesions in these patients, arteriography from the level of the renal arteries to the toes should be performed and pressure gradients of aortic and iliac stenoses determined. Resting gradients of 10 mmHg or more across stenoses should be considered for treatment.

Gadolinium-enhanced magnetic resonance angiography (MRA) has been successfully substituted for conventional angiography as a guide to planning distal reconstruction.[13] Gadolinium can also be used as a contrast agent for the performance of conventional angiography and has the advantage of visualizing small distal vessels without the risk of renal toxicity. Duplex ultrasonography is also being evaluated as an imaging modality to select lesions amenable to specific treatments.

H Lesions most amenable to angioplasty are well delineated, short, noncalcified, symmet-

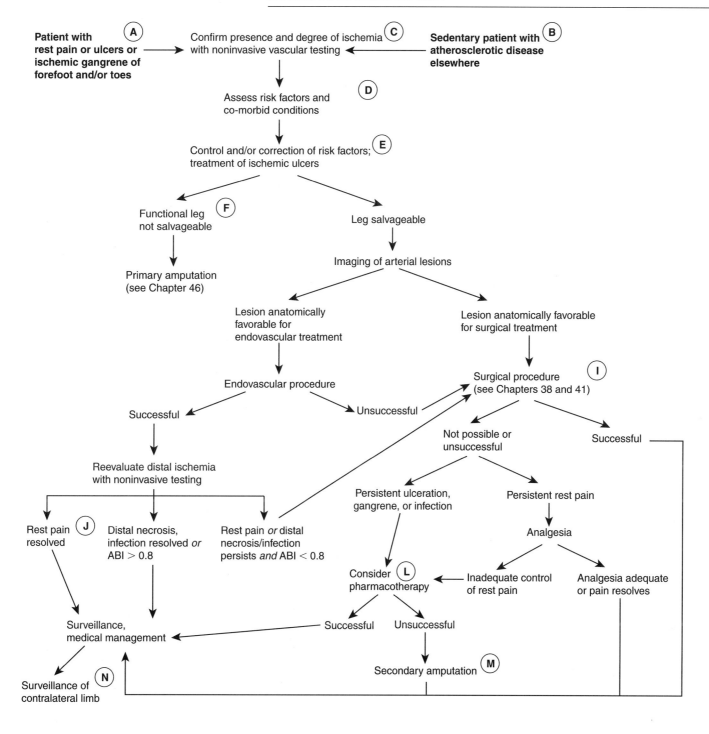

ric iliac stenoses with good outflow. The technical success rate for treatment of these lesions is 79% to 98% and the 5-year patency rates range from 56% to 85% with a 30-day mortality of 0.8% for balloon angioplasty and 1.0% for stent procedures.[14–16] Stents appear to be useful for longer stenoses, occlusions, or external iliac lesions, but long-term follow-up is required to substantiate this impression. Isolated iliac lesions are rarely the sole cause of CLI and, if present, are usually associated with significant occlusive lesions in distal segments. Therefore, while percutaneous transluminal angioplasty (PTA) should be performed for such lesions when found, the overall role and effectiveness of iliac PTA/stenting in these patients is much more limited than in patients with claudication. In most patients with CLI, surgical revascularization is required. Similarly, a short femoropopliteal stenosis or occlusion may be considered for PTA but is rarely found in patients with CLI who have more diffuse disease. In the absence of good outflow and a short stenosis, PTA is of little benefit in patients with CLI who usually require surgical revascularization.[17]

(I) Aortobifemoral bypass is an appropriate procedure for many patients with aortoiliac occlusive disease. This procedure is associated with an overall mortality rate of 3.3%, a morbidity rate of 8.3%, and a 10-year patency of 81.8% (meta-analysis[18]). In the presence of a minimally diseased contralateral aortoiliofemoral arterial tree, unilateral reconstruction is acceptable and may be desirable. A unilateral aortofemoral or iliofemoral bypass may afford better long-term patency than a femorofemoral crossover graft because of unappreciated disease in the donor limb of a crossover graft.[19] Any patent, uncompromised proximal vessel, including the iliac and common, superficial, deep femoral, and popliteal arteries, may serve as the inflow vessel for distal arterial reconstruction. Autogenous vein grafts give excellent results. Prosthetic grafts may be used if autogenous vein is not available, and their patency may be improved by vein cuffs (see Chapters 38 and 41).

(J) Patients who present with recent-onset or only occasional rest pain may experience relief with relatively small incremental increases in distal flow and perfusion pressure. In the setting of hemodynamically significant aortoiliac disease successfully treated, rest pain is relieved in the majority of patients, although some may experience claudication upon ambulation. In the presence of distal tissue necrosis and/or distal infection, a higher perfusion pressure and pulsatile flow to the foot are usually necessary. Therefore, if necrosis and infection persist and the ABI is below 0.8, an infrainguinal bypass procedure should be considered.[20]

(K) All endovascular and surgical interventions for the treatment of CLI should be subject to periodic surveillance to detect deterioration in function. At intervals, patients should be evaluated by history, physical examination, and resting and postexercise ABIs to determine the onset of new symptoms or signs suggestive of recurrent ischemia. Additionally, lower extremity vein bypass grafts should undergo duplex scanning of the entire length of the graft to identify stenotic lesions[21, 22] (see Chapter 42).

(L) Pharmacotherapy for patients with CLI is directed at promoting healing of the areas of distal necrosis and infection. Though many agents have been tried, few have been found to be of use. In some studies, prostanoids have helped to promote healing of ulcers and to reduce the incidence of amputation in the short term.[23] Results have been mixed, however, and these agents are currently not approved for use in the United States. Most agents are more beneficial in patients with only rest pain or superficial ulcers. Topical platelet-derived growth factor may also stimulate healing of ulcers.[24] Gene-induced angiogenesis is being evaluated as a potential treatment in such patients but is only experimental at this time.

(M) Secondary amputation should be performed when endovascular or surgical intervention has failed and reintervention is no longer possible or when the limb continues to deteriorate because of infection or necrosis despite a patent graft. The goals of secondary amputation are (1) relief of ischemic pain; (2) complete removal of diseased, infected, and necrotic tissue; and (3) construction of a stump suitable for ambulation with a prosthesis (see Chapter 46).

(N) Continued surveillance of the contralateral extremity is essential. Progression of arterial occlusive disease causes the loss of the contralateral extremity in approximately 10% of patients each year.[25]

REFERENCES

1. Rutherford RB, Baker JD, Ernst C, et al: Recommended standards for reports dealing with lower extremity ischemia (rev). J Vasc Surg 1997;26:517–538.
2. Dormandy J, Belcher G, Broos P, et al: A prospective study of 713 below-knee amputations for ischaemia. Br J Surg 194;81:33–37.
3. McDermott MM, Feinglass J, Slavensky R, Pearce WH: The ankle-brachial index as a predictor of survival in patients with peripheral vascular disease. J Gen Intern Med 1994;9:445–449.
4. Taylor LM, DeFrang RD, Harris EJ, Porter JM: The association of elevated plasma homocysteine with progression of symptomatic peripheral arterial disease. J Vasc Surg 1991;13:128–136.
5. Alexandrova NA, Gibson WC, Norris JW, Maggisano R. Carotid artery stenosis in peripheral vascular disease. J Vasc Surg 1996; 23:645–649.
6. Nehler MR, Krupski W: Cardiac complications and screening. In Rutherford RB (ed): Vascular Surgery, 5th ed. Philadelphia, WB Saunders, 2000.
7. Ad Hoc Committee on Reporting Standards: Suggested standards for reports dealing with lower extremity ischemia. J Vasc Surg 1986;4:80–94.
8. Criqui MH, Langer RD, Fronek A, et al: Mortality over a period of 10 years in patient with peripheral arterial disease. N Engl J Med 1992;326:381–386.
9. Hirsch AT, Treat-Jacobson D, Lando HA, Hatsukami DK: The role of tobacco cessation, antiplatelet and lipid-lowering therapies in the treatment of peripheral arterial disease. Vasc Med 1997;2:243–251.
10. Kannel WB: Risk factors for atherosclerotic cardiovascular outcomes in different arterial territories. J Cardiovasc Risk 194;1:333–339.

CHRONIC CRITICAL LIMB ISCHEMIA

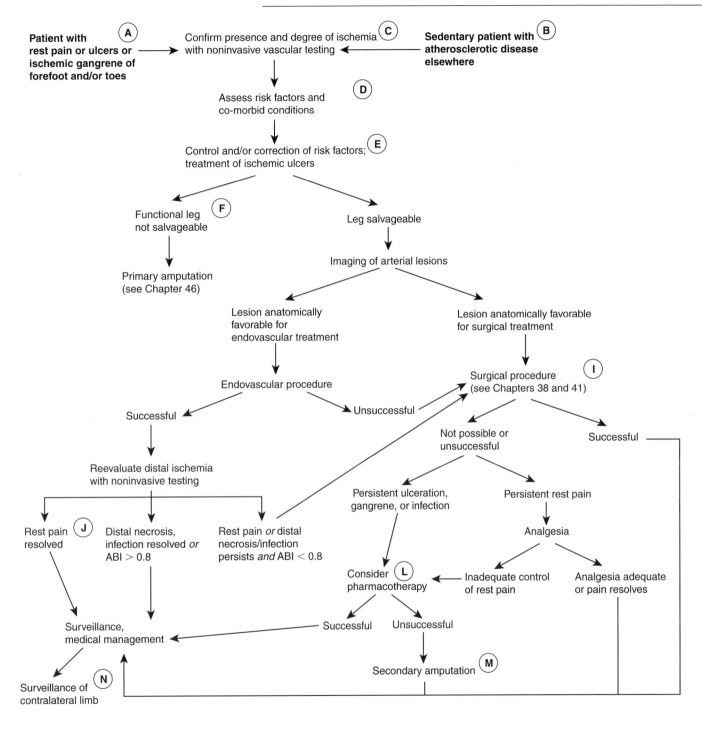

Chronic Critical Limb Ischemia (continued)

11. Taylor LM, Yeager RA, Moneta GL, et al: The incidence of perioperative myocardial infarction in general vascular surgery. Vasc Surg 1992;15:52–61.
12. Isakov E, Budoragin N, Shenav S, et al: Anatomic sites of foot lesions resulting in amputation among diabetics and non-diabetics. Am J Phys Med Rehabil 1995;74:130–133.
13. Cambria R, Kaufman JA, L'Italien GJ, et al: Magnetic resonance angiography in the management of lower extremity arterial occlusive disease: A prospective study. J Vasc Surg 1997;25:380–389.
14. Gupta AK, Ravimandalam K, Roa VRK, et al: Total occlusions of the iliac arteries: Results of balloon angioplasty. Cardiovasc Intervent Radiol 1993;16:165–177.
15. Blum U, Gabelman A, Redecker M, Noeldge G, et al: Percutaneous recanalization of iliac artery occlusions: Results of a prospective study. Radiology 1993;189:536–540.
16. Bosch JL, Hurink MGM: Meta-analysis of the results of percutaneous transluminal angioplasty and stent placement for aortoiliac occlusive disease. Radiology 1997;204:87–96.
17. Jeans WD, Armstrong S, Cole SEA, et al: Fate of patients undergoing transluminal angioplasty for lower-limb ischemia. Radiology 1990;177:559–564.
18. deVries SO, Hunink MGM: Results of aortic bifurcation grafts for aortoiliac occlusive disease: A meta-analysis. J Vasc Surg 1997;26:558–569.
19. Ricco JB: Unilateral iliac artery occlusive disease: A randomized multicenter trial examining direct revascularization versus crossover bypass. Ann Vasc Surg 1992;6:209–219.
20. Berstein EF, Rhodes GA, Stuart SH, et al: Toe pulse-reappearance time in prediction of aortofemoral bypass success. Ann Surg 1981;193:201–205.
21. Lundel A, Lindblad B, Bergqvist D, Hansen F: Femoropopliteal-crural graft patency is improved by an intensive surveillance program: A prospective, randomized study. J Vasc Surg 1995;21:26–33.
22. Winter-Warnars HAO, van der Graaf Y, Mali WPM: Ankle-arm index, angiography, and duplex ultrasonography after recanalization of occlusions in femoropopliteal arteries: Comparison of long-term results. Cardiovasc Intervent Radiol 1996;19:234–238.
23. European Working Group on Critical Leg Ischemia: Second consensus document on chronic arterial leg ischaemia. Circulation 1991;84:S1–S26.
24. Wieman TJ: Clinical efficacy of becaplermin (rhPDGF-BB) gel. Am J Surg 1998;176:74S–79S.
25. Dawson I, Hajo van Brockel J, Pesch-Batenburg J, et al: Late outcomes of limb loss after failed infrainguinal bypass. J Vasc Surg 1995;21:613–622.

Chapter 36 begins on the following page

Chapter 36 Acute Limb Ischemia

ROBERT B. RUTHERFORD, MD

(A) In the initial evaluation, *current symptoms* are explored relative to the presence and severity of acute limb ischemia (ALI), and *background information* is gathered that may indicate the etiologic mechanism and the presence of significant concurrent disease. Specifically, suddenness *and* time of onset of pain, weakness or numbness, and their location, intensity, and change over time should be elucidated.

A *past history* of claudication, coronary disease or arrhythmias, atherosclerosis elsewhere or its risk factors, clotting problems, or recent percutaneous interventions or diagnostic procedures should be sought. Age, longevity outlook, and anesthetic risk bear on decision making.

The *physical examination* should be directed toward the pulses and skin color and temperature and should focus primarily on sensory or motor deficits, which are the key to staging ALI and further decision making. Comparison with the opposite extremity is extremely valuable.

Doppler interrogation of the ankle and pedal vessels is a valuable adjunct. If clearly audible *arterial* signals are present, limb viability is sufficient to allow delay for transfer or referral,[1] arteriography, or fuller evaluation and treatment of causative factors and co-morbidities.

(B) Although the emphasis here is on native artery or graft thrombosis or embolism, other less common causes of ALI should be considered, such as thrombosed aneurysm (especially popliteal artery), dissection, popliteal entrapment or cyst, and spontaneous thrombosis associated with hypercoagulability, arteritis, or severe vasospasm (e.g., secondary to ergotism). In addition, several conditions may mimic ALI: (1) heart failure superimposed on chronic occlusive arterial disease, (2) early stages of deep venous thrombosis, and (3) acute compressive neuropathy.

(C) The Society for Vascular Surgery/International Society for Cardiovascular Surgery (SVS/ISCVS) *revised* reporting standards[2] stratify ALI into four classes on the basis of severity and perceived limb threat, with their names imparting obvious prognostic and therapeutic implications:

Class I. Limb viable
Class IIa. Limb marginally threatened
Class IIb. Limb immediately threatened
Class III. Irreversible changes in limb

In brief, their differentiating characteristics are:

Class I. No persisting pain, no motor or sensory deficits, Doppler distal arterial signals clearly audible
Class IIa. Additionally, numbness and paresthesias or limited (digital) sensory loss and no audible Doppler signals
Class IIb. In addition, persisting ischemic pain, greater sensory loss, and *any* motor deficit
Class III. Profound anesthesia and paralysis:
early. Limbs with these latter findings soon after the onset of ischemia should be managed like those in *Class IIb*, for differentiation is impossible.
late. Limbs with muscle rigor, marbling of the skin, and/or without detectable venous flow, even with compressive maneuvers, can be considered to have major irreversible changes.

The main implications of this stratification is that there is time for formal angiography and other key diagnostic tests, and even catheter-directed thrombolysis, in *class I* and *class IIa*; patients with *class IIb* or *early class III* should be taken directly to the operating room for immediate revascularization. *Late class III* patients predictably undergo major tissue loss or neuromuscular damage that precludes salvage of a painless functional foot.

(D) All patients should receive heparin therapy as soon as the diagnosis of ALI is made to prevent further clot propagation and to control possible embolic sources. This measure may be delayed briefly, if surgical exploration is truly imminent, to allow performance of spinal or epidural anesthesia, if desired, before anticoagulation.

(E) Patients with ALI have significant co-morbidities and are at high risk when revascularization is done emergently. As long as the limb is classified as viable according to the criteria as listed (and stays this way under close surveillance), revascularization would be safer if it were carried out more deliberately with good preprocedural planning and full evaluation of risk and institution of control measures. On the other hand, if clot removal is to be an integral part of revascularization and if revascularization is deemed likely to be necessary in any event, the sooner the patient can be stabilized and revascularization can be carried out, the better. Timing here is a matter of judgment, balancing benefit against risk.

(F) The choice between endovascular versus operative treatment is usually dictated by the severity of ischemia and the perceived immediate limb threat. The time to revascularization with regional thrombolysis averages 6 to 8 hours, but improved perfusion may occur earlier. However, time to surgical revascularization combines actual operative time with time getting into an available operating room suite. Thus, this decision is not as absolute as this scheme might imply.

(G) Catheter-directed thrombolysis (CDT) holds the theoretical advantages, when time allows, of (1) gentler clot removal, (2) frequent angiographic control, and (3) clearing out and visualizing the distal runoff vessels and the involved segment, thereby revealing the underlying lesion. Thus, *when time allows,* this is the preferred initial treatment. However, there are other considerations in choosing between CDT and thromboembolectomy: (1) the location and extent of clot, (2) type of clot (embolus or thrombus), (3) native artery or graft (especially a vein graft), (4) contraindications to thrombolysis, and (5) operative risk. These considerations constitute the basis for selected exceptions to the tendency to choose thrombolysis when time allows, in class I and class IIa cases. For example, a thin patient with a proximal embolus can be well treated with femoral embolectomy under local anesthesia without considering other factors heavily. In fact, because of the lack of predeveloped collaterals, patients with emboli usually present with immediate limb-threatening ischemia, which in turn dictates emergency operation. In contrast, arterial thromboses characteristically present with less severe ischemia and allow time for arteriography and CDT. This natural dichotomy is fortunate, for it matches disease presentation with best therapy in most cases.

(H) An absolute time limit cannot be imposed for this decision. Permanent neuromuscular damage can begin in 4 to 6 hours, but salvage can be achieved in limbs with profound ischemia for up to 12 hours. However, this is the general time frame in which surgical revascularization is justified, even in advanced cases. In such cases, fasciotomy is likely to be necessary (see Chapters 66 and 47). Better markers of irreversible tissue damage are needed.

(I) Delayed amputation holds the same advantages mentioned earlier for delayed revascularization (i.e., control of co-morbidities and risk factors), beyond which there is little advantage to waiting. The decision to delay amputation must also be tempered by the need to control pain and to avoid systemic consequences of circulating byproducts of ischemia and tissue necrosis. Myoglobinuria and acute tubular necrosis are tangible risks of delay.

(J) The techniques of CDT—and its contraindications—are well established.[3] Achieving catheter access is a major key to success, and failure to achieve this in almost 25% of cases has adversely affected its performance in randomized trials.[4, 5] The current unavailability of urokinase has resulted in the use of tissue-type plasminogen activator (tPA) and other newer agents; therefore, new data to support the continued use of CDT

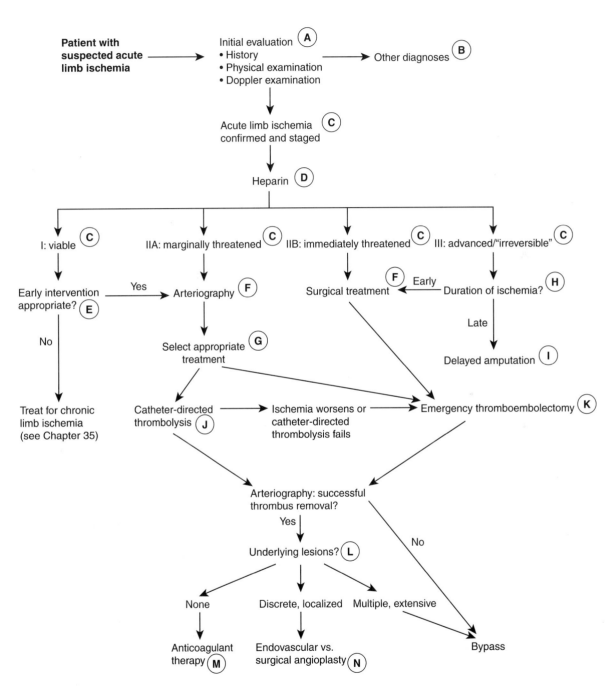

are needed. Furthermore, percutaneous mechanical thrombectomy (PMT), with devices like the Angiojet, is being actively evaluated in this setting. Many PMT techniques still require additional thrombolysis to complete adequate clot removal, but by speeding up the process of clot removal, they may further narrow the choice between endovascular and surgical techniques for patients with class II ALI.

(K) Modem thromboembolectomy,[6] carried out under fluoroscopic control with the use of a C-arm imaging system with freeze and tracking capabilities, has improved outcomes and is less likely to leave residual clot, which can be visualized and retrieved by additional passes of a balloon catheter embolectomy or cleared with intraoperative thrombolytic therapy. Otherwise, inadequate clot removal may occur in as high as one third of cases, and the underlying lesion, in cases of native artery or graft thrombosis, cannot be identified or appropriately treated. Improvements in perioperative monitoring and care, rather than technical advances, have reduced mortality and morbidity rates, but operative risk remains high for emergency revascularization in ALI.[7]

(L) Just as control of the source lesion in arterial embolism is critically important, so is proper treatment of the underlying lesion that precipitates arterial thrombosis. The difference in outcome when an underlying lesion is corrected and when it is not (i.e., cannot be treated or no lesion is demonstrated) is striking.[8] Treatment of the underlying lesion should involve a procedure that produces durable results at a reasonable risk and should not be automatically linked with the method of clot removal, such as by percutaneous transluminal angioplasty (PTA) after thrombolysis or surgical reconstruction after thromboembolectomy. An accurate comparison of different methods of clot removal in most studies is complicated by differing treatment of the underlying lesion. For example, poor patient risk or limited longevity may justify choosing a less durable endovascular treatment of the underlying lesion, but the understandable tendency to make this choice is probably one of the reasons that CDT failed in clinical trials against surgery, when judged in terms of overall late outcome.[4,5] Appropriate choices are also discussed in Chapters 38 and 41.

(M) One reason for finding "no underlying lesion" is complete removal of an embolus; another is spontaneous thrombosis of an artery (caused by hypercoagulability or arteritis) or of a graft (typically a prosthetic graft with a high minimum threshold velocity). In each case, anticoagulant therapy is indicated for an indefinite period of time. Embolic sources may occasionally be corrected or removed, but in most cases long-term anticoagulant therapy is needed. Failure to institute such therapy results in a high recurrence rate and mortality.[9]

(N) Discrete, localized atherosclerotic plaques are the anatomic lesions for which PTA is most generally accepted as the initial treatment of choice. However, some other localized lesions are not as amenable to durable control by balloon dilatation, for example, anastomotic-neointimal hyperplasia in prosthetic grafts and vein valve or venovenostomy strictures in vein grafts. Patch angioplasty, vein interposition grafts, or short extension grafts bring more durable results in this case and should be employed, especially if surgical exploration has already been completed to deal with the acute occlusion.

REFERENCES

1. Lavenson GS, Rich NK, Baugh JH: Value of ultrasonic flow detector in the management of peripheral vascular disease. Am J Surg 1970;120:522–526.
2. Rutherford RB, Baker JD, Ernst C, et al: Recommended standards for reports dealing with lower extremity ischemia. J Vasc Surg 1997;26:517–538.
3. Verstraete M, Verhaeghe R, Belch J, et al: Thrombolysis in the management of lower extremity occlusion: A consensus document. Am J Cardiol 1998;81:207–218.
4. The STILE Investigators: Results of a prospective randomized trial evaluating surgery versus thrombolysis for ischemia of the lower extremity. Ann Surg 1994;220:251–268.
5. Ouriel K, Veith FJ, Sasahara AA: Thrombolysis or peripheral arterial surgery: Phase I results. J Vasc Surg 1996; 23:64–73.
6. Parsons RE, Marin ML, Veith FJ, et al: Fluoroscopically assisted thromboembolectomy: An improved method for treating acute arterial lesions. Ann Vasc Surg 1996;10: 201.
7. Ouriel K, Shortell CK, De Weese JA, et al: A comparison of thrombolytic therapy with operative revascularization in the initial treatment of acute peripheral artery ischemia. J Vasc Surg 1994;19:1021–1030.
8. McNamara TO, Bomberger RA, Merchant RF: Intraarterial urokinase as the initial therapy for acutely ischemic lower limbs. Circulation 1991;83(Suppl):106–119.
9. Elliot JP, Hagerman JK, Szilagyi DE, et al: Arterial embolization: Problems of source, multiplicity, recurrence and delayed treatment. Surgery 1980;88:833.

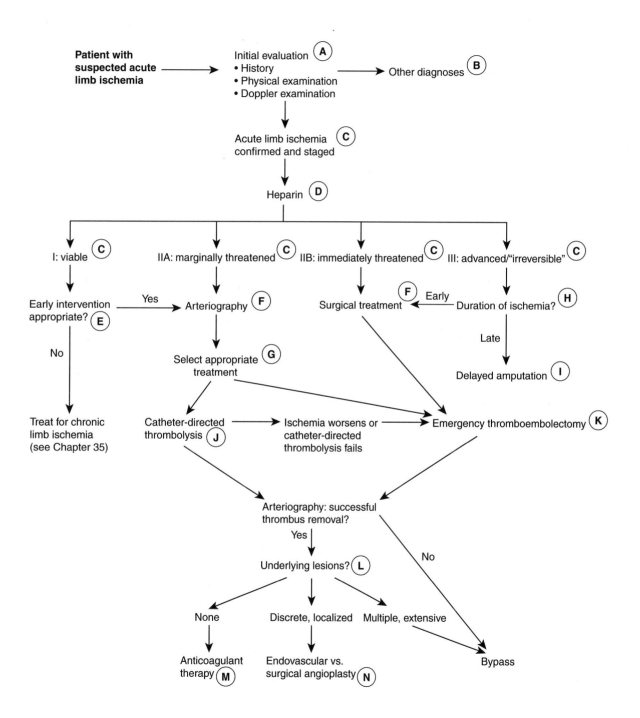

Chapter 37 Atheroembolism

JEFFREY L. KAUFMAN, MD

(A) Atheroembolism refers to microscopic, cholesterol-laden debris that originates from unstable plaque in proximal arteries.[1,2] Because of their small size, atheroemboli are not trapped until they reach the very distal circulation, typically the skin of the lower extremities. Classically, patients with lower extremity atheroemboli present with focal toe ischemia despite palpable pedal pulses, the so-called "blue toe syndrome."[3] In contrast, most emboli that arise from mural thrombus (either cardiac or aneurysmal) are larger and are trapped in more proximal arteries, resulting in more diffuse ischemia. Atheroemboli can originate from the arterial wall within an aneurysm, but the pathogenesis is plaque disruption rather than dislodgment of aneurysmal thrombus.

(B) Patients with atheroemboli to the legs usually present with sudden onset of cyanosis of a toe or more extensive areas of skin, in an irregular, splotchy pattern.[4] If there is bilateral involvement, it is usually asymmetric and a proximal, aortic source is suggested. Because atheroembolic lesions are usually painful, their timing can be established. When the lesions are focal in a patient with normal pulses, the diagnosis is straightforward. However, if multiple, sequential atheroemboli occur, differentiating more diffuse causes of ischemia can be more difficult. Furthermore, although continuously patent arteries are usually required for atheroemboli to reach the foot, they can also traverse well-developed collateral circulation in a patient without palpable pedal pulses, further confounding the diagnosis.

A careful history to identify concomitant vascular disease is important.[5] Examination should focus on possible sources of atheroemboli, including palpation for aneurysms and auscultation to detect bruits associated with preocclusive stenoses. More extensive proximal atheroemboli can affect skin from the lower abdomen to the feet, causing a livedo reticularis pattern. Visceral or renal injury can also result from proximal emboli and must be excluded. Eosinophilia may be found if atheroemboli are extensive. Vascular laboratory testing with segmental Doppler pressure measurements is helpful to localize the level of any hemodynamically significant stenoses.

(C) The principal differential diagnosis for atheroembolism is more diffuse atherosclerotic occlusive disease causing localized foot ischemia. However, patients with localized foot ischemia lack pedal pulses, whereas most patients with atheroemboli have such pulses, as noted earlier. Isolated toe ischemia, often occurring after local trauma, is common in diabetic patients with arterial occlusive disease. Buerger's disease often presents with focal ischemic foot changes but is also characterized by absent pedal pulses. The late effects of frostbite can appear similar to those of atheroembolism on physical examination, and a careful history is therefore required. Chronic pulmonary disease or venous disease may lead to distal cyanosis, but this color blanches with elevation, whereas skin changes from atheroemboli usually do not. Connective tissue disorders may occasionally be manifested by distal cyanosis, as can treatment with β blockers, but this pattern is usually symmetric. Sympathetic dystrophy following mild injury can cause cyanotic discoloration, but such discoloration is usually more generalized, rather than splotchy, and symmetric across the toes.

(D) Although atheroemboli are often spontaneous, plaque disruption can also result from arterial catheter manipulation or from arterial clamping or manipulation during surgery.[6,7] These events are usually manifested during or immediately after such procedures, but plaque disruption has occurred as many as 6 weeks later. If such emboli are minor and nonrepetitive, conservative treatment is initially recommended, since the likelihood of recurrent atheroemboli is presumably lower than with initially spontaneous emboli. If these emboli are massive or multiple, however, more thorough evaluation and potential treatment is indicated.

(E) Medical management of atheroemboli consists primarily of antiplatelet therapy, usually with aspirin.[8] In patients who experience atheroemboli while already taking aspirin, more potent antiplatelet agents, such as ticlopidine or clopidogrel, should be considered. There are no data to support the use of warfarin anticoagulation therapy to prevent atheroemboli. In fact, paradoxical embolism from presumed plaque hemorrhage and disruption in the thoracic aorta has been reported as the cause of visceral and peripheral atheroembolism related to warfarin therapy. Medical management also includes control and treatment of generalized atherosclerotic risk factors.

(F) Appropriate management of ischemic foot lesions from atheroemboli depends on the extent of tissue injury. In mild cases, expectant treatment with pain control is sufficient. However, pain can be severe, and the patient may benefit from consultation with a pain specialist. Intermittent chemical sympathetic blockade or even surgical sympathectomy has been recommended in severe cases. With more extensive tissue loss, it is best to wait until the nonviable tissue is clearly demarcated in order to minimize the extent of amputation required.

If pain or local infection do not necessitate amputation, allowing mummification with autoamputation may salvage the most tissue. Usually, patients with atheroemboli have sufficient circulation so that local amputations will heal. However, careful assessment is necessary because some patients with proximal occlusive disease and atheroembolism through collateral vessels may require arterial reconstruction to facilitate amputation healing. In these cases, toe pressure and transcutaneous oxygen tension measurement can aid clinical decision making.

Occasionally, atheroemboli to the more proximal leg may result in local skin or subcutaneous necrosis that may call for local excision and skin grafting. Healing of any amputation requiring skin flaps can be problematic as a result of microvascular injury of otherwise normal-appearing tissue after atheroembolism. Gentle surgical technique is therefore of great importance in these procedures.

(G) Appropriate treatment of atheroembolism requires the embolic source to be localized as precisely as possible. Patients with bilateral lower extremity atheroemboli almost always have a proximal, aortic source, especially if these lesions occur simultaneously. Rarely, patients may experience bilateral emboli from separate lesions within each leg, but these rarely occur simultaneously. Thus, the initial diagnostic evaluation for patients with bilateral emboli should focus on the aorta. In patients with unilateral emboli, the source may also be aortic, especially if only a single event has occurred. Thus, although the initial evaluation of unilateral atheroemboli is usually focused on the ipsilateral leg, complete evaluation of the aorta should be performed if no dominant lesion is found within the affected leg or if any other evidence suggests aortic disease.

(H) Physical examination and Doppler segmental pressures should help to localize a dominant atherosclerotic plaque if an associated stenosis or aneurysm exists. Often, however, the source of atheroemboli is a nonstenotic plaque that can be detected only by arterial imaging. Color duplex ultrasonography can visualize the iliac, femoral, popliteal, and tibial arteries noninvasively, and a good-quality, negative scan can avoid the need for arteriography. If this technique is not available or if it cannot yield adequate images of the iliac arteries, conventional arteriography, performed from the contralateral groin to avoid catheter manipulation of potential atheroembolic sites, is recommended.

(I) For patients with a suspected aortic origin of atheroemboli, complete aortic imaging with computed tomography (CT) or magnetic resonance imaging or angiography (MRI/MRA) is recommended as the initial step. CT and MRI/MRA

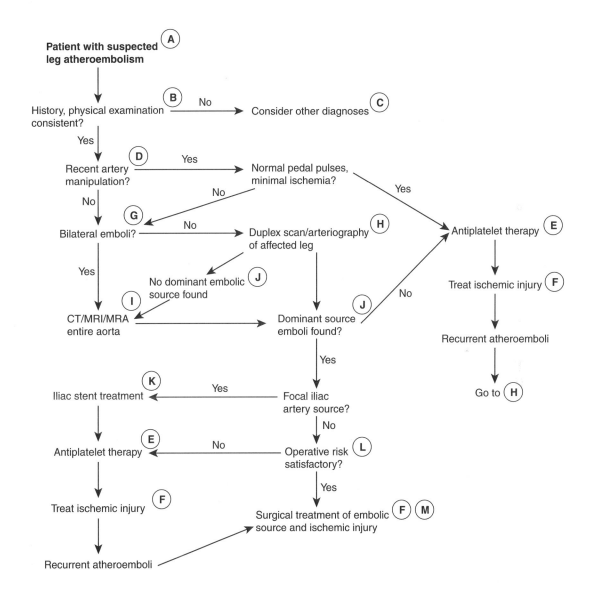

allow one to avoid catheter manipulation of the potential atheroembolic site, and they provide excellent detail, especially if a technique such as spiral CT scanning is employed. Subsequent arteriography, via a transaxillary approach to avoid catheter manipulation of the atheroembolic source when appropriate, may be required for preoperative planning, but spiral CT or MRA can often eliminate this potentially hazardous step. Occasionally, the proximal aorta can be the source of atheroemboli to the legs. Transesophageal echocardiographic studies may be helpful in delineating these lesions.

(J) In some patients with atheroemboli, careful arterial imaging reveals diffuse, atherosclerotic changes but no dominant stenotic, ulcerative, or aneurysmal lesion. In such cases, nonoperative management with antiplatelet therapy is the best immediate option. When a likely, dominant source for the atheroemboli is found, however, it is desirable to eliminate this source from the circulation to prevent future emboli.

(K) Traditionally, the elimination of an atheroembolic source involved surgical excision or exclusion of that arterial segment.[9] However, experience with balloon angioplasty and stent placement for isolated iliac artery lesions has demonstrated that this procedure is associated with a low incidence of procedural emboli and has appeared adequate to prevent future embolic events. The mechanism of this activity is unclear but appears to involve stabilization of the plaque by stent placement. Covered stents have been used anecdotally in this setting, but sufficient experience is lacking to recommend them over conventional stents. More diffuse iliac disease is better treated with surgical bypass.

(L) For patients with an identified source of atheroemboli, in which surgical elimination of the source is possible, operative risk must be balanced against the risk of future emboli. Although the natural history of spontaneous atheroemboli is not precisely known, recurrence is likely and tissue loss often ensues. Thus, for patients considered to have a satisfactory operative risk, depending on the scope of the required surgical procedure, operative exclusion of the embolic source is recommended.

For patients with high operative risk or with a less obvious source of atheroembolism, medical management with antiplatelet therapy is preferred, with future reevaluation recommended if recurrent emboli occur. Suprarenal aortic atheroembolism is particularly virulent, often leading to renal and visceral ischemia and death.[10] Thus, surgical treatment of these lesions is desirable, even though the surgical procedure is more complicated and poses a higher risk.

For high-risk patients with suprarenal aortic lesions causing atheroemboli, some success has been reported with axillobifemoral bypass and iliac artery ligation for prevention of further leg atheroembolism.[11] Unfortunately, this treatment does not preclude pelvic, renal, or visceral atheroemboli, but it may be the only option if recurrent lower extremity atheroemboli persist in high-risk patients with aortic lesions. In the future, covered aortic stent grafts may represent a less invasive treatment for disease not involving the visceral aortic segment, but this approach has not been tested.

(M) Surgical treatment to exclude the source of arterial atheroemboli must be tailored to the anatomic location and the underlying pathologic process. In general, bypass grafting with exclusion of the involved arterial segment is used.[12-14] For localized disease, especially involving the aorta, endarterectomy is a useful option.

Finally, in the unusual case in which an aneurysm is the cause of atheroemboli, conventional aneurysm repair is performed, thus excluding the embolic source. For high-risk patients with aortic atheroemboli (see L), axillobifemoral bypass with iliac artery ligation has been used with some success.

REFERENCES

1. Kempczinski RF: Lower-extremity arterial emboli from ulcerating atherosclerotic plaques. JAMA 1979;241:807–810.
2. Khatibzadeh M, Mitusch R, Stierle U, et al: Aortic atherosclerotic plaques as a source of systemic embolism. J Am Coll Cardiol 1996;27:664–669.
3. Karmody AM, Powers SR, Monaco VJ, et al: "Blue toe" syndrome: An indication for limb salvage surgery. Arch Surg 1976;111:1263–1268.
4. Fisher DF, Clagett GP, Brigham RA, et al: Dilemmas in dealing with the blue toe syndrome: Aortic versus peripheral source. Am J Surg 1984;148:836–839.
5. Dahlberg PJ, Frecentese DF, Cogbill TH: Cholesterol embolism: Experience with 22 histologically proven cases. Surgery 1989;105:737–746.
6. Saklayen MG, Gupta S, Suryaprasad A, et al: Incidence of atheroembolic renal failure after coronary angiography: A prospective study. Angiology 1997;48:609–613.
7. Kolh PH, Torchiana DF, Buckley MJ: Atheroembolization in cardiac surgery: The need for preoperative diagnosis. J Cardiovasc Surg (Torino) 1999;40:77–81.
8. Morris-Jones W, Preston FE, Greaney M, Chatterjee DK: Gangrene of the toes with palpable peripheral pulses: Response to platelet suppressive therapy. Ann Surg 1981; 193:462–466.
9. McFarland RJ, Taylor RS, Woodyer AB, Eastwood JB: The femoropopliteal segment as a source of peripheral atheroembolism. J Cardiovasc Surg (Torino) 1989;30:597–603.
10. Kaufman JL, Stark K, Brolin RE: Disseminated atheroembolism from extensive degenerative atherosclerosis of the aorta. Surgery 1987;102:63–70.
11. Kaufman JL, Saifi J, Chang BB, et al: The role of extraanatomic exclusion bypass in the treatment of disseminated atheroembolism syndrome. Ann Vasc Surg 1990; 4:260–263.
12. Keen RR, McCarthy WJ, Shireman PK, et al: Surgical management of atheroembolism. J Vasc Surg 1995;21:773–780.
13. Baumann DS, McGraw D, Rubin BG, et al: An institutional experience with arterial atheroembolism. Ann Vasc Surg 1994;8:258–265.
14. Sharma PV, Babu SC, Shah PM, Nassoura ZE: Changing patterns of atheroembolism. Cardiovasc Surg 1996;4:573–579.

ATHEROEMBOLISM

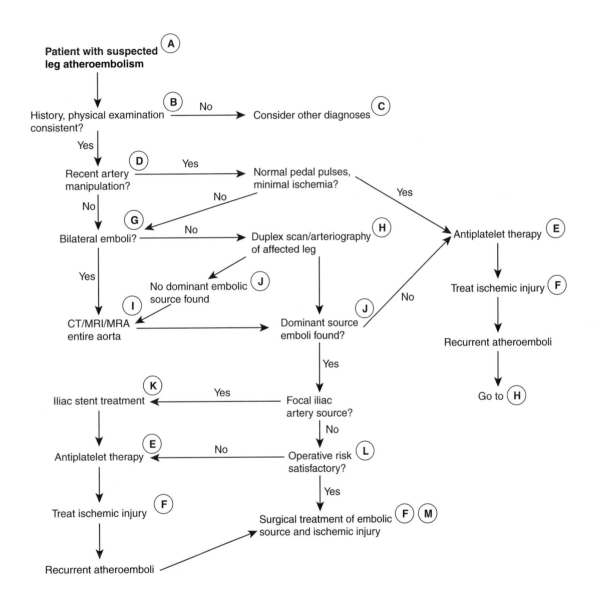

Chapter 38 **Aortoiliac Disease**

JACK L. CRONENWETT, MD

(A) To select appropriate treatment for symptomatic aortoiliac occlusive disease, it is first necessary to assess the extent and location of disease, which can range from unilateral, focal iliac stenosis to total aortic occlusion. History and physical examination, with attention to femoral pulses, can often determine whether unilateral or bilateral disease is present. Occult, subcritical iliac stenoses, however, may be overlooked without more definitive testing.

Catheter-directed arteriography has traditionally been used to obtain detailed anatomic information regarding the extent and location of occlusive disease, with the use of oblique views to detect posterior plaque hidden in the anteroposterior projection. Advantages of this technique are that endovascular treatment can often immediately follow with the same catheter access used and the hemodynamic significance of questionable stenoses can be determined with the use of pull-back pressure gradients.[1] Less invasive initial evaluation relies on duplex ultrasound scanning or magnetic resonance angiography (MRA), which can help select conservative versus endovascular versus open surgical treatment, avoiding catheter-directed arteriography in some cases.

(B) Often the key decision for treatment of iliac occlusive disease is whether to use endovascular or surgical therapy. Because of reduced morbidity and mortality, endovascular treatment is preferred when a "satisfactory" result is likely. In general, endovascular treatment is most successful and durable for localized iliac disease in the common iliac segment.[2] More diffuse iliac disease, especially when bilateral or involving the external iliac segments or with long occlusion, is less successfully treated by endovascular methods.[3-5] Thus, for patients with *unilateral* iliac disease, "focal" lesions are best managed with endovascular treatment whereas "diffuse" disease is best managed surgically. Obviously, this disease extent is a continuum, for which decision making needs to be individualized for each patient and according to the experience of individual centers.

For patients with *bilateral* iliac disease, endovascular treatment is appropriate for the common iliac segments. However, when this disease involves the common *and* external iliac arteries bilaterally, endovascular treatment is so unlikely to yield durable results that surgical treatment is preferred.[3, 6]

(C) Common iliac artery stenoses usually respond to balloon angioplasty alone, with stent placement reserved for unresponsive lesions, evidenced by residual pressure gradients, or angioplasty complicated by local arterial dissection.[2] Treatment of the proximal common iliac artery often requires simultaneous, bilateral "kissing" balloon angioplasty to avoid injury or encroachment on the contralateral iliac orifice. Common iliac artery occlusions and external iliac artery disease are more frequently treated with primary stent placement, although better studies to identify appropriate candidates for stent placement are still needed.[7]

(D) Following balloon angioplasty or stent placement, the technical result is assessed with both arteriography and pull-back pressure measurements. A residual pressure gradient predicts worse patency and should lead to a search for additional stenoses, with appropriate angioplasty or stent treatment.[8] Intravascular ultrasound can be used to judge stent-artery wall apposition and has been shown to improve the durability of stent treatment in one study.[9]

(E) If unilateral iliac endovascular treatment is unsuccessful or if diffuse disease is not amenable to endovascular treatment, surgical options must be assessed. Unilateral iliofemoral bypass is our first choice if the proximal common iliac artery is not diseased, including absence of severe calcification, as assessed by arteriography or computed tomography. In general, we avoid unilateral aortofemoral bypass, believing that bilateral reconstruction is preferred if aortic exposure and cross-clamping are required. Femoral-femoral bypass has comparable patency but requires an ideal contralateral iliac system and places the contralateral femoral artery and leg at some risk. However, femoral-femoral bypass can be performed with less anesthesia and the risk of neurogenic sexual dysfunction from pelvic dissection can be avoided. Thus, the choice between iliofemoral and femoral-femoral bypass depends on several factors, not the least often being surgeon experience.[10]

(F) Although most patients considered for iliofemoral bypass are appropriate operative candidates for a low, retroperitoneal approach to the pelvis for this operation, extensive, previous surgery or radiation may make this approach less attractive. Very-high-risk patients may be better candidates for groin-incision-only femoral-femoral bypass.

(G) Patients with unilateral iliac disease can be treated with femoral-femoral bypass if the contralateral "donor" iliac artery is adequate. Although a normal femoral pulse is reassuring in this regard, it is insensitive to subcritical iliac stenoses and difficult to evaluate in obese patients.

Arteriography is usually used to assess both iliac arteries, but it also may underestimate posterior plaque. Duplex scanning is now being used more commonly to evaluate the iliac arteries, with an increase in focal velocity needed to indicate a stenosis. The adequacy of a donor iliac artery is best assessed, however, by pressure measurement in the contralateral femoral artery and comparison with systemic pressure, both at rest and after infusion of a vasodilator, such as 30 mg papaverine.[1] Vasodilator infusion increases blood flow (unless outflow is severely restricted) to simulate the increased flow that results after a femoral-femoral bypass. This should unmask a subcritical stenosis that might reduce the durability of subsequent femoral-femoral bypass.

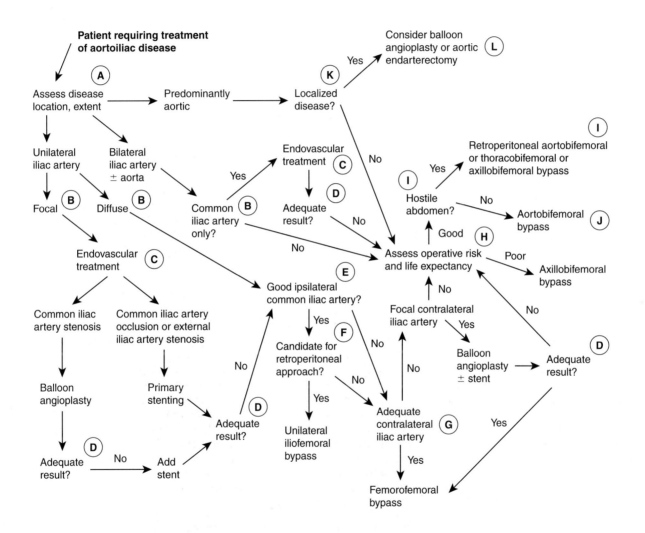

In general, a resting gradient greater than 5 mmHg or an enhanced gradient of 15 mm Hg should prompt treatment of the donor iliac lesion prior to femoral-femoral bypass or performance of a bilateral revascularization.[1] This decision may depend on several factors, such as patient operative risk, focal versus diffuse contralateral iliac stenosis, and patient preference.

Pretreatment of contralateral, localized iliac stenosis does not reduce long-term patency of femoral-femoral bypass.[11] However, the influence of more diffuse contralateral iliac disease has not been tested. In such cases, bilateral surgical reconstruction is usually favored.

(H) Patients with diffuse bilateral iliac disease or severe aortic disease are best treated with surgical reconstruction. Initial assessment requires a determination of operative risk for potential aortofemoral bypass, since this is the most durable but also the most invasive procedure. Cardiac disease (see Chapter 1) and renal insufficiency are primary determinants of operative risk, with secondary factors including pulmonary disease, advanced age, and malnutrition. Life expectancy should also be estimated, because the less durable but less invasive axillobifemoral bypass is more appropriate when life expectancy is poor.

(I) Patients with satisfactory operative risk and good life expectancy are candidates for transabdominal aortobifemoral bypass unless they have a "hostile" abdomen, usually from multiple previous operations or intestinal stomas. In such patients, a retroperitoneal approach to the abdominal aorta may be preferred. Alternatively, a transthoracic approach to the descending thoracic aorta can provide good inflow and is attractive in younger patients with good pulmonary function.[12] If these options are not available or if the patient is at higher risk, axillobifemoral bypass is also possible. For most patients, however, bilateral aortoiliac disease is optimally treated with transabdominal, aortobifemoral bypass, which is considered the "gold standard."

(J) The proximal anastomosis for an aortobifemoral bypass is constructed in the infrarenal location with either an *end-end* or an *end-side* configuration. Occasionally, the location of iliac occlusive disease and pelvic collateral circulation may dictate the best approach. Thus, patients with predominantly external iliac artery disease and with patent common and internal iliac arteries are best treated with an end-side proximal anastomosis to preserve internal iliac perfusion. Similarly, an end-side anastomosis may be a good method to preserve flow though a distal accessory renal artery or a large inferior mesenteric artery.

In most patients with predominantly distal aortic and common iliac artery disease, an end-end proximal anastomosis provides a better hemodynamic configuration, with resultant internal iliac perfusion retrograde through the external iliac arteries. In many cases, the choice of proximal anastomotic configuration is a matter of surgeon preference, since neither has proved to have clear superiority when both are applicable.

(K) In younger patients, aortoiliac disease may be localized to the distal aorta, although often at least the proximal common iliac arteries are involved. When the dominant occlusive lesion is in the aorta with minimal iliac disease, however, more localized aortic treatment can be considered.

(L) Balloon angioplasty can be performed to treat localized stenoses of the distal aorta, although the results are not as durable as surgical bypass in the relatively small series that have been reported.[13] Either bilateral, "kissing" balloons or one large balloon, depending on the proximity to the iliac orifices, can be used. In general, this technique is applicable only to a small proportion of patients, with truly localized, early atherosclerotic lesions. Aortic endarterectomy, often extended into the proximal common iliac arteries, is appropriate for patients with localized disease that is too extensive for balloon angioplasty. Often at surgery, however, the iliac disease is more diffuse than expected, so that aortobifemoral bypass is preferred. Although extensive endarterectomy of the aortoiliac system can be performed, it is more difficult and time-consuming than bypass and is rarely performed.

REFERENCES

1. Flanigan DP, Ryan TJ, Williams LR, et al: Aortofemoral or femoropopliteal revascularization? A prospective evaluation of the papaverine test. J Vasc Surg 1984;1(1):215.
2. Pentecost MJ, Criqui MH, Dorros G, et al: Guidelines for peripheral percutaneous transluminal angioplasty of the abdominal aorta and lower extremity vessels: A statement for health professionals from a special writing group of the Councils on Cardiovascular Radiology, Arteriosclerosis, Cardio-Thoracic and Vascular Surgery, Clinical Cardiology, and Epidemiology and Prevention, the American Heart Association. Circulation 1994;89(1):511.
3. Ballard JL, Sparks SR, Taylor FC, et al: Complications of iliac artery stent deployment [see comments]. J Vasc Surg 1996;24(4):545.
4. Johnston KW: Iliac arteries: Reanalysis of results of balloon angioplasty. Radiology 1993;186(1):207.
5. Strecker EP, Boos IB, Hagen B: Flexible tantalum stents for the treatment of iliac artery lesions: Long-term patency, complications, and risk factors. Radiology 1996;199(3):641.
6. Powell R, Fillinger M, Walsh D, et al: The durability of endovascular treatment of diffuse iliac occlusive disease. J Vasc Surg 2000;31:1178–1184.
7. Bosch JL, Hunink MG: Meta-analysis of the results of percutaneous transluminal angioplasty and stent placement for aortoiliac occlusive disease [erratum in Radiology 1997;205(2):584]. Radiology 1997;204(1):87.
8. Nawaz S, Cleveland T, Gaines P, et al: Aortoiliac stenting, determinants of clinical outcome. Eur J Vasc Endovasc Surg 1999;17(4):351.
9. Arko F, Mettauer M, McCollough R, et al: Use of intravascular ultrasound improves long-term clinical outcome in the endovascular management of atherosclerotic aortoiliac occlusive disease. J Vasc Surg 1998;27(4):614.
10. Harrington ME, Harrington EB, Haimov M, et al: Iliofemoral versus femorofemoral bypass: The case for an individualized approach. J Vasc Surg 1992;16(6):841.
11. Perler BA, Williams GM: Does donor iliac artery percutaneous transluminal angioplasty or stent placement influence the results of femorofemoral bypass? Analysis of 70 consecutive cases with long-term follow-up. J Vasc Surg 1996;24(3):363.
12. Criado E, Johnson G Jr, Burnham SJ, et al: Descending thoracic aorta-to-iliofemoral artery bypass as an alternative to aortoiliac reconstruction. J Vasc Surg 1992;15(3):550.
13. Odurny A, Colapinto RF, Sniderman KW, et al: Percutaneous transluminal angioplasty of abdominal aortic stenoses. Cardiovasc Intervent Radiol 1989;12(1):1.

AORTOILIAC DISEASE

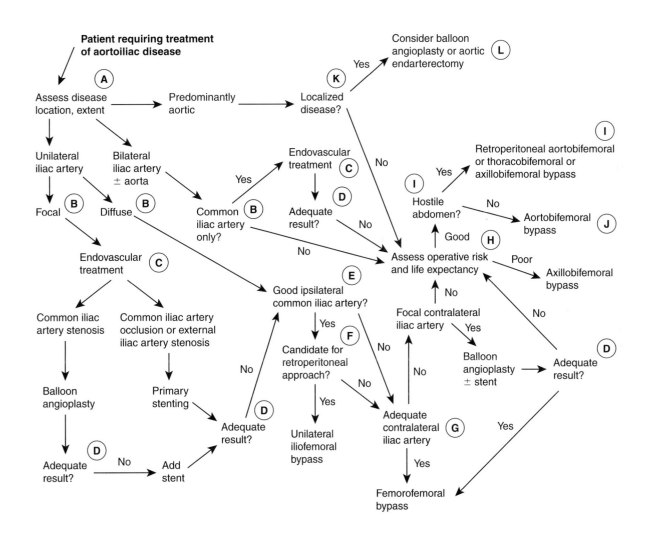

Chapter 39 Aortic Graft Limb Thrombosis

THOMAS F. REHRING, MD • DAVID C. BREWSTER, MD

(A) Aortofemoral bypass is one of the most durable arterial reconstructive procedures performed by vascular surgeons, with a 5-year patency of 85% to 95%.[1-3] Nevertheless, graft limb thrombosis is the most frequent late complication and is estimated to occur in up to 10% to 20% of graft limbs, depending on length of follow-up.[2, 4-6] The average time from graft implantation to limb thrombosis ranges from 34 to 60 months.[6-8] The diagnosis is suspected by sudden or progressive onset of ischemic symptoms, decreased or absent pulses, and reductions in ankle pressures and/or pulse volume recordings compared with baseline values. The duplex scan, showing no flow in the ipsilateral graft limb, is confirmatory.

(B) *Early* graft limb occlusion is arbitrarily defined as an occlusion presenting within 30 days of operation. As a rule, this type of occlusion arises from technical complications rendered at the original operation, commonly at the distal anastomosis. Such technical mishaps occur in 1% to 2% of grafts placed and include intimal flaps, anastomotic stenoses, and graft kinking or torsion.[9, 10]

Occasionally, failure to flush thrombus from the lumen of the graft before completion of the distal anastomosis can also lead to early thrombosis. Because operation is required to deal with these technical defects, catheter-directed thrombolytic therapy is not used in this case even if sufficient time has passed since operation to make it relatively safe. Other than standard preoperative evaluation and control of patient risk factors for operation, little further diagnostic workup is required.

Vascular diagnostic laboratory confirmation of the event suffices; preoperative arteriography is rarely needed in early thromboses. The patient is given systemic heparin therapy and transported to the operating room, and thrombectomy is performed. An anatomic or technical cause for the graft occlusion is corrected if found. In the absence of an anatomic or a technical etiologic mechanism, other possible causes of the thrombosis may be (1) graft thrombogenicity, (2) poor runoff, (3) periods of hypotension or hypoperfusion, or (4) a hypercoagulable state. Such conditions must be individually managed to prevent rethrombosis.

(C) *Late* graft limb occlusion (>30 days) is generally secondary to neointimal fibroplasia or progression of disease at the *distal* anastomotic site. Conversely, impaired inflow is a distinctly unusual cause of graft limb thrombosis and is more likely to cause failure of the entire graft. However, a relatively low aortic anastomosis can lead to proximal progression of atherosclerosis (as well as the kinking or torsion of a graft limb as noted earlier) encroaching onto one limb of a bifurcation graft. In rare instances, a thrombosed pseudoaneurysm at the distal anastomosis can cause graft limb thrombosis.

(D) Individual surgeons differ on timing and indications for arteriography. We believe that preoperative visualization is of great importance in planning and facilitating treatment. Therefore, it is only the rare patient with *immediately threatened limb ischemia* (Society for Vascular Surgery/International Society for Cardiovascular Surgery [SVS/ISCVS] category IIb[11]) in whom we would *not* perform preoperative angiography. Even in cases of irreversible ischemia (SVS/ISCVS category III), preoperative delineation of inflow and runoff vessels may assist in planning for (or limiting) amputation. In patients with less threatening ischemia (SVS/ISCVS categories I, IIa), catheter-directed thrombolysis is an option under certain circumstances (see H).

(E) Retrograde thrombectomy of the occluded graft limb is successful in up to 90% of cases and results have proved relatively durable if adequate outflow exists.[7, 8, 12-15] Although it is more likely to be successful in graft occlusions of short duration, successful thrombectomy of occlusions greater than 6 months' duration have been documented.[7]

The technique we use is as follows. We open and extend the original femoral incision to provide satisfactory exposure (particularly of the profunda femoris artery [deep femoral artery]). The femoral arteries and graft limb are identified and surrounded with vessel loops. Systemic heparin is administered if anticoagulation therapy has not already been given to the patient.

A balloon catheter thrombectomy is performed through a transverse incision on the hood of the graft. Cross-embolization into the contralateral limb may be avoided by several maneuvers. First, the embolectomy catheter should be passed in progressive 5-cm increments, thus allowing systemic pressure to "blow out" the organized proximal plug, which is typically present in late thromboses and the removal of which is the key to successful thrombectomy. Second, digital compression of the contralateral femoral artery pulsation at the groin may reduce flow through the uninvolved limb, encouraging thrombotic debris to be flushed out the thrombectomized limb.

Heparinized saline flushes are used judiciously. We inspect distal anastomoses from within and look for impairment of profundal and superficial femoral outflow. The management of outflow revision is detailed later (see G).

We strip the organized proximal plug, or residual parts of it, in the form of adherent fibrin and pseudointima using a ring stripper or adherent clot catheter. To use the ring stripper or loop endarterectomy catheter, we first pass a deflated balloon embolectomy catheter through the ring, advance it retrograde into the graft limb, and inflate it in the graft body to occlude flow and prevent cross-embolization. The ring stripper is advanced until it engages the balloon. The balloon is deflated slightly, and both stripper and balloon are removed as a unit, bringing adherent thrombus, pseudointima, and debris with them.

AORTIC GRAFT LIMB THROMBOSIS

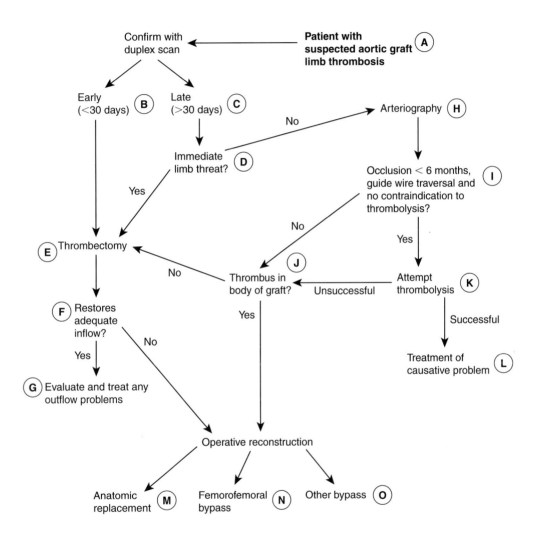

Aortic Graft Limb Thrombosis (continued)

(F) Completion angiography or angioscopy should be performed to assess the technical adequacy of the maneuvers just described. We prefer to achieve this with retrograde flush aortography injected by hand through a large-bore catheter. This may be supplemented with aortic, iliac, and femoral "pull-down" pressures using intraoperative pressure monitoring once flow has been restored. Unexplained peak-to-peak systolic or mean pressure gradients at or above 20 mmHg are significant and require further investigation or intervention. Preoperative placement of calf pulse volume recording cuffs can be helpful in documenting the restoration of pulsatile flow.

(G) Most unilateral aortic graft limb occlusions are attributable to a compromise of graft outflow. Therefore, once adequate inflow has been established and confirmed, attention should be turned to graft runoff, especially the profunda femoris artery. In nearly all cases of late occlusion, outflow can be augmented by local endarterectomy, profundaplasty, or both. To achieve adequate outflow in this setting, we frequently divide the graft limb, perform a patch closure of the arteriotomy, and interpose a new segment of prosthetic material from the end of the transected graft to the profunda distal to the diseased portion. Another option is to perform a profunda endarterectomy with anastomosis of the long beveled tip of the graft over the profunda arteriotomy.

If the profunda femoris artery appears atretic or extensively diseased, we may consider a concomitant distal reconstruction. Preoperative angiography may delineate the feasibility of this procedure; however, we have found that several intraoperative criteria can facilitate this judgment. If the profunda femoris artery accepts a 4-mm probe and measures 20 to 25 cm in length with a catheter, the runoff will generally support aortic graft flow. If not, simultaneous distal bypass to the popliteal or tibial level will likely be necessary. Resorting to a distal bypass is required in 14% to 32%.[7,15] Use of a distal bypass should be routinely considered in tertiary reoperative procedures for graft limb occlusion.

(H) In the absence of profound limb ischemia, arteriography should be obtained to assist in planning operative strategy. If performed, a contralateral femoral artery (or graft limb) access is preferred to brachial or axillary approaches if it is possible that thrombolytic agents may be utilized (see I).

Attention to specific anatomic details is important; such details include biplanar visualization of the abdominal aorta and the proximal anastomosis to evaluate inflow and delineate anastomotic integrity. If graft limb occlusion is identified, the extent of thrombus in the limb and body of the graft should be noted (see J). The status of the contralateral limb should also be studied as a potential donor site for a femorofemoral bypass.

Finally, we inspect the appearance of reconstituted distal runoff vessels (including oblique views of the pelvis) to determine the need and feasibility for concomitant distal bypass grafting as an option. However, lack of visualization of distal arteries should not preclude operative exploration, since adequate recipient vessels may be found in the absence of radiologic visualization.

(I) The role of thrombolysis in this setting remains somewhat controversial, and many surgeons prefer a direct operative approach in all cases. Arguments for proceeding directly to the operating room include:

- The rapidity of reestablishing inflow
- The high success rate of thrombectomy
- The usual necessity of operative intervention regardless of the outcome of thrombolysis
- The ease of performing outflow augmentation (e.g., profundaplasty) (see G) through the same incision

In addition, the risk of complications from thrombolysis such as hemorrhage, and even further thrombosis, must be considered.

In some cases, however, it may be advantageous to attempt graft thrombolysis. With clearing of the clot, characterization of the causative lesion may direct the choice between an endovascular and an open approach and may possibly point to a simpler operation. This may be particularly attractive in the high-risk patient. Lysis is likely to be successful in relatively fresh clot when the entire occlusion can be traversed with a guide wire. Of course, no contraindications to lytic therapy can be present (e.g., recent cerebrovascular accident, intracranial neoplasm, active internal bleeding, recent major surgery). Consideration must also be given to the graft material because knitted polyester (Dacron) prostheses may develop significant transgraft hemorrhage in response to lytic therapy.

(J) If the arteriogram reveals thrombus extending proximally from the occluded graft limb into the body of the graft rather than being confined to the graft limb itself, thrombectomy is frequently unsuccessful. This is particularly true of old, layered thrombus. In general, the thrombus is loosened, but not removed, by balloon catheter, resulting in subsequent reocclusion or thromboembolism of the contralateral limb. In this situation, it is advisable to proceed directly to arterial reconstruction.

(K) Thrombolysis is initiated by placement of an intra-arterial working sheath to facilitate catheter exchanges. A multiple side-hole catheter and guide wire are introduced coaxially. The thrombus is crossed with the guide wire and gently macerated. The multiple side-hole catheter is then placed across the thrombus and a direct bolus of lytic agent given with a pulsed-spray technique. A continuous infusion of the lytic agent is then administered along with systemic anticoagulation. Generally, lysis begins distally and gradually moves proximally. Frequent monitoring of the patient is necessary to detect evidence of worsening ischemia and complications of lytic therapy.

(L) Thrombolysis achieves relief of clot burden in nearly all cases, but only in rare circumstances does it alone prove sufficient treatment for an occluded aortic graft limb (e.g., in a low-flow or hypercoagulable state in which no local causative lesion is involved).[8] More commonly, lysis of the

AORTIC GRAFT LIMB THROMBOSIS

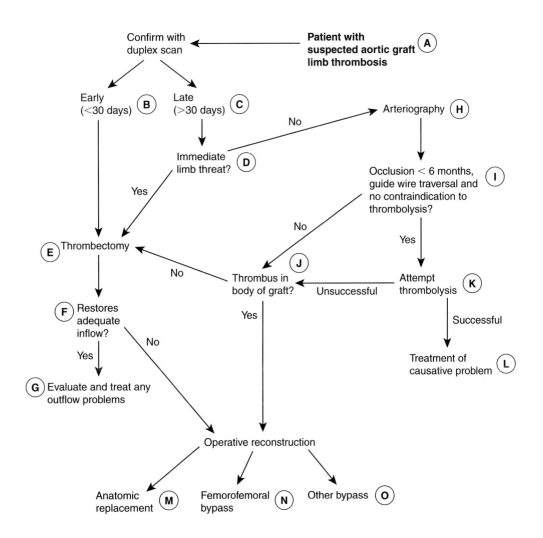

thrombus can uncover a specific abnormality responsible for the graft limb thrombosis. The surgeon may then proceed with the appropriate operative or endovascular approach for the particular underlying lesion, such as balloon angioplasty, stenting, atherectomy, or stent graft placement.[16-18] In most such cases, however, surgical options must be considered.

(M) Insertion of an entirely new aortofemoral graft limb was once touted as the most definitive and durable method of reconstruction in unilateral graft limb occlusions.[14,19] This procedure may be carried out through a retroperitoneal lower abdominal or flank approach or through the original transperitoneal incision. The entire occluded graft limb is exposed to the graft bifurcation. The graft body is tangentially clamped and the occluded limb transected. Following this, a new graft is tunneled posterior to the ureter to the common femoral or profunda femoris artery.

Although this approach certainly establishes inflow, it may prove quite taxing on both surgeon and patient. Reoperation in the retroperitoneum may incur major venous lacerations as well as injuries to the ureter or duodenum. Operative mortality may approach 10% in this population.[5] Furthermore, the long-term results may be no better than with other methods of reconstruction.[7,12] Therefore, unless preoperative angiography has revealed proximal occlusive disease at or above the aortic anastomosis, a direct approach with complete graft replacement is rarely necessary.

(N) If reliable inflow through the contralateral limb is present, a transpubic femorofemoral crossover bypass is generally the procedure of choice. The graft may originate from the hood of the donor graft limb and may be anastomosed at the contralateral profundal outflow tract. Quite satisfactory outcomes may be achieved, and an intra-abdominal procedure is avoided. Thus, femorofemoral graft insertion is generally the procedure of choice if thrombectomy is not feasible or unsuccessful. This procedure helps avoid a laparotomy in a reoperative field and has acceptable long-term function with 5-year secondary patencies approximating 85% in modern series.[20]

Ideally, preoperative angiography will have confirmed satisfactory flow in the contralateral limb. If any doubt exists, on-table angiograms or intraoperative pressures may be of assistance in documenting acceptability.

(O) Infrequently, other sources of inflow may be required to avoid an infected or hostile field. In such cases, inflow from the axillary artery or thoracic artery has been utilized.[21]

REFERENCES

1. Hallett JW Jr, Marshall DM, Petterson TM, et al: Graft-related complications after abdominal aortic aneurysm repair: Reassurance from a 36-year population-based experience. J Vasc Surg 1997;25:277–284; discussion, 285–286.
2. Littooy FN, Steffan G, Steinam S, et al: An 11-year experience with aortofemoral bypass grafting. Cardiovasc Surg 1993;1:232–238.
3. Szilagyi DE, Elliott JP Jr, Smith RF, et al: A thirty-year survey of the reconstructive surgical treatment of aortoiliac occlusive disease. J Vasc Surg 1986;3:421–436.
4. Brewster DC: Aortic graft limb occlusion. In Ernst CB, Stanley JC (eds): Current Therapy in Vascular Surgery, 3rd ed. St. Louis, Mosby–Year Book, 1995, pp 419–426.
5. Brewster DC: Surgery of late aortic graft occlusion. In Bergan JJ, Yao JST (eds): Surgery of the Aorta. Philadelphia, WB Saunders, 1989, pp 519–538.
6. Haiart DC, Callam MJ, Murie JA, et al: Reoperations for late complications following abdominal aortic operation. Br J Surg 1991;78:204–206.
7. Brewster DC, Meier GH 3rd, Darling RC, et al: Reoperation for aortofemoral graft limb occlusion: Optimal methods and long-term results. J Vasc Surg 1987;5:363–374.
8. Erdoes LS, Bernhard VM, Berman SS: Aortofemoral graft occlusion: Strategy and timing of reoperation. Cardiovasc Surg 1995;3:277–283.
9. Ameli FM, Provan JL, Williamson C, Keuchler PM: Etiology and management of aorto-femoral bypass graft failure. J Cardiovasc Surg (Torino) 1987;28:695–700.
10. Naylor AR, Ah-See AK, Engeset J: Graft occlusion following aortofemoral bypass for peripheral ischaemia. Br J Surg 1989;76:572–575.
11. Rutherford RB, Baker JD, Ernst C, et al: Recommended standards for reports dealing with lower extremity ischemia: Revised version. J Vasc Surg 1997;26:517–538.
12. Nevelsteen A, Suy R: Graft occlusion following aortofemoral Dacron bypass. Ann Vasc Surg 1991;5:32–37.
13. Frisch N, Bour P, Berg P, et al: Long-term results of thrombectomy for late occlusions of aortofemoral bypass. Ann Vasc Surg 1991;5:16–20.
14. Colburn MD, Moore WS: Reoperative approach for failed aortofemoral, axillofemoral, and femorofemoral bypasses. Semin Vasc Surg 1994;7:139–151.
15. Agrifoglio G, Lorenzi G, Castelli PM, et al: Thrombectomy for late graft limb occlusion: Our experience in 182 consecutive cases. J Cardiovasc Surg (Torino) 1990;31:617–620.
16. Marin ML, Veith FJ, Sanchez LA, et al: Endovascular aortoiliac grafts in combination with standard infrainguinal arterial bypasses in the management of limb-threatening ischemia: Preliminary report. J Vasc Surg 1995;22:316–324; discussion, 324–325.
17. Enon B, Reigner B, Lescalie F, et al: In situ thrombolysis for late occlusion of suprafemoral prosthetic grafts. Ann Vasc Surg 1993;7:270–274.
18. Ohki T, Marin ML, Veith FJ, et al: Endovascular aortounifemoral grafts and femorofemoral bypass for bilateral limb-threatening ischemia. J Vasc Surg 1996;24:984–987.
19. Drury JK, Leiberman DP, Gilmour DG, Pollock JG: Operation for late complications of aortic grafts. Surg Gynecol Obstet 1986;163:251–255.
20. Nolan KD, Benjamin ME, Murphy TJ, et al: Femorofemoral bypass for aortofemoral graft limb occlusion: A ten-year experience. J Vasc Surg 1994;19:851–856; discussion, 856–857.
21. Cormier JM, Marzelle J, Albrand JJ, et al: Lower-limb revascularization from the supracoeliac aorta through a transcrural approach. Cardiovasc Surg 1993;1:44–47.

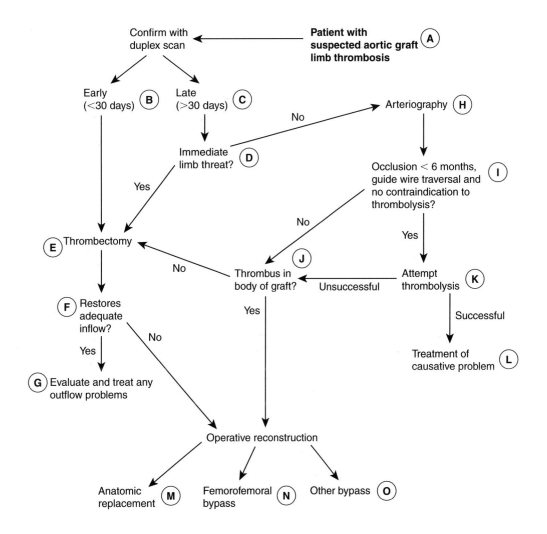

Chapter 40 Aortic Graft Infection

MARK R. JACKSON, MD • G. PATRICK CLAGETT, MD

A The reported incidence of aortic graft infection (AGI) is related to the site of graft implantation, specifically whether a femoral anastomosis is performed. The incidence of AGI for aortoiliac graft placement is approximately 0.5% to 1.0%, and increases to about 1.5% to 3.0% for aortofemoral grafts.[1] The clinical presentation of AGI ranges from overt signs, such as purulent drainage from a sinus tract overlying a femoral limb of an aortobifemoral bypass, to a more subtle presentation, characterized by fever of unknown origin and vague constitutional symptoms. Malaise and chronic fatigue are almost uniformly present. Unexplained gastrointestinal bleeding in a patient with an aortic prosthetic graft can indicate a graft-enteric fistula (see Chapter 25).

Early presentation of AGI within weeks of graft implantation is generally secondary to *Staphylococcus aureus* or gram-negative bacteria. *Late* presentation (months to years later), with graft complications such as false aneurysm formation, cutaneous drainage tracts, and perigraft fluid without systemic sepsis, is generally due to *Staphylococcus epidermidis*.

Physical examination must include inspection of the surgical incisions for sinus tracts or other evidence of infection. Palpation of the abdomen and groins (aortofemoral grafts) sometimes demonstrates pseudoaneurysm formation. Petechial lesions in the feet can indicate septic emboli. Evidence of other remote infections should be sought because this can cause hematogenous seeding of the aortic graft.

Laboratory studies commonly reveal leukocytosis and an elevated erythrocyte sedimentation rate, but these findings are not specific. Blood specimens as well as specimens of any drainage should be obtained for culture to identify the causative organism. Appropriate antibiotic treatment should be initiated.

B Regardless of the degree of clinical manifestations that suggest AGI, diagnostic imaging studies are necessary to evaluate whether inflammation, false aneurysm, perigraft fluid, or gas is present. In many centers, computed tomography (CT) is the initial imaging test of choice. In a blinded, retrospective review of 55 cases, CT was found to be 94% sensitive and 85% specific for AGI using operative findings as the "gold standard."[2] CT findings suggesting AGI included ectopic gas, perigraft fluid, and pseudoaneurysm formation.

Other investigators from the same institution previously reported success using magnetic resonance imaging (MRI), with AGI correctly diagnosed on the basis of MRI in 14 of 16 cases.[3] MRI was found to be useful in differentiating perigraft fluid and inflammatory changes from subacute or chronic hematoma.

Indium 111–labeled white blood cell scanning is often used to detect perigraft inflammation associated with AGI. Several studies indicate high sensitivity (86% to 100%) and specificity (85% to 100%), but false-negative and false-positive results have been reported.[4,5] Another limitation of this modality is the presence of false-positive results in the early postoperative period (1 to 12 months).[6]

Arteriography is important in planning reconstruction options required after partial or complete removal of an infected prosthesis. If autogenous revascularization using superficial femoropopliteal veins (deep veins) (SFPV) is being considered, venous duplex ultrasonography is necessary to determine the diameter, patency, and quality of these veins.

C In the absence of clear evidence for AGI, other etiologic mechanisms of an infectious problem should be evaluated and the patient carefully observed. If no other cause of infection can be found, selected patients with possible AGI may need to undergo diagnostic surgical exploration in the absence of positive imaging findings. This scenario is most often encountered in patients suspected of having a graft-enteric fistula when no other source of gastrointestinal bleeding is identified and in patients with apparently bland anastomotic false aneurysms. The finding at surgery of tissue incorporation of the graft generally rules out graft infection. Conversely, nonincorporation of the prosthesis is considered evidence of infection, with *S. epidermidis* likely to be present if purulence is absent.[7]

D If CT scanning or other testing indicates infection of the body of the aortic graft, the entire graft must be removed. This is usually also the case when both limbs of a graft are involved, since involvement of the body of the graft is quite likely even if it is not demonstrated on preoperative images. Occasionally, localized infections of both groins can be treated without total graft excision if a nonvirulent organism is the cause (see E). If only the distal portion of one limb is involved, the body of the graft can be potentially saved if the involved limb can be removed without contaminating the remainder of the graft.

E Microbiology culture has an important role in the diagnosis and treatment of graft infection. It is important to use ultrasonic processing of graft cultures to disrupt potential bacterial biofilm from the infected prosthesis. This is a much more sensitive technique than standard broth culture technique, in which bacteria can remain undetected in the biofilm.[8] Most prosthetic graft infections are caused by coagulase-negative staphylococci (CNS), specifically *S. epidermidis*. These organisms are not virulent and generally do not cause perigraft tissue invasion or bacteremia. CNS exist on the surface of the graft in a biofilm that protects the organisms from host defense mechanisms. It is important to differentiate CNS graft infection from infection caused by more virulent organisms, since the former is more amenable to local treatment with in situ graft replacement.[9]

Specimens may be obtained preoperatively from sinus tracts, blood, or ultrasound-controlled

AORTIC GRAFT INFECTION

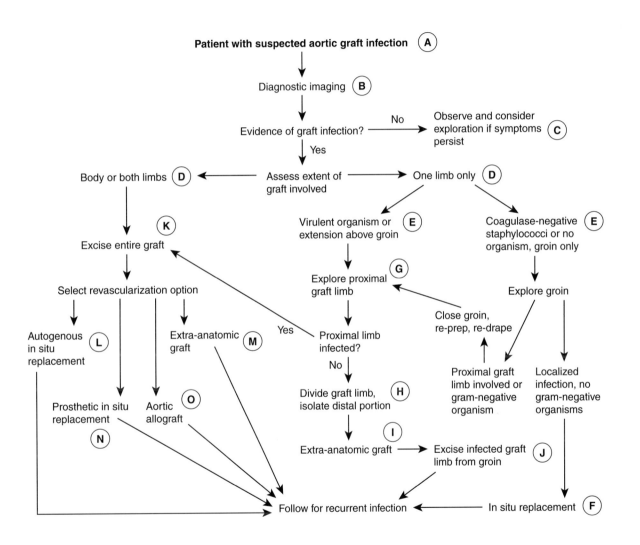

aspiration of localized fluid collections in the groin, but often preoperative identification is not possible. In general, more virulent organisms (e.g., *S. aureus, Pseudomonas*) tend to be associated with more cellulitis and systemic signs of infection, whereas CNS infection is usually subtle and is often detected only on exploration of an apparently noninfected groin pseudoaneurysm.

Assessment of the extent of isolated graft limb involvement is also important. If imaging shows fluid extending above the groin into the retroperitoneum, local treatment via the groin is probably not possible.

(F) In the presence of a CNS graft infection confined to the groin, Bandyk and associates recommend in situ replacement with polytetrafluoroethylene (PTFE) material after removal of the infected distal graft limb via the groin and débridement of any infected surrounding tissue.[8] The proximal anastomosis is performed to the tissue-incorporated segment of the divided aortofemoral graft limb, usually approached through the groin incision. Intravenous antibiotics are continued for 14 to 28 days, followed by 6 to 12 weeks of oral antibiotics. Using this approach, Bandyk and associates successfully treated 11 patients with infected aortic grafts without recurrent graft infection during follow-up ranging from 5 to 50 months (mean, 21 months). Despite these encouraging results, recurrent graft infection involving the proximal aortic segment remains a risk, and careful follow-up is required.

(G) When AGI appears confined to the distal portion of a single limb of an aortobifemoral graft and the infection is more virulent than that caused by CNS, excision of the involved limb with preservation of the remainder of the graft may still be possible; however, great care must be taken not to contaminate the noninfected, proximal portion of that graft limb. In such cases, the first step is to confirm that the proximal portion of the infected limb is not involved in the infectious process. The surgeon accomplishes this step by exposing the graft limb, usually through a separate retroperitoneal incision, and checking for the presence of graft infection.

(H) If the graft is well incorporated in the proximal portion, the limb is divided. The surgeon isolates the distal part of the limb by carefully closing retroperitoneal tissue over that distal portion of the limb so that this portion can be later removed via the infected groin incision without infecting the proximal portion. In most cases, revascularization of the leg is necessary.

(I) Revascularization is usually done with an extra-anatomic graft through uninfected tissue planes. This can be accomplished with a transobturator bypass to the mid-superficial femoral artery or a lateral approach from the pelvis to the profunda or superficial femoral artery (SFA), with autogenous vein or PTFE. These grafts originate from the noninfected proximal segment of the exposed retroperitoneal aortic graft limb. Recurrent graft infection, however, remains a risk with partial graft excision. In a review of 106 patients treated in this manner, there was a 44% incidence of recurrent infection that often involved the remaining aortic graft.[9] Thus, careful follow-up is necessary.

(J) After completing the extra-anatomic revascularization and closing and bandaging all incisions, the surgeon excises the infected distal portion of the aortofemoral graft limb via a new groin incision, which is then left open to heal secondarily in the presence of infection. Ideally, the femoral artery should be closed in such a way that SFA–profunda artery continuity is maintained, if both arteries are patent, to optimize the revascularization. If an autogenous vein patch rather than primary closure or SFA-profunda artery direct anastomosis is required, the extent and severity of infection need to be considered, since a vein patch may disrupt in the presence of severe infection.

(K) Excision of an infected aortic graft is a technically demanding procedure for the surgeon, with significant risk to the patient. Care must be taken to avoid injury to adherent intestine and ureters. If the proximal anastomosis is very near the renal arteries, suprarenal-celiac clamping may be required. Rarely, extra-anatomic renal revascularization is necessary (hepato-spleno-renal) if the pararenal aorta is involved by the infectious process.

(L) There are several options for revascularization after excision of an infected aortic graft. We prefer to use the SFPV for autogenous, in situ aortic revascularization, which we described in 1993.[10] Complete excision of the infected prosthesis as a single-stage procedure is performed. In our experience with the neo-aortoiliac system (NAIS) reconstruction for AGI using this method, the mortality rate was low (7.3%), only 5% of patients required amputation at 30 days, and the 5-year limb salvage rate was 86%.[11] The 5-year primary and secondary graft patency rates were 83% and 100%, respectively.

Our NAIS experience in patients with failed or infected extra-anatomic bypass performed after removal of infected aortic prostheses has also been favorable.[12] Problems related to extra-anatomic bypass, prosthetic infection, and aortic stump blow-out are avoided with NAIS reconstruction. Venous morbidity after SFPV harvest is surprisingly low.[13]

(M) Many still consider extra-anatomic revascularization after aortic graft excision the standard operation for AGI. A major question that arises when this surgical option is chosen is that of sequencing the operations. At the Cleveland Clinic, there was no difference in operative or 1-year mortality rates whether graft excision and extra-anatomic bypass were combined or staged.[14] Amputation rates, however, were significantly lower (7% versus 41%) with a staged approach. Others, however, have found a trend toward lower mortality when extra-anatomic bypass preceded graft excision, either at the same operation (sequenced) or at a second operation (staged).[15]

AORTIC GRAFT INFECTION

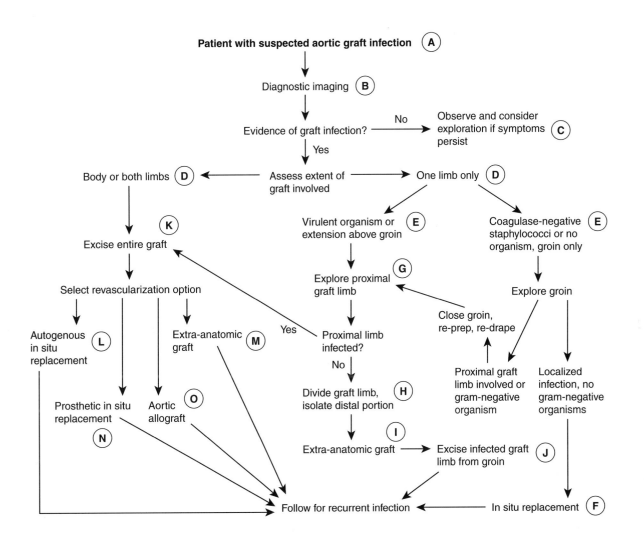

On the basis of these studies, it is generally advisable to consider staging graft excision as a separate operation after extra-anatomic bypass when this approach is used. Persistent infection in the aortic stump can cause subsequent, fatal stump blow-out[13]—a complication that is avoided with an in-line NAIS revascularization. Other limitations of axillobifemoral revascularization in these patients are lower patency rates than are associated with aortic-based revascularization and subsequent graft infection, which occurs in approximately 20% of cases.[15,16] In some patients, the extent of groin cellulitis and inadequacy of potential distal targets for extra-anatomic revascularization preclude this approach.

(N) The third revascularization option after aortic graft excision is in situ prosthetic replacement. This method was the initial treatment for AGI after the introduction of aortic prosthetic grafts, but it fell into disfavor because of the high risk of graft reinfection.[17] This approach is perhaps most appealing in the emergency management of graft-enteric fistula with life-threatening gastrointestinal hemorrhage, a circumstance in which revascularization cannot precede graft excision and in which the time needed for deep vein harvest (for NAIS revascularization) might be problematic. In a report of 20 such cases in 1987, 3 resulted in reinfection of the graft, causing early recurrent rupture or false aneurysm involving the proximal anastomosis.[18]

Rifampin-impregnated polyester (Dacron) grafts have been shown in animal models of graft infection and in a small case series to be a potential alternative allowing for in situ prosthetic revascularization.[19,20] These grafts, however, are not commercially available, and the reported experience is limited.

Given the limitation imposed by the risk of recurrent graft infection and the availability of alternative methods of in situ autogenous revascularization, in situ prosthetic replacement should not be regarded as the treatment of choice for AGI. It is best considered a "bridge" procedure for the emergency treatment of AGI when circumstances mitigate against the initial use of more standard options. In this manner, in situ prosthetic replacement might allow initial "damage control" surgery, followed by graft excision and NAIS revascularization, or extra-anatomic bypass and graft excision as separate procedures.

(O) Finally, aortic allograft replacement, another option, has been successfully used to treat aortic prosthetic infections.[21-23] The main advantages of this approach include convenience and decreased operating time obviating the need to harvest and prepare autogenous conduits. However, allografts are subject to reinfection and short-term and long-term deterioration, often with disastrous consequences. Many consider in situ allograft aortic replacement to be a bridge procedure until a more definitive reconstruction can be undertaken.[22,23]

REFERENCES

1. Bandyk DF, Bergamini TM: Infection in prosthetic vascular grafts. In Rutherford RB (ed): Vascular Surgery, 5th ed. Philadelphia, WB Saunders, 2000, pp 733–751.
2. Low RN, Wall SD, Jeffrey RB, Sollitto RA, et al: Aortoenteric fistula and perigraft infection: Evaluation with CT. Radiology 1990;175:157–162.
3. Olofsson PA, Auffermann W, Higgins CB, et al: Diagnosis of prosthetic aortic graft infection by magnetic resonance imaging. J Vasc Surg 1988;8:99–105.
4. Lawrence PF, Dries DJ, Alazraki N, Albo D: Indium 111–labeled leukocyte scanning for detection of prosthetic vascular graft infection. J Vasc Surg 1985;2:165–173.
5. Brunner MC, Mitchell RS, Baldwin JC, et al: Prosthetic graft infection: Limitations of indium white blood cell scanning. J Vasc Surg 1986;3:42–48.
6. Sedwitz MM, Davies RJ, Pretorius HT, Vasquez TE: Indium 111–labeled white blood cell scans after vascular prosthetic reconstruction. J Vasc Surg 1987;6:476–481.
7. Padberg FT, Smith SM, Eng RHK: Accuracy of disincorporation for identification of vascular graft infection. Arch Surg 1995;130:183–187.
8. Bandyk DF, Bergamini TM, Kinney EV, et al: In situ replacement of vascular prostheses infected by bacterial biofilms. J Vasc Surg 1991;13:575–583.
9. Bunt TJ: Treatment options for graft infections. In Bunt TJ (ed): Vascular Graft Infections. Armonk, NY, Futura Publishing, 1994.
10. Clagett GP, Bowers BL, Lopez-Viego MA, et al: Creation of a neo-aortoiliac system from lower extremity deep and superficial veins. Ann Surg 1993;218:239–249.
11. Clagett GP, Valentine RJ, Hagino RT: Autogenous aorto-iliac/femoral reconstruction from superficial femoral–popliteal veins: Feasibility and durability. J Vasc Surg 1997;25:255–270.
12. Gordon LL, Hagino RT, Jackson MR, et al: Complex aortofemoral prosthetic infections: The role of autogenous superficial femoropopliteal vein reconstruction. Arch Surg 1999;134:615–621.
13. Wells JK, Hagino RT, Bargmann KM, et al: Venous morbidity after superficial femoral–popliteal vein harvest. J Vasc Surg 1999;29:282–291.
14. O'Hara PJ, Hertzer NR, Beven EG, Krajewski LP: Surgical management of infected abdominal aortic grafts: Review of a 25-year experience. J Vasc Surg 1986;3:725–731.
15. Reilly LM, Stoney RJ, Goldstone J, Ehrenfeld WK: Improved management of aortic graft infection: The influence of operation sequence and staging. J Vasc Surg 1987;5:421–431.
16. Yeager RA, Moneta GL, Taylor LM, et al: Improving survival and limb salvage in patients with aortic graft infection. Am J Surg 1990;159:466–469.
17. Lawrence PF: Management of infected aortic grafts. Surg Clin N Am 1995;75:783–797.
18. Walker WE, Cooley DA, Duncan JM, et al: The management of aortoduodenal fistula by in situ replacement of the infected abdominal aortic graft. Ann Surg 1987;205:727–732.
19. Colburn MD, Moore WS, Chvapil M, et al: Use of an antibiotic-bonded graft for in situ reconstruction after prosthetic graft infections. J Vasc Surg 1992;16:651–658; discussion, 658–660.
20. Torsello G, Sandmann W, Gehrt A, Jungblut RM: In situ replacement of infected vascular prostheses with rifampin-soaked vascular grafts: Early results. J Vasc Surg 1993;17:768–773.
21. Kieffer E, Bahnini A, Koskas F, et al: In situ allograft replacement of infected infrarenal aortic prosthetic grafts: Results in forty-three patients. J Vasc Surg 1993;17:349–356.
22. Bahnini A, Ruotolo C, Koskas F, Kieffer E: In situ fresh allograft replacement of an infected aortic prosthetic graft: Eighteen months' follow-up. J Vasc Surg 1991;14:98–102.
23. Nevelsteen A, Feryn T, Lacroix H, et al: Experience with cryopreserved arterial allografts in the treatment of prosthetic graft infections. Cardiovasc Surg 1998;6:378–383.

AORTIC GRAFT INFECTION

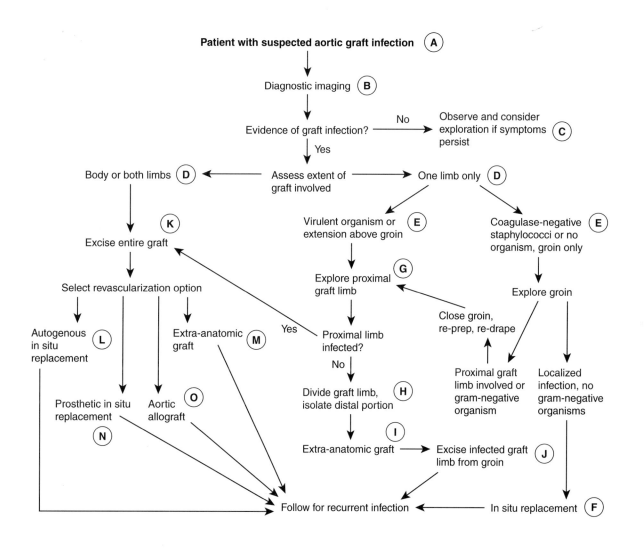

Chapter 41 Infrainguinal Occlusive Disease

M. C. DONALDSON, MD • ANTHONY D. WHITTEMORE, MD

(A) Imaging studies are generally reserved until it is clear that the patient is a candidate for revascularization from the standpoint of indications and safety. Percutaneous selective contrast arteriography remains the standard for clarifying vascular anatomy. Nonetheless, other less invasive imaging methods are available and have become increasingly valuable with refinement and experience. These alternatives allow directed screening to help plan the best management, whether endovascular, surgical, or conservative. Arteriography can thus be used selectively to confirm the anatomic diagnosis, often combined at the same sitting with catheter-guided therapeutic intervention when appropriate.

Among the alternative methods, duplex ultrasound is widely available in virtually all noninvasive vascular laboratories and can be used to clarify the arterial anatomy from the common femoral level into the popliteal and, to some extent, into the tibial vessels.[1,2] Duplex imaging differentiates long segment superficial femoral artery (SFA) occlusion from focal stenosis possibly amenable to percutaneous therapy. Some laboratories also have imaging capability of the iliac arteries.

Magnetic resonance angiography (MRA) is another safe, noninvasive means of identifying patterns of disease. With proximal occlusions, MRA may be a satisfactory substitute for arteriography, although in smaller distal arteries the anatomic definition may be inadequate for confident surgical planning.[3,4]

Spiral (helical) computed tomography (CT) also has potential, although it calls for intravenous contrast injection and experience is still limited.

(B) Focal femoropopliteal lesions are potentially amenable to percutaneous endovascular therapy. Alternatively, a localized surgical approach, such as profundaplasty or SFA endarterectomy, may be possible. The lesions best suited for percutaneous transluminal angioplasty (PTA) are short, concentric stenoses (<2 cm) with nearly normal adjacent artery lumen, most commonly found at the adductor tendon insertion among claudicants. Eccentric short stenoses, multiple short stenoses, or single relatively longer stenoses (2 to 4 cm) are also feasible.

Occlusions do not behave as favorably as stenoses. Nonetheless, short occlusions (<5 cm) may be successfully treated with PTA. For example, patency following PTA of short SFA stenosis among claudicants with good runoff (two to three vessels into calf) is roughly 60% at 5 years. Patency after PTA for short SFA occlusion is closer to 35% among claudicants with good runoff.[5,6] Use of stents below the groin does not improve long-term results.[7]

Extensive femoropopliteal lesions involve long segments (>5 cm) with diffuse disease, multiple stenoses, or occlusion or absence of a reconstituted popliteal artery above or below the knee. Patients with this distribution of disease do not do as well with percutaneous therapy and are best managed with surgical bypass.

(C) "Good" runoff refers to angiographic reconstitution of two to three crural vessels in direct continuity with the distal popliteal artery. Under the best circumstances, one or two of these vessels also cross the ankle joint into the foot to fill the plantar arches.[8] "Poor" runoff refers to angiographic reconstitution of one vessel in continuity with the distal popliteal artery or no vessel in continuity (the "isolated popliteal segment"), reconstitution of a distal tibial artery that may run across the ankle joint into the foot, or other combinations of tibial artery reconstitution without popliteal patency or pedal artery reconstitution.

(D) In general, PTA would be the initial approach among most patients with focal disease and good runoff, regardless of estimated surgical risk. Patients with less favorable anatomy might be offered PTA to minimize morbidity if surgical risk were estimated to be high, if therapeutic goals were strictly palliative and directed at healing of a superficial ulcer, or if longevity were estimated to be short, as in patients with end-stage renal disease.[9]

(E) Bypass is the preferred method of revascularization for all patients except (1) those with focal femoropopliteal disease and good runoff or (2) selected patients with less favorable anatomy and limited palliative goals in the face of estimated high surgical morbidity. However, a bypass into an extremely limited runoff bed using poor conduit with expectation of no more than 25% 1-year patency may simply add morbidity with little durable benefit to the patient. Under such circumstances, conservative nonoperative therapy or a definitive amputation may be more sensible.

Primary amputation should be reserved for patients with:

1. Extensive foot necrosis extending proximal to the metatarsal bones.
2. Sepsis that involves the tarsal bones, ankle, or soft tissues of the calf with severe systemic illness.
3. Debilitated and bedridden patients with no ambulatory potential.

The surgical risk of major amputation is at least as high as for bypass. In some cases, the inability to perform a bypass may lead the surgeon to reconsider PTA even if the lesions are not optimal, but this choice must be carefully individualized.

(F) Bypass to the above-knee popliteal artery is optimal when the entire popliteal artery is free of disease, with good distal runoff. When the pattern of disease involves poor runoff below the knee but allows a distal anastomosis above the knee, autogenous vein graft is preferred. Vein grafts to an isolated popliteal artery are associated with 65% 5-year patency rates.[10,11] Alternatively, even though a vein graft anastomosis can be positioned above the knee in patients with poor runoff, it is usually preferable to select a more distal location in order to obtain direct flow into the foot unless sufficient vein length is not available.

G Prosthetic grafts implanted above the knee joint with good runoff are associated with a 60% 5-year cumulative patency rate.[12, 13] It has been suggested that polytetrafluorethylene (PTFE) and polyester (Dacron) perform equally well in this position.[14] Vein graft results are superior to prosthetic results and may be preferred in all locations, including the above-knee femoropopliteal position. A strategy using above-knee prosthetic early in the course of disease, reserving the vein for bypass to more distal levels later, has some appeal but remains to be validated.[15] If the ipsilateral greater saphenous vein (GSV) is not available, however, a prosthetic graft is often selected over an alternative vein in this setting.

H Autogenous vein, using ipsilateral GSV and ectopic sources such as the contralateral greater saphenous vein, lesser saphenous vein, arm vein, or even joining residual or duplicated GSV from the ipsilateral or contralateral leg, has remained the most effective conduit for infrainguinal revascularization.[16, 17] Duplex ultrasound surveillance can be used to "map" superficial veins and to characterize size, length, and quality of potential venous conduits. This information greatly facilitates surgical planning and reduces morbidity related to venous exploration at the time of surgery.[18]

In some instances, physical examination may suffice to clarify presence of an adequate autogenous conduit and vein mapping may not be necessary. A history of previous vein harvesting does not necessarily mean that there is no residual conduit of value, since accessory or parallel veins can exist.[19]

I Among autogenous conduits, ipsilateral GSV, when adequate, is preferred. Assessment of conduit quality is in part a subjective judgment. In general, any vein with a distended internal diameter less than 3 mm is more likely to develop stenosis early in its course. A vein with focal or diffuse sclerosis is unsuitable until modified to excise the involved segments. Veins with dupli-

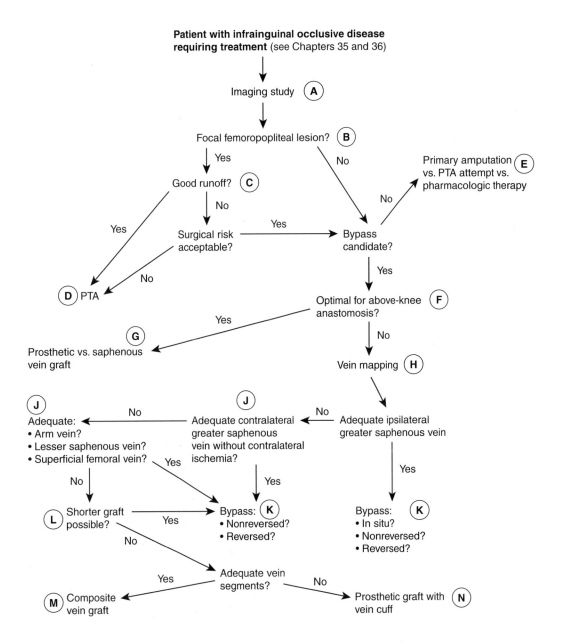

cated segments are best modified by eliminating the smaller of the two channels. Veins with diffuse dilation associated with varicosities may be used, provided they are not grossly enlarged (>8 mm) or thin-walled, and veins with focal varicosity or aneurysm may be modified by excision of the involved segments.

(J) The contralateral GSV is generally the next choice after ipsilateral GSV unless significant contralateral ischemia exists, which unfortunately is often the case. Most concur with use of arm vein as the next choice, starting with the nondominant extremity when possible.[20, 21]

Because arm vein harvest generally necessitates the use of general anesthesia, this method may be less desirable in some patients. The lesser saphenous (LSV) vein would then be considered, a less favorable choice because of the relative difficulty of harvesting and the higher likelihood of sclerosis and calcification.[22] The LSV might be preferred when the distal popliteal artery is used for inflow for bypass to a tibial or pedal vessel. Residual or duplicated segments of GSV are often of excellent quality and can serve well even when spliced to create an autogenous composite conduit.[23]

The superficial femoral vein (SFV) has been used with good results and surprisingly little postoperative morbidity related to impaired venous outflow.[24, 25]

Another option to consider is SFA endarterectomy, either as a definitive procedure or as a procedure to provide a more distal inflow site for a short bypass to the tibial or pedal level.[26-28]

(K) Choice of bypass technique for autogenous vein is largely a matter of technical rather than intrinsic biologic considerations. The in situ GSV has a good size match between the proximal vein graft and donor artery and the distal vein graft and the recipient artery, particularly in the tibial and pedal locations. The in situ vein also is uniquely amenable to recent technical advances, which allow a minimally invasive approach to infrainguinal bypass.[29]

Use of a nonreversed orientation may be preferred for greater flexibility in moving the vein proximally or distally to accommodate inflow from sources other than the common femoral artery and outflow into a variety of distal vessels not easily reached by in situ vein.[30] Both in situ and nonreversed, translocated grafts require perfection of valve cusp incision technique. Reversed vein bypass has proved as effective and durable as the other techniques.[31] A technical challenge unique to reversed vein is creation of a satisfactory anastomosis to a heavily diseased common femoral artery using the small distal end of the vein.

(L) If adequate vein length is not available, it may be possible to shorten the required graft length with the use of a more distal location for the proximal anastomosis. Results of bypass to infrapopliteal arteries from hemodynamically normal arteries distal to the common femoral artery are very acceptable.[32-34] Distal inflow from the popliteal artery may be satisfactorily improved under selected circumstances by PTA or endarterectomy of focal proximal SFA or popliteal disease. In some cases, a more proximal site for the distal anastomosis can be selected, such as an isolated popliteal artery.

(M) Spliced segments of autogenous vein of good quality provide superior patency compared with prosthetic grafts below the knee and are preferred when a single segment of vein is not available.

(N) Prosthetic grafts include PTFE, Dacron, human umbilical vein, and cryopreserved venous homografts.[35, 36] Prosthetic grafts can be inserted with short operative times and minimal wound morbidity; for this reason, they are occasionally selected over vein grafts in very-high-risk patients. However, they are generally reserved for the small percentage of patients in whom no autogenous vein is available. Prosthetic graft patency is markedly inferior to autogenous vein when the distal anastomosis is below the knee.[12, 13, 35-37]

In some series, human umbilical vein performs better than PTFE below the knee[38] and is preferred by some despite aneurysmal degeneration over time. Anticoagulation therapy appears to prolong patency among patients with below-knee prosthetic grafts[39] and is also helpful among patients after high-risk autogenous bypass.[40, 41] There is increasing evidence that a vein "cuff" between the prosthetic graft and the distal anastomosis improves patency. Different modifications have been suggested, including the Miller cuff, Wolfe boot, and Taylor patch, but all use the same concept.[42-45] A randomized trial showed no effect of vein cuffs on above-knee PTFE graft patency; for below-knee femoropopliteal bypass, however, the 2-year graft patency rate was 52% with a cuff and only 29% without.[46]

Addition of an arteriovenous fistula distal to a prosthetic anastomosis does not appear to improve patency.[47] Composite prosthetic-vein grafts have not shown superiority over prosthetic grafts alone. Composite-sequential grafts, with a prosthetic anastomosis to the above-knee popliteal artery and a venous jump graft to a distal runoff vessel, have the theoretical advantage of increased proximal graft flow by virtue of two distal anastomoses but have not shown clinical superiority.

REFERENCES

1. Moneta GL, Yeager RA, Lee RW, Porter JM: Noninvasive localization of arterial occlusive disease: A comparison of segmental Doppler pressures and arterial duplex mapping. J Vasc Surg 1993;17(3):578–582.
2. Thompson MM, Sayers RD, Beard JD, et al: The role of pulse-generated run-off, Doppler ultrasound and conventional arteriography in the assessment of patients prior to femorocrural bypass grafting. Eur J Vasc Surg 1993;7(1): 37–40.
3. Baum R, Rutter C, Sunshine J, et al: Multicenter trial to evaluate vascular magnetic resonance angiography of the lower extremity. JAMA 1995;274:875–880.
4. Cambria R, Kaufman J, Gertler J, et al: Magnetic resonance angiography in the management of lower extremity occlusive disease: A prospective study. J Vasc Surg 1997;25:380–389.
5. Hunink MG, Donaldson MC, Meyerovitz MF, et al: Risks and benefits of femoropopliteal percutaneous balloon angioplasty. J Vasc Surg 1993;17(1):183–192; discussion, 192–194.

6. Johnston K: Femoral and popliteal arteries: Reanalysis of results of balloon angioplasty. Radiology 1992;183:767.
7. White G, Liew S, Waugh R, et al: Early outcome and intermediate follow-up of vascular stents in the femoral and popliteal arteries without long-term anticoagulation. J Vasc Surg 1995;21:270–281.
8. Rutherford R, Baker J, Ernst C, et al: Recommended standards for reports dealing with lower extremity ischemia: Revised version. J Vasc Surg 1997;26:517–538.
9. Whittemore AD, Donaldson MC, Mannick JA: Infrainguinal reconstruction for patients with chronic renal insufficiency. J Vasc Surg 1993;17(1):32–39; discussion, 39–41.
10. Kaufman JL, Whittemore AD, Couch NP, Mannick JA: The fate of bypass grafts to an isolated popliteal artery segment. Surgery 1982;92:1027–1031.
11. Kram HB, Gupta SK, Veith FJ, et al: Late results of two hundred seventeen femoropopliteal bypasses to isolated popliteal artery segments. J Vasc Surg 1991;14:386–390.
12. Quinones-Baldrich W, Prego A, Ucelay-Gomez R, et al: Long-term results of infrainguinal revascularization with polytetrafluoroethylene: A ten-year experience. J Vasc Surg 1992;16:209–217.
13. Whittemore AD, Kent KC, Donaldson MC, et al: What is the proper role of polytetrafluoroethylene grafts in infrainguinal reconstruction? J Vasc Surg 1989;10(3):299–305.
14. Abbott W, Green R, Matsumoto T, et al: Prosthetic above-knee femoropopliteal bypass grafting: Results of a multicenter randomized prospective trial. J Vasc Surg 1997;25:19–28.
15. Quinones-Baldrich W, Busuttil R, Baker J, et al: Is the preferential use of polytetrafluoroethylene grafts for femoropopliteal bypass justified? J Vasc Surg 1988;8:219–228.
16. Donaldson MC, Whittemore AD, Mannick JA: An argument in favor of all-autogenous tissue for vascular bypasses below the inguinal ligament. Adv Surg 1991;24:69–90.
17. Donaldson MC, Whittemore AD, Mannick JA: Further experience with an all-autogenous tissue policy for infrainguinal reconstruction. J Vasc Surg 1993;18(1):41–48.
18. Ligush J, Reavis S, Preisser J, Hansen K: Duplex ultrasound scanning defines operative strategies for patients with limb-threatening ischemia. J Vasc Surg 1998;28:482–491.
19. Rutherford R, Sawyer J, Jones D: The fate of residual saphenous vein after partial removal or ligation. J Vasc Surg 1990;12:422–428.
20. Andros G, Harris R, Salles-Cunha S, et al: Arm veins for arterial revascularization of the leg: Arteriographic and clinical observations. J Vasc Surg 1986;4:416–427.
21. Balshi J, Cantelmo N, Menzoian J, LoGerfo F: The use of arm veins for infrainguinal bypass in end-stage peripheral vascular disease. Arch Surg 1989;124:1078.
22. Chang B, Paty P, Shah D, Leather R: The lesser saphenous vein: An underappreciated source of autogenous vein. J Vasc Surg 1992;15:152–157.

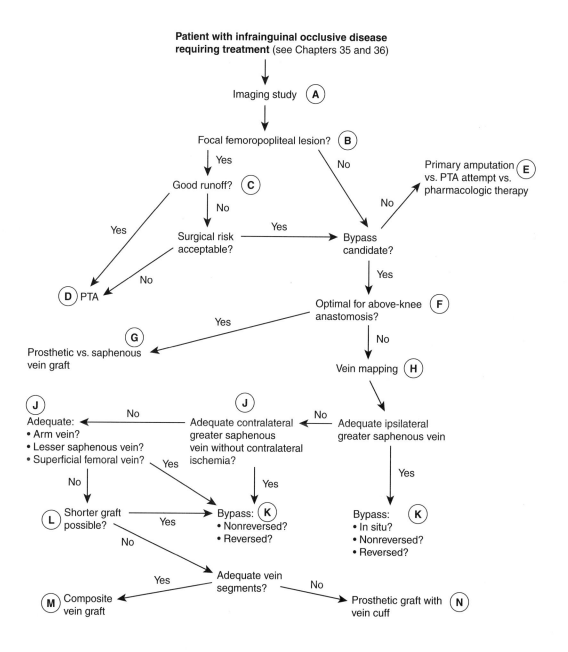

Infrainguinal Occlusive Disease (continued)

23. Belkin M, Donaldson MC, Whittemore AD: Composite autogenous vein grafts. Semin Vasc Surg 1995;8(3):202–208.
24. Coburn M, Ashworth C, Francis W, et al: Venous stasis complications of the use of the superficial femoral and popliteal veins for lower extremity bypass. J Vasc Surg 1993;17(6):1005–1008; discussion, 1008–1009.
25. Schulman M, Badhey M, Yatco R: Superficial femoral–popliteal veins and reversed saphenous vein as primary femoropopliteal bypass grafts: A randomized comparative study. J Vasc Surg 1987;6:1–10.
26. Inahara T, Scott C: Endarterectomy for segmental occlusive disease of the superficial femoral artery. Arch Surg 1981;116:1547.
27. Taylor SM, Langan EM 3rd, Snyder BA, Crane MM: Superficial femoral artery eversion endarterectomy: A useful adjunct for infrainguinal bypass in the presence of limited autogenous vein. J Vasc Surg 1997;26(3):439–445; discussion, 445–446.
28. van der Heijden FHWM, Eikelboom BC, van Reedt Dortland RWH, et al: Long-term results of semiclosed endarterectomy of the superficial femoral artery and the outcome of failed reconstructions. J Vasc Surg 1993;18:271–279.
29. Rosenthal D, Tucker JG, Atkins CP, et al: Extraluminal endoscopic-assisted ligation of venous tributaries for infrainguinal in situ saphenous vein bypass: A preliminary report. Cardiovasc Surg 1996;4(4):512–514.
30. Belkin M, Knox J, Donaldson MC, et al: Infrainguinal arterial reconstruction with nonreversed greater saphenous vein. J Vasc Surg 1996;24(6):957–962.
31. Taylor LM, Edwards JM, Porter JM: Present status of reversed vein bypass grafting: Five-year results of a modern series. J Vasc Surg 1990;11:193–206.
32. Rosenbloom M, Walsh J, Schuler J, et al: Long-term results of infragenicular bypasses with autogenous vein originating from the distal superficial femoral and popliteal arteries. J Vasc Surg 1988;7:691–696.
33. Wengerter K, Yang P, Veith F, et al: A twelve-year experience with the popliteal-to-distal artery bypass: The significance and management of proximal disease. J Vasc Surg 1992;15:143–151.
34. Veith F, Gupta S, Samson R, et al: Superficial femoral and popliteal arteries as inflow sites for distal bypass. Surgery 1981;90:980.
35. Leseche G, Penna C, Bouttier S, et al: Femorodistal bypass using cryopreserved venous allografts for limb salvage. Ann Vasc Surg 1997;11(3):230–236.
36. Shah RM, Faggioli GL, Mangione S, et al: Early results with cryopreserved saphenous vein allografts for infrainguinal bypass. J Vasc Surg 1993;18(6):965–969; discussion, 969–971.
37. Veith F, Gupta S, Ascer E, et al: Six-year prospective multicenter randomized comparison of autologous saphenous vein and expanded polytetrafluoroethylene grafts in infrainguinal arterial reconstruction. J Vasc Surg 1986;3:104–114.
38. Dardik H, Miller N, Dardik A, et al: A decade of experience with the glutaraldehyde-tanned human umbilical cord vein graft for revascularization of the lower limb. J Vasc Surg 1988;7:336.
39. Flinn W, Rohrer M, Yao J, et al: Improved long-term patency of infragenicular polytetrafluoroethylene grafts. J Vasc Surg 1988;7:685.
40. Kretschmer G, Wenzl E, Piza F, et al: The influence of anticoagulant treatment on the probability of function in femoropopliteal vein bypass surgery: Analysis of a clinical series (1970 to 1985) and interim evaluation of a controlled clinical trial. Surgery 1987;102:453.
41. Sarac T, Huber T, Back M, et al: Warfarin improves the outcome of infrainguinal vein bypass grafting at high risk for failure. J Vasc Surg 1998;28:446–457.
42. Miller J, Foreman R, Ferguson L, Faris I: Interposition vein cuff for anastomosis of prosthesis to small artery. Aust N Z J Surg 1984;54:283.
43. Morris GE, Raptis S, Miller JH, Faris IB: Femorocrural grafting and regrafting: Does polytetrafluoroethylene have a role? Eur J Vasc Surg 1993;7(3):329–334.
44. Taylor R, Loh A, McFarland R, et al: Improved technique for polytetrafluoroethylene bypass grafting: Long-term results using anastomotic vein patches. Br J Surg 1992;79:348–354.
45. Smout JD, Wolfe JH: Venous boot construction for a distal prosthetic bypass. Semin Vasc Surg 2000;13(1):53–57.
46. Stonebridge PA, Prescott RJ, Ruckley CV, for The Joint Vascular Research Group: Randomized trial comparing infrainguinal polytetrafluoroethylene bypass grafting with and without vein interposition cuff at the distal anastomosis. J Vasc Surg 1997;26(4):543–550.
47. Hamsho A, Nott D, Harris PL: Prospective randomised trial of distal arteriovenous fistula as an adjunct to femoro-infrapopliteal PTFE bypass. Eur J Vasc Endovasc Surg 1999;17(3):197–201.

Chapter 42 begins on the following page

Chapter 42 Infrainguinal Graft Surveillance

DENNIS F. BANDYK, MD

(A) Bypass grafts constructed of either autologous vein or prosthetic material tend to develop stenotic lesions during the first weeks to months after implantation into the arterial circulation. Observational studies that use duplex scanning to image infrainguinal bypasses have confirmed that strictures develop in approximately 20% of vein grafts and 5% to 10% of prosthetic grafts during the first 1 to 2 postoperative years.[1-6] Most lesions are the result of myointimal hyperplasia and, when present, are associated with a threefold increase in graft occlusion, accounting for 80% of graft failures.

Prospective clinical trials have confirmed the efficacy of duplex ultrasound surveillance after infrainguinal vein bypass with a 25% improvement in 3-year patency (78% versus 53%),[1-4] but a similar benefit has not been demonstrated after prosthetic bypass grafting.[6] When a progressive graft stenosis that reduces flow is identified, prophylactic repair is recommended.

Graft revision by balloon percutaneous transluminal angioplasty (PTA), vein patch angioplasty, or interposition replacement of the abnormal graft segment is safe (30-day mortality and graft failure rates below 1%) and is associated with an excellent 80% assisted primary patency. Delay until graft occlusion occurs both complicates the graft revision procedure by requiring thrombectomy and is associated with a poor outcome, with primary patency as low as 25% and secondary patency below 50% at 3 years. For this reason, duplex ultrasound surveillance is recommended for all infrainguinal vein grafts. Whether prosthetic grafts can benefit from surveillance is unclear. For this reason, the algorithm in this chapter considers infrainguinal vein grafts only.

(B) Surveillance after infrainguinal vein grafting begins in the operating room. Color duplex ultrasonography is preferred over arteriography because it provides an evaluation of bypass graft hemodynamics in addition to imaging. The goal of testing is to verify that the arterial reconstruction has no stenosis and that it has sufficient blood flow for patency and improvement of limb perfusion.

A variety of bypass graft abnormalities can be detected with duplex ultrasonography, including:

- Vein conduit stenosis or fibrosis
- Inadequate vein valve lysis
- Small-caliber conduit
- Anastomotic stenosis
- Inflow-outflow artery obstruction or stenosis
- Clamp injury
- Formation of fibrin-platelet aggregates
- Low graft velocity caused by inadequate runoff arteries

Detection and correction of bypass graft abnormalities reduce the incidence of early graft thrombosis and the need for secondary interventions for residual stenosis.[7]

A color duplex scanner with a 7- to 10-MHz linear array scan head is used to image the entire vein bypass and both anastomoses and to assess the inflow and outflow arteries. Both antegrade and retrograde flow in the runoff artery of a distal end-to-side anastomosis should be observed. Papaverine HCl (30 to 45 mg) can be injected directly into the distal graft segment to augment blood flow if resting measurements are borderline. Recorded velocity spectra (at a 60-degree Doppler angle) should indicate low outflow resistance with antegrade flow throughout the pulse cycle. Patent vein side branches after in situ saphenous vein bypass grafting can be located by B-mode imaging with distal graft compression. Ligation of vein side branches larger than 1.5 mm in diameter is recommended.

Graft velocity spectra with calculation of peak systolic velocity (PSV) should be obtained from normal graft segments at the high thigh, above-knee, below-knee, and distal graft segments. At these locations, PSV is used to identify a "low flow" graft and serves as a baseline value for subsequent postoperative duplex assessments.

If duplex ultrasound scanning is not available, intraoperative arteriography should be used to verify a technically adequate result after infrainguinal vein bypass. In general, stenoses greater than 50% diameter reducing are hemodynamically significant and warrant repair.

(C) PSV should be less than 150 cm/sec in the proximal anastomosis and less than 200 cm/sec in the inflow femoral or external iliac artery. Anastomotic abnormalities should be revised. Inflow stenoses can often be treated with intraoperative angioplasty or stenting, since these stenoses are usually focal if they have not been detected and repaired preoperatively (see Chapter 38 on alternative procedures to treat aortoiliac disease).

(D) The average PSV of a vein bypass should be greater than 40 cm/sec. If intraoperative velocity is lower, graft thrombosis is more likely. Adequate blood pressure and cardiac output should be ensured. Papaverine can be administered to potentially augment flow (and velocity) by decreasing peripheral resistance. If no cause can be found (including poor outflow; see E), long-term anticoagulation therapy with warfarin (and aspirin) should be considered because graft thrombosis is likely in the setting of low flow.

(E) Low graft velocity due to poor outflow is associated with low or absent diastolic flow, characteristic of a high resistance outflow bed. If no focal velocity increase is detected at the distal anastomosis (PSV in the distal anastomosis should be less than 180 cm/sec), this is likely due to an inadequate outflow artery. In such cases, intraoperative arteriography may be useful to define an alternate distal target artery, for graft revision, or for an additional jump-graft. If this is not possible, anticoagulation therapy should be strongly considered (see D). Some surgeons have successfully used a distal arteriovenous fistula in this setting to

INFRAINGUINAL GRAFT SURVEILLANCE

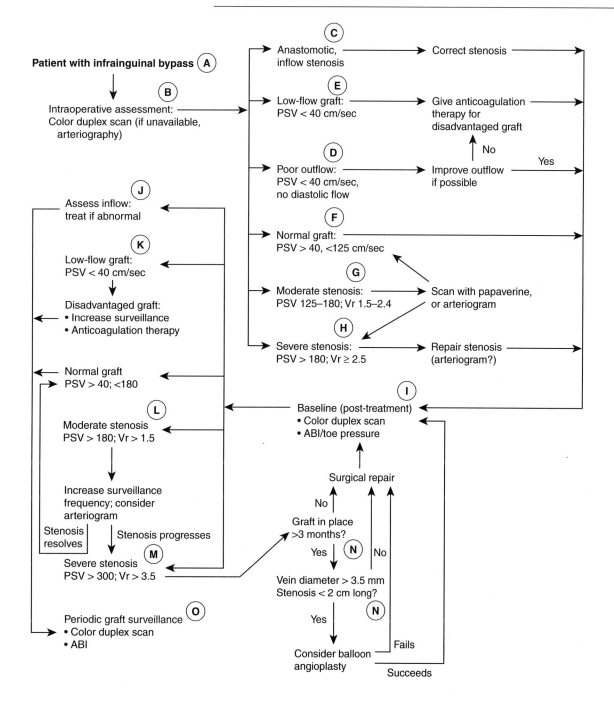

Infrainguinal Graft Surveillance (continued)

improve graft patency, but this practice has not been widely adopted.

(F) PSV in a normal vein bypass 3 to 5 mm diameter should be 70 + 20 (SD) cm/sec in the distal graft segment. At sites of valve lysis, PSV should be less than 150 cm/sec and the velocity ratio (Vr), the ratio of PSV at valve site compared with adjacent normal vein, should be less than 2.0. In other areas, the PSV should be less than 125 cm/sec, with a Vr less than 1.4. Such grafts warrant no further action except routine postoperative surveillance.

(G) The significance of duplex ultrasound–detected residual stenosis is based on real-time color Doppler imaging of a focal abnormality with the velocity spectra features of a moderate or severe stenosis. Velocity spectra of a moderate stenosis (PSV 125 to 180 cm/sec) may be the result of revascularization hyperemia, small caliber, or spasm in addition to a real stenosis. The decision to proceed with repair can be based on a repeated evaluation after papaverine administration to reduce spasm or a diagnostic arteriogram to identify more than 50% diameter reduction stenosis or lumen filling defect. If a decision is made not to treat a moderate stenosis, very careful postoperative surveillance is indicated.

(H) A severe, focal vein graft stenosis (PSV > 180 cm/sec; Vr > 2.5 requires graft revision. Critical stenoses (PSV > 300 cm/sec; Vr > 4) are typical of platelet aggregation. Vein patch angioplasty or segmental interposition is required, supplemented with anticoagulation therapy and/or dextran as indicated. Some surgeons use intraoperative arteriography before repair of duplex detected stenoses to confirm this finding.

(I) The importance of postoperative, predischarge scanning relates to the type and findings of the intraoperative assessment. If duplex testing has been performed and demonstrates a *normal* bypass graft (i.e., no stenosis, low outflow resistance graft flow pattern, PSV in the expected range [40 to 100 cm/sec], and excellent augmentation of distal limb perfusion), the likelihood of detecting a graft abnormality is low (<3%).[7] This might suggest that a predischarge scan is not necessary if intraoperative findings were normal. However, the predischarge study is performed in a vascular laboratory setting in an unanesthetized patient with closed wounds and as such serves as an important baseline for future surveillance. Therefore, our policy is to perform a predischarge graft evaluation in all cases.

The most common problems detected in a predischarge study include:

- Graft entrapment caused by tunneling or torsion
- Patent vein side-branch (in situ bypass)
- Residual stenosis of moderate severity

Intraoperative test results should be available for comparison with the predischarge graft testing. This testing should include (1) measurement of ankle-brachial systolic pressure index (ABI) and (2) color duplex scanning to record graft velocity spectra along the length of the bypass and to image the bypass graft for stenoses.

After in situ grafting, duplex scanning should also be used to detect and grade the hemodynamic significance of any residual vein side branch arteriovenous fistulas. This same study is performed as a baseline study following any subsequent graft interventions.

(J) Inflow stenoses that were subcritical preoperatively may become apparent with the increased flow associated with a new infrainguinal bypass. The femoral pulse should be assessed and the femoral duplex waveform inspected for abnormalities (monophasic velocity spectral waveform or prolonged acceleration time [>250 msec]). If an inflow stenosis is suspected, additional imaging (arteriography, MRA, or duplex scanning) should be performed and appropriate treatment given (see Chapter 38).

(K) The identification of low-flow bypass graft postoperatively (PSV < 40 cm/sec throughout a vein bypass) indicates a disadvantaged vein graft. If arteriography has not already been performed intraoperatively, an arteriogram may help to localize a treatable cause, such as an inadequate outflow artery. If no mechanical problem can be treated, my colleagues and I use warfarin anticoagulation therapy at a dosage to keep the International Normalized Ratio at 1.6 to 2, coupled with antiplatelet therapy (enteric-coated aspirin 325 mg/day).

(L) When a moderate vein graft stenosis (PSV >180 but < 300 cm/sec; Vr > 1.5 but < 3.5) is detected by postoperative duplex scanning, increased surveillance frequency is indicated (see P). Of these stenoses, which result from intimal hyperplasia, 30% to 35% resolve, 10% to 12% remain stable, but 50% to 60% progress.[5, 8, 9] Borderline or multiple lesions should be evaluated by arteriography, especially if the postoperative ABI and graft PSV are not in the expected range.

(M) It is recommended that all severe (>75%: PSV > 300 cm/sec; Vr > 3.5) stenoses be considered for repair by either percutaneous balloon angioplasty or by an open surgical procedure (vein patch angioplasty, interposition grafting, vein graft replacement). Repair of a non–flow-limiting stenosis should be considered when average PSV in the graft is below 40 cm/sec or when exercise testing demonstrates a decrease of more than 20% in resting ankle pressure. Some surgeons routinely use arteriography to confirm vein graft stenoses, but my practice has been to use duplex scanning alone unless the values are borderline or there are multiple lesions.

If a low-flow state has developed in a vein graft but duplex scanning has not identified a graft or outflow stenosis, arteriography should be performed to evaluate the inflow, outflow, and the entire bypass for a possible "missed" lesion. After repair of a graft defect, the surveillance program should begin again at time zero, with the first follow-up scan at 4 weeks.

(N) The use of endovascular treatment by balloon PTA for acquired vein graft stenosis is

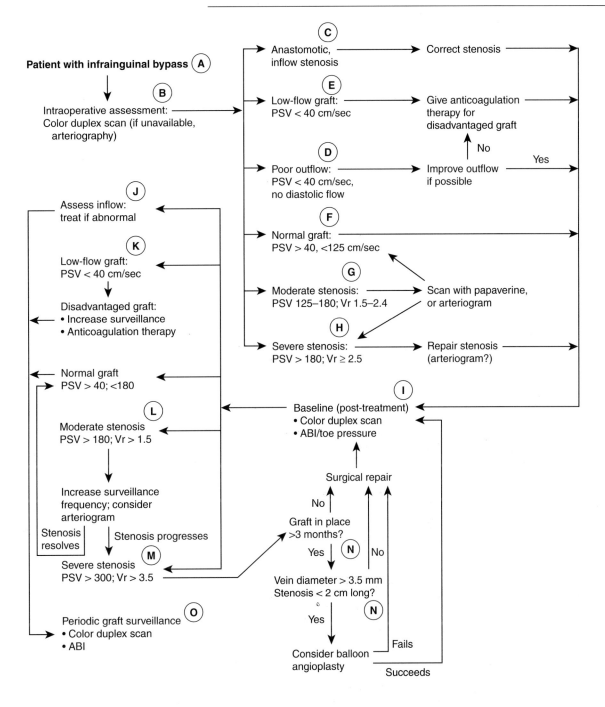

controversial. Surgical options of vein-patch angioplasty, interposition grafting, and jump-grafting are preferred by some surgical groups, whereas others have recommended selective PTA for graft revision. I have selected vein graft stenosis for treatment by PTA based on duplex scan findings of stenosis severity, lesion length, vein caliber, and appearance time.[10] Duplex scan features of the stenosis judged suitable for endovascular treatment include vein diameter greater than 3.5 mm, stenosis length less than 2 cm, and appearance time more than 3 months after bypass placement.

Surveillance of more than 500 infrainguinal vein bypasses using duplex scanning identified graft lesions that met the criteria for repair in 22% of patients. When these selection criteria were used for PTA versus open surgery, overall stenosis-free patency was identical (63%) at 2 years for open surgical repair compared with endovascular PTA.[11] Overall, assisted graft patency was 91% at 1 year and 80% at 3 years.

Following either surgical or PTA repair, the surveillance protocol should be reinstituted at the initial time sequence with a new baseline study just like the predischarge evaluation described earlier (see I).

O For accurate interpretation of graft surveillance studies, the vascular technologist and evaluating physician require information indicating the type of infrainguinal bypass including location of anastomotic sites, graft type, and previous surveillance test interpretation. The patient should be interviewed for symptoms of recurrent limb ischemia (claudication distance, recurrent skin lesions). Limb pressures (ABI, toe pressure) should be measured and compared to prior levels. A decrease in ABI of more than 0.15 or toe pressure of less than 30 mmHg are considered significant and indicate development of an occlusive lesion.

Duplex scan imaging is performed as in the predischarge evaluation to evaluate the aortoiliac segment, the bypass itself, and the outflow arteries for occlusive or aneurysmal lesions. PSV is recorded from nonstenotic graft segments at three to four levels (high thigh, above-knee, below-knee, distal graft segment) and compared with prior values. A decrease in PSV of more than 30 cm/sec is considered significant and warrants a detailed investigation for an occlusive lesion, including arteriography, if the average PSV has fallen to less than 40 cm/sec.

Vein graft surveillance studies are classified into four categories that dictate the need for intervention, additional testing such as arteriography, or the time interval to the next surveillance study. At the University of South Florida, my associates and I found that the following duplex scan criteria correlate stenosis severity with arteriographic diameter reduction:

1. *<20% stenosis:* Vr < 1.5; mild spectral broadening in systole; PSV < 150 cm/sec.
2. *20% to 50% stenosis:* Vr 1.5 to 2.5; spectral broadening throughout systole; no change in waveform configuration across stenosis; PSV > 150 cm/sec.
3. *50% to 75% stenosis:* Vr > 2.5; severe spectral broadening in systole with reversed flow components; PSV > 180 cm/sec.
4. *>75% stenosis:* Vr > 3.5; severe lumen reduction and "flow jet" present by color Doppler imaging; PSV > 300 cm/sec; and end-diastolic flow velocity (EDV) in flow jet > 40 cm/sec.

The frequency of vein graft surveillance depends on (1) the time since initial surgery and (2) whether the graft is considered disadvantaged because of low flow or whether it is more likely to result in problems because of previous revisions or other conditions such as small caliber, arm vein, and multiple venovenostomies. For optimal vein grafts with a normal predischarge duplex scan, the recommended postoperative surveillance intervals are 4 to 6 weeks, 3 months, and 6 months for 2 years, followed by annual scans.

For disadvantaged grafts or those with lesser abnormalities not justifying immediate intervention, the 6-month intervals are shortened to 3 months for the first 2 years. Detection of any change in PSV or Vr that might suggest a developing stenosis should also result in an increased surveillance frequency, and after treatment of a stenosis, the surveillance protocol should restart but with appropriately shorter intervals between evaluations.

REFERENCES

1. Bandyk DF, Schmitt DD, Seabrook GR, et al: Monitoring the functional patency of in situ saphenous vein bypass: The impact of a surveillance program and elective revision. J Vasc Surg 1989;9:289–296.
2. Mills JL, Fujitani RM, Taylor SM: The characteristics and anatomic distribution of lesions that cause reversed vein graft failure: A five-year prospective study. J Vasc Surg 1993;17:195–206.
3. Idu MM, Blankenstein JD, De Gier P, et al: Impact of a color-flow duplex surveillance program on infrainguinal vein graft patency: A five-year experience. J Vasc Surg 1993;17:42–53.
4. Mills JL, Bandyk DF, Gahtan V, Esses GE: The origin of infrainguinal vein graft stenosis: A prospective study based on duplex surveillance. J Vasc Surg 1995;21:16–25.
5. Gupta AK, Bandyk DF, Cheanvechai D, Johnson BL: Natural history of infrainguinal vein graft stenosis relative to by pass grafting technique. J Vasc Surg 1997;25:211–225.
6. Lundell A, Lindblad B, Bergqvist D, Hansen F: Femoropopliteal-crural graft patency is improved by an intensive surveillance program: A prospective randomized study. J Vasc Surg 1995;21:26–33.
7. Johnson BL, Bandyk DF, Back MR, et al: Intraoperative duplex monitoring of infrainguinal vein bypass procedures. J Vasc Surg 2000;4:678–690.
8. Westerband A, Mills JL, Kistler S, et al: Prospective validation of threshold criteria for intervention in infrainguinal vein grafts undergoing duplex surveillance. Ann Vasc Surg 1997;11:44–48.
9. Caps T, Cantwell-Gab K, Bergelin RO, Strandness DE: Vein graft lesions: Time of onset and rate of progression. J Vasc Surg 1995;22:466–475.
10. Gonsalves C, Bandyk DF, Avino AJ, Johnson BL: Duplex features of vein graft stenosis which predict successful percutaneous transluminal angioplasty. J Endovascular Surgery 1999; 6:66–72.
11. Avino AJ, Bandyk DF, Gonsalves AJ, et al: Surgical and endovascular intervention for infrainguinal vein graft stenosis. J Vasc Surg 1999;29:60–71.

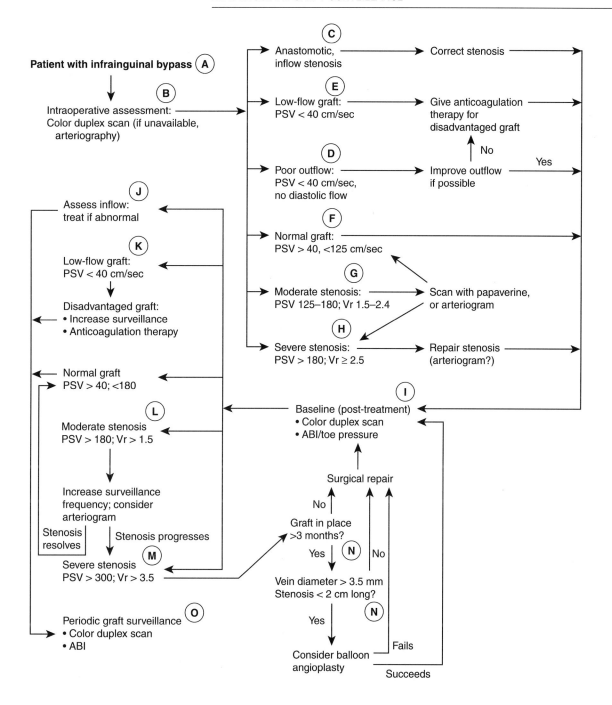

Chapter 43 Infrainguinal Graft Thrombosis

DANIEL B. WALSH, MD

A Infrainguinal graft thrombosis is suspected based on recurrent ischemic symptoms (see Chapter 36) and loss of distal or graft pulses. Duplex ultrasound surveillance is useful for differentiating occlusion from severe stenosis.

B In most cases, when the original infrainguinal graft has been placed for critical limb ischemia, graft thrombosis again leads to limb threat; however, if an ulcer or amputation has healed or when the initial indication is only claudication, revascularization may not be required. Considerable clinical judgment is required in these cases, since delay in treatment may precipitate irreversible tissue injury and may limit thrombolytic options. However, long-term patency following infrainguinal graft thrombosis is generally poor, such that unnecessary intervention should not be undertaken.[1] If present, claudication should be managed as discussed in Chapter 34.

C Heparin should be administered to inhibit thrombus propagation after the diagnosis of graft thrombosis. Anticoagulation therapy can be delayed briefly in order to establish epidural anesthesia (which may improve short-term bypass patency).[2]

The urgency of treatment of infrainguinal graft thrombosis and the utility of additional diagnostic studies must be decided at the initial presentation. As with other causes of acute ischemia, extremity neurologic status is the primary determinant of the timing of treatment (see Chapter 36). If there is no paralysis or anesthesia, diagnostic studies that are helpful in decision making and that may provide alternative therapeutic maneuvers may be pursued, with close monitoring for signs of worsening ischemia. If extremity neurologic function is severely compromised, other studies, including risk assessment, the search for causes of graft thrombosis, assessment of inflow and outflow status, and the search for a suitable vein graft, is not be possible, and blind exploration supplemented by intraoperative imaging will be necessary. In such cases, all potential donor sites for venous conduit should be included in the sterile surgical field.

D If the severity of ischemia is mild enough to allow time for thorough investigation, a number of studies are worthwhile. The availability of vein for use as a new bypass conduit or patch material is critical in determining revascularization options and should be assessed by physical examination and duplex ultrasound surveillance. The quality of ipsilateral and contralateral leg vein, as well as arm vein, should be determined.

As time allows, initial evaluation should also investigate possible causes of graft thrombosis. If not previously studied, a potential hypercoagulable state should be investigated with appropriate blood studies (see Chapter 3).[3] Less common causes of hypercoagulability, such as sepsis, malignancy, and increased blood viscosity from dehydration or polycythemia should be considered.

Cardiac decompensation associated with hypotension is another possible cause of graft thrombosis that should be evaluated. Cardiac assessment is also valuable in determining the risks associated with various therapeutic options. When time permits, other potential operative risk factors, such as pulmonary and renal dysfunction, should be assessed.

E In addition to systemic causes, local causes of graft thrombosis due to inflow lesions should be evaluated. Inflow may be evaluated with femoral artery pressure measurement, duplex ultrasound, and/or arteriography.

Femoral artery pressure measurement may be unreliable if most limb outflow has been through the graft, which is now occluded. For that reason, arterial pressure should be rechecked at the proximal graft anastomosis after restoring graft patency to exclude an inflow stenosis. A pressure gradient of 10 mmHg at rest (compared with systemic pressure), or 15–20 mmHg after intra-arterial administration of a vasodilator, suggests an inflow stenosis that should be evaluated with arteriography and probably treated (see Chapter 38).

F After adequate inflow is established, the next steps are governed by the nature of the graft conduit, either prosthetic or vein. For prosthetic grafts, the ease of surgical thrombectomy makes this option preferred over thrombolysis in most cases. Indications for thrombolysis of a prosthetic graft are usually patient-specific, such as high operative risk and multiple previous explorations leading to technically difficult surgical procedures with higher risk of infection.

After graft thrombectomy, whether by thrombolysis or surgery, the graft and the outflow arteries are evaluated with arteriography to identify a possible cause of graft failure. It is usually difficult to adequately image outflow arteries before restoring graft patency. Considerations are as follows:

1. If no problem is found with the inflow, the graft, or the outflow, a hypercoagulable state is presumed and anticoagulation therapy is continued indefinitely.
2. If an outflow problem occurs at an above-knee popliteal anastomosis, a prosthetic patch or graft extension above the knee may be possible.
3. If an outflow problem is found in the popliteal artery below the knee, the availability of venous conduit determines the next step.
4. If there is sufficient vein for a below-knee bypass, this bypass should be performed. If not, the outflow lesion may be able to be treated directly, either by balloon angioplasty or surgical vein patch arterioplasty.
5. As a last resort, the above-knee prosthetic bypass may be extended to a below-knee artery beyond the outflow stenosis using a vein cuff at the distal anastomosis, which was beneficial below the knee in a randomized trial.[4]

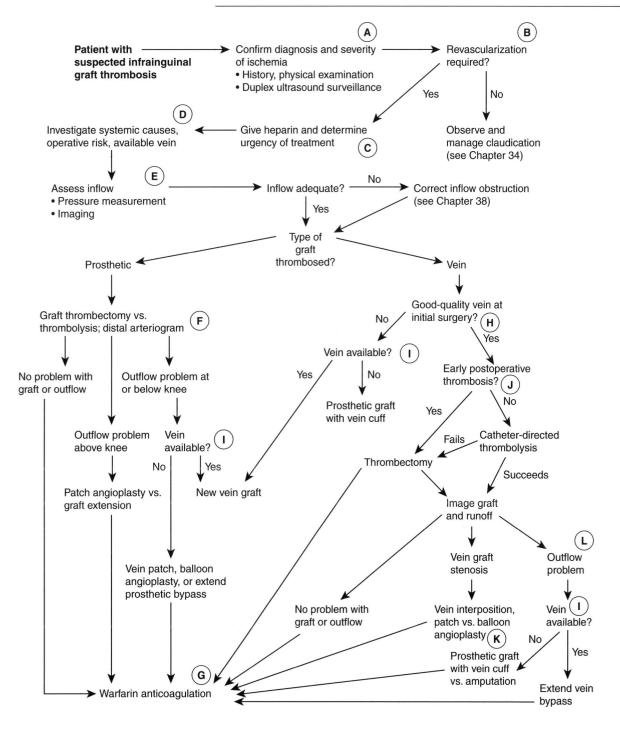

Infrainguinal Graft Thrombosis (continued)

(G) In most cases, once an infrainguinal graft has thrombosed, it is considered to be disadvantaged in terms of future patency. In this situation, chronic warfarin anticoagulation therapy appears to improve long-term patency.[5] This is especially true if no hemodynamic cause for graft thrombosis has been detected. If a definite local cause of graft thrombosis has been identified and corrected, anticoagulation agents may be withheld or used only temporarily.

(H) Based on personal experience, the management of vein graft thrombosis is determined primarily by the quality of vein as assessed at the initial operation and by the timing of postoperative graft thrombosis. If the quality of the initial venous conduit was poor, it is very unlikely that this vein can be salvaged. Thus, therapeutic attempts should focus on replacement with a new venous conduit; if a new venous conduit is unavailable, a prosthetic conduit using a vein cuff at the distal anastomosis is recommended.

Other adjunctive techniques to improve infrainguinal prosthetic graft patency, such as a distal arteriovenous fistula have been suggested, but have not proved satisfactory. If the quality of the initial vein graft was good, attempts at thrombectomy or thrombolysis are justified, even though long-term patency is poor, since alternative venous conduit is usually limited.

(I) Potential venous conduit for a new infrainguinal bypass should be evaluated with duplex ultrasound vein mapping. Rarely is sufficient ipsilateral greater saphenous vein still available. Although contralateral greater saphenous vein is the next ideal option, many patients have substantial contralateral ischemia or diabetes, which increases the probability that they will need their contralateral saphenous vein for future use in that leg.[6] Accordingly, I usually use arm vein for reoperative infrainguinal bypass, although lesser saphenous vein is another, albeit less accessible, option.

(J) If a thrombosed vein graft has been in place less than 2 weeks, surgical thrombectomy should generally be employed because of the danger of hemorrhagic complications from percutaneous thrombolysis. If the vein graft was placed more than 2 weeks previously, percutaneous thrombolysis is usually safe and is probably less injurious to the vein graft than balloon thrombectomy. Obviously, other potential contraindications for thrombolytic treatment must be considered. Unfortunately, patency of vein grafts that have thrombosed in the early postoperative period is poor, regardless of treatment.[1]

(K) Treatment of an intrinsic vein graft defect should be determined by the characteristics of the vein and the stenosis:

1. If the vein diameter is large and the stenosis is short, balloon angioplasty with duplex ultrasound verification of the technical result provides acceptable patency.[7]
2. If the stenosis is long (>2 cm) or the vein diameter small (<3 mm in diameter), treatment with either a vein patch angioplasty or a segmental vein interposition is preferred.

Availability of venous conduit determines which of the surgical options is technically possible and most easily accomplished. I prefer a vein interposition with replacement of the stenotic segment if possible.

(L) If the cause for vein graft thrombosis is a stenosis in the outflow artery, the treatment response is determined by the availability of venous conduit:

1. If there is adequate venous conduit available, the graft is extended beyond the outflow stenosis.
2. If the vein graft cannot be extended, endovascular or surgical vein patch arterioplasty of a localized outflow stenosis should be considered.
3. If there is no possibility of local repair of the outflow problem and if there is insufficient vein to extend the bypass, a possible option is replacement or extension of the vein graft with a prosthetic conduit using a distal anastomotic vein cuff; however, my experience with distal prosthetic conduit after vein graft thrombosis has been universally poor. In this situation, amputation may be a more realistic alternative.

REFERENCES

1. Nackman GB, Walsh DB, Fillinger MF, et al: Thrombolysis of occluded infrainguinal vein grafts: Predictors of outcome. J Vasc Surg 1997;25(2)512–521.
2. Perler BA, Christopherson R, Rosenfeld BA, et al: The influence of anesthetic method on infrainguinal bypass graft patency: A closer look. Am Surg 1995;61(9)784–789.
3. Donaldson MC, Belkin M, Whittemore AD, et al: Impact of activated protein C resistance on general vascular surgical patients. J Vasc Surg 1997;25:1054–1060.
4. Stonebridge PA, Prescott RJ, Ruckley CV, for the Joint Vascular Research Group: Randomized trial comparing infrainguinal polytetrafluoroethylene bypass grafting with and without vein interposition cuff at the distal anastomosis. J Vasc Surg 1997;26(4)543–550.
5. Sarac TP, Huber TS, Back MR, et al: Warfarin improves the outcome of infrainguinal vein bypass grafting at high risk for failure. J Vasc Surg 1998;28: 446–457.
6. Tarry WC, Walsh DB, Fillinger MF, et al: The fate of the contralateral leg following infrainguinal bypass. J Vasc Surg 1998;27:1039–1048.
7. Avino AJ, Bandyk DF, Gonsalves AJ, et al: Surgical and endovascular intervention for infrainguinal vein graft stenosis. J Vasc Surg 1999;29:60–70.

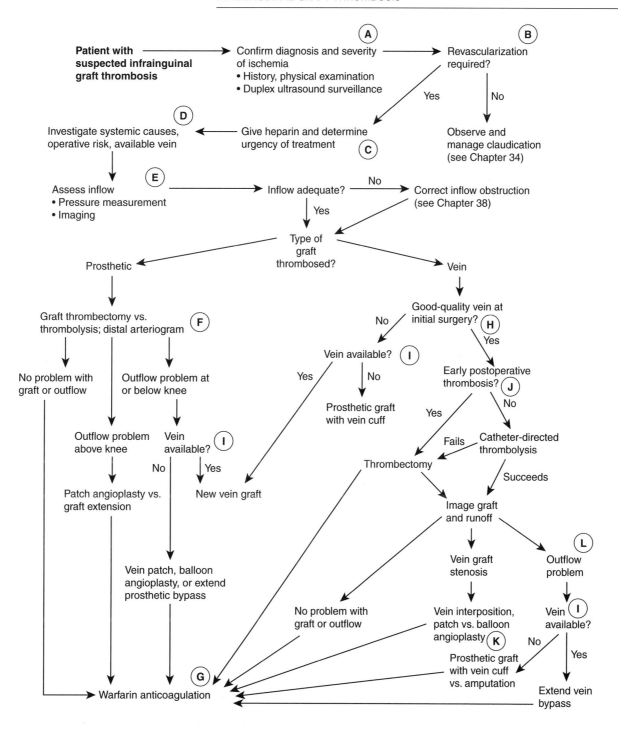

Chapter 44 Infrainguinal Prosthetic Graft Infection

KEITH D. CALLIGARO, MD

A Infrainguinal arterial graft infections can present in a variety of ways, including incisional drainage, erythema, fever, malaise, stable pseudoaneurysm, or hemodynamic instability secondary to bleeding.[1] The manner of presentation determines the surgical strategy to treat these complications and the urgency required to intervene.[2] The most crucial presentation is hemorrhage resulting in hemodynamic instability.

B Patients with an expanding hematoma or hemodynamic instability secondary to hemorrhage should be brought immediately to the operating room for control of bleeding without obtaining any preoperative studies that might otherwise help to determine the extent of infection or to plan secondary revascularization. Proximal and distal control of the bleeding site is the first step in managing hemorrhage caused by an infected arterial graft.

If the hemorrhage is from a disrupted anastomosis, inflow and outflow arteries must be expeditiously dissected free or controlled with balloon occlusion catheters. If bleeding is from the body of the graft, control of the proximal and distal graft should be obtained.

If the hemorrhage is secondary to a disrupted infected anastomosis, the safest course of action to prevent recurrent bleeding is ligation or oversewing of all inflow and outflow arteries. Oversewing only the residual wall of the artery involved with anastomotic hemorrhage or placing a patch on the artery is more likely to result in rupture in the future. All infected graft and soft tissue should be completely excised (see I later).

After the hemorrhage is controlled and the patient is hemodynamically stable, attention can then be turned to saving the threatened limb. Intravenous heparin should be administered. The wounds should be packed with antibiotic-soaked dressings and covered with isolation dressings. At this point, limb viability should be assessed by clinical and Doppler examination.

C If the graft has been placed because of claudication, mild rest pain, or a superficial ischemic ulcer that has now healed, the threatened limb may have adequate collateral circulation to remain viable. Frequent assessment of the limb should be carried out in the postoperative period. Even if the patient experiences mild but bearable rest pain postoperatively, the best strategy is to wait until the infectious process has resolved before proceeding with secondary revascularization.

D If the limb is not viable after graft excision, the surgeon is faced with a potentially difficult secondary revascularization strategy because emergent control of bleeding prevented obtaining an arteriogram before surgery. In some cases, arteriography performed in the radiology suite may be necessary to determine a suitable outflow artery if the limb can survive for the time required to perform this study and then to perform a secondary bypass. If the limb cannot survive for this extended period of time, arteriography must be performed in the operating room. Contrast material can be injected through the graft remnant before complete graft removal or, preferably, arteriography can be performed at a site remote from the infection.

Last, the surgeon may need to perform a cutdown on a potential outflow artery that is expected to be patent on the basis of the course of the original graft, an arteriogram performed before the original bypass, or the presence of Doppler signals.

E If secondary revascularization is possible, the bypass is best tunneled through a sterile route.[2,3] Although some authors have reported good results with placement of an autologous graft such as vein or endarterectomized occluded superficial femoral artery through the original graft site, placement of a new graft through uninfected tissue usually leads to less recurrent infection.[4]

F If secondary revascularization is not possible because of lack of a suitable conduit or outflow artery or if the patient is too critically ill to tolerate another lengthy operation, amputation should be performed to prevent adverse consequences, such as metabolic acidosis and hyperkalemia.

G When a patient presents with stable manifestations of an infected infrainguinal graft, namely sepsis, a stable pseudoaneurysm, or wound drainage, preoperative testing can be performed to better plan the operative strategy. Intravenous antibiotics should be started after blood and wound specimens are obtained for culture. Computed tomography (CT), magnetic resonance imaging (MRI), or ultrasound scanning can reveal the extent of graft infection. My colleagues and I generally prefer CT scanning because we are most familiar with this highly accurate modality.[5]

A sinogram can be useful if a sinus tract extends from the skin to the graft. A white blood cell scan is rarely needed because clinical findings or one of the other imaging studies usually reveal the extent of infection. An arteriogram should routinely be performed preoperatively to best determine the method of secondary revascularization.

H If the infected graft causes systemic sepsis, preoperative testing should be performed expeditiously and the graft excised the day of presentation unless the patient demonstrates rapid clinical improvement with intravenous antibiotics. There is no role for graft preservation when the infected graft is causing sepsis because the graft itself is seeded with bacteria and must be removed.[2,3]

I In the presence of systemic sepsis or an occluded graft, or if more than a focal infection is involved, excision of the *entire* infected graft and associated infected soft tissue should be performed. Similarly, disrupted grafts with hemorrhage should be removed and the surrounding infected tissue débrided. (see B). If the graft is patent and limb threat is likely to result after graft excision, revascularization with a new graft tunneled via a sterile route can be considered before excision of the infected graft.

The appropriate sequence of graft excision and replacement should be individualized according to these priorities: (1) treat life-threatening infection, (2) prevent infection of the new graft, and (3) avoid prolonged leg ischemia; however, sometimes these priorities are unavoidably in conflict. If a new graft is placed before the infected graft is excised, the incisions should be covered with adhesive dressings to avoid contamination with the infected graft. The new graft is then removed.

If maintaining patency of an underlying artery involved with the infected graft anastomosis is critical to achieving limb salvage, healing an amputation, or otherwise providing important collateral circulation (e.g., to the deep femoral artery), preserving flow through the artery can sometimes be achieved after infected graft excision by placing an autologous tissue patch via vein or an endarterectomized segment of occluded superficial femoral artery[1, 2, 4]; however, autologous patch ruptures have been reported.[2] For this reason, another possible option is to oversew a small 2- to 3-mm prosthetic graft remnant when the anastomosis is intact. The oversewn prosthetic remnant serves as a patch and maintains patency of the underlying artery.[2, 6] With this technique, the original anastomosis does not need to be taken down and dissecting the underlying arteries that may be encased in dense scar tissue can be avoided.

Virulence of the involved bacteria and extent of local infection must be balanced against the need for preserving the artery when one is making this decision. If the underlying artery is not essential to achieve limb salvage or to heal an amputation, such as an infrapopliteal artery that is occluded proximally, ligating or oversewing the vessel is the most appropriate measure to prevent future arterial disruption from persistent or recurrent infection.

J An infected infrainguinal graft that is not associated with systemic sepsis or unstable bleeding has the potential to be treated by complete or partial graft preservation, depending on

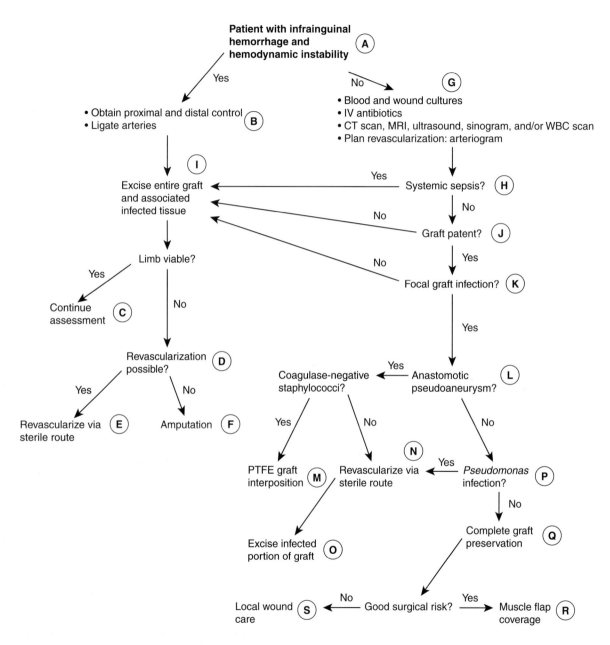

the patency status of the graft. If the infected graft is occluded, there is no advantage of preserving the graft, which should be removed.

(K) A patent but infected infrainguinal graft that is not causing sepsis or bleeding can potentially be treated by graft preservation. If the entire graft is involved with the infectious process, as demonstrated by pus or fluid tracking along its length, or if the entire graft is poorly incorporated by surrounding tissue, total graft excision is indicated. However, focal infection of a patent infrainguinal graft that is not causing sepsis or unstable bleeding is best treated by preservation of part or all of the graft.

(L) An infected, stable pseudoaneurysm involving the anastomosis of an infrainguinal graft must be excised and should not be treated by repairing the disrupted anastomosis. Revascularization strategies are determined by the virulence of the causative organism.

(M) A stable pseudoaneurysm that arises due to coagulase-negative *Staphylococcus epidermidis* (CNS) can be treated by excision of the infected segment of graft and replacement with a new polytetrafluoroethylene (PTFE) interposition graft.[7] In many instances, these organisms cannot be obtained for culture from the clear fluid surrounding the graft but, instead, can be isolated only by graft sonication. Bandyk has reported excellent results with this strategy.[7]

(N) An infected graft pseudoaneurysm caused by organisms other than CNS should not be treated by in situ replacement with a prosthetic graft for fear of recurrent infection. The new graft can be tunneled through extra-anatomic sterile fields, and the remaining segment of uninfected graft can be used as an inflow or outflow conduit. As long as the infection involves only a focal segment of graft, as determined by preoperative imaging studies and intraoperative findings of graft incorporation and negative Gram stains, using the remaining part of the graft greatly simplifies secondary revascularization.

(O) Once the secondary revascularization is completed and the wounds are closed, the infected graft, pseudoaneurysm, and surrounding tissue should be excised (see I for details concerning possible preservation of continuity of the involved artery).

(P) *Pseudomonas* is a particularly aggressive organism that is associated with high rates of anastomotic disruption and poor wound healing.[8,9] When *Pseudomonas* is the cause of a focal graft infection, a secondary bypass should be tunneled through a sterile field and anastomosed to an uninfected segment of the original graft. The infected segment of graft should then be excised, with care taken to avoid contamination of the newly placed graft segment.

(Q) A patient who presents with a focal infection of a patent infrainguinal graft with an intact anastomosis, without sepsis and without *Pseudomonas* as a causative organism, may be treated by complete graft preservation. When these criteria are fulfilled, several authors have documented equivalent patient survival and improved limb salvage rates using this strategy compared with traditional total graft excision.[2,3,10,11] Advantages of this management include avoiding the need for secondary revascularization and obviating the need for placement of a patch on the underlying artery. Repeated and aggressive excision of all infected tissue and at least 6 weeks of appropriate intravenous antibiotics are mandatory to achieve a successful outcome.

(R) For good-risk patients who can tolerate another major operation, placement of an autologous muscle flap over the exposed graft after healthy granulation tissue has formed may lead to higher successful graft preservation rates and shorter hospital stays.[12,13]

(S) For poor-risk patients, allowing the wound to heal by delayed secondary intention with formation of granulation tissue has proved successful in approximately 75% of patients.[3,12] Failure to heal or to control infection adequately would require additional débridement and, probably, complete graft excision (see I).

REFERENCES

1. Bunt TJ: Synthetic vascular graft infections: I. Graft infections. Surgery 1983;93:733–746.
2. Samson RH, Veith FJ, Janko GS, et al: A modified classification and approach to the management of infections involving peripheral arterial prosthetic grafts. J Vasc Surg 1988;8:147–153.
3. Calligaro KD, Veith FJ, Schwartz ML, et al: Selective preservation of infected prosthetic arterial grafts: Analysis of a 20-year experience with 120 extracavitary-infected grafts. Ann Surg 1994;220:461–469.
4. Ehrenfeld WK, Wilbur BG, Olcott CN, Stoney RJ: Autogenous tissue reconstruction in the management of infected prosthetic grafts. Surgery 1979;85:82–92.
5. Mark AS, McCarthy SM, Moss AA, Price D: Detection of abdominal aortic graft infection: Comparison of CT and indium-labeled white blood cell scans. Am J Roentgenol 1985;144:315–318.
6. Calligaro KD, Veith FJ, Valladares JA, et al: Prosthetic patch remnants to treat infected arterial grafts. J Vasc Surg 2000;31:253–259.
7. Bandyk DF, Bergamini TM, Kinney EV, et al: In situ replacement of vascular prostheses infected by bacteria biofilms. J Vasc Surg 1991;13:575–583.
8. Geary KJ, Tomkiewica AM, Harrison HN, et al: Differential effects of a gram-negative and gram-positive infection on autogenous and prosthetic aortic grafts. J Vasc Surg 1990;11:339–347.
9. Calligaro KD, Veith FJ, Schwartz RP, et al: Are gram-negative bacteria a contraindication to selective preservation of infected prosthetic arterial grafts? J Vasc Surg 1992;16:337–346.
10. Cherry KJ, Roland CF, Pairolero PC, et al: Infected femorodistal bypass: Is graft removal mandatory? J Vasc Surg 1992;15:295–305.
11. Kikta MJ, Goodson SF, Bishara RA, et al: Mortality and limb loss with infected infrainguinal bypass grafts. J Vasc Surg 1987;5:566–571.
12. Calligaro KD, Veith FJ, Sales CM, et al: Comparison of muscle flaps and delayed secondary intention wound healing for infected lower extremity arterial grafts. Ann Vasc Surg 1994;8:31–37.
13. Mixter RC, Turnipseed WD, Smith DJ Jr, et al: Rotational muscle flaps: A new technique for covering infected vascular grafts. J Vasc Surg 1989;9:472–478.

INFRAINGUINAL PROSTHETIC GRAFT INFECTION

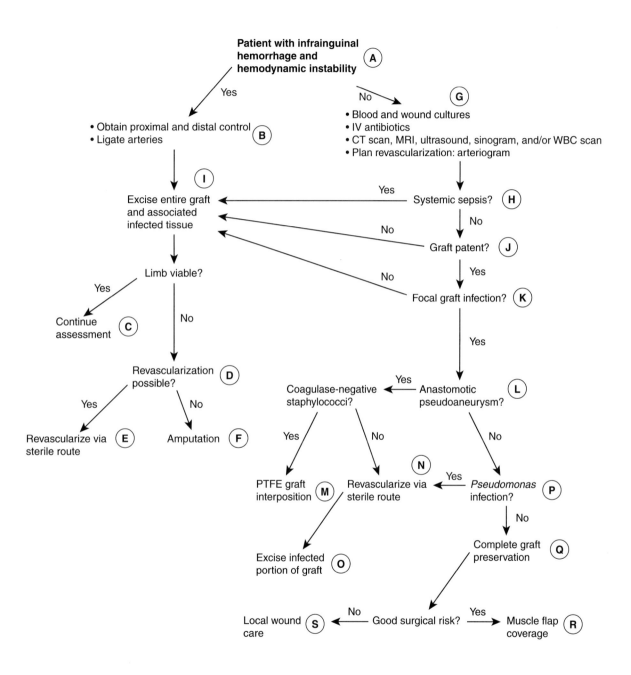

Chapter 45 Diabetic Foot Infections

JONATHAN B. TOWNE, MD

(A) Foot infections in patients with diabetes mellitus tend to be serious, even limb-threatening, because of factors that impede prompt detection and because of defects in the patient's immune defense system. Lesions that progress to infection are usually directly attributable to diabetic neuropathy, because infection can rapidly develop and progress even without the patient's awareness that it is present. Thus, when infections occur in diabetic patients in whom significant neuropathy has developed, these patients are more likely to progress to an advanced state before clinical presentation and more likely to present with significant tissue destruction.

(B) Careful physical examination of the foot is crucial for planning the appropriate management of infection in diabetic patients. The extent of cellulitis is determined, and underlying abscess is assessed by palpation for tenderness or crepitus from gas-producing bacteria. Most of the lymphatic drainage of the foot goes though the plantar space. Thus, most deep abscesses involve the plantar space, where careful examination is essential.

Because of coexisting sensory neuropathy, the patient commonly cannot sense pain in the foot, which would serve as an early warning sign of infection in the normally innervated patient. The degree of neuropathy should be documented. Arterial status should be initially checked by pulse examination, followed up with vascular laboratory measurements as needed. It is important to evaluate coexisting medical problems, especially cardiac and renal disease, in diabetic patients with foot infection. Because many of these patients will require operative therapy, it is important to determine their cardiac status as soon as possible.

(C) A diabetic patient with a septic foot can represent a medical emergency if blood glucose levels are uncontrolled. Occasionally, patients can present in septic shock. Thus, initial laboratory testing should include a white blood cell count, blood glucose, electrolytes, blood urea nitrogen/creatinine, urinalysis, and electrocardiogram. If there is evidence of septicemia or cardiac instability, a Swan-Ganz catheter is inserted to monitor fluid resuscitation. Generally, 8 to 12 hours is required to prepare such a patient for surgery if these measures are needed. During this interval, hyperglycemia is controlled, cardiovascular instability is corrected, and an adequate blood level of antibiotics is achieved.

(D) Although the treatment of polymicrobial diabetic foot infections relies on empirical selection of antibiotics, microbiologic studies should be performed to identify (1) organisms resistant to standard regimens and (2) unusual virulent organisms that may require specific antimicrobial therapy. Initial antibiotic therapy should empirically employ drugs that cover the wide spectrum of microorganisms typically involved in these soft tissue foot infections. A semisynthetic penicillin with a β-lactamase inhibitor covers most aerobic and anaerobic organisms.[1]

The quinolones are ideal for the treatment of diabetic foot infections; however, the antimicrobial spectra of these agents vary greatly, depending on the generation. *Second-generation* quinolones exhibit excellent gram-negative facultative activity but should never be used alone in the treatment of an acute diabetic foot infection because they demonstrate little activity against gram-negative anaerobic populations. Clindamycin or metronidazole should be added to provide more effective anaerobic coverage for the microbial flora encountered in a diabetic foot infection.

Fourth-generation quinolones are agents with excellent aerobic and anaerobic coverage against both gram-positive and gram-negative pathogens encountered in serious foot infections.[2]

(E) Patients with diabetic foot infections must be assessed for healing potential based on their arterial status. Sometimes dependent rubor caused by profound ischemia of the foot can be confused with cellulitis and vice versa. Pulse palpation may be difficult in the presence of swelling caused by local infection. For this reason, noninvasive testing is useful, although diabetic patients pose unique problems for the application of noninvasive diagnostic tests that are usually used to quantitate lower extremity arterial flow.

Because of increased vessel wall calcification in medium-sized and small arteries, it is difficult to compress the vessels with a cuff when arterial segmental limb pressures are measured. This problem is most marked with long-standing insulin-dependent diabetes and produces erroneously high pressure readings. Because calcification of the digital vessels is less pronounced than in proximal metatarsal, plantar, and tibial vessels, great or second toe pressures can be measured accurately.[3] Unfortunately, some diabetics have lost one or more toes, or these toes may be the site of infection or open foot lesions. These noninvasive tests can be of great value in assessing the vascular supply of the foot and evaluating the healing potential of local amputations or ulcerations.

Holstein and Lassen reported successful healing of local amputations when toe pressures were greater than 30 mmHg.[4] Only 9% of toe amputations healed when the digital pressure was 20 mmHg or less, whereas the amputation sites of all 33 patients with pressures greater than 30 mmHg healed. Barnes reported successful healing in patients whose digital pressures were greater than 25 mmHg.[5]

Pulsatile plethysmographic waveforms are a good index of healing and transcutaneous oxygen tension (TcO_2) measurements are also useful in assessing healing potential in diabetic patients with calcified distal arteries and falsely elevated arterial pressure measurements. A TcO_2 above 30 mmHg is predictive of healing.

(F) In addition to physical examination, roentgenograms of the foot, especially magnifica-

DIABETIC FOOT INFECTIONS

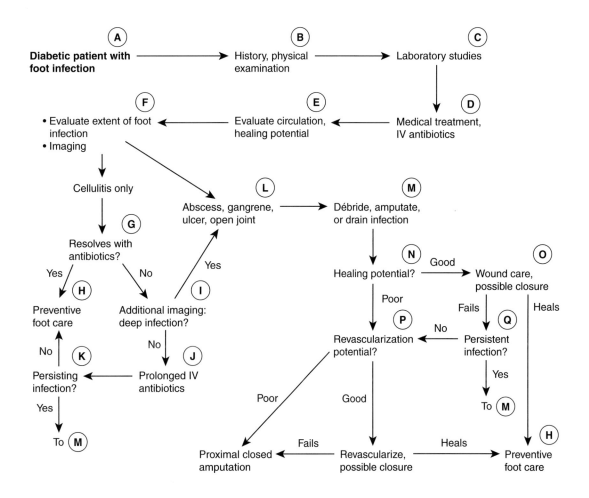

tion views, are helpful in assessing the extent of foot infection:

1. They can determine whether advanced osteomyelitis is present. However, radiography is often insensitive for detecting early bone involvement. Shults and colleagues found positive bone cultures and negative radiographs in 48% of diabetic patients with foot ulcers.[6]
2. They can demonstrate gas in the soft tissues of both the foot and lower leg. This is often the first clue that the patient has a significant deep infection warranting urgent surgical care.

Although bone scans are sometimes employed to detect chronic osteomyelitis, they are seldom indicated in the initial evaluation of acute foot infection in a diabetic patient.

MRI is sensitive for detecting deep abscesses and can be used in cases of persisting foot infection when the diagnosis cannot be made by clinical assessment.

(G) When no underlying deep infection is detected, diabetic patients with cellulitis alone are managed with intravenous antibiotic therapy. If the cellulitis does not improve in several days, there should be concern that a deep infection is present or that antibiotic coverage is not adequate. In this circumstance, the choice of antibiotic should be reviewed (see D) and a reevaluation for deep infection, performed by careful examination and additional imaging, is required.

(H) The need for careful foot care to avoid infection in diabetic patients with insensate feet cannot be overemphasized. Podiatry evaluation is often helpful, with regular follow-up for patients with recurrent problems. It is especially important for patients to wear proper shoes, most commonly extra-depth shoes with total contact orthotic inserts to distribute weight evenly. This avoids overloading the often-protruding metatarsal heads on the plantar aspect of the foot.

(I) The most frequent cause of persisting infection is the involvement of devitalized tissue in a closed space that has not been adequately drained. Repeating foot films and looking for gas in the tissues can sometimes detect this situation. MRI, which demonstrates high tissue contrast, is very sensitive for detection of soft tissue infections. Early changes are detected with low signal intensity on T1-weighted images and high signal intensity on T2-weighted images. In addition to study of bone structure, MRI allows the evaluation of the soft tissue and localization of infection.[7]

Osteomyelitis is another cause of persisting cellulitis and may become evident only on later plain radiographs, owing to the inflammatory hyperemia and subsequent deossification. Diagnostic findings include focal osteopenia and disturbances in the cortex and medullary bone. The process is not evident until significant amounts of bone have been resorbed, which usually takes 2 to 3 weeks from the onset of infection.[8]

Technetium phosphate bone scans are also useful, since they can detect osteomyelitis within days of onset, long before changes can be observed on conventional radiographs. Scintigraphic findings are associated with focal hyperemia. Gallium scanning localizes osseous infection because granulocytes or bacteria take up the tracer. Indium-labeled white blood cells studies are specific for infection because radiolabeled leukocytes are not incorporated into areas of active bone metabolism.[9] Scans normalize when the infection resolves.

(J) If no underlying deep infection or osteomyelitis can be detected despite further evaluation, aggressive antibiotic therapy should be continued. Patients should be carefully monitored for any sign of worsening cellulitis, however, which would suggest a deep infection and the need for surgical drainage.

(K) In the rare case in which cellulitis or other signs of local infection persist despite prolonged intravenous antibiotics but no deep infection or osteomyelitis can be positively identified, surgical exploration or even digital amputation may be necessary to identify a possible abscess or to eliminate possible osteomyelitis.

(L) When foot infection is associated with an abscess, an open ulcer, gangrene, or an open joint, surgical treatment in addition to aggressive antibiotic therapy is required. For small shallow ulcers, simple débridement may suffice, but these ulcers commonly involve deeper structures when they are carefully inspected, especially the joint space under neurotrophic, "mal perforans" ulcers.

(M) Initial surgical treatment involves drainage of infection and removal of devitalized tissue while the surgeon attempts to preserve as much potentially viable tissue as possible, especially if subsequent arterial reconstruction can improve circulation and potentially save marginal tissue. However, the principal requirement is to eliminate the source of infection and sepsis, which in advanced cases may require major, open amputation. For example, if there is extensive gas in the foot with systemic sepsis, a guillotine amputation done at the supramalleolar level is usually required. Patients with severe hindfoot ischemia may also require open ankle amputation.

For patients with a good blood supply or for patients who are potential revascularization candidates, a foot salvage procedure may be considered. The initial procedure consists of an extensive débridement of infected necrotic tissues, which must be excised without regard for subsequent reconstruction of the foot. This procedure often includes several digits and metatarsals and occasionally extends to the level of the tarsal bones. All pockets of purulent material must be opened widely.

In cases of plantar space infection, extensive drainage with longitudinal incisions on the plantar aspect of the foot along the tendon sheaths provides drainage and may allow ultimate foot salvage. The amount of devitalized infected tissue is generally much greater than the amount estimated on initial examination of the foot. The best indication of the need for amputation above the malleolar level is pain in the calf, which is accompanied by gas in late cases.

DIABETIC FOOT INFECTIONS

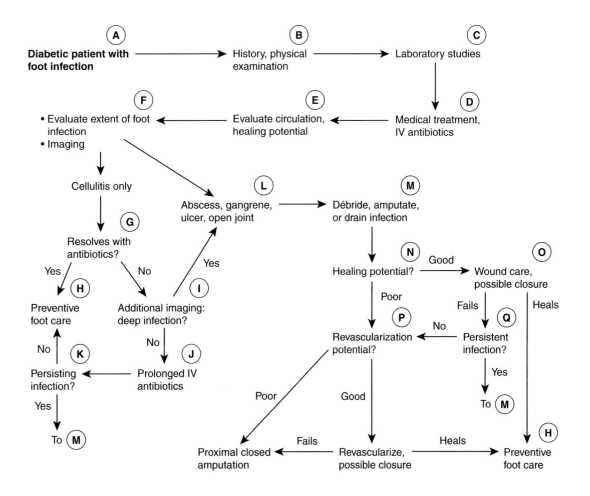

Diabetic Foot Infections *(continued)*

At the conclusion of the débridement, all necrotic and devitalized tissue should be removed; in the well-vascularized patient, all wound surfaces should be bleeding. In general, I prefer to leave the cartilage intact over exposed bones to prevent spread of infection into the marrow cavity.

For less severe infection of the distal foot, the extent of débridement must be individualized. If the infection involves a joint, healing is nearly impossible and the joint needs to be excised.

Most commonly involved are the interphalangeal joints (IP) and the metatarsophalangeal (MP) joints. With the interphalangeal joint, an open toe amputation is the optimal procedure. For MP joint involvement, excision of the joint with preservation of the adjacent bone is often sufficient, leaving the toe in place. This results in a better appearance of the foot and makes obtaining adequate footwear easier and less expensive.

An effective treatment for patients with a "mal perforans" ulcer is to excise the MP joint through a dorsal incision and to allow the ulcer and the plantar aspect of the foot to granulate in secondarily. The advantages to this technique are that it (1) removes the septic focus and (2) eliminates the pressure point.

(N) Once infection has been treated, the main residual problem with healing usually relates to inadequate blood supply. The initial assessment of healing potential (see *E*) must now be adjusted, depending on the extent of the soft tissue defect and the progress of healing in the open wound observed in the first few days after surgery:

1. If the wound shows no sign of new granulation tissue or shows regression (e.g., tissue necrosis at the periphery), arterial status is carefully reassessed with the probability of revascularization considered.
2. If signs of healing are present and circulation appears adequate, local wound care is continued with the best closure technique considered (see *O*).

(O) After surgical débridement, postoperative wound care, often aided by whirlpool therapy, is employed. In some patients, infection clears after surgery and local wound care but there is not sufficient blood supply to heal the wounds despite an initial assessment of adequate healing potential. In this case, revascularization options must be assessed.

If infection clears and circulation is adequate, secondary wound closure should be considered. Although the foot wounds generally granulate well, there is often a need for additional skin coverage in order to shorten the period of recovery. This can be accomplished by the application of split-thickness skin grafts.

Before skin grafts are applied, quantitative specimens are obtained for culture to ensure that the bacterial count is 10^5 grams per tissue or less. If the bacterial count is greater than 10^5, my practice is to apply mafenide acetate (Sulfamylon) cream to decrease the surface bacterial count. In resistant cases, however, excision of the granulation tissue may be necessary.

My associates and I generally do not perform formal transmetatarsal amputations unless the medial three toes have been previously removed. In some cases, healing by secondary intention, although more delayed, may be selected, depending on the size of the wound, its effect on ambulation, and other factors.

(P) Arteriography is performed to assess revascularization potential unless the patient is an unacceptable candidate for bypass surgery because of medical risk or nonambulatory status. Alternative imaging methods, such as duplex ultrasound scans and magnetic resonance angiography, may be appropriate in selected cases.

(Q) Postoperatively, wound care must be vigilant. Any purulent material on the dressing generally indicates an incompletely drained abscess pocket, which must be widely opened and débrided, usually in the operating room. Pain in the heel or just above the ankle may be the only symptom of a proximal extension of the infectious process. If healing does not occur but no residual infection is present, arterial status should be carefully assessed and revascularization performed if appropriate.

REFERENCES

1. Grayson ML, Gibbons GW, Habershaw DV, et al: Use of ampicillin/sulbactam versus imipenem/cilastatin in the treatment of limb-threatening foot infections in diabetic patients. Clin Infect Dis 1994;18:683–693.
2. DiPirro JT, Edmiston CE, Bohnen JMA: Pharmacodynamics of antimicrobial therapy in surgery. Am J Surg 1996;171:615–622.
3. Ferrier TM: Comparative study of arterial disease in amputated lower limbs from diabetics and nondiabetics. Med J Aust 1967;1:5.
4. Holstein P, Lassen NA: Healing of ulcers on the feet correlated with distal blood pressure measurements in occlusive arterial disease. Acta Orthop Scand 1980;51:995.
5. Barnes RW: Discussion of Gibbons GW, Wheelock FC Jr, Siembieda C, et al: Noninvasive prediction of amputation levels in diabetics. Arch Surg 1979;114:1253.
6. Shults DW, Hunter GC, McIntyre KE, et al: Value of radiographs and bone scans in determining the need for therapy in diabetic patients with foot ulcers. Am J Surg 1989;158:525.
7. Erdman WA, Tamburro F, Jayson HT, et al: Osteomyelitis: Characteristics and pitfalls of diagnosis with MR imaging. Radiology 1991;180:533.
8. Crim JR, Seeger LL: Imaging evaluation of osteomyelitis. Crit Rev Diagn Imaging 1994;35:201–256.
9. Newman GL, Waler J, Palestro CJ, et al: Unsuspected osteomyelitis in diabetic foot ulcers. JAMA 1991;266:1246–1251.

DIABETIC FOOT INFECTIONS

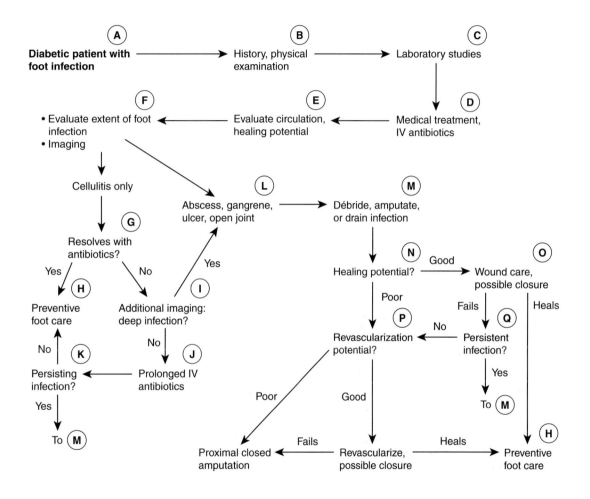

Chapter 46 Amputation Level

ROBERT E. CARLIN, MD • BLAIR A. KEAGY, MD

(A) It is estimated that at least 115,000 lower extremity amputations are performed in the United States each year.[1,2] The indication for many lower extremity amputations is end-stage ischemia caused by peripheral arterial occlusive disease (PAOD). When one is determining at which level to perform an amputation, the knee joint should be preserved whenever possible. In one series, 71% of patients who underwent below-knee amputation (BKA) were successfully rehabilitated[3]; in a separate series, however, only 30% of patients who underwent above-knee amputation (AKA) were successfully rehabilitated.[4]

Using clinical judgment alone, one can expect approximately 80% of below-knee amputations to heal and 90% to 95% of above-knee amputations to heal.[5] Objective testing, as described later, should be used as a *supplement* to clinical judgment in an effort to improve amputation healing rates.

(B) Patients with dry gangrene of the toes do not require immediate surgical amputation. In patients with nonreconstructible PAOD, it is best to allow complete demarcation of dry gangrene before proceeding with toe amputation. Because healing of the amputation site may be difficult, a dedicated wound care program should be initiated and continued as long as possible.

(C) Ischemia with wet gangrene of the foot demands immediate attention. Patients may become extremely ill, especially if they have diabetes mellitus. All patients should be started immediately on broad-spectrum intravenous antibiotics; if the patient is hyperglycemic, this condition should also be addressed immediately.

The first decision to make is a clinical one: Is enough of the foot viable to preserve ambulatory function? This may involve consideration of amputation levels from the transmetatarsal to the Symes level. In some cases, the decision can be made easily on the basis of the amount of tissue loss or extent of infection. In other cases, the decision is not as clear-cut, and in these circumstances we recommend an attempt to salvage the foot if the procedure does not result in increased patient morbidity and mortality.

(D) Patients with chronic critical ischemia typically present with rest pain, tissue loss, or both. When revascularization is not possible, either because of lack of conduit or lack of a distal "target" vessel for bypass, more information is required before the suitable level of amputation can be determined.

(E) Patients with acute ischemia may sometimes present late with septic complications from a nonviable limb. Such patients are often elderly, diabetic, and usually with some degree of underlying cardiac or renal dysfunction, making an emergency amputation a high-risk procedure. Indeed, emergency above-knee amputation in the setting of uncontrolled sepsis has been accompanied by a 46% mortality rate.[6] Careful preoperative evaluation and optimization lead to a reduction in mortality in this group of high-risk patients.

(F) In one randomized study, there was a 21% incidence of wound complications in patients undergoing amputation with a one-stage technique (amputation with delayed skin closure). In contrast, there was a 0% incidence of wound complications with the two-stage technique (ankle guillotine followed by formal amputation). Furthermore, duration of hospitalization was longer for the one-stage group than for the two-stage group.[7]

(G) After initial clinical assessment, more objective information may be required to determine the lowest amputation level that will heal. Objective tests such as Doppler systolic calf pressure, transcutaneous oxygen tension ($tcPO_2$), and digital photoplethysmography (PPG) are available in most institutions and provide valuable adjunctive information. The objective tests are not infallible, of course, and should therefore be combined with clinical judgment.

(H) Dry ice cryoamputation may be used as a means of halting the deleterious effects of progressive gangrene, thus delaying operative intervention. During the period of cryoamputation, efforts may be made at maximizing the patient's condition prior to definitive, elective surgery. One large study demonstrated 0% mortality for patients undergoing cryoamputation before definitive amputation and 14% mortality for the same patients after definitive amputation.[8] For these reasons, we suggest that in severely ill patients cryoamputation represents a good alternative to any surgical amputation or débridement procedure that would require an anesthetic.

(I) This decision box should not be interpreted as posing the question: Is there enough tissue to actually perform a forefoot amputation? Instead, the decision box refers to any possibility of a forefoot amputation *healing* at a level that would preserve ambulation function (i.e., preserve a functional foot).

(J) Measurement of Doppler systolic calf pressure is an easy test to perform and should be applied to patients who may be candidates for below-knee amputation. Although a range of Doppler systolic calf pressures has been reported, one study demonstrated 100% healing of below-knee amputations when the systolic calf pressure was above or at 70 mmHg.[9] However, a calf pressure below 70 mmHg should not be an absolute contraindication to below-knee amputation, because the same study reported a 91% healing rate for below-knee amputation when the systolic calf pressure was above 50 mmHg.[9] Therefore, in patients with a calf pressure below 70 mmHg, an additional test ($tcPO_2$) may provide useful information.

(K) Transcutaneous oximetry is a reproducible, noninvasive tool that can be used to measure

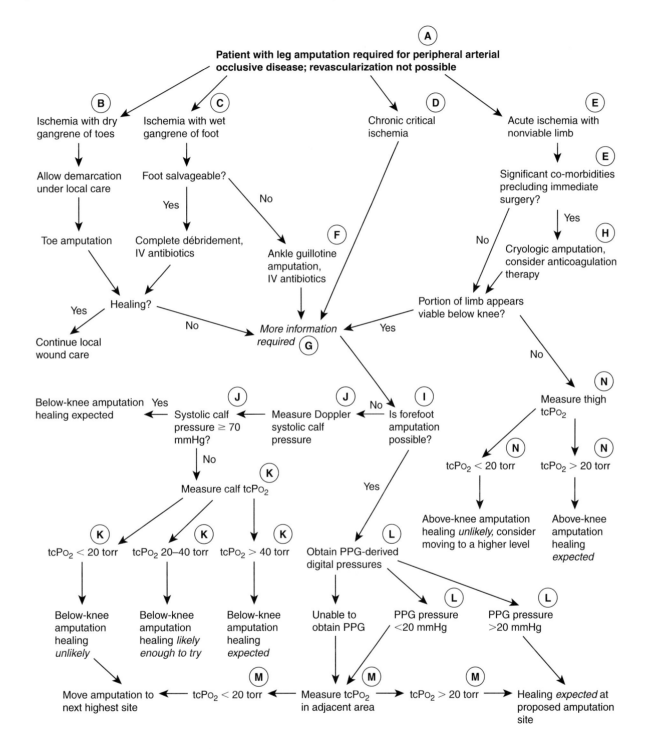

Amputation Level (continued)

calf $tcPO_2$. An oxygen sensor should be placed approximately 10 cm below the knee both anteriorly (over the tibialis anterior muscle) and posteriorly (over the gastrocnemius muscle).

Although there is no single critical value of oxygen tension above which below-knee amputation healing always occurs, several predictive ranges are commonly accepted. One study demonstrated universal healing when the $tcPO_2$ was above 40 mmHg and universal amputation failure when the $tcPO_2$ was below 20 mmHg.[10] In the same study, however, approximately 75% of amputations healed when the $tcPO_2$ was between 20 and 40 mmHg.[10] Another study found that 96% of below-knee amputations healed when the $tcPO_2$ was above 20 mmHg.[11] We recommend performing below-knee amputation if the $tcPO_2$ is above 20 mmHg and moving to a higher amputation level if the $tcPO_2$ is below 20 mmHg.

(L) Measurement of PPG-derived digital pressures is a noninvasive test that utilizes special digital cuffs. A PPG sensor detects digital systolic blood pressure after the digital cuff is deflated from suprasystolic levels. One can measure a transmetatarsal pressure in a similar fashion by applying a cuff at the midmetatarsal level with the PPG sensor at the distal forefoot level. Measuring the PPG-derived digital pressure in a toe adjacent to a necrotic digit or to necrotic tissue can help to predict forefoot amputation healing.

In one study, uniform healing of digit and forefoot amputations occurred when the PPG-derived digital or transmetatarsal pressures were above 20 mmHg.[12] Most studies have shown little to no healing potential if these pressures are below 20 mmHg. If PPG is below 20 mmHg or if PPG pressure cannot be obtained, we recommend obtaining a $tcPO_2$.

(M) As mentioned, transcutaneous oximetry is a noninvasive tool that can also be used to measure the $tcPO_2$ of the forefoot. An oximetric sensor is placed on the dorsum of the mid to distal forefoot. Again, there is no absolute value above which a forefoot amputation always heals, although one study demonstrated 100% healing of forefoot amputations if the $tcPO_2$ was above 20 mmHg and 0% healing if the $tcPO_2$ was below 20 mmHg.[13]

(N) Although approximately 90% to 95% of above-knee amputations can be expected to heal based on clinical judgment alone, measuring the $tcPO_2$ of the anterior and posterior thighs (at the proposed level of incision) may help to increase the healing rate. In one series, healing was 100% when the $tcPO_2$ was above 20 mmHg and 0% when the $tcPO_2$ was below 20 mmHg.[13] If the $tcPO_2$ is below 20 mmHg at the low thigh level, the proposed incision should be moved to the mid or upper thigh level. The obvious difficulty arises if the $tcPO_2$ is below 20 mmHg at the upper thigh level. There is no good solution in this instance, and we would attempt a high above-knee amputation.

We again emphasize that when determining an amputation level, one should use the objective tests discussed in this chapter as adjuncts to clinical experience in an effort to improve overall amputation healing rates.

REFERENCES

1. Yao JST: Choice of amputation level. J Vasc Surg 1988;8:544–545.
2. Ernst CB, Rutkow IM, Cleveland RJ, et al: Vascular surgery in the United States. J Vasc Surg 1987;6:611–621.
3. Castronuovo Jr JJ, Deane LM, Deterling Jr RA, et al: Below-knee amputation: Is the effort to preserve the knee joint justified? Arch Surg 1980;115:1184–1187.
4. Couch NP, David JK, Tilney NL, et al: Natural history of the leg amputee. Am J Surg 1977;133:469–473.
5. Keagy BA, Schwartz JA, Kotb M, et al: Lower extremity amputation: The control series. J Vasc Surg 1986;4:321–326.
6. Gorman JF, Rosenberg JC: Dry ice refrigeration for above-knee amputations. Am J Surg 1967;113:241–245.
7. Fisher DF, Clagett GP, Fry RE, et al: One-stage versus two-stage amputation for wet gangrene of the lower extremity: A randomized study. J Vasc Surg 1988;8:428–433.
8. Hunsaker RH, Schwartz JA, Keagy BA, et al: Dry ice cryoamputation: A twelve-year experience. J Vasc Surg 1985;2:812–816.
9. Barnes RW, Shanik GD, Slaymaker EE: An index of healing in below-knee amputation: Leg blood pressure by Doppler ultrasound. Surgery 1976;79:13–20.
10. Bacharach JM, Rooke TW, Osmundson PJ, et al: Predictive value of transcutaneous oxygen pressure and amputation success by use of supine and elevation measurements. J Vasc Surg 1992;15:558–563.
11. Kram HB, Appel PL, Shoemaker WC: Multisensor transcutaneous oximetric mapping to predict below-knee amputation wound healing: Use of a critical PO_2. J Vasc Surg 1989;9:796–800.
12. Schwartz JA, Schuler JJ, O'Connor RJA, et al: Predictive value of distal perfusion pressure in the healing of amputation of the digits and the forefoot. Surg Gynecol Obstet 1982;154:865–869.
13. Malone JM, Anderson GG, Lalka SG, et al: Prospective comparison of noninvasive techniques for amputation level selection. Am J Surg 1987;154:179–184.

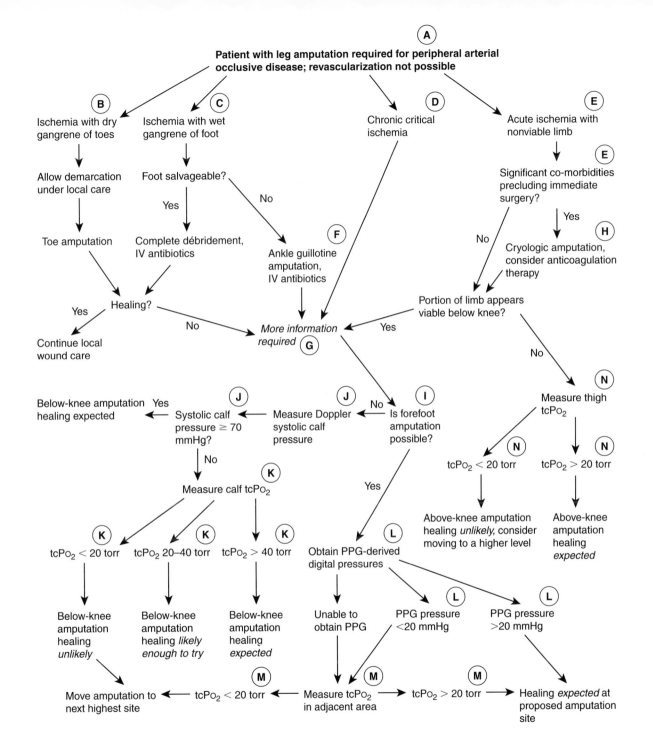

Chapter 47 Compartment Syndromes

WILLIAM D. TURNIPSEED, MD

(A) Compartment syndrome is a clinical condition that results in compromised perfusion to neuromuscular structures within confined myofascial spaces of the upper or lower extremities. The underlying pathologic process is compartmental hypertension.[1]

(B) *Acute compartment syndrome* (ACS) may result from blunt or penetration injury, long-bone fractures, prolonged vascular ischemia, severe soft tissue crush injury, chemical or thermal burns, and extrinsic muscle compression. As a consequence, major vascular and orthopedic reconstructions are often necessary to achieve limb salvage and preserve function. Compartment problems often develop when (1) patients experience long periods (e.g., >6 hours) of ischemia after acute arterial occlusion, (2) popliteal arterial and venous injuries occur simultaneously, or (3) venous ligation or failed venous repair occurs in conjunction with acute arterial vascular reconstructions.

The most common cause of amputations in patients with acute arterial injury results from compartment syndromes that develop because of a delay in diagnosis or incomplete compartment release. Unfortunately, patients who experience neuromuscular dysfunction prior to acute compartment release almost always have significant dysfunction postoperatively. The diagnosis of ACS should be suspected when limb swelling, motor-sensory dysfunction, vasomotor instability, or a combination of these symptoms occurs in conjunction with blunt or penetration injury of an extremity.[2]

(C) In patients with *chronic (exertional) compartment syndrome* (CCS), exercise increases intramuscular pressure to a point at which pain develops from venous hypertension and calf muscle swelling, leading to ischemia. Clinical symptoms are not uniformly reproducible and often mimic those of other musculoskeletal ailments associated with overuse injury. CCS usually occurs in well-conditioned athletes, particularly runners. Uncommon causes include intramuscular hemorrhage secondary to blunt trauma, venous hypertension, and soft tissue tumor expansion.

(D) ACS may be difficult to diagnose unless serial evaluations are made by the same clinical observer. Progressive motor and sensory limb dysfunction associated with provocative trauma (i.e., blunt or penetrating injury, chemical or thermal burns), tense global swelling, edema of compartment muscles, disproportionate muscle pain with passive extension, decreased peripheral pulses, and slow capillary refill may develop in sequence over time, making the diagnosis more obvious on repetitive examinations. The diagnosis is difficult to confirm in comatose or confused patients, and compartment pressure measurements may be required for confirmation.

(E) The diagnosis of CCS is based on clinical history. Symptoms are long-standing and most prevalent in the distribution of the anterolateral, the deep posterior, or the superficial posterior compartment, respectively. Although symptoms may abate with rest, they quickly return when exercise is resumed. Symptoms do not improve with physical therapy or anti-inflammatory medications.

The most prevalent complaint is claudication, which differs from the symptoms associated with chronic arterial occlusive disease, in that exercise distances are long and only isolated muscle groups are affected in CCS. These symptoms occur without clinical evidence of arterial or venous insufficiency. Muscle tightness and swelling in specific myofascial compartments are often diagnostic and may persist for hours after exercise. Bilateral symptoms are common. Paresthesias are uncommon and usually occur in patients with symptomatic anterior compartment complaints.[3] Unlike acute compartment syndromes, CCS rarely causes permanent neuromuscular injury because discomfort restricts patient activity enough to prevent prolonged elevation of compartment pressures.

(F) The diagnosis of compartment syndrome is confirmed by measurement of compartment pressures. These measurements can be performed with a number of techniques, including the wick catheter,[4] the Whiteside needle method,[5] and a hand-held computerized needle transducer (Striker Corporation, Kalamazoo, Mich.). Normal extremity resting pressures are less than 15 mmHg.[2] Venous duplex ultrasound assessment of tibial vein flow (spontaneity and augmentation) can be useful in monitoring dynamic changes during the evolution of the ACS. Loss of venous augmentation correlates with increasing compartment pressure. Laboratory blood chemistry values, such as creatine phosphokinase (CPK) and myoglobin, herald the critical ischemic muscle injury sometimes associated with acute compartment syndromes.

(G) Abnormal circulatory changes begin to occur when compartment pressures exceed 25 mmHg. The first change is loss of phasic flow in peripheral veins. Venous flow augmentation ceases when pressures exceed 30 mmHg. When acute pressure measurements exceed 60 mmHg, ischemic symptoms uniformly develop. ACS, however, may develop at much lower pressures in patients who experience hypovolemic shock or who have chronic arterial occlusive disease. When borderline pressure measurements (≤30 mmHg) are detected in patients at risk for development of ACS, serial pressure measurements may be required.

Indwelling catheters or repetitive needle sticks can be used to obtain serial pressures. When patients describe increasing pain in the distribution of affected muscle compartments or when paresthesias develop, immediate surgical intervention is indicated. In obtunded or comatose patients, loss of tibial venous flow augmentation on duplex ultra-

COMPARTMENT SYNDROMES

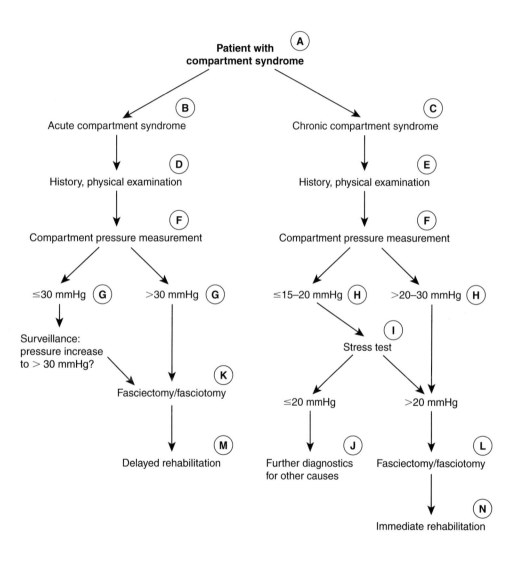

sound testing, compartment pressure increases above 30 mmHg, or significant rises in CPK or myoglobin levels should prompt immediate surgical intervention.

(H) In patients with long-standing clinical symptoms, resting pressures between 16 mm and 20 mmHg are suggestive of CCS, whereas pressures exceeding 20 mmHg are markedly abnormal and uniformly consistent with this diagnosis.

(I) When symptomatic patients have borderline resting compartment pressures (16 to 20 mmHg), measurements should be repeated after a treadmill or running stress test. My colleagues and I prefer to let patients run outside the clinic and return when symptoms develop. Claudication distances can be quite long, often requiring prolonged exercise time on a treadmill, which can cause a severe bottleneck in traffic through a busy diagnostic laboratory. Compartment pressures normally increase after exercise (two or three times the resting pressure) but return to baseline values quickly, within 10 minutes or less after exercise. Symptomatic patients with borderline pressures commonly exhibit postexercise increases in compartment pressure that persist for prolonged periods (>20 minutes) before returning to baseline values.

(J) Noninvasive tests should be selectively used to rule out vascular disorders that might mimic CCS or to detect early circulatory changes in patients at risk of ACS. Premature artherosclerosis, popliteal entrapment syndrome, and chronic venous insufficiency can produce symptoms similar to those of CCS.

Resting and postexercise pulse volume recordings (PVRs) provide plethysmographic and segmental pressure data that can be used to screen for intrinsic arterial occlusive disease and for popliteal entrapment in patients who have chronic symptoms but whose compartment pressures are within normal range. Color flow duplex scanning can be used to screen for venous occlusions or valvular incompetence in patients with chronic symptoms and to monitor changes in arterial or venous limb perfusion in patients at risk for ACS.

Magnetic resonance imaging or computed tomography has been useful in identifying soft tissue tumors or hemorrhage uncommonly associated with CCS. Electromyography and nerve conduction tests are appropriate when chronic peripheral neuropathy or nerve impingement is suspected. Bone scans may be diagnostic for periostitis or shin splints when tibial pain is associated with overuse injury.[2]

(K) When clinical signs and symptoms of ACS develop, early decompression with open fasciotomy or fasciectomy may avert ischemic complications and prevent permanent disability or amputation. Acute compartment symptoms most commonly occur in muscles below the knee. Several techniques for lower extremity compartment release have been described. The double-incision technique of Mubarak and Owen[6] is the most widely used procedure. An incision is made on the anterolateral and medial surfaces of the lower leg, with fasciotomy or fasciectomy being used to release muscles of the anterior, lateral, posterior superficial, and posterior deep compartments.

Other methods of surgical decompression of the distal lower extremity include fibulectomy with fasciotomy[7] and four-compartment fasciotomy without the use of fibulectomy. Both techniques are performed through an incision placed on the posterolateral surface of the leg. When the lateral approach is used, the intermuscular septum must be incised to release the deep posterior compartment muscles when the fibula is not to be removed. The posterior superficial compartment is released by excision of the lateral gastrocnemius fascia. An epimysiotomy of individual deep posterior compartment flexor muscles may be necessary as well.

Unlike surgery for CCS, the surgical treatment of ACS requires that skin and underlying subcutaneous tissues be opened along the entire length of the muscle compartment. Acute swelling and edema may limit the ability of skin and subcutaneous tissues to stretch adequately, resulting in a secondary compartment syndrome as underlying muscles begin to swell.

When ACS develops from blunt injury and long-bone fracture, open compartment release converts closed fractures into open ones, requiring rigid stabilization with intramedullary nails or external fixators. Fasciotomy incisions should be placed so as to allow skin and muscle coverage of vascular or orthopedic repairs that might be required.

Acute compartment syndromes affecting muscles of the thigh are uncommon and usually result from crush injury or high-velocity vehicular accidents. Affected patients commonly have multiple orthopedic and abdominal visceral injuries and suffer mortality rates exceeding 50%. Renal failure commonly results from myoglobinuria unless aggressive treatment with fluids, diuretics, and alkalizing agents is administered.

The anterior and posterior compartments of the thigh are most commonly involved in acute injuries. The anterior compartment contains the quadriceps muscle along with the femoral nerve, artery, and vein. The posterior compartment contains the hamstring muscles and the sciatic nerve. Both compartments can be released through a laterally placed thigh incision. Fasciotomy should be performed even for open fractures, so that adequate muscle decompression may be obtained.

ACS in the upper extremity is much less common and is usually associated with supracondylar fractures, comminuted forearm fractures, and crush or thermal injuries. The forearm, which is most commonly involved, has two compartments (volar and dorsal). The median and ulnar nerves and their respective arteries as well as the flexors of the forearm and hand occupy the volar compartment, whereas the dorsal compartment contains the wrist and finger extensors. Compartment release should be performed when pressures exceed 30 mmHg.

Volar fasciotomy is performed by means of a curvilinear incision from the medial epicondyle to the midpalm. The dorsal release, if indicated, is

COMPARTMENT SYNDROMES

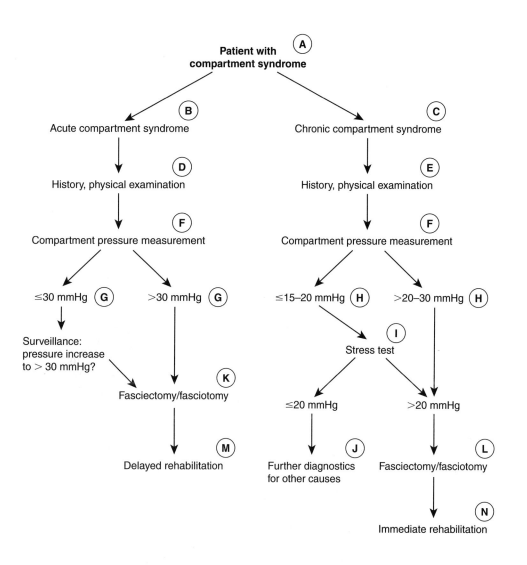

made with a straight dorsal incision from the elbow to the midarm. Epimysiotomy of the involved muscles is usually necessary. Hand swelling may require further decompression to ensure protection of intrinsic muscles and neurovascular structures of the digits. Decompression of the hand is performed through straight incisions on the dorsum over the second and fourth metacarpals. Incisions over the first or fifth metacarpal may be necessary to decompress the thenar or hypothenar space, respectively.

Closure of open fasciotomies must be delayed until limb swelling resolves and frequently requires split-thickness skin grafting. Skin grafts should not be placed until (1) limb swelling has receded, (2) sepsis is controlled, and (3) life-threatening organ dysfunction has been stabilized.

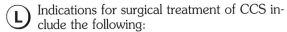 Indications for surgical treatment of CCS include the following:
- Persistent symptoms during athletic activity despite aggressive medical management
- Progression of claudication symptoms to a point that daily activities are affected
- Development of paresthesias
- Presence of resting compartment pressures exceeding 30 mmHg

Extended subcutaneous fasciotomy is the most commonly utilized surgical technique for treating chronic compartment syndromes of the anterolateral and posterior superficial compartments. Compartment fascia is incised with subcutaneous passage of scissors or cutting devices between proximal and distal incisions along the compartment.

Open fasciectomy is an alternative technique performed through linear incisions placed over the anterior lateral or medial surface of the leg, depending on whether the anterior or posterior muscle groups are to be released. A window of fascia is removed from muscles within the compartment, and extended subcutaneous fasciotomy is performed under direct vision so that the entire length of the affected muscle is decompressed.

Open fasciectomy is associated with fewer postoperative complications and fewer recurrences compared with blind subcutaneous fasciotomy. Intraoperative and early postoperative complications occur in 11% of patients with fasciotomy and in 5% of patients with open fasciectomy. The recurrence rate with open fasciectomy is much lower than that recorded in the literature for fasciotomy (2% versus 20%). All compartment releases, except the proximal deep posterior compartment release, can be performed with the use of local anesthesia.[2]

M Recovery from ACS is frequently complicated by morbidity associated with catastrophic orthopedic and soft tissue injuries. Patients may need prolonged physical therapy because of orthopedic rehabilitation requirements and delayed recovery of neuromuscular function.

N Early mobilization and weight bearing are important in the rehabilitation of patients with CCS. Patients are instructed to rest for 48 hours after discharge. They are encouraged to ambulate after that, discarding crutch support as soon as a comfortable heel-strike gait can be achieved. The patients are reevaluated 1 week after surgery. If the wounds have healed completely, patients begin nonimpact training exercises, such as swimming, stationary biking, and the use of a stair-climbing machine. This regimen is maintained for 3 weeks. One month after surgery, if the patients are doing well, they are advanced to the injured runner's program commonly employed in sports rehabilitation. Our success rate in returning symptomatic patients to effective daily life and athletic performance exceeds 98% with proper patient selection.

REFERENCES

1. Bourne RB, Rorabeck CH: Compartment syndromes of the lower leg. Clin Orthop 1989;240:97–104.
2. Turnipseed WD: Compartment syndrome. In Yao JST, Pearch WH (eds): Advances in the Treatment of Ischemic Extremities. Norwalk, Conn, Appelton & Lange, 1994, pp 557–573.
3. Turnipseed WD, Detmer DE, Girdley F: Chronic compartment syndrome: An unusual cause for claudication. Ann Surg 1989;210:557–562.
4. Mubarak SJ, Owen CA, Hargens AR, et al: Acute compartment syndromes: Diagnosis and treatment with the aid of the wick catheter. J Bone Joint Surg Am 1978;60:1091–1095.
5. Whitesides TE Jr, Haney TC, Morimoto K, et al: Tissue pressure measurements as a determinant for need of fasciotomy. Clin Orthop 1975;113:43–51.
6. Mubarak SJ, Owen CA: Double-incision fasciotomy of the leg for decompression in compartment syndromes. J Bone Joint Surg Am 1977;59:184–187.
7. Ernst CB, Kaufer H: Fibulectomy-fasciotomy: An important adjunct in the management of lower extremity arterial trauma. J Trauma 1971;11:365–380.

COMPARTMENT SYNDROMES

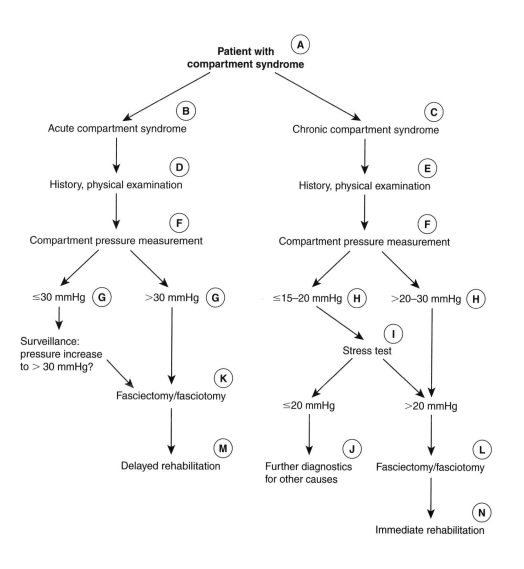

Chapter 48 Popliteal Artery Entrapment Syndrome and Popliteal Cystic Adventitial Disease

LEWIS LEVIEN, MB, BCh, PhD(Med)

(A) In most patients who present to the vascular surgeon with infrainguinal arterial disease causing claudication, the underlying disease process is peripheral atherosclerotic occlusive disease (PAOD). In the subgroup of patients younger than 40 years of age, however, nonatherosclerotic causes, including popliteal artery entrapment syndrome (PAES) and popliteal cystic adventitial disease (PCAD), are more common.[1-4]

(B) In the absence of the usual atherosclerotic risk factors (hypertension, diabetes, hyperlipidemia, and smoking) or homocystinemia, vasculitis, and a family history of premature atherosclerosis, PAES and PCAD should be evaluated as potential causes of claudication in patients who present between the ages of 40 and 55 years. In patients older than 55 years, new-onset claudication is most commonly caused by atherosclerosis.[2, 5, 6]

(C) In the initial stages of both PAES and PCAD, the pedal pulses are usually present at rest because the arterial lumen remains patent and degenerative changes in the arterial wall have not yet resulted in localized stenosis or occlusion.[7, 8] With long-standing symptoms, however, occlusion may have occurred, making the differentiation from other causes of arterial occlusion more difficult.

(D) When symptoms of claudication are due to PAES, although pulses may be present at rest, "stress maneuvers" usually result in significant narrowing of the popliteal artery with consequent reduction or elimination of the distal pulses.[9, 10] Forced plantiflexion of the foot against resistance with the knee extended usually provokes a reduction in popliteal artery flow. Less commonly, passive forced dorsiflexion or active dorsiflexion against resistance with the knee extended may be required to recruit the entrapment mechanism and result in diminished distal pulses.

These stress maneuvers are therefore an integral part of any diagnostic evaluation, be it clinical examination or one of the many diagnostic tests commonly employed to support the clinical diagnosis of PAES, including continuous-wave Doppler ultrasonography, duplex ultrasound evaluation of the popliteal artery, magnetic resonance imaging (MRI), and arteriography.[11-14]

Reduction of distal pulses and flows may occur with these stress maneuvers in up to a third of normal, asymptomatic individuals. Therefore, the demonstration of such a reduction should not be regarded as absolute proof of the presence of PAES.[15] Even in symptomatic individuals, the clinical finding of a reduction of pulses with stress maneuvers should be supported by positive noninvasive tests. One should try to elicit a drop in ankle pressure followed by duplex imaging of the popliteal artery to localize the site of arterial constriction.

(E) Arteriography with stress maneuvers demonstrates the position of the narrowed segment in PAES and gives an indication of the type (I to V) of PAES present. The type of PAES can also be determined on MRI or reconstruction of computed tomography (CT) scans. However, arteriography or magnetic resonance arteriography (MRA) is required to accurately determine the presence of luminal degeneration, aneurysm formation, or distal emboli. If arteriography does not disclose PAES, it usually defines other abnormalities, such as PCAD, atherosclerosis, and popliteal aneurysm. My colleagues and I prefer to perform arteriography in all cases of suspected PAES in which either the clinical findings or noninvasive test results indicate compression with stress maneuvers.[2, 16, 17]

(F) In the absence of alterations in distal pulses and/or blood flow in the popliteal artery with the performance of stress maneuvers, the probability of PAES is low. Another diagnosis for the calf pain, such as compartment syndrome, should be considered. In most cases, this process ultimately results in arteriography anyway and excludes the diagnosis of PAES.

(G) In the presence of PCAD with normal pulses at rest, a popliteal bruit and reduction of distal pulses may be found with extremes of flexion of the knee joint. Such findings are virtually diagnostic of PCAD,[18] but their absence does not exclude this diagnosis.

(H) Imaging of the popliteal fossa with duplex ultrasound surveillance, CT, or MRI confirms the presence of an adventitial cyst and may add valuable information about the relationship of the cyst to the arterial lumen.[18]

(I) Although PCAD has a very characteristic appearance on arteriography (symmetric narrowing or scimitar sign), most cases can be diagnosed by the imaging techniques described previously. Therefore, the role of arteriography in PCAD is to demonstrate the extent of the cystic degeneration and the degree of luminal involvement to permit planning of the operative intervention.[18, 19] MRA or duplex ultrasound scanning may be substituted at centers with good experience in the use of these alternative imaging techniques.

(J) PAES is commonly a bilateral condition. If the popliteal artery has undergone occlusion, careful evaluation of the contralateral limb (see D and E) may demonstrate PAES.[2] A positive evaluation mandates bilateral evaluation.

(K) An arteriogram, MRA image, or duplex scan that demonstrates a focal popliteal occlusion with totally normal proximal and distal arteries suggests PAES or PCAD as the cause of the occlusion. Similarly, in the absence of any degenerative disease of the proximal and distal vessels, the find-

POPLITEAL ARTERY ENTRAPMENT SYNDROME AND POPLITEAL CYSTIC ADVENTITIAL DISEASE

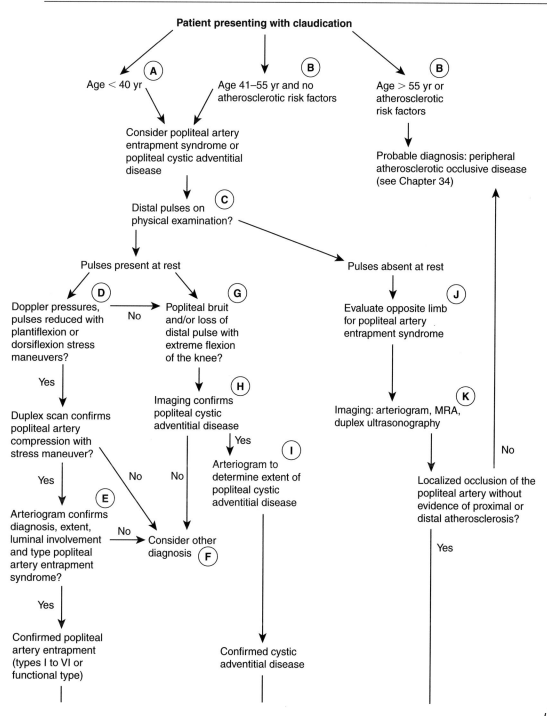

Illustration continued on page 231

ing of either a localized poststenotic popliteal aneurysm or focal popliteal abnormality associated with distal emboli strongly suggests the presence of PAES.[2,6] My preference is to use arteriography for this imaging, although MRA or duplex ultrasound scanning is used in some centers.

(L) Symptomatic PAES that is associated with types I to V vascular entrapment but in which the lumen of the entrapped artery has not developed significant stenosis or aneurysmal change is best treated with division of the entrapment mechanism (i.e., at the medial head of the gastrocnemius muscle in type I or II entrapment or abnormal muscular tendinous or fibrous bands in type III or IV). The functional type of PAES[20] that is associated with severe symptoms and high-grade compression of the popliteal artery with stress maneuver may warrant division of the muscular portion of the medial head of gastrocnemius, even though the anatomic arrangement of the structures in the popliteal fossa appears relatively normal.[2]

(M) When PAES of any type is associated with substantial luminal irregularity, thromboembolic manifestations, or aneurysmal degeneration, the degenerative process caused by the recurrent trauma of prolonged entrapment has resulted in extensive replacement of the normal arterial wall by fibrous tissue. Vein graft replacement of these arteries is required because lesser procedures, which retain the damaged flow surface, are associated with poor long-term patency.[7,8]

(N) Focal popliteal artery narrowing caused by PCAD can be restored to normal through simple excision of the cyst (cystectomy) in most cases.[18,19,21] When the flow surface has degenerated as a result of prolonged thrombosis or when it is not possible to restore a normal flow surface satisfactorily because of extensive involvement of the popliteal artery, a saphenous vein graft replacement of the entire involved segment is indicated.[22]

(O) If, on exploration of an occluded popliteal artery, focal PCAD is encountered as the cause of the occlusion, replacement with a saphenous vein graft should be performed unless simple cyst removal restores a popliteal artery of normal caliber.

(P) If, on exploration of an occluded popliteal artery, PAES is encountered as the cause of the occlusion, replacement with a saphenous vein graft should always be performed because thrombectomy carries a poor long-term patency rate. Similarly, angioplasty of the thrombosed segment is not associated with acceptable long-term patency.

If, on exploration of an occluded popliteal artery, no evidence of PAES or PCAD is found, the patient should be regarded as having a coagulopathy (see Chapter 3 for evaluation) or atherosclerotic occlusive disease (see Chapter 34 for treatment).

REFERENCES

1. Murray A, Halliday M, Croft RJ: Popliteal artery entrapment syndrome. Br J Surg 1991;78:1414–1419.
2. Levien LJ, Veller MG: Popliteal artery entrapment syndrome: More common than previously recognised. J Vasc Surg 1999;30:587–598.
3. Rich NM, Collins GJ, McDonald PT, et al: Popliteal vascular entrapment—its increasing interest. Arch Surg 1979;114:1377–1384.
4. di Marzo L, Cavallaro A, Sciacca V, et al: Surgical treatment of popliteal artery entrapment syndrome: A ten year experience. Eur J Vasc Surg 1991;5:59–64.
5. Persky JM, Kempczinski RF, Fowl RJ: Entrapment of the popliteal artery. Surg Gynecol Obstet 1991;173:84–90.
6. Fowl RJ, Kempczinski RF: Popliteal artery entrapment. In Rutherford RB (ed): Vascular Surgery, 5th ed. Philadelphia, WB Saunders, 2000, pp 1087–1093.
7. di Marzo L, Cavallaro A, Sciacca V, et al: Natural history of entrapment of the popliteal artery. J Am Coll Surg 1994;178:553–556.
8. Levien LJ: Popliteal artery thrombosis caused by popliteal entrapment syndrome. In Greenhalgh RM, Powell JT (eds): Inflammatory and Thrombotic Problems in Vascular Surgery. London, WB Saunders, 1997, pp 159–168.
9. McDonald PT, Easterbrook JA, Rich NM, et al: Popliteal artery entrapment syndrome: Clinical, noninvasive and angiographic diagnosis. Am J Surg 1980;139:318–325.
10. Greenwood LH, Yrizanny JM, Hallett JW: Popliteal artery entrapment: Importance of the stress runoff for diagnosis. Cardiovasc Interv Radiol 1986;9:93–99.
11. Di Marzo L, Cavallaro A, Sciacca V, et al: Diagnosis of popliteal artery entrapment syndrome: The role of duplex scanning. J Vasc Surg 1991;13:434–438.
12. Rizzo RJ, Flinn WR, Yao JST, et al: Computed tomography for evaluation of arterial disease in the popliteal fossa. J Vasc Surg 1990;11:112–119.
13. Fujiwara H, Sugano T, Fujii N: Popliteal artery entrapment syndrome: Accurate morphological diagnosis utilizing MRI. J Cardiovasc Surg 1992;33:160–162.
14. McGuinnes G, Durham JD, Rutherford RB, et al: Popliteal artery entrapment: Findings at MR imaging. J Vasc Interv Radiol 1991;2:241–245.
15. Erdoes LS, Devine JJ, Berhard BM, et al: Popliteal vascular compression in a normal population. J Vasc Surg 1994;20:978–986.
16. Bouhoutsos J, Daskalakis E: Muscular abnormalities affecting the popliteal vessels. Br J Surg 1981;68:501–506.
17. Turnipseed WD, Pozniak M: Popliteal entrapment as a result of neurovascular compression by the soleus and plantaris muscles. J Vasc Surg 1992;15:285–294.
18. Levien LJ, Bergan JJ: Adventitial cystic disease of the popliteal artery. In Rutherford RB (eds): Vascular Surgery, 5th ed. Philadelphia, WB Saunders, 2000, pp 1079–1087.
19. Rignault DP, Pailler JL, Lunel F: The "functional" popliteal artery entrapment syndrome. Int Angiol 1985;4:341–343.
20. Flanigan DP, Burnham SJ, Goodreau JJ, Bergan JJ: Summary of cases of adventitial cystic disease of the popliteal artery. Ann Surg 1979;189:165–175.
21. Ishikawa K: Cystic adventitial disease of the popliteal artery and of other stem vessels in the extremities. Jpn J Surg 1987;17:221–229.
22. Hiertonn T, Karacagil S, Bergqvist D: Long term follow-up of autologous vein grafts: 40 years after reconstruction for cystic adventitial disease. Vasa 1995;24:250–252.

POPLITEAL ARTERY ENTRAPMENT SYNDROME AND POPLITEAL CYSTIC ADVENTITIAL DISEASE

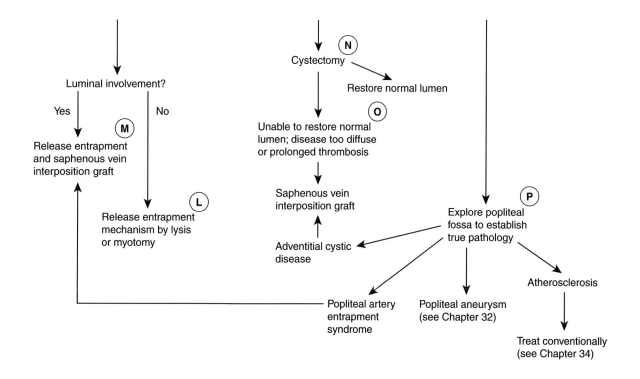

Chapter 49 Upper Extremity Ischemia

MARK D. MORASCH, MD • WILLIAM H. PEARCE, MD

A Compared with lower extremity ischemia, upper limb ischemia is uncommon. Surgical correction of upper extremity arterial disease accounts for less than 5% of all vascular interventions. Although atherosclerosis causes the vast majority of symptomatic lower extremity ischemia, upper limb ischemia can result from multiple causes.

B Particular attention to patient history often defines the etiology of symptoms, whereas close examination usually provides an anatomic diagnosis that pinpoints the site of obstruction. The medical history must include occupational and athletic activities and detailed inquiries into medical co-morbidities, pharmacologic treatments, and prior irradiation. Presenting symptoms and signs can include Raynaud's phenomenon, ischemic rest pain or intermittent limb claudication, and digital gangrene. Patients with proximal disease may also describe central neurologic symptoms resulting from emboli or steal phenomena. A history of bilaterality strongly suggests a nonatherosclerotic cause.

Physical examination must include careful palpation for pulses and auscultation for bruits. Palpation over the clavicle may detect a cervical rib or a subclavian aneurysm. Each of these maneuvers should be repeated with the arm in stressed positions of abduction and external rotation, with particular attention given to pulse changes or positional changes in a bruit. Allen's test and careful inspection of the hand for pulsatile masses, excessive calluses, muscle wasting, and evidence of microemboli complete the examination.

C Several noninvasive tests are available to further delineate upper extremity disease. The most useful tests are systolic Doppler pressure measurements combined with spectral waveform analysis. These tests identify the level of stenosis or occlusion. It is important that these studies be performed bilaterally and include digital indices. Measurements are usually obtained through insonation of the axillary, brachial, radial, and ulnar arteries in their most superficial anatomic positions. The palmar arches are best heard at the midthenar and hypothenar regions, the common digital arteries at the base of the finger, and the proper digital arteries along the shaft of each finger.

Segmental pressures are measured with an inflatable cuff placed on the upper arm and on the forearm. These measurements are normally within 10 mmHg of the measurements on the other arm. Additionally, a drop of 20 to 30 mmHg between upper arm and forearm cuff measurements indicates interval disease. A 2.5-mm cuff can also be placed at the base of each digit. Disease within or distal to the palmar arch is signified by a pressure gradient between fingers of more than 15 mmHg or a drop from wrist to digit measurement greater than 30 mmHg.

The diagnosis of Raynaud's disease is made after exclusion of other organic causes but can be suggested on the basis of results of cold immersion tests. Raynaud's disease is discussed further in Chapter 69.

When bilateral hand ischemia is present, a systemic cause is likely and certain serologic and immunologic tests should be obtained at this point. Erythrocyte sedimentation rate (ESR) and antinuclear antibody (ANA) measurements are the most sensitive for detecting forms of arteritis and connective tissue disorders, respectively. Because these tests are used primarily for screening purposes, more specific serologic testing should follow when the ESR or ANA value suggests disease.

D If physical examination and noninvasive testing reveal an occlusive lesion, arteriography demonstrating the entire upper extremity arterial vasculature from the aortic arch to the digital vessels is indicated. If extrinsic compression from structures in the thoracic outlet is suspected, provocative arm positioning should be performed with separate injections of contrast material. If patient history suggests a systemic disorder and bilateral disease is suspected from the physical findings, the arteriogram should include both upper extremities.

Intra-arterial vasodilators can reverse distal vasospasm during arteriography. Anatomic variation is commonplace in the upper extremity (see classic descriptions of anatomy and radiography by Coleman and Anson[1] and Janevski[2]). In instances of traumatic injury or in clear-cut cases of acute cardioembolic obstruction of the brachial artery, patients with critical ischemia should proceed directly to surgery without a diagnostic arteriogram.

E Proximal occlusive lesions are defined as those occurring above the elbow. The most common sites of atherosclerotic involvement are the proximal innominate and subclavian arteries. These lesions can be associated with radiographic evidence of steal from the vertebral circulation (subclavian steal) or carotid circulation (innominate steal). Symptomatic steal from supra-aortic trunk disease is an indication for treatment.[3] Arteriography can also demonstrate proximal occlusive disease secondary to thoracic outlet syndrome, arteritis (radiation-induced, Takayasu's, giant cell, polymyalgia rheumatica) or fibromuscular dysplasia (FMD). In addition, emboli that originate in the heart or within aneurysms of the upper extremity are not uncommon.

F Distal occlusive lesions involve the arteries below the elbow. Distal lesions tend to predominate in the arteries of the wrist and hand. Collagen vascular diseases, including scleroderma, systemic lupus erythematosus, polyarteritis nodosa, and dermatomyositis, can manifest as chronic symptoms ranging from Raynaud's phenomenon to digital gangrene. Buerger's disease is a separate entity characterized by occlusion of the larger arteries in the distal forearm and hand in

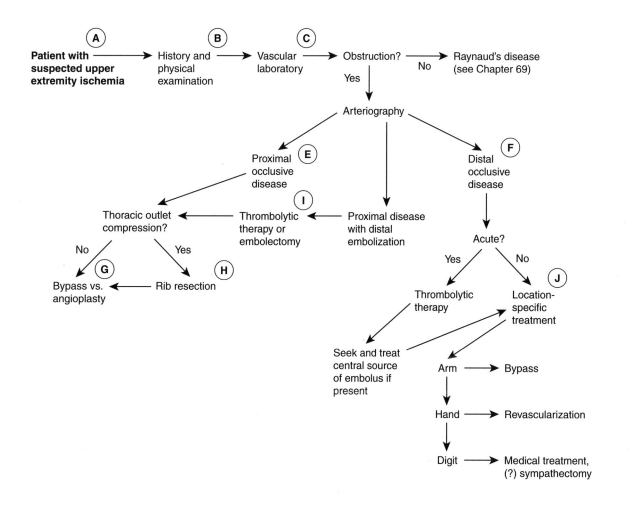

Upper Extremity Ischemia (continued)

patients who present with a heavy smoking history and digital gangrene. Patients with chronic renal failure, particularly those with diabetes, can experience a calciphylactic arteriopathy characterized by circumferential accumulation of mineralized calcium within the media of the arteries below the elbow that leads to distal ischemia and digital gangrene. Although both upper extremities may not have symptoms, the disease states previously listed lead to bilateral findings on arteriography. Unilateral causes of distal arterial occlusion include vibration white finger, hypothenar hammer syndrome, catheter injury, dialysis access steal, and accidental arterial drug injection.

(G) The treatment of proximal upper extremity occlusions must be appropriately tailored for the specific cause. Symptomatic atherosclerotic occlusive disease involving the proximal subclavian artery is usually best treated via cervical reconstruction based on ipsilateral carotid inflow. Subclavian transposition and short prosthetic bypass grafts have excellent long-term patency rates, in excess of 90% after 5 years.[4] Angioplasty and possible stent treatment of proximal atherosclerotic lesions have also been shown to have excellent early results, although long-term follow-up is lacking.[5] Vascular occlusions that result from the various forms of arteritis are best treated with surgical bypass reconstruction. Steroid therapy is an important adjuvant when systemic symptoms are present and should be completed, if possible, prior to surgery for arteritis.

(H) Thoracic outlet syndrome (TOS) is the most common disorder causing proximal arterial symptoms in young adults. Arterial compression can occur between the highest rib and the clavicle, within the interscalene triangle, over the insertion of the pectoralis minor muscle, or with the humeral head in extreme external rotation. Arterial complications of TOS, including aneurysm formation, thrombosis, and distal embolization, require surgical intervention, usually in the form of interposition vein bypass and decompressive resection of the first rib. We prefer a supraclavicular approach, although transaxillary rib resection can also be used. When distal embolization has occurred as a result of arterial TOS, both thrombolytic therapy and surgical embolectomy can be used to restore the distal vasculature.

(I) Emboli and thromboses can be treated either surgically or with intra-arterial thrombolytic therapy. After elimination of an occluding embolus, a completion arteriogram is necessary to confirm outflow patency. In the case of an embolic occlusion, it is equally important that the proximal source be aggressively sought. When TOS generally and subclavian aneurysms, axillary artery intimal injury, or branch aneurysms from repetitive humeral head compression specifically are responsible for distal embolization, additional surgical intervention is required.

(J) Distal occlusive lesions can also result from a number of different causes, and treatment should be tailored for the specific nature of disease. When arteriography demonstrates occlusion of the radial and ulnar arteries with reconstitution of a proximal palmar arch, reversed vein bypass has been shown to be beneficial. When short-segment occlusion of the distal radial or ulnar arteries is encountered, local endarterectomy and vein patch angioplasty usually suffice.

Ulnar artery aneurysms that develop as a result of repetitive trauma require resection and either direct reanastomosis or interposition vein grafting to prevent distal embolization. The results of reconstruction to the level of the wrist are also excellent, and major amputations are rarely required.[6] If a digital artery occlusion cannot be treated with thrombolytic therapy, particularly in instances related to connective tissue disorders, the treatment is usually supportive.

If distal vasoreactivity remains intact, patients may benefit from vasodilator therapy or cervicothoracic sympathectomy, although this treatment remains controversial. Smoking cessation is imperative.

REFERENCES

1. Coleman SS, Anson BJ: Arterial patterns in the hand based upon a study of 650 specimens. Surg Gynecol Obstet 1961;113:409–442.
2. Janevski BK: Angiography of the Upper Extremity. The Hague, Martinus Nijhoff, 1982.
3. Morasch MD, Berguer R: Supra-aortic trunk revascularization. In Yao JST, Pearce WH (eds): Modern Trends in Vascular Surgery. Stamford, Conn, Appleton & Lange, 1999.
4. Berguer R, Morasch MD, Kline RA, et al: Cervical reconstruction of the supra-aortic trunks: A 16-year experience. J Vasc Surg 1999;29:239–248.
5. Brunkwall J, Bergentz SE: Long-term results of arterial reconstruction of the upper extremity. In Yao JST, Pearce WH (eds): The Ischemic Extremity: Advances in Treatment. Norwalk, Conn, Appleton & Lange, 1995, pp 211–227.
6. Nehler MR, Dalman RL, Harris EJ, et al: Upper extremity arterial bypass distal to the wrist. J Vasc Surg 1992;6:633–640.

UPPER EXTREMITY ISCHEMIA

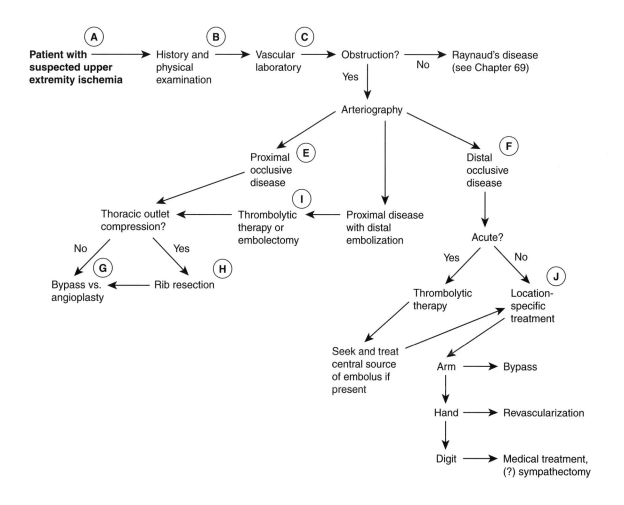

RENOVASCULAR DISEASE

Chapter 50 Renovascular Occlusive Disease: Evaluation

JAMES M. WONG, MD • KIMBERLEY J. HANSEN, MD

(A) The estimated prevalence of renovascular hypertension in the general population is low (~3%); however, in select populations with severe hypertension, especially at the extremes of age, renovascular disease (RVD) is common. In 78% of hypertensive children younger than 5 years of age, the cause is renovascular.[1] Among adults 60 years of age or older with severe hypertension, 50% have RVD. When combined with renal insufficiency (i.e., *ischemic nephropathy*), the prevalence of RVD exceeds 70%.[2]

Although an abdominal bruit in a hypertensive, young white female strongly suggests renovascular hypertension, physical signs are unreliable and their absence cannot rule out RVD. Severe hypertension (diastolic blood pressure ≥ 105 mmHg), particularly at the extremes of age or when combined with renal insufficiency, should prompt the search for a renovascular cause. In the complete absence of hypertension, renal insufficiency should not be attributed to RVD.

(B) Screening studies used to define the presence of RVD may be either anatomic or functional (Table 50–1). The authors advocate the use of anatomic screening studies, particularly renal duplex sonography (RDS). Although the performance of RDS is dependent on a skilled sonographer, it is free of nephrotoxic risk, minimal preparation (an overnight fast) is required, and no change in medications is necessary. The primary limitation of RDS is that it does not reliably identify branch or polar renal artery disease as an etiologic mechanism of hypertension.[3] However, when RDS is used to screen for RVD causing renal insufficiency, negative findings exclude ischemic nephropathy.

Magnetic resonance imaging/angiography (MRI/MRA) and computed tomography (CT) may offer accurate main renal artery assessment; however, cost (MRI/MRA), contrast exposure (CT), and resolution (MRI/MRA and CT) have limited their widespread application.[4,5]

Despite favorable reported results,[6] we have not found captopril renography to be a useful screening study because baseline renographic findings are abnormal in most contemporary patients with critical stenosis.

(C) Patients with negative screening results are managed medically. Hypertensive children and young adults are considered for angiography despite negative screening results to search for branch or polar RVD.

(D) Cut-film angiography provides the best renal artery image (Table 50–2). Intra-arterial digital subtraction angiography (IADSA) permits the use of lower amounts of contrast medium.[7] Carbon dioxide angiography has also been a useful alternative in patients with severe renal dysfunction, but it does not provide adequate information in cases of renal artery occlusion.[8] Intravenous DSA (IVDSA) is no longer recommended.[9]

(E) Hypertension is a prerequisite for renal artery intervention. Where unilateral RVD is associated with medically controlled hypertension, functional studies (i.e., renal vein renin assays [RVRA]) are advisable to establish a causal relationship between hypertension and the renovascular lesion. Exceptions include children, young patients, and adults with poorly controlled hyperten-

TABLE 50–2
Imaging Studies*

	IADSA†	Carbon Dioxide Angiography‡	IVDSA§
Sensitivity	90%	83%	88%
Specificity	98%	99%	90%

*Compared with conventional angiography.
†Data from Kim D, et al: Angiology 1991;42:345–357.[7]
‡Data from Schreier DZ, et al: Arch Surg 1996;131:503–508.[8]
§Data from Havey RJ, et al: JAMA 1985;254:388–393.[9]
IADSA, intra-arterial digital subtraction angiography; IVDSA; intravenous digital subtraction angiography.

TABLE 50–1
Screening Studies

	RDS*	MRI/MRA†	Spiral CT‡	Captopril Renography§
Sensitivity	93%	100%	90%	91%
Specificity	98%	89%	97%	94%

*Data from Hansen KJ, et al: J Vasc Surg 1990;12:227–236[3]
†Data from Snidow JJ, et al: Radiology 1996;198:725–732[4]
‡Data from Kim TS, et al: J Vasc Interv Radiol 1998;9:553–559.[5]
§Data from Setaro JF, et al: Hypertension 1991;18:289–298.[6]
CT, computed tomography; MRA, magnetic resonance angiography; MRI, magnetic resonance imaging; RDS, renal duplex sonography.

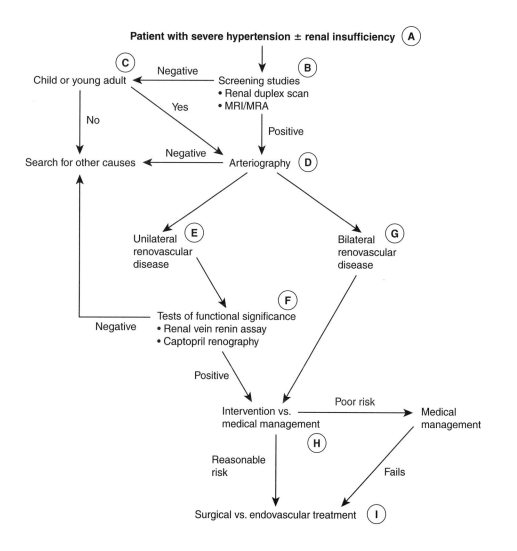

TABLE 50-3
Functional Studies

	RVRA*	Plasmin Renin†	Captopril Renography‡
Sensitivity	74%	27%	91%
Specificity	100%	95%	94%

*Data from Dean RH, et al: Curr Probl Surg 1997;34:209–316.[2]
†Data from Grim CE, et al: Ann Intern Med 1979;91:617–622.[10]
‡Data from Setaro, JF, et al: Hypertension 1991;18:289–298.[6]
RVRA, renal vein renin assay.

sion who should undergo empirical intervention without functional studies.

(F) With proper patient preparation, RVRA with simultaneous dual-catheter sampling can establish the relationship between unilateral RVD and hypertension (Table 50–3). A positive study is indicated by a renal vein renin ratio at or greater than 1.5 after sodium restriction and removal from all antihypertensive medications except calcium-channel blocking agents or sodium nitroprusside.[2]

With rare exception, hypertension can be controlled with bed rest, calcium channel agents, and diuretics. Peripheral plasma renin levels have proved unreliable.[10] Captopril renography has been reported to be predictive of hypertension response after intervention; however, it is adversely influenced by associated renal insufficiency and intrinsic parenchymal disease.[6]

(G) Management of patients with bilateral RVD depends on the severity of hypertension and the associated renovascular lesions:

1. When only one lesion is severe (i.e., ≥ 80% stenosis), the patient is evaluated and treatment is given as for unilateral disease.
2. When both lesions are moderate (i.e., 60% to 80% stenosis), empirical intervention is indicated when hypertension is severe.
3. Patients with severe bilateral RVD (i.e., ≥ 80% stenosis) and hypertension of any degree are considered for empirical intervention, especially when renal insufficiency is present.[2]

(H) Optimal management of RVD is controversial. However, the rationale for intervention is to reduce the incidence of adverse cardiovascular events and renal failure. Patients with significant and independent risk factors for cardiovascular mortality and dialysis-dependence are considered poor candidates for intervention. Risk factors include:

1. Clinical congestive heart failure secondary to systolic dysfunction.
2. Long-standing diabetes mellitus.
3. Uncorrectable renal insufficiency.

In these patients, medical management is the best option.

Although reduced hypertension in adults has not been associated with improved survival in contemporary studies, improved renal function after intervention is associated with a significant and independent improved survival and decreased dialysis. Correlates of improved excretory renal function in response to surgical repair include severe hypertension, global renal ischemia, severe stenosis (≥80%) or renal artery occlusion, and rapid deterioration of renal function. Kidney size is not predictive of function response.

Management of the occluded renal artery depends on the level of function of the affected kidney. Nephrectomy is reserved for kidneys with minimal function with unreconstructible RVD causing severe hypertension.[11]

(I) Surgical or endovascular intervention is chosen according to the etiology and the anatomic location of the renal artery lesion. Although endovascular intervention is an attractive alternative to surgery, long-term blood pressure and renal function improvement and anatomic results have not been established.

On the basis of the available data, percutaneous transluminal renal angioplasty (PTRA) with or without stenting for ostial atherosclerotic lesions does not yield equivalent blood pressure or renal function response as compared with surgical repair. The authors preferentially select PTRA for optimal lesions (i.e., nonostial atherosclerotic lesions and fibromuscular lesions of the medial fibroplasia type limited to the main renal artery). In addition, PTRA may be considered in selected high-risk patients with other suboptimal lesions. Methods of surgical intervention are discussed in Chapter 51.

REFERENCES

1. Lawson JD, Boerth R, Foster JH, Dean RH: Diagnosis and management of renovascular hypertension in children. Arch Surg 1977;112:1307–1316.
2. Dean RH, Benjamin ME, Hansen KJ: Surgical management of renovascular hypertension. Curr Probl Surg 1997;34:209–308.
3. Hansen KJ, Tribble RW, Reavis SW, et al: Renal duplex sonography: Evaluation of clinical utility. J Vasc Surg 1990;12:227–236.
4. Snidow JJ, Johnson MS, Harris VJ, et al: Three-dimensional gadolinium-enhanced MR angiography for aortoiliac inflow assessment plus renal artery screening in a single breath hold. Radiology 1996;198:725–732.
5. Kim TS, Chung JW, Park JH, et al: Renal artery evaluation: Comparison of spiral CT angiography to intra-arterial DSA. J Vasc Interv Radiol 1998;9:553–559.
6. Setaro JF, Saddler MC, Chen CC, et al: Simplified captopril renography in diagnosis and treatment of renal artery stenosis. Hypertension 1991;18:289–298.
7. Kim D, Porter DH, Brown R, et al: Renal artery imaging: A prospective comparison of intra-arterial digital subtraction angiography with conventional angiography. Angiology 1991;42:345–357.
8. Schreier DZ, Weaver FA, Frankhouse J, et al: A prospective study of carbon dioxide-digital subtraction vs. standard contrast arteriography in the evaluation of the renal arteries. Arch Surg 1996;131:503–508.
9. Havey RJ, Krumlovsky F, delGreco F, Martin HG: Screening for renovascular hypertension: Is renal digital-subtraction angiography the preferred test? JAMA 1985;254:388–393.
10. Grim CE, Luft FC, Weinberger MH, Grim CM: Sensitivity and specificity of screening tests for renal vascular hypertension. Ann Intern Med 1979;91:617–622.
11. Oskin TC, Hansen KJ, Deitch JS, et al: Chronic renal artery occlusion: Nephrectomy versus revascularization. J Vasc Surg 1999;29:140–149.

RENOVASCULAR OCCLUSIVE DISEASE: EVALUATION

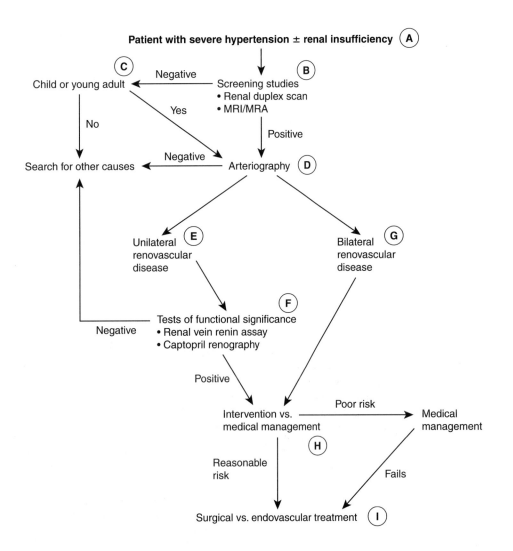

Chapter 51 Renovascular Occlusive Disease: Treatment

JAMES C. STANLEY, MD • GILBERT R. UPCHURCH, JR., MD

Pediatric Renovascular Occlusive Disease

(A) Ostial stenoses represent the most common renal artery occlusive lesion in the pediatric age group.[1] These are true hypoplastic vessels, associated with multiple renal arteries in 80% of patients, and perirenal abdominal aortic coarctation in approximately 20% of patients. The latter type is often observed in children with von Recklinghausen's disease. Treatment involves aortic reimplantation (see E) or aortorenal bypass with an internal iliac artery graft (see F).

(B) Main renal artery stenoses in the midportion of the vessel are relatively uncommon.[1] They likely represent a postinflammatory or post-traumatic narrowing with secondary intimal fibroplasia. Rare lesions may represent persistent fetal musculoelastic intimal rests. These lesions are usually unilateral. Treatment is most often by aortorenal bypass with an internal iliac artery graft (see F).

(C) Segmental renal artery stenoses in children are focal or web-like and may represent a sequelae of neonatal embolization accompanying umbilical catheter exchange transfusion.[1] These are usually solitary lesions, except those seen in association with rubella, when multiple diffuse segmental narrowings are present. Treatment, when other than a simple web, usually involves an aortorenal bypass with an internal iliac artery graft (see F) or reimplantation into an adjacent renal artery (see G).

(D) Intrarenal webs are extremely uncommon, occurring usually as solitary stenoses in second-order branches.[1] They often exhibit poststenotic dilatations. Treatment usually involves reimplantation to an adjacent renal artery (see G) and operative dilation, percutaneous angioplasty (PTA), or renal ablation (see H) in selected cases.

(E) Aortic reimplantation is appropriate treatment for ostial lesions and is the preferred method in contemporary practice.[1] The renal artery beyond the stenosis is transected and subsequently spatulated anteriorly and posteriorly in order to create a generous perimeter with which to reimplant it in an end-to-side manner as a patch into the aorta. For occasional patients with a hostile aorta, the right renal artery may be reimplanted into the superior mesenteric artery. Tension-free anastomoses can be ensured by simple mobilization of the kidney medially if necessary. The anastomosis should be at least 8 mm in length, with interrupted cardiovascular sutures preferred, to provide for later growth.

(F) Aortorenal bypass with an internal iliac artery graft is appropriate treatment of many pediatric renovascular lesions except intrarenal webs.[1,2] These autologous arterial grafts are favored over vein grafts which have a known predisposition to aneurysmal degeneration.[3] If vein grafts are the only available conduit, they should be surrounded at the time of placement with a loosely fabricated knit support.[4] Nonanatomic bypass with a splenorenal end-to-end anastomosis is not favored in children because of early postoperative thromboses and the potential development of celiac artery narrowings over ensuing years.[1,2]

The internal iliac artery, when removed for use as a free graft, should be excised with its distal branches so that they can be spatulated to provide for a generous aortic anastomosis. The latter anastomosis is completed with interrupted or continuous cardiovascular sutures. To complete the graft-to-renal artery anastomosis, it is also important that the iliac artery graft be spatulated posteriorly and the distal transected renal artery spatulated anteriorly to provide for a generous ovoid anastomosis.

(G) Spatulation of segmental arteries beyond their stenoses with reimplantation onto an adjacent segmental or main renal artery is an appropriate revascularization technique in selected patients; interrupted fine cardiovascular sutures are used. Routine ex vivo repairs are not suggested but may be used, when needed, to allow completion of the revascularization in complex cases.[2]

(H) Operative dilatation via rigid metal dilators or PTA, unlike the situation in adults, is appropriate only for simple segmental web-like lesions in children.[1] Use of a silicone lubricant during intraoperative dilation and cautious use of dilators and balloons no greater than 1 mm, the size of the presumed normal renal artery being treated, are recommended. In rare cases, transcatheter alcohol ablation (infarction) of the renal parenchyma beyond a stenosis successfully eliminates the renin-producing tissue and eliminates the hypertensive state.

(I) Secondary nephrectomy is appropriate when the primary intervention (see D to H) is unsuccessful and the cause of the failure is not reversible by re-revascularization.[1,5] This eventuality has been reported in slightly fewer than 10% of pediatric patients but may occur in nearly 30% of patients needing reoperation.

(J) Irreparable ischemic atrophy, such as that accompanying a chronically occluded renal artery with evidence of only a few millimeters of viable cortex, as well as the occasional kidney labeled "hypoplastic" (although such a label may reflect an earlier ischemic vascular process), may be treated by primary nephrectomy if the remaining contralateral kidney is normal.[1]

(K) Primary nephrectomy is uncommon. It is usually performed in a subcapsular manner to minimize troublesome bleeding from perinephric vessels. An initial nephrectomy is usually performed when little renal function can be ascribed to the kidney (see J) and occasionally when the attempted primary intervention proves impossible.[1]

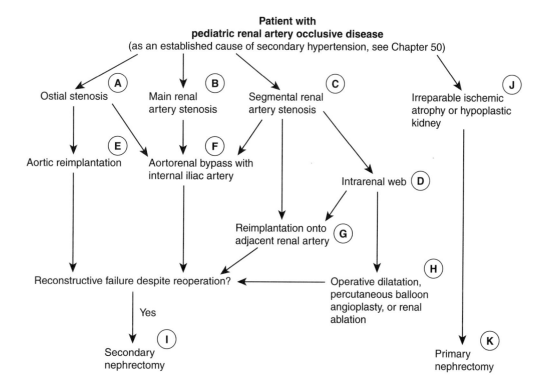

Renovascular Occlusive Disease: Treatment (continued)

Adult Fibrodysplastic Renovascular Occlusive Disease

(A) Intimal fibroplasia accounts for 5% of all dysplastic renal artery lesions. It is most commonly encountered in younger patients, and there is no gender predilection.[6-9] Mesenchyme-like cells encroaching into the vessel lumen above an intact internal elastic lamina are characteristic of this disease. The disease process is usually unilateral. Once a pressure gradient exists, the disease is very progressive.

Those rare stenoses appearing as a thin, discrete web may be treated by PTA (see D), although the more common focal hourglass stenoses are usually treated operatively (see E to H).

(B) Medial fibrodysplasia accounts for 85% of all dysplastic renal artery lesions and invariably affects women.[9,10] The average age at recognition is in the 30s. This disease has a "string of beads" arteriographic appearance, with serial webs of dysplastic media projecting into the lumen, which alternate with mural aneurysms due to medial thinning. Bilateral disease occurs in 60% of patients, including 10% to 15% in whom the lesions are functionally important and warrant treatment. In 25% of patients, the disease extends into the segmental arteries.

PTA (see D) is usually successful when the disease is unassociated with macroaneurysms or extension into the segmental branches. Operative therapy (see E) is recommended in the latter circumstances.

(C) Perimedial dysplasia accounts for 10% of dysplastic renal artery disease and affects predominantly women a decade older than those with medial fibrodysplasia.[6-9] This disease is bilateral in 10% of patients. It is characterized by serial stenoses composed of excessive elastin in the perimedial-subadventitial region, without intervening mural aneurysms. Segmental disease is uncommon. An occasional isolated focal stenosis may respond favorably to PTA (see D), but failed treatment due to recoil of the excess elastic tissue is common. Most of these lesions are treated operatively (see E).

(D) PTA is successful in treating nearly 85% of patients with medial fibrodysplasia (see B) and in carefully chosen patients with focal weblike lesions due to intimal fibroplasia (see A) or perimedial dysplasia (see C).[10-12] Recurrence rates in the latter two categories range from 10% to 20%, compared to a 5% restenosis rate with medial fibrodysplasia. Although operative dilation can be performed, it is usually undertaken only in conjunction with a simultaneous bypass procedure.

(E) Operative therapy, whether performed in situ or ex vivo, is undertaken in two basic modes with either (1) an aortorenal bypass or (2) a nonanatomic bypass.[6,7,13] In situ revascularizations are preferred in treating the majority of fibrodysplastic lesions, in that disruption of preexisting collateral vessels does not accompany this reconstructive procedure. However, ex vivo revascularizations are appropriate in certain patients with complex disease, especially that affecting multiple segmental vessels or when associated with aneurysmal disease of these smaller arteries.[14]

(F) Age of the patient and the status of the aorta become important determinants in the choice of an in situ operation. In patients younger than 21 years of age, vein grafts are avoided because of the potential for late aneurysmal degeneration.[3] Internal iliac artery grafts are favored in younger patients and in occasional older patients.

(G) Vein grafts are favored in most patients older than 21 years in whom the aorta is relatively normal. In patients with no suitable vein, synthetic conduits of polytetrafluoroethylene (PTFE, Teflon) or polyester (Dacron) may be used, but these materials are not favored over autologous grafts in younger patients.

(H) When an aorta is encased in scar tissue from previous surgery or when clamping of the aorta would be hazardous because of ventricular dysfunction, a nonanatomic revascularization in the form of a hepatorenal, splenorenal, or iliorenal reconstruction is appropriate.[15] A normal, undiseased celiac artery is necessary for a hepatorenal or splenorenal bypass.

Proper exposure of the renal artery, careful procurement of autologous grafts, and creation of generous anastomoses contribute to long-term successful outcomes. Salutary results are expected in 85% to 90% of patients treated by operation for hypertension secondary to fibrodysplastic renal artery occlusive disease, with cure rates approaching 75% to 80%.[6,7,13]

(I) Secondary nephrectomy may be necessary to provide adequate blood pressure control in patients whose primary operation has failed when attempts at re-revascularization have been unsuccessful.[5]

(J) In rare circumstances, a kidney initially appears to be hypoplastic or to exhibit irreparable ischemic atrophy. When the contralateral kidney appears normal, a primary nephrectomy (see K) may be performed.

(K) The surgeon usually begins primary nephrectomy by making a small incision with the electrocautery a few centimeters in length on the anterior capsular surface of the lower pole of the kidney and then uses his or her finger, performing a blunt dissection of the kidney from its capsule. A second incision over the vascular pedicle close to the renal pelvis allows identification and transection of the artery and vein as well as the ureter. Small nonparenchymal vessels entering the renal capsule may then be electrocoagulated from within. This technique avoids disturbing the adrenal gland and perinephric adnexa as well as the multitude of nonparenchymal collateral vessels in the surrounding adipose tissue.

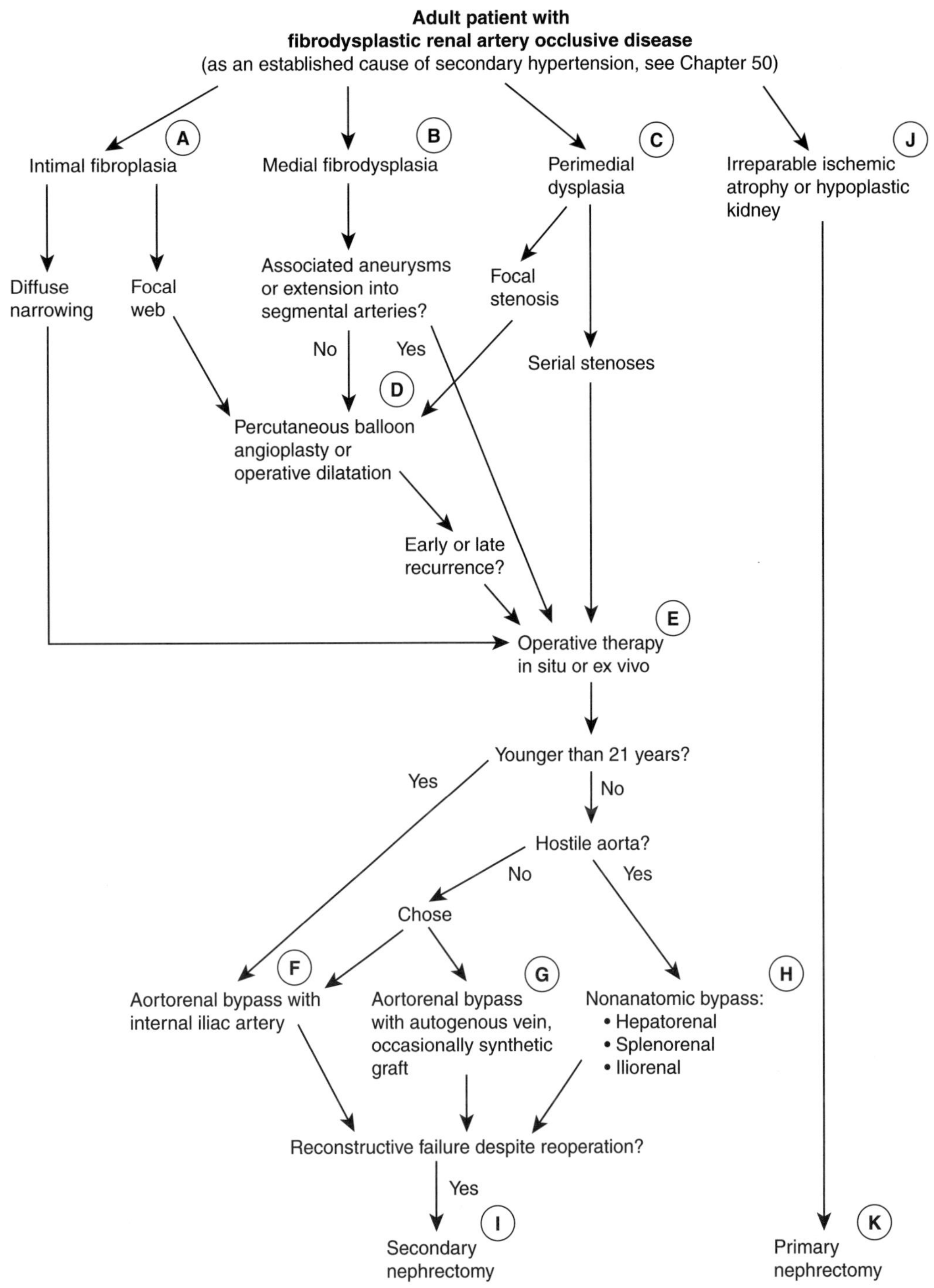

RENOVASCULAR OCCLUSIVE DISEASE: TREATMENT

Adult patient with fibrodysplastic renal artery occlusive disease
(as an established cause of secondary hypertension, see Chapter 50)

- (A) Intimal fibroplasia
  - Diffuse narrowing
  - Focal web
- (B) Medial fibrodysplasia
  - Associated aneurysms or extension into segmental arteries?
    - No
    - Yes (D)
- (C) Perimedial dysplasia
  - Focal stenosis
  - Serial stenoses
- (J) Irreparable ischemic atrophy or hypoplastic kidney

Percutaneous balloon angioplasty or operative dilatation
→ Early or late recurrence?

(E) Operative therapy in situ or ex vivo
→ Younger than 21 years?
- Yes
- No → Hostile aorta?
  - No → Chose
  - Yes

(F) Aortorenal bypass with internal iliac artery

(G) Aortorenal bypass with autogenous vein, occasionally synthetic graft

(H) Nonanatomic bypass:
- Hepatorenal
- Splenorenal
- Iliorenal

Reconstructive failure despite reoperation?
→ Yes

(I) Secondary nephrectomy

(K) Primary nephrectomy

Renovascular Occlusive Disease: Treatment (continued)

Arteriosclerotic Renal Artery Occlusive Disease

(A) Arteriosclerotic stenoses of the renal artery are common in older people and are the most common cause of renovascular hypertension and ischemic nephropathy.[7, 16–21] Men are affected twice as often as women. Management of this disease remains controversial as to the best method of therapy as well as to the expected long-term results.

Although considerable clinical experience with arteriosclerotic renal artery disease exists, the failure to categorize these patients (unilateral versus bilateral stenoses, aortic spillover versus intrinsic renal artery stenoses, and normal versus abnormal renal function) in most published reports has contributed to many misunderstandings. Nevertheless, certain accepted practices are recognized by most clinicians.[6, 7]

(B) Unilateral isolated renal artery stenosis affects fewer than 20% of patients with arteriosclerotic renovascular disease.[7] In the case of normal renal function, PTA with or without stenting (see D) may be performed in lieu of operative therapy (see E),[11, 12, 19] although with abnormal renal function surgical treatment is favored.[16, 17]

(C) Unilateral and bilateral ostial aortic spillover stenoses account for approximately 80% of arteriosclerotic renovascular lesions.[7] The ratio of unilateral-to-bilateral spillover stenoses is 1 to 3. These lesions represent complex plaque with mural hemorrhage, calcification, numerous cholesterol crystals, and accumulation of mural thrombus. Intrarenal disease, as an extension of the aortic spillover disease, is not rare but is uncommon. Isolated arteriosclerotic segmental disease is uncommon, affecting fewer than 5% of these patients, most of whom are diabetic.[7]

In the case of unilateral disease and normal renal function, either PTA or operative therapy (see D and E) provides acceptable results. In the presence of abnormal renal function, operative therapy (see E) is thought to be safer and more durable. In the case of bilateral disease, regardless of renal function status, operative therapy (see E) is slightly advantageous over PTA (see D) because of its greater long-term durability.[17]

(D) PTA, in particular with stent placement for ostial disease, provides a salutary outcome regarding blood pressure control in approximately 65% of patients with arteriosclerotic renovascular hypertension.[11, 12] There is negligible mortality. A continuing problem with this therapy remains restenosis, which occurs in 15% to 40% of patients. When restenosis is severe enough to warrant operation (see E), it frequently results in secondary nephrectomy (see I) and a much poorer outcome than that following primary renal revascularization.[7, 22]

One group of patients deserves particular mention, namely those with diabetes who have first-order and second-order branch disease. PTA is not favored in this group because of a high incidence of restenosis and the renal toxicity associated with the use of iodinated contrast material in patients with Kimmelstiel-Wilson diabetic nephropathy. Unfortunately, satisfactory therapeutic alternatives do not exist in this subset of renovascular hypertensive patients.

(E) Operative therapy for arteriosclerotic renovascular disease must consider the status of the aorta. A nonanatomic bypass (see F) is appropriate in the case of a hostile aorta from intrinsic disease nontreatable without inordinate patient risks or in instances of very poor cardiac function in which aortic cross-clamping would be hazardous.[15]

In patients with treatable abnormal aortic aneurysms or severe aortoiliac occlusive disease, a concomitant aortic reconstruction and an aortorenal bypass (see G) or endarterectomy (see H) are appropriate.[7, 16, 23–25] These last two options also exist in the case of a normal aorta, with an aortorenal bypass (see G) favored in the treatment of renal artery disease when unilateral, and aortorenal endarterectomy (see H) favored for treatment of multiple renal arteries to the same kidney, or for treatment of bilateral disease. For some very-high-risk patients, PTA may be appropriate when surgical treatment would otherwise be preferred.

(F) Nonanatomic bypass is an important means of renal revascularization in certain patients (see E) if flow within the donor artery is normal.[15] This mandates that there be no stenotic disease of the celiac artery in the case of hepatorenal or splenorenal bypasses and no pressure gradients across the aorta or proximal iliac arteries in the case of iliorenal bypasses.

(G) Aortorenal bypass is the most common remedy for arteriosclerotic renovascular disease.[7, 23] Reversed saphenous vein is the favored conduit for bypass of small renal arteries or for multiple vessel reconstructions. For reconstruction of a large poststenotic renal artery, especially when the graft is originating from a concurrently placed synthetic aortic prosthesis, use of a PTFE or Dacron graft is acceptable.

(H) Many surgeons prefer aortorenal endarterectomy, especially when it is undertaken in concert with an aortic reconstructive operation.[25] This form of renal revascularization is generally considered more technically demanding than a nonanatomic bypass (see F) or a conventional bypass (see G).[24] It is often performed through an axial aortotomy extending from the level of the superior mesenteric artery to the infrarenal aorta or through the transected aorta at the time of the aortic reconstruction.[26]

The axial transaortic approach has particular applicability for treatment of bilateral and multiple renal artery ostial stenoses as well as for coexistent celiac and superior mesenteric arterial stenoses. A direct renal arteriotomy with endarterectomy has certain advantages in the treatment of complex disease extending into early branchings of the renal artery, but it is performed much less often than transaortic endarterectomy.

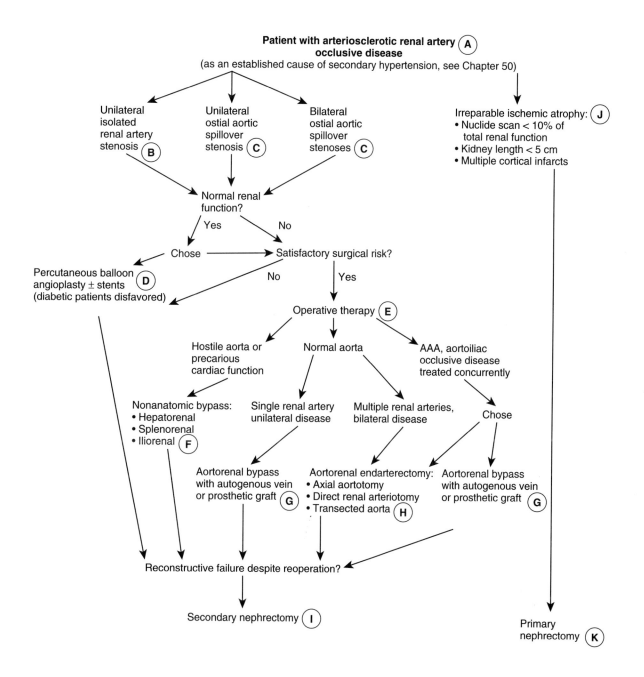

Renovascular Occlusive Disease: Treatment (continued)

The best anatomic exposure for renal revascularization depends on the procedure being undertaken.[26] In general, a transverse supraumbilical or vertical midline incision provides adequate access to the involved vasculature. A thoracoabdominal approach may be necessary when one is undertaking concomitant revascularization of the celiac and superior mesenteric arteries. All patients should receive systemic anticoagulation with heparin therapy before renal blood flow is interrupted. Similarly, a diuresis should be established with the administration of mannitol or, in the case of an azotemic patient, with loop diuretics. The outcome of surgical revascularization for arteriosclerotic renovascular disease is good, with hypertension cured in approximately 20% and improved in 60%. Operative mortality approaches 2%.[6, 7, 17]

(I) Secondary nephrectomy is performed in a manner previously noted (see first algorithm, K). This should be done only after failed reconstruction is deemed impossible to salvage with reoperation.[5, 27]

(J) Irreparable ischemic atrophy or injury in some patients may be a consequence of advanced arteriosclerotic occlusive disease. It is most likely to exist when:
1. Nuclide scanning reveals that the kidney is contributing less than 10% of total renal function.
2. Kidney length is less than 5 cm.
3. Extensive cortical infarction is evident.

In such circumstances, especially if serum creatinine levels are below 3 mg/dL, a primary nephrectomy (see K) is appropriate. Renal revascularization is unlikely to improve either blood pressure control or renal function in these patients.

(K) Primary nephrectomy is performed in some patients when operative or catheter-based procedures are not possible and only when a benefit is expected after removal of the kidney,[28] especially regarding blood pressure control.[21] The technique of primary intracapsular nephrectomy is the same as with secondary nephrectomy (see I).

REFERENCES

1. Stanley JC, Zelenock GB, Messina LM, et al: Pediatric renovascular hypertension: A thirty-year experience of operative treatment. J Vasc Surg 1995;21:212–227.
2. Novick AC, Straffon RA, Stewart BH, et al: Surgical treatment of renovascular hypertension in the pediatric patient. J Urol 1982;119:794–753.
3. Stanley JC, Ernst CB, Fry WJ: Fate of 100 aortorenal vein grafts: Characteristics of late graft expansion, aneurysmal dilatation and stenosis. Surgery 1973;74:931–944.
4. Berkowitz HD, O'Neill JA Jr: Renovascular hypertension in children: Surgical repair with special reference to the use of reinforced vein grafts. J Vasc Surg 1989;9:46–55.
5. Stanley JC, Whitehouse WM Jr, Zelenock GB, et al: Reoperation for complications of renal artery reconstructive surgery undertaken for treatment of renovascular hypertension. J Vasc Surg 1985;2:133–144.
6. Stanley JC: The evolution of surgery for renovascular occlusive disease. Cardiovasc Surg 1994;2:195–202.
7. Stanley JC: Surgical treatment of renovascular hypertension. Am J Surg 1997;174:102–110.
8. Stanley JC, Gewertz BL, Bove EL, et al: Arterial fibrodysplasia: Histopathologic character and current etiologic concepts. Arch Surg 1975;110:551–556.
9. Stanley JC, Wakefield TW: Arterial fibrodysplasia. In Rutherford RB (ed): Vascular Surgery, 5th ed. Philadelphia, WB Saunders, 2000, pp 387–408.
10. Messina LM, Stanley JC: Renal artery fibrodysplasia and renovascular hypertension, In Rutherford RB (ed): Vascular Surgery, 5th ed. Philadelphia, WB Saunders, 2000, pp 1650–1664.
11. Martin LG, Rees CR, O'Bryant T: Percutaneous angioplasty of the renal arteries. In: Rutherford RB (ed): Vascular Surgery, 5th ed. Philadelphia, WB Saunders, 2000, pp 1611–1639.
12. Slonim SM, Dake MD: Radiographic evaluation and treatment of renovascular disease. In Strandness DE Jr, VanBreda A (eds): Vascular Disease: Surgical and Interventional Therapy. New York, Churchill Livingstone, 1994, pp 721–741.
13. Stanley JC, Fry WJ: Renovascular hypertension secondary to arterial fibrodysplasia in adults: Criteria for operation and results of surgical therapy. Arch Surg 1975;110:922–928.
14. vanBockel JH, vanSchilfgaarde R, Felthius W, et al: Long-term results of in situ and extracorporeal surgery for renovascular hypertension caused by fibrodysplasia. Surgery 1982;92:642–645.
15. Khauli RB, Novick AC, Ziegelbaum M: Splenorenal bypass in the treatment of renal artery stenosis: Experience with sixty-nine cases. J Vasc Surg 1985;2:547–551.
16. Hansen KJ, Thomason RB, Craven TE, et al: Surgical management of dialysis-dependent ischemic nephropathy. J Vasc Surg 1995;21:197–211.
17. Hansen KJ, Staff SM, Sands RD, et al: Contemporary surgical management of renovascular disease. J Vasc Surg 1992;16:319–331.
18. Messina LM, Zelenock GB, Yao KA, et al: Renal revascularization for recurrent pulmonary edema in patients with poorly controlled hypertension and renal insufficiency: A distinct subgroup of patients with arteriosclerotic renal artery occlusive disease. J Vasc Surg 1992;15:73–82.
19. Palmaz JC: The current status of vascular intervention in ischemic nephropathy. J Vasc Interv Radiol 1998;9:439–543.
20. Chaikof EL, Smith RB III, Salam AA, et al: Ischemic nephropathy and concomitant aortic disease: A ten-year experience. J Vasc Surg 1994;19:135–148.
21. Whitehouse WM Jr, Kazmers A, Zelenock GB, et al: Chronic total renal artery occlusion: Effects of treatment on secondary hypertension and renal function. Surgery 1981;89:753–763.
22. Wong JM, Hansen KJ, Oskin TC, et al: Surgery after failed percutaneous renal artery angioplasty. J Vasc Surg 1999;30:468–483.
23. Cambria RP, Brewster DC, L'Italien G, et al: Simultaneous aortic and renal artery reconstruction: Evolution of an eighteen-year experience. J Vasc Surg 1995;21:916–925.
24. Dougherty MJ, Hallett JW Jr, Naessens J, et al: Renal endarterectomy vs. bypass for combined aortic and renal reconstruction: Is there a difference in clinical outcome? Ann Vasc Surg 1995;9:87–94.
25. Stoney RJ, Messina LM, Goldstone J, et al: Renal endarterectomy through the transected aorta: A new technique for combined aortorenal atherosclerosis—a preliminary report. J Vasc Surg 1989;9:224–233.
26. Stanley JC, Messina LM, Wakefield TW, et al: Renal artery reconstruction. In Bergan JJ, Yao JST (eds): Techniques in Arterial Surgery. Philadelphia, WB Saunders, 1990, pp 247–263.
27. Hansen KJ, Deitch JS, Oskin TC, et al: Renal artery repair: Consequence of operative failures. Ann Surg 1998;277:678–690.
28. Oskin TC, Hansen KJ, Deitch JS, et al: Chronic renal artery occlusion: Nephrectomy versus revascularization. J Vasc Surg 1999;29:140–149.

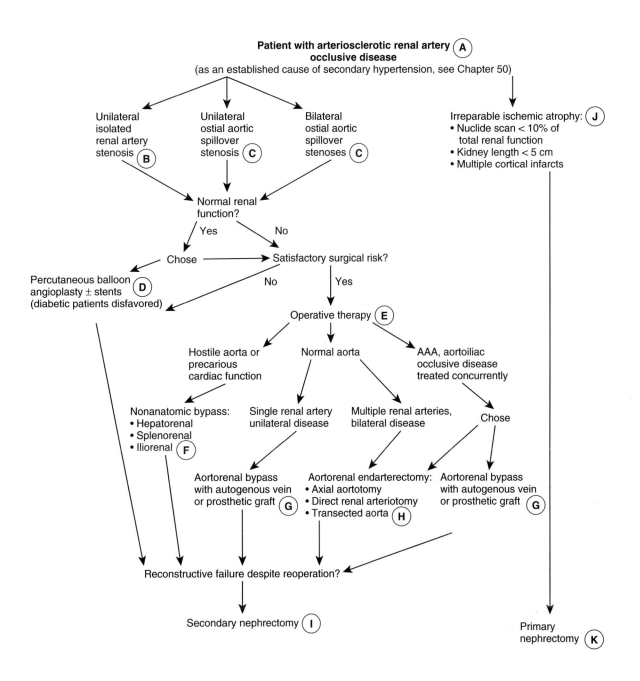

Chapter 52 Acute Mesenteric Ischemia

TINA R. DESAI, MD • BRUCE L. GEWERTZ, MD

(A) Initial clinical evaluation, including history and physical examination and routine laboratory evaluation, separates patients into two groups:

1. Patients presenting with an acute surgical abdomen, often with tachycardia, and quickly progressing to fever, leukocytosis, hemoconcentration, and acidosis.
2. Patients presenting with slower symptom progression, including vague abdominal pain and heme-positive stools.

Patients presenting acutely with severe abdominal pain out of proportion to physical findings, tachycardia, and gut emptying with heme-positive liquid stool, may be suspected to have acute embolic occlusion of the superior mesenteric artery (SMA). Mesenteric artery thrombosis tends to present less dramatically. Particular attention should be paid to historical clues and risk factors, including:

1. Atrial fibrillation.
2. Previous arterial embolic events.
3. A history of chronic mesenteric ischemia symptoms (postprandial abdominal pain, weight loss, "food fear").
4. Hypercoagulable states.
5. Medications that may be associated with non-occlusive mesenteric ischemia (digitalis, vasopressors).

Other findings suggesting acute mesenteric ischemia include:

1. Unexplained abdominal distention.
2. Colonoscopic finding of isolated right colon ischemia.
3. Acidosis without identifiable cause.

Laboratory studies, including white blood cell count and concentrations of lactic acid, serum amylase, hemoglobin, and creatine phosphokinase, may be suggestive but are not specific. An aggressive diagnostic approach is essential to identify patients before the onset of intestinal gangrene.

(B) Patients presenting early with acute or subacute symptoms should undergo prompt fluid resuscitation and preliminary evaluation, including plain abdominal films and possibly abdominal computed tomography (CT) scans. These initial studies may allow exclusion of alternate diagnoses or may be suggestive of mesenteric ischemia.

Abdominal radiographic findings of bowel wall thickening, "thumbprinting," pneumatosis intestinalis, or ileus are consistent with a diagnosis of mesenteric ischemia. Normal abdominal films, however, do not rule out mesenteric ischemia and can be expected in up to 25% of patients with this diagnosis.[1]

Abdominal CT scan, particularly with intravenous (IV) contrast enhancement, may demonstrate bowel wall thickening.[2] High-resolution scans with IV contrast can demonstrate patency or occlusion of the SMA and celiac arteries and may be diagnostic. Filling defects in the superior mesenteric vein (SMV) or portal vein, massive bowel wall thickening, and ascites are diagnostic of mesenteric venous thrombosis.

(C) Arteriography remains the definitive diagnostic study for acute mesenteric ischemia and also offers treatment options, especially for nonocclusive ischemia.[3] It should be performed expediently after rapid preliminary evaluation and resuscitation. Lateral and anteroposterior views of the abdominal aorta, with selective cannulation of the celiac, superior mesenteric, and inferior mesenteric arteries, are often required.

(D) Patients with delayed presentation whose abdominal findings indicate advanced peritonitis and deteriorating hemodynamic and metabolic status require urgent laparotomy without preoperative arteriography but with concomitant aggressive resuscitation.

(E) Urgent laparotomy usually reveals frankly gangrenous bowel segments with adjacent ischemic segments. Obviously, gangrenous bowel should be resected to prevent perforation and enteric contamination of the peritoneal cavity and to minimize systemic toxicity; ischemic segments should be preserved until revascularization is complete so that they can be reevaluated for potential improvement. The final decision to perform reanastomosis after resection should be delayed until revascularization is complete and depends on the appearance of previously ischemic segments, hemodynamic stability of the patient, and the presence of co-morbidities. Intravenous antibiotics should be administered perioperatively.

(F) Intraoperative assessment of the underlying cause of the mesenteric ischemia focuses on assessment of the arterial inflow and the appearance of the bowel. First, the SMA is palpated at the root of the small bowel mesentery. In addition to pulse quality, Doppler signal quality can be assessed. The pattern of ischemic bowel may also indicate the cause, since SMA embolism often spares the proximal jejunum. This may be confirmed by palpating a pulse in the proximal SMA but not distally, because emboli tend to lodge near its middle colic branch.

SMA thrombosis usually produces more diffuse ischemia involving the proximal jejunum, and there is no palpable pulse in the proximal SMA. With mesenteric venous thrombosis, the bowel is congested, cyanotic, and edematous. The pattern of ischemic bowel in nonocclusive disease is variable; it may be patchy or diffuse, but a pulse can usually be felt in the SMA associated with a high-resistance Doppler signal.

Exposure of the celiac artery is occasionally necessary, depending on the pattern of ischemia noted, and can be executed by opening the gastrohepatic ligament and dividing the diaphragmatic crus. Following the anterior surface of the aorta caudally from this location reveals the celiac artery

ACUTE MESENTERIC ISCHEMIA

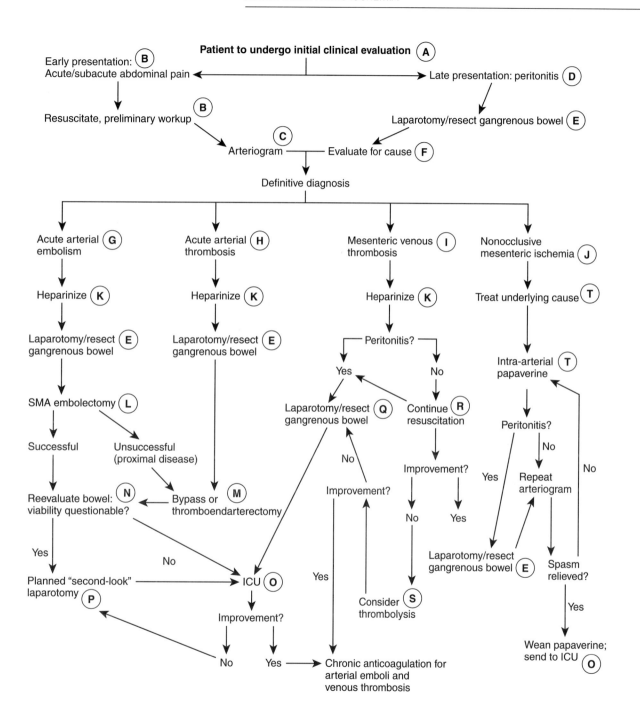

origin. Occasionally, intraoperative duplex or arteriography may be helpful.

(G) *Arterial embolism* is the most common cause of acute mesenteric ischemia, responsible for 30% to 50% of cases.[4] Historical features may include an absence of chronic ischemic symptoms and the presence of a potential source of embolism, such as atrial fibrillation, myocardial infarction, left ventricular aneurysm, mitral stenosis, or congestive heart failure. A history of peripheral arterial embolization (present in 20% of patients) should raise suspicion.

The embolus usually lodges 3 to 10 cm from the origin of the SMA, near the origin of the middle colic artery.[5] Distal thrombosis and reactive vasoconstriction may further contribute to the ischemic insult. Up to 20% of patients have synchronous emboli in other peripheral arteries.[4]

Intraoperative evaluation is aided by the use of a Doppler probe to identify the location of the embolus. In patients with embolic occlusions, the native mesenteric vessels usually feel soft and normal in quality. Intraoperative arteriography, especially of the distal mesenteric circulation, may be necessary to ensure complete embolus or thrombus extraction.

(H) *Acute mesenteric arterial thrombosis* occurs in the setting of a preexisting high-grade mesenteric arterial stenosis. The pattern of symptoms depends on the number and distribution of occluded vessels (usually at least two of the three mesenteric vessels are diseased) and the adequacy of collateral circulation. Twenty percent to 50% of patients have a history of antecedent chronic mesenteric ischemia symptoms (postprandial abdominal pain, weight loss, "food fear").[6] Symptoms often appear gradually, producing a subacute presentation rather than the abrupt onset of pain associated with embolism.

Arteriography is diagnostic and shows occlusion at the SMA origin. Associated stenosis or occlusion of the celiac or inferior mesenteric arteries (IMA) may also be evident. Intraoperative palpation of the SMA near its origin reveals an atherosclerotic vessel with proximal occlusion. Atherosclerotic disease of the celiac or inferior mesenteric arteries may also be appreciated.

(I) *Mesenteric venous thrombosis*, an uncommon cause of acute mesenteric ischemia, is associated with hypercoagulable states, portal hypertension, visceral infections, acute pancreatitis, malignancy, and trauma. The pathophysiologic derangements are related to bowel wall edema, hypovolemia, and increased outflow resistance and hemoconcentration compromising arterial inflow. Symptoms are produced by a massive influx of fluid into the bowel wall and lumen.

The diagnosis is suggested by diffuse bowel wall thickening and mesenteric venous or portal venous filling defect on CT scan. In atypical cases, selective mesenteric arteriography with venous phase imaging may be helpful. These studies can reveal reflux of contrast back into the aorta with injection, a prolonged arterial phase, vasospasm, extravasation of contrast into the bowel lumen, and visualization of venous thrombus or nonvisualization of the venous phase.[7]

Duplex ultrasound surveillance of the mesenteric and portal veins can also be diagnostic when these veins are visualized. The intraoperative appearance is of thickened edematous bowel loops, venous congestion, and ascites.

(J) *Nonocclusive mesenteric ischemia* occurs in the absence of anatomic arterial or venous obstruction during periods of low mesenteric flow due to poor cardiac output with excessive compensatory mesenteric vasoconstriction. The ischemia is usually limited to the SMA distribution. Risk factors include advanced age, cardiac failure, sepsis, hypovolemia, hypotension, and the administration of vasopressors or digitalis.

The symptom complex is often atypical, and a high index of suspicion is necessary to make the diagnosis. Arteriography shows multiple areas of narrowing and irregularity in the major branches of the SMA ("string of sausage sign"). Mortality is high as a result of concurrent medical problems.[8]

(K) Once the diagnosis of occlusive mesenteric ischemia is made, early anticoagulation therapy with IV heparin (100 units/kg) is essential to prevent propagation of thrombus.

(L) SMA embolectomy requires exposure of the SMA at the root of the mesentery. The transverse colon is retracted cephalad and the ligament of Treitz is mobilized to expose the root of the small bowel mesentery. An SMA pulse may be felt proximal to the embolus; Doppler interrogation may assist in identifying the site of obstruction.

After the SMA is mobilized and controlled at this location, a transverse arteriotomy is made and balloon-tipped embolectomy catheters are passed retrograde and antegrade. Vasodilators and heparin solution can be flushed distally. The transverse arteriotomy is closed with interrupted sutures. If the SMA is small or proximal arterial disease is suspected, a longitudinal arteriotomy is created, allowing patch angioplasty or bypass from the aorta. Successful embolectomy restores pulsatile flow through the SMA and its branches.

(M) SMA revascularization is the mainstay of treatment of acute mesenteric ischemia in the settings of failed embolectomy or arterial thrombosis superimposed on atherosclerotic disease. Although at least two mesenteric vessels are usually diseased, revascularization of additional mesenteric arteries is generally impractical in these critically ill patients.

An infrarenal aortic or iliac inflow source with limited cross-clamping of the aorta is usually safest. Prosthetic conduits may be used in the absence of bowel gangrene or contamination, but the greater saphenous vein is preferable in the presence of perforation. SMA thromboendarterectomy with vein patch may be feasible in selected cases, but extensive disease may preclude this approach. In general, the simplest, shortest procedure for revascularization is preferred in these ill patients.

(N) Reevaluation of bowel viability after reinstitution of mesenteric blood flow is essential. This is accomplished by simple inspection for color and peristalsis, Doppler evaluation, and fluorescein injection with ultraviolet lamp examina-

ACUTE MESENTERIC ISCHEMIA

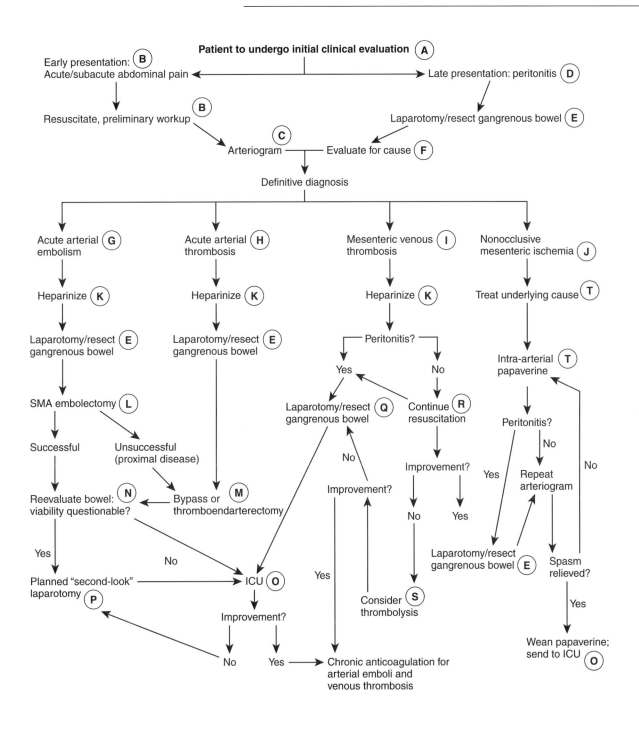

Acute Mesenteric Ischemia (continued)

tion. None of these techniques is definitive; in most cases, a "second look" laparotomy is indicated in 24 to 48 hours if bowel viability is in question after revascularization.[9]

(O) Postoperative multiorgan system failure with pulmonary insufficiency (adult respiratory distress syndrome) and elevation of liver enzymes is common after reperfusion of acutely ischemic bowel. Prolonged ventilatory support is occasionally necessary.[10]

(P) Second-look laparotomy is indicated in patients who deteriorate during their early postoperative course and in those whose bowel viability was questioned at the original operation. It is usually performed within 24 to 48 hours of the initial operation. The bowel and the mesenteric flow are reexamined, and additional nonviable bowel segments are resected.

(Q) In patients with mesenteric venous thrombosis requiring exploration for peritonitis, extensive bowel resection is common. In one large series, short-gut syndrome was reported in more than 20% of patients.[5] Mesenteric venous thrombectomy is occasionally attempted but is rarely practical. It may be considered in patients with remaining viable bowel and a proximal acute thrombus in the SMV, but this situation is infrequently encountered.

(R) Mesenteric venous thrombosis is frequently accompanied by large fluid shifts, electrolyte imbalances, and decreased intravascular volume requiring continued monitoring and aggressive fluid resuscitation. Central venous or pulmonary arterial catheters are often helpful.

(S) Systemic thrombolytic therapy has been advocated for patients with mesenteric venous thrombosis who do not improve or who gradually worsen.[11, 12] There are no large series to support this modality, but it should be considered in patients who do not improve with heparin anticoagulation and volume replacement measures.

(T) Treatment of the underlying cause of poor cardiac output is central to the treatment of nonocclusive mesenteric ischemia, since there is no underlying abnormality of the mesenteric vessels. Attempts are made to discontinue all α-adrenergic medications and digitalis. Optimizing cardiac performance is critical, with the specific techniques dependent on the underlying problem.

After angiographic diagnosis of nonocclusive mesenteric ischemia, an intra-arterial catheter can be placed in the SMA for prolonged vasodilator infusion. Intra-arterial papaverine infusion is begun at a rate of 30 to 60 mg/hr for 24 to 48 hours.[13] Continuous hemodynamic monitoring is required during infusion. Repeated arteriography can be performed early after initiation of papaverine to ensure resolution of spasm. If clinical improvement is seen, another arteriogram may be obtained before cessation of papaverine. If peritonitis ensues, laparotomy is necessary while attempts are continued to relieve vasospasm through papaverine administration, raising ambient room temperature, and using warm saline lavage.

REFERENCES

1. Smerud MJ, Johnson CD, Stephens DH: Diagnosis of bowel infarction: A comparison of plain films and CT scans in 23 cases. AJR Am J Roentgenol 1990;154:99–103.
2. Wolf EL, Sprayregen S, Bakal CW: Radiology in intestinal ischemia: Plain film, contrast, and other imaging studies. Surg Clin North Am 1992;72:107–124.
3. Bakal CW, Sprayregen S, Wolf EL: Radiology in intestinal ischemia: Angiographic diagnosis and management. Surg Clin North Am 1992;72:125–141.
4. Kaleya RN, Boley SJ: Acute mesenteric ischemia: An aggressive diagnostic and therapeutic approach. 1991 Roussel Lecture. Can J Surg 1992;35:613–623.
5. McKinsey JF, Gewertz BL: Acute mesenteric ischemia. Surg Clin North Am 1997;77:307–318.
6. Kaleya RN, Boley SJ: Acute mesenteric ischemia. Crit Care Clin 1995;11:479–512.
7. Rhee RY, Gloviczki P, Mendonca CT, et al: Mesenteric venous thrombosis: Still a lethal disease in the 1990s. J Vasc Surg 1994;20:688–697.
8. Howard TJ, Plaskon LA, Wiebke EA, et al: Nonocclusive mesenteric ischemia remains a diagnostic dilemma. Am J Surg 1996;171:405–408.
9. Ballard JL, Stone WM, Hallett JW, et al: A critical analysis of adjuvant techniques used to assess bowel viability in acute mesenteric ischemia. Am Surg 1993;59:309–311.
10. Harward TR, Brooks DL, Flynn TC, Seeger JM: Multiple organ dysfunction after mesenteric artery revascularization. J Vasc Surg 1993;18:459–467; discussion, 467–469.
11. Miyazaki YY, Shinomura S, Kitamura S, et al: Portal vein thrombosis associated with active ulcerative colitis: Percutaneous transhepatic recanalization. Am J Gastroenterol 1995;90:1533–1534.
12. Poplausky MR, Kaufman JA, Geller SC, Waltman AC: Mesenteric venous thrombosis treated with urokinase via the superior mesenteric artery. Gastroenterology 1996;110:1633–1635.
13. Stoney RJ, Cunningham CG: Acute mesenteric ischemia. Surgery 1993;114:489–490.

ACUTE MESENTERIC ISCHEMIA

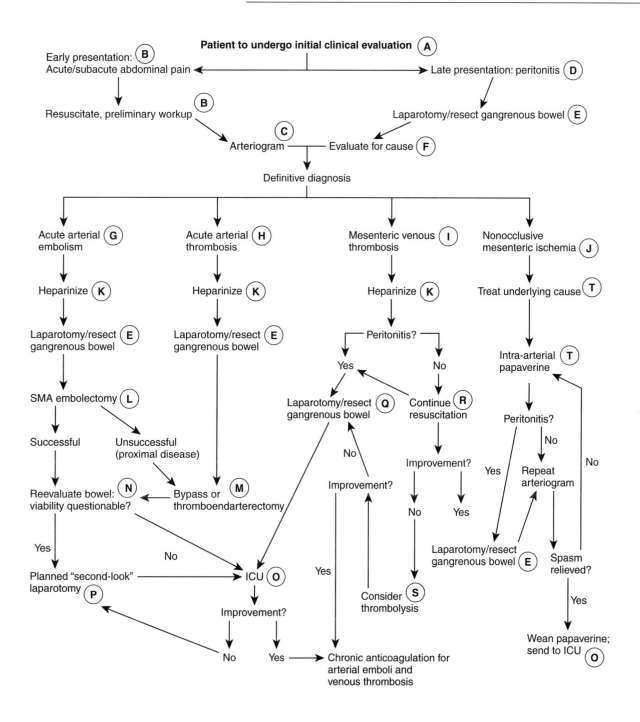

Chapter 53 Chronic Mesenteric Ischemia

PETER R. NELSON, MD • ROBERT M. ZWOLAK, MD, PhD

A In contrast to symptomatic peripheral arterial occlusive disease, which affects predominantly men, chronic mesenteric ischemia (CMI) is more common in women. A bimodal distribution has been described, with one peak in the fifth and sixth decades in heavy smokers (≥50 pack-years) and a second in the sixth and seventh decades in patients with the typical constellation of cardiovascular risk factors (coronary artery disease, peripheral vascular disease, dyslipidemia, hypertension).

Symptomatic CMI is relatively rare. Autopsy studies suggest the prevalence of a >50% mesenteric arterial stenosis to be 6% to 10%, with the majority being asymptomatic. Initial symptoms can be vague and may go unnoticed. As disease progresses, the hallmark of CMI is postprandial midabdominal and epigastric pain, 10 to 15 minutes following a large meal, lasting 1 to 4 hours in duration. Intermittent symptoms have typically been present for an average of 18 months before an accurate diagnosis is made.

With advanced disease, the patient may complain of continuous midabdominal pain and voluntarily reduces food intake (sitophobia), resulting in a significant weight loss of 10 to 15 kg or more.[1] Diarrhea may be seen as a result of villous atrophy. Ischemic gastritis is uncommon but, when present, carries a dismal prognosis.[2] Physical examination is of limited value in the evaluation of CMI, but suggestive findings include evidence of weight loss, evidence for peripheral vascular occlusive disease, and an abdominal bruit.

B Duplex ultrasonography is the initial noninvasive diagnostic study of choice. In the authors' practice, the workup for all patients begins with a mesenteric duplex ultrasound examination, followed by conventional arteriography if duplex findings are positive. Like all duplex ultrasound examinations, this modality is technologist-dependent, but it has a high degree of accuracy and can be performed successfully in a large percentage of cases.[3-6]

Diagnostic thresholds have been published for peak systolic velocity (PSV) and end-diastolic velocity (EDV). For the superior mesenteric artery (SMA), a PSV ≥275 cm/sec demonstrated a sensitivity of 92% and a specificity of 96% for a ≥70% angiographic stenosis.[4] An EDV of ≥45 cm/sec had a sensitivity of 90% and a specificity of 91% for a stenosis of ≥50%.[6] For the celiac artery, a PSV ≥200 cm/sec demonstrated sensitivity of 90% and specificity of 91% for a stenosis ≥70%.[4] Retrograde hepatic arterial flow is 100% predictive of a severe celiac artery stenosis or occlusion. Celiac artery EDV ≥55 cm/sec had 93% sensitivity and 100% specificity for a ≥50% stenosis.

Duplex ultrasonography can also accurately identify anatomic anomalies that can influence study interpretation and give helpful information for operative planning.[6] Magnetic resonance angiography (MRA) with gadolinium may also be a second safe, noninvasive method to investigate the mesenteric vasculature, but accuracy data are limited.[7,8]

C Timely duplex examination in symptomatic patients may allow for a more efficient process of diagnosis and definitive management before occurrence of an acute event. Despite the increasing accuracy of mesenteric duplex examination, however, conventional arteriography has been the standard for operative planning for CMI.[9,10] Both anteroposterior and lateral arteriographic projections are essential to fully evaluate typical atherosclerotic lesions of the mesenteric vasculature. Digital subtraction techniques can be used to reduce contrast load while still providing adequate imaging.

SMA involvement is nearly universal in patients with symptomatic CMI, combined with celiac artery involvement in up to 90%, inferior mesenteric artery (IMA) involvement in up to 90%, and bilateral hypogastric involvement in as many as 60%.[11] Selective arterial catheterization may be necessary to further delineate proximal disease or to detect more distal arterial disease if the celiac and SMA origins do not appear significantly narrowed, but a high-quality biplane aortogram is usually sufficient.

D Single-vessel mesenteric vascular disease rarely results in symptomatology. If SMA occlusion is the only finding on arteriography, however, collateral flow from the celiac artery and IMA may not be adequate to prevent significant gut ischemia. A patient with a solitary SMA occlusion and clear-cut symptoms of CMI should be considered for single-vessel SMA revascularization.

Similarly, isolated celiac artery stenosis is found in the median arcuate ligament syndrome.[12] If all other causes of abdominal pain have been exhausted, patients with this rare entity may be successfully treated with an operation to release the celiac artery compression caused by the median arcuate ligament and diaphragmatic crura. In some cases of median arcuate ligament syndrome, celiac endarterectomy, patch angioplasty, or bypass is necessary. In more straightforward cases, the repair may be approached laparoscopically. These generally young patients can achieve complete resolution of their debilitating symptoms with dramatic improvement in their quality of life.[13,14]

E Development of symptoms is thought to be due to the progression of disease in at least two of the three visceral branches to severe stenosis or occlusion such that collateral circulation is no longer sufficient to maintain adequate gut perfusion. With an overall prevalence of mesenteric vascular disease of 6% to 10% but an incidence of symptomatic intestinal ischemia much less than that,[1] the issue of management of incidentally discovered, asymptomatic mesenteric arterial disease is raised.

Although the true natural history of such incidental, asymptomatic lesions is not known, in one report 86% of patients with three-vessel mesenteric atherosclerosis experienced vague abdominal symptoms or frank mesenteric ischemia, or they died during a 2.6-year mean follow-up interval.[15] These authors suggest that prophylactic treatment of asymptomatic patients with advanced mesenteric atherosclerosis should be considered, particularly at the time of aortoiliac reconstruction for occlusive or aneurysmal disease, but no consensus has been reached.[15] The subsequent discussion applies to incidental as well as symptomatic disease.

(F) Ideally, a standard thorough preoperative risk assessment should be considered in patients with symptomatic CMI. Investigation of coronary artery or cerebrovascular disease should be undertaken in this high-risk population. Patients with symptomatic CMI are routinely malnourished; however, preoperative hyperalimentation has not been of significant benefit and it introduces the risk of catheter-related sepsis.[16] In addition, with the typical urgent presentation of patients with advanced disease, preoperative evaluation or nutritional support should not stand in the way of definitive surgical revascularization.

(G) The experience with percutaneous transluminal angioplasty (PTA) is limited to a small number of series describing experiences in 5 to 28 patients.[17–20] The limited availability of data probably represents the infrequent presentation of these patients in daily practice, compounded by a hesitancy to consider percutaneous treatment in the typical situation of far advanced multiple-vessel stenosis and occlusion. Like angioplasty of other major abdominal aortic branches (i.e., renal), PTA seems to be most applicable to short-segment, focal, nonostial lesions with stenting reserved for an inadequate angiographic result.

Initial primary technical success rates of 80% to 95% have been described with corresponding clinical responses of 67% to 100%.[17–20] PTA may be considered a primary approach in patients unfit for surgical arterial revascularization. However, the predominant ostial nature of mesenteric arterial disease, combined with the high incidence of occlusion and frequency of long-segment lesions, precludes the use of PTA as a primary therapeutic option in most reasonable-risk patients with CMI.

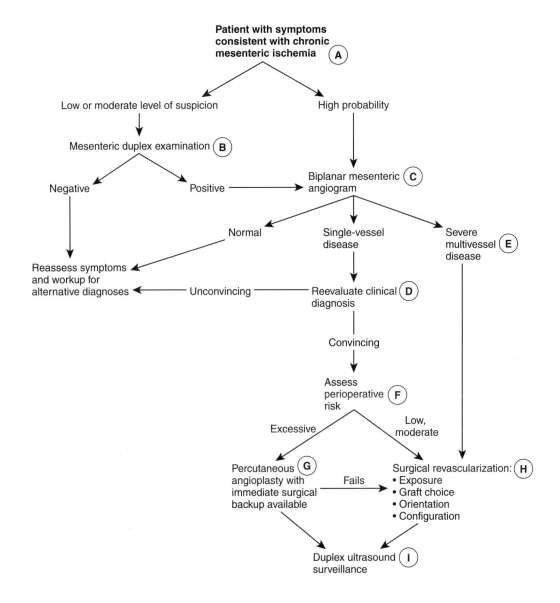

In the authors' practice, surgical revascularization is the primary approach, whereas exceptionally high-risk surgical candidates may undergo an initial attempt at percutaneous treatment.

(H) There is no clearly superior technique for mesenteric revascularization, and the approach should be individualized for each patient. Five decisions confront the vascular surgeon concerning mesenteric revascularization:

1. *Endarterectomy versus bypass.*
2. *Route of exposure.*
3. *Choice of conduit:* saphenous vein or prosthetic graft.
4. *Route of the bypass graft:* antegrade from the supraceliac aorta, or retrograde from the infrarenal aorta or iliac artery.
5. *Number of vessels* to revascularize.

Overall, the following outcomes have been reported[9, 11, 20–23]:

1. Perioperative mortality, 0 to 10% (mainly from graft failure).
2. Patency (3 to 5 years), 65% to 89%.
3. Symptom-free survival, 70% to 86%.
4. Overall 5-year survival, 64% to 79%.

General technical considerations, regardless of surgical procedure or approach, include:

1. Preservation of the IMA if it represents the primary collateral circulation.
2. Dissection of the celiac trunk from its origin to its splenic, hepatic, and left gastric branches.
3. Dissection of the SMA for at least 2 to 3 cm beyond the stenosis or occlusion.

Patients receive a full regimen of anticoagulation therapy, and mannitol is administered for renal protection before suprarenal aortic cross-clamping.

Endarterectomy was the first described approach to mesenteric revascularization, and subsequent excellent results have been described. When performed by experts, transaortic endarterectomy may offer comparable patency to antegrade mesenteric bypass. It is limited to selected patients with ostial mesenteric arterial occlusive lesions and is contraindicated in patients with aneurysmal dilatation of the pararenal or infrarenal aorta. Performed through a trap-door aortotomy, it offers the advantage of simultaneous endarterectomy when disease extends to the renal arteries, but it is technically more demanding and less versatile than arterial bypass for more extensive mesenteric disease.[25]

In choosing conduit, many favor synthetic polyester (Dacron) or polytetrafluoroethylene (PTFE) grafts for what typically are short, high-flow bypasses. For large vessel bypass, ease of use, size match, and resistance to compression outweigh the small additional risks of graft infection. However, synthetic grafts are contraindicated in patients with intestinal infarction or perforation because the risk of graft infection in this setting is prohibitive.

Early patency rate for saphenous vein grafts and prosthetic grafts are similar at 95% and 89%, respectively,[9] but long-term (3-year) patency may be superior for prosthetic grafts (78% to 89% versus 29% to 69% for autogenous grafts).[24] Analysis of data comparing synthetic to autogenous conduit should be performed with caution, however, since numbers of autogenous conduits in various reports are generally low and may represent sicker patients with marginal bowel viability in which synthetic material was considered to be contraindicated.

Despite individual bias, no statistical advantage has been demonstrated for either antegrade bypass from the supraceliac aorta or retrograde bypass from the infrarenal aorta or iliac artery with comparable early patency rates of 93% and 95%, respectively.[9] Antegrade bypass has the theoretical advantage of more anatomic flow with less turbulence from a typically normal uninvolved segment of supraceliac aorta. It allows for shorter grafts with less kinking but requires more extensive exposure and employs a supraceliac aortic clamp with the risk of renal ischemia.[10, 11, 25, 26] The exposure can be approached either anteriorly through the lesser sac or via medial visceral rotation or by a left retroperitoneal approach, which provides excellent access to the supraceliac donor aorta and the mesenteric branches.

Retrograde bypass from the infrarenal aorta lends itself to easier, more familiar exposure and is a technically simpler operation without concern for renal ischemia. Its limitations include (1) reverse flow configuration with more turbulence, (2) longer grafts, (3) a higher risk of kinking or compression, and (4) increased difficulty with extensive infrarenal aortic atherosclerosis.[27]

Some authors suggest that single-vessel SMA revascularization simplifies the operation and provides adequate perfusion with good technical and clinical results.[23] Others describe a correlation between improved outcome and the greater number of vessels that are revascularized.[11, 26] Some suggest that complete revascularization may not be possible in as many as 75% of patients. Complete revascularization, when possible, appears to give improved recurrence-free survival but possibly at the expense of a greater rate of perioperative complications.[24]

In general, if the decision is made to expose the supraceliac aorta for inflow, antegrade bypass to both the celiac artery and SMA is preferable. If a retrograde iliac-mesenteric bypass is chosen for ease, a single graft to the SMA may be reasonable to simplify the procedure and to avoid extensive dissection of the suprarenal aorta.

We generally favor an antegrade bypass, taking advantage of the supraceliac aorta as the inflow source exposed through a transperitoneal or retroperitoneal approach. Prosthetic material is used, and multivessel revascularization is performed.

(I) Mesenteric arterial bypass, irrespective of operative approach, is a durable form of revascularization. Predictors correlated with graft failure following revascularization include[22, 24]:

1. Advanced age.
2. Widespread atherosclerotic disease.

3. Male gender.
4. A short duration of preoperative symptoms.

Reliance on recurrence of symptoms may be an inaccurate and misleading method of follow-up.[9] Objective assessment is important to accurately record visceral bypass patency rates. Duplex ultrasound surveillance is a noninvasive, sensitive, objective method offering standardized annual follow-up after mesenteric bypass.[9, 22, 24] This is our practice. Reintervention is important for patients with symptomatic recurrence and may be selectively indicated for patients with asymptomatic recurrence.

REFERENCES

1. Stanley JC: Chronic mesenteric ischemia. In Longo WE, Peterson GJ, Jacobs DL (eds): Intestinal Ischemia Disorders. St. Louis, Quality Medical Publishing, 1999, pp 189–205.
2. Casey KM, Quigley TM, Kozarek RA, Raker EJ: Lethal nature of ischemic gastropathy. Am J Surg 1993;165:646–649.
3. Bowersox JC, Zwolak RM, Walsh DB, et al: Duplex ultrasonography in the diagnosis of celiac and mesenteric artery occlusive disease. J Vasc Surg 1991;14:780–786; discussion, 786–788.
4. Moneta GL, Lee RW, Yeager RA, et al: Mesenteric duplex scanning: A blinded prospective study. J Vasc Surg 1993;17:79–84; discussion, 85–86.
5. Harward TR, Brooks DL, Flynn TC, Seeger JM: Multiple organ dysfunction after mesenteric artery revascularization. J Vasc Surg 1993;18:459–467; discussion, 467–469.
6. Zwolak RM, Fillinger MF, Walsh DB, et al: Mesenteric and celiac duplex scanning: A validation study. J Vasc Surg 1998;27:1078–1087; discussion, 1088.
7. Li KC: MR angiography of abdominal ischemia. Semin Ultrasound CT MR 1996;17:352–359.
8. Meaney JF, Prince MR, Nostrant TT, Stanley JC: Gadolinium-enhanced MR angiography of visceral arteries in patients with suspected chronic mesenteric ischemia. J Magn Reson Imaging 1997;7:171–176.
9. McMillan WD, McCarthy WJ, Bresticker MR, et al: Mesenteric artery bypass: Objective patency determination. J Vasc Surg 1995;21:729–740; discussion, 740–741.
10. Moawad J, Gewertz BL: Chronic mesenteric ischemia: Clinical presentation and diagnosis. Surg Clin North Am 1997;77:357–369.
11. Johnston KW, Lindsay TF, Walker PM, Kalman PG: Mesenteric arterial bypass grafts: Early and late results and suggested surgical approach for chronic and acute mesenteric ischemia. Surgery 1995;118:1–7.

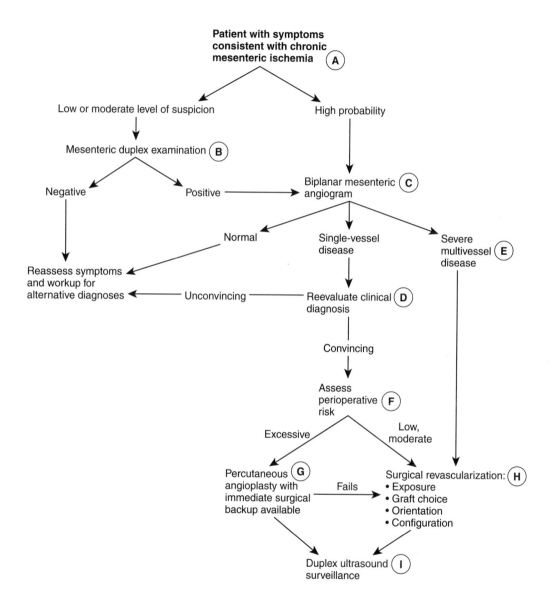

Chronic Mesenteric Ischemia (continued)

12. Carey JP, Stemmer EA, Connolly JE: Median arcuate ligament syndrome: Experimental and clinical observations. Arch Surg 1969;99:441–446.
13. Bech FR: Celiac artery compression syndromes. Surg Clin North Am 1997;77:409–424.
14. Takach TJ, Livesay JJ, Reul GJ Jr, Cooley DA: Celiac compression syndrome: Tailored therapy based on intraoperative findings [erratum in J Am Coll Surg 1997;184:439]. J Am Coll Surg 1996;183:606–610.
15. Thomas JH, Blake K, Pierce GE, et al: The clinical course of asymptomatic mesenteric arterial stenosis [see comments]. J Vasc Surg 1998;27:840–844.
16. Mueller C, Borriello R, Perlov-Antzis L: Parenteral nutrition support of a patient with chronic mesenteric artery occlusive disease. Nutr Clin Pract 1993;8:73–77.
17. Nyman U, Ivancev K, Lindh M, Uher P: Endovascular treatment of chronic mesenteric ischemia: report of five cases. Cardiovasc Intervent Radiol 1998;21:305–313.
18. Rose SC, Quigley TM, Raker EJ: Revascularization for chronic mesenteric ischemia: Comparison of operative arterial bypass grafting and percutaneous transluminal angioplasty. J Vasc Interv Radiol 1995;6:339–349.
19. Allen RC, Martin GH, Rees CR, et al: Mesenteric angioplasty in the treatment of chronic intestinal ischemia. J Vasc Surg 1996;24:415–421; discussion, 421–423.
20. Kasirajan K, O'Hara PJ, Gray BH, et al: Chronic mesenteric ischemia: Open surgery versus percutaneous angioplasty and stenting. J Vasc Surg 2001;33:63–71.
21. Mateo RB, O'Hara PJ, Hertzer NR, et al: Elective surgical treatment of symptomatic chronic mesenteric occlusive disease: Early results and late outcomes. J Vasc Surg 1999;29:821–831; discussion, 832.
22. Moawad J, McKinsey JF, Wyble CW, et al: Current results of surgical therapy for chronic mesenteric ischemia. Arch Surg 1997;132:613–618; discussion, 618–619.
23. Gentile AT, Moneta GL, Taylor LM Jr, et al: Isolated bypass to the superior mesenteric artery for intestinal ischemia. Arch Surg 1994;129:926–931; discussion, 931–932.
24. Kihara TK, Blebea J, Anderson KM, et al: Risk factors and outcomes following revascularization for chronic mesenteric ischemia. Ann Vasc Surg 1999;13:37–44.
25. Rapp JH, Reilly LM, Qvarfordt PG, et al: Durability of endarterectomy and antegrade grafts in the treatment of chronic visceral ischemia. J Vasc Surg 1986;3:799–806.
26. McAfee MK, Cherry KJ Jr, Naessens JM, et al: Influence of complete revascularization on chronic mesenteric ischemia. Am J Surg 1992;164:220–224.
27. Taylor LM, Moneta GL, Porter JM: Treatment of chronic intestinal ischemia. In Rutherford RB (ed): Vascular Surgery, 5th ed. Philadelphia, WB Saunders, 2000, pp 1532–1540.

VENOUS DISEASE

Chapter 54 Subclavian-Axillary Vein Thrombosis

ROBERT B. RUTHERFORD, MD • SCOTT HURLBERT, MD

(A) Of the patients with primary subclavian-axillary vein thrombosis (SAVT), 100% present with swelling, 82% have venous engorgement, 73% have pain, and 55% have cyanosis.[1] These figures and the abrupt onset in a typical patient (usually <30 years old, male gender, history of unusual arm activity or positioning and involvement of the dominant upper extremity) make the clinical diagnosis accurate. With secondary thrombosis, due mainly to indwelling venous catheters, the onset is more gradual and the signs and symptoms are more subtle. However, the realization that most patients with long-term indwelling catheters suffer some degree of thrombosis should create a high index of suspicion, and loss of access is a common presentation. Duplex ultrasound scanning confirms the diagnosis in questionable cases, with venography reserved for patients requiring intervention.

(B) In prospective trials, the incidence of SAVT associated with indwelling catheters has varied from 8% to 46%[2] but symptoms were recorded in only 0% to 29%. Since the advent of frequent use of indwelling catheters, secondary thromboses outnumber primary thromboses by 2:1 to 3:1. Most patients with secondary SAVT have serious intercurrent diseases, often with limited longevity.

(C) Because of milder symptoms, limited longevity, and reduced activity due to chronic intercurrent disease, most patients with secondary SAVT are treated conservatively. Thrombectomy does not succeed in the face of the more chronic and inflammatory process. Thrombolysis may succeed initially, as reported in cancer chemotherapy patients,[3,4] but follow-up is not documented. Normally, other access sites are chosen after catheter-induced SAVT, and the process itself is treated conservatively, there being little risk of pulmonary embolism (PE). Only in patients with limited access sites with a continuing need for access can thrombolytic therapy be justified. If it succeeds, access is resumed. If it fails, conservative therapy is applied as needed and other access sites are sought.

(D) Of patients with primary SAVT, as many as 10% may progress to PE and only 1% develop venous gangrene (usually patients with an underlying coagulopathy). However, fewer than 10% of thrombi recanalize spontaneously. The extent of the thrombus is characteristically more extensive than with secondary SAVT, which develops gradually and rarely progresses beyond the major collaterals. This fact and the fact that most patients with primary SAVT actively use the arm for work or sport explain why the majority of patients with "effort thrombosis" (65%) subsequently have moderate to severe symptoms. This is not diminished by initial treatment with anticoagulants.[1] Because symptoms are a result of obstruction, not reflux, the amount of swelling and discomfort is related directly to the degree of arm use.

(E) Because they tend to be young and healthy, patients with primary SAVT are better able to tolerate intervention and have more to gain from it over time, thanks to its good success and durability. Furthermore, these patients are more incapacitated by obstructive symptoms from persisting thrombus than most patients with secondary SAVT. The two important patient characteristics, in the decision of whether to choose thrombolysis, are (1) an ongoing need for *active* use of the involved arm and (2) a healthy, active patient with no serious underlying diseases or contraindications to thrombolysis.

(F) Conservative treatment consists of (1) anticoagulant therapy (heparin initially, then warfarin for 3 to 6 months), (2) avoidance of excessive use of the involved arm, (3) elevation of that arm to combat swelling, and (4) the use of elastic support (i.e., a gauntlet) when effective. Patients with secondary SAVT generally respond well and may need little treatment beyond the initial episode. Conservative therapy alone is only occasionally indicated for primary SAVT (see E).

(G) Standard contraindications for thrombolytic therapy are observed but are infrequently present in the typically healthy, young patient with primary SAVT. If thrombolysis is contraindicated but intervention is indicated, surgical thombectomy should be considered as an alternate means of clot removal.

(H) Catheter-directed thrombolytic therapy has become accepted as the first step in interventional treatment of primary SAVT. The interventionalist obtains access in the major inflow vein below the clot, often via the antecubital fossa, with advancement into the thrombus, lacing it with boluses of the lytic agent, before beginning a continuous infusion. Frequent monitoring venograms, with repositioning of the catheter, improve success. Postlysis venography usually visualizes and directs definitive treatment of any underlying lesions. Subsequent therapy depends on:

1. The extent of clot clearance.
2. Demonstration of or, in some cases, reasonable presumption of *extrinsic* compression at the thoracic outlet.
3. Residual *intrinsic* narrowing.

If there is no significant lysis after proper catheter positioning and 24 hours has passed (see I), thrombectomy should be considered. If there is partial lysis but a long residual clot remains, again thrombectomy might be considered if the thrombosis is acute. Most such cases, however, represent delay in referral or treatment, resulting in organized clot, and should be considered for additional intervention only after a trial of conservative therapy (see F).

(I) Surgical thrombectomy, when combined with thoracic outlet decompression, is effective and durable.[5] Thrombectomy may be carried out following any of the standard approaches to

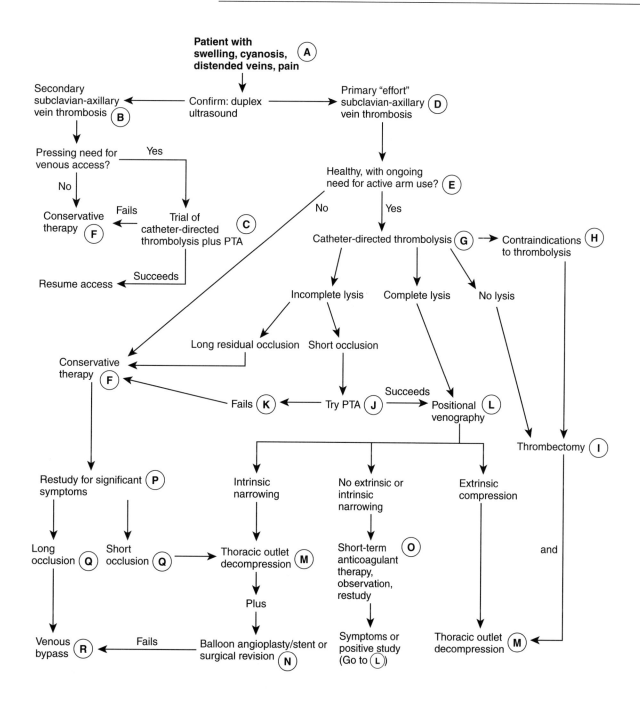

Subclavian-Axillary Vein Thrombosis (continued)

first rib resection, but it is important to place the transverse venotomy low enough to leave adequate room for proximal control. The transaxillary and supraclavicular approaches to first rib removal leave limited exposure of the vein.

We prefer a subclavicular approach in this setting, much like that used for axillofemoral bypass but with division of the insertion of the pectoralis minor muscle to provide wider access. The arm is prepared and draped into the field via a stockinet so it may be manipulated as needed during first rib removal and thrombectomy. Venous thrombectomy catheters can be used proximally but are normally not needed because (1) after first rib removal, a finger can be inserted into the thoracic outlet and (2) after ensuring that there are no associated congenital bands and the outlet is widely decompressed, the surgeon can simply feel the upper extent of the clot and gently stroke it down and out through the venotomy. This technique not only provides more complete clot removal but also adds to the security of proximal control. The distal clot can usually be massaged out by firm stroking cephalad along the inner aspect of the upper arm. Occasionally, wrapping an elastic bandage aids in clot extrusion.

If thrombectomy is delayed or cannot be completed satisfactorily, the incision can be extended medially into a partial upper sternotomy (see N) and the confluence of the subclavian and internal jugular veins can be exposed without claviculectomy; the residual obstruction can then be corrected under direct vision, followed by local revision and patch angioplasty. A surgical approach has the advantage of removing the clot and correcting the underlying cause of thrombosis in one operation or patient admission. Intraoperative venography may be used to assess the adequacy of thrombectomy and to confirm the need for thoracic outlet decompression if the latter is not obvious (see L).

(J) If catheter-directed thrombolysis clears all but the final superior segment of the occlusion and if a catheter can be passed, percutaneous transluminal angioplasty (PTA) should be tried, since only older residual thrombus may be there. If an underlying stenosis remains after most of the clot has been cleared, PTA alone cannot suffice and stenting *prior to thoracic outlet decompression* will not be durable. Therefore, treatment at this point should proceed as outlined for complete lysis: investigation of and appropriate treatment of the underlying lesions (see L). Additional lysis or a short period of anticoagulation to avoid rethrombosis during the next therapeutic step is commonly advised, but a few days to a week appears adequate, not 1 to 3 months, as originally recommended.

(K) If the catheter cannot pass a short residual proximal clotted segment or if PTA does not open the segment, it is recommended that the gains of thrombolysis be consolidated with a period of anticoagulation therapy and that close observation for symptoms be continued. This is because short residual occlusions (e.g., above the cephalic vein) are well tolerated if rethrombosis can be avoided.

(L) After the clot has been fully lysed or the final segment has been opened by PTA, venography should be performed to visualize any residual intrinsic narrowing and to demonstrate any extrinsic compression. The latter may require positioning to mimic the repetitive thoracic outlet compression, causing intimal trauma and, ultimately, thrombosis. The findings can be categorized as (1) extrinsic compression, (2) intrinsic narrowing, (3) both, or (4) neither. If extrinsic compression is demonstrated, or if there is an intrinsic stenosis that can be presumed to have been caused by it, thoracic outlet decompression is required to prevent rethrombosis.

(M) Thoracic outlet decompression, usually achieved by first rib removal (although congenital bands may be present and are removed concomitantly), is presumed to be a necessary part of treatment in most patients with primary SAVT. Evidence of thoracic outlet obstruction or some underlying anatomic cause of thrombosis has been found in 75% to 100% of surgical cases, although this high figure (average, 92%)[1] is obviously subject to selection bias. However, ignoring the likelihood of an underlying thoracic outlet syndrome is the reason why thrombolysis alone, in earlier series, was not very successful.[6] Thoracic outlet decompression is required, no matter how an intrinsic venous stenosis is managed.

(N) When residual intrinsic narrowing is significant, thoracic outlet decompression must be *combined* with either surgical revision (e.g., vein patch angioplasty) or endovascular treatment (PTA/stent). Usually, balloon angioplasty is tried first, which may occasionally be sufficient but usually is not desirable. If the stenosis persists, either stent placement or surgical revision is recommended. Stenting *without* thoracic outlet decompression results in deformed or crushed stents, whether Palmaz[7] or Wallstent.[8] Thus, using a stent does not avoid operation, because first rib removal is still necessary, but it does simplify the surgical procedure.

If long-term follow-up shows durability of stenting for residual venous stenoses, it will prevail. In the meantime, it is appropriate to treat with stenting in centers with good experience with this approach. If future reports show that stents fail despite concomitant thoracic outlet decompression, surgical venous angioplasty will regain popularity. Fortunately, it is no longer necessary to perform claviculectomy to gain the necessary additional exposure to deal with intrinsic narrowing at the same time as first rib removal. Molina has described a ministernotomy approach to facilitate this exposure without removing the head of the clavicle.[9]

A variety of staging strategies are being explored:

1. Lysis and stenting, followed by thoracic outlet decompression during the same patient admission.

SUBCLAVIAN-AXILLARY VEIN THROMBOSIS

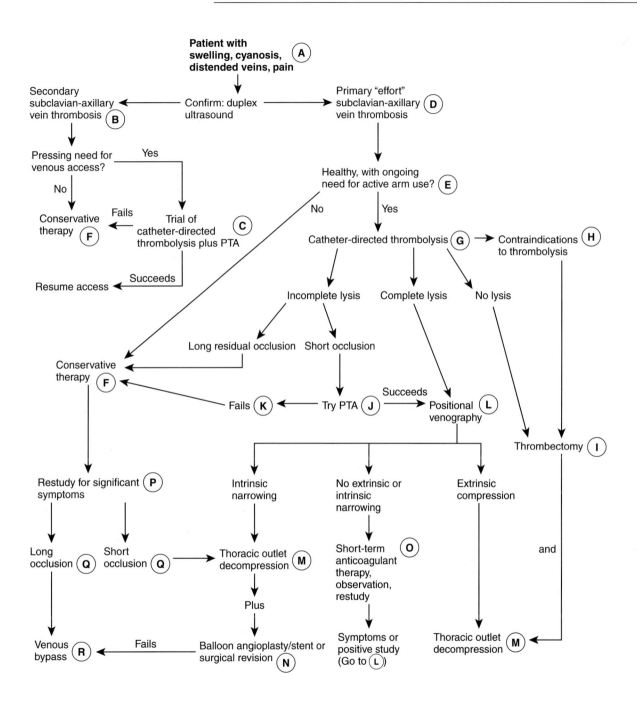

2. Lysis, followed by thoracic outlet decompression the same day, followed by later venography and stenting of any residual stenosis.[10]
3. Lysis, followed by thoracic outlet decompression and surgical revision of any intrinsic lesion at the same operation.[11,12]

Each of these strategies subjects the physician to pressures to limit hospital stay, to reduce the number of admissions, and to shorten the time before the patient can return to full activities. Because of the relative infrequency of primary SAVT and the recent development of these newer strategies, no comparable long-term data are yet available to settle the issue of which is the best approach.

(O) Occasionally, neither stenosis nor evidence of extrinsic compression can be demonstrated by postlysis venography. Many presume that thoracic outlet compression is responsible even if it cannot be demonstrated. However, because of the possibility that the repetitive effort or prolonged positioning in these cases is more significant than some anatomic abnormality, it seems appropriate to order anticoagulation and to observe such patients while activity is restricted for 3 months. A positional venogram is then obtained again, in all possible positions that might cause compression. If results are positive, thoracic outlet decompression is performed; if results are still negative, the patient is released to return to full activities.

(P) Patients with residual occlusions after incomplete lysis who are given a trial of conservative therapy initially (see F) and who exhibit disabling symptoms deserve restudy and consideration for a revascularization procedure. The extent of the stenosis or occlusion determines treatment. In many instances, reconstruction is impossible because of lack of suitable, patent inflow and outflow sites to allow venous bypass, although there are some patients who can be benefited.

(Q) Although the cutoff point is admittedly arbitrary, patients with short occlusions (e.g., 2 to 5 cm) may still benefit from the approaches described earlier under initial treatment (see I, J) or surgical angioplasty and may be reentered into the algorithm at M.[13] Patients with longer occlusions require venous bypass.

(R) Internal jugular vein turndown and transposition to the subclavian vein near the cephalic vein entry have the best success of the venous bypasses.[14] Unfortunately, the transposed vein does not reach very far distally (not much beyond the cephalic vein entry point) and is thus applied primarily to relatively short, chronic residual occlusions without good collateralization. Patients with longer occlusions, who are more symptomatic and need bypass the most, usually require a longer vein graft. Because most saphenous vein segments are smaller in diameter than the recipient vessels and because flow in the resting state may not support patency, a temporary arteriovenous fistula is recommended at the time of venous bypass, for at least 3 months, or until duplex ultrasound monitoring confirms adequate enlargement. Unfortunately, longer bypasses are not associated with good patency and the patency of prosthetic grafts, even with a permanent arteriovenous fistula, is quite low. All of these factors support aggressive early thrombolytic treatment of appropriately selected patients. It is also unfortunate that many primary care physicians still routinely treat all patients with primary SAVT with only anticoagulant therapy initially and refer patients with persisting symptoms too late for optimal interventional therapy.

REFERENCES

1. Hurlbert SN, Rutherford RB: Primary subclavian-axillary vein thrombosis. Ann Vasc Surg 1995;9:217–223.
2. Hurlbert SN, Rutherford RB: Subclavian-axillary vein thrombosis. In Rutherford RB (ed): Vascular Surgery, 5th ed. Philadelphia, WB Saunders, 2000.
3. Haire WD, Lieberman RP, Edney J, et al: Hickman catheter-induced thoracic vein thrombosis. Cancer 1990;66:900–908.
4. Seigel EL, Jew AC, Delcore R, et al: Thrombolytic therapy for catheter-related thrombosis. Am J Surg 1993;166:716–719.
5. Adams JT, DeWeese JA: "Effort" thrombosis of the axillary and subclavian veins. J Trauma 1971;11:923–930.
6. Glanz S, Gordon DH, Lipkowitz GS, et al: Axillary and subclavian vein stenosis: Percutaneous angioplasty. Radiology 1988;168:371–373.
7. Bjarnason H, Hunter DW, Crain MR, et al: Collapse of a Palmaz stent in the subclavian vein. Am J Radiol 1993;160:1123–1124.
8. Meier GH, Pollak JS, Rosenblatt M, et al: Initial experience with venous stents in exertional axillary-subclavian vein thrombosis. J Vasc Surg 1996;24:974–983.
9. Molina JE: A new surgical approach to the innominate and subclavian vein. J Vasc Surg 1998;27:576–581.
10. Chang BB, Kreienberg PB, Darling RC III, et al: One stage definitive therapy for Paget-Schroetter syndrome: A multidisciplinary approach. Presented at the 44th Annual Meeting of the North American Chapter of the International Society for Cardiovascular Surgery, Chicago, 1996 (submitted).
11. Molina JE: Surgery for effort thrombosis of the subclavian vein. J Thorac Cardiovasc Surg 1992;103:341–346.
12. Lee MC, Belkin M, Mannick JA, et al: Early operative intervention following thrombolytic therapy for primary subclavian vein thrombosis: An effective treatment aproach. J Vasc Surg 1998;27:101–108.
13. Molina JE: Need for emergency treatment in subclavian vein effort thrombosis. J Am Coll Surg 1995;181:414–420.
14. Sanders RJ, Cooper MA: Surgical management of subclavian vein obstruction, including six cases of subclavian vein bypass. Surgery 1995;118:856–863.

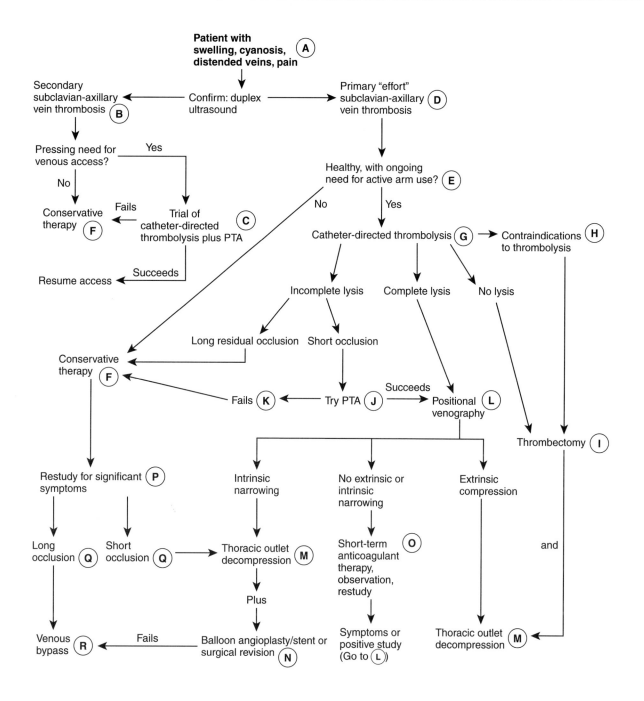

Chapter 55 Superficial Phlebitis

JOHN J. SKILLMAN, MD

(A) In hospitalized patients, superficial phlebitis is usually catheter-induced, whereas among outpatients it is usually spontaneous, although it may be associated with intravenous (IV) drug abuse. Spontaneous phlebitis usually occurs in the distal lower extremity in tributaries of the greater saphenous vein.

Predisposing factors include recent childbirth, operative procedure, minor trauma, varicose veins, or simply venous stasis that might result from a long automobile or airplane trip. Patients with no apparent explanation or risk factors (idiopathic) deserve close surveillance for malignancy and screening for hypercoagulable state. Recurrent phlebitis, especially with a positive family history, suggests an underlying hypercoagulable state.

Superficial phlebitis presents as a painful erythematous streak overlying a superficial vein. A palpable, tender thrombus, or cord, can usually be appreciated on physical examination. Differentiation from more diffuse cellulitis depends primarily on the local distribution of erythema over the vein.

(B) In its minor form, catheter-induced phlebitis commonly develops when needles or plastic cannulas are left in place for 2 to 3 days or longer. This inflammatory phlebitis can be caused either by direct mechanical or chemical irritation of the vein by the catheter[1] or by infused solutions and drugs that may injure the vascular endothelium.[2] When this condition is detected, the catheter should be removed as the first step in treatment of catheter-induced phlebitis.

Catheter-induced phlebitis can be more significant if a central vein is involved, in which case deep vein thrombosis (DVT) rather than superficial phlebitis exists. Generally in such instances, the catheter should still be removed. In exceptional circumstances, when patients have limited venous access sites, an attempt may be made at preserving the catheter via thrombolytic treatment, without removing the catheter (see Chapter 54).

(C) Although superficial phlebitis is nearly always an inflammatory rather than an infectious process, it can be complicated by bacterial infection when it is catheter-induced or associated with IV drug abuse. In the early stages of an infectious phlebitis, differentiation may be difficult. More diffuse erythema and pain as well as systemic signs such as fever, elevated white blood cell count, or bacteremia may signal the development of an infected thrombus. A wide variety of gram-positive and gram-negative bacteria may be implicated in infectious phlebitis.

The experience of Pruitt and coauthors[3-5] suggests that suppurative thrombophlebitis occurs more frequently in immunocompromised patients, such as patients with major burns, in whom *Staphylococcus aureus* is the most common organism. However, these infections are often polymicrobial and also involve gram-negative organisms (including *Pseudomonas aeruginosa* and the *Klebsiella-Enterobacter-Serratia* group) and yeast. It is thought that skin microorganisms responsible for infectious and suppurative phlebitis are introduced at the time of catheter insertion and that these organisms later gain access to the intraluminal vein by migration along the catheter from the surface of the skin.[6] Proteinaceous material (fibrin and fibronectin) is deposited around the IV catheter and forms a scaffold to which organisms (particularly gram-positive cocci) can adhere.[7,8] Glycoproteins produced by these bacteria add to the host-produced protein scaffold to form a biofilm in which these organisms can proliferate.[9] In burn patients, Pruitt and coworkers found that physical signs to aid in the diagnosis were uncommon[3,5,10] and that exploration of the vein was often necessary to establish a diagnosis.

A subsequent report regarding burn patients by Hammond and coworkers[11] indicated that the most common symptom of suppurative phlebitis was pain (in 83%) followed by a temperature higher than 39°C (in 63%).

(D) When infectious phlebitis is suspected, IV antibiotics should be initiated. Gram-positive coverage is essential and should be broadened if the initial response is poor, if the patient is immunocompromised, or if circumstances suggest multiple organisms.

(E) Although antibiotic treatment may be successful in treating an infected site of catheter-based phlebitis, this result would be unlikely if a true abscess were present, especially in a more central vein. For this reason, it is important to detect an abscess by examining for fluctuance over the vein, air in the soft tissue, or purulent discharge after "milking" the vein toward the previous puncture site.

(F) Catheter-induced superficial phlebitis in a peripheral vein is unlikely to progress to DVT. When more proximal catheter-induced phlebitis is present, a duplex ultrasound scan should be performed to determine whether a DVT is present.[12] Phlebitis associated with a subclavian, jugular, or femoral vein catheter by definition involves a deep vein, and its extent should be determined by duplex scanning or phlebography if necessary.

Spontaneous superficial phlebitis nearly always involves the lower extremities and is more likely to be associated with DVT. For this reason, some authors recommend routine duplex scanning in these patients with superficial phlebitis to exclude DVT.[13] Others reserve this scanning for patients in whom the superficial phlebitis extends above the knee, especially as it approaches the saphenofemoral junction. In such patients, a DVT may be found in 17%.[14]

The common association of varicose veins with superficial phlebitis was noted more than 50 years ago by Edwards.[15] However, most thrombosed varicosities involve only short segments of saphenous tributaries and are associated with deep venous thrombosis in only 2.6% of patients.[13] Clearly, if signs of DVT accompany superficial phlebitis, duplex ultrasound scanning should be performed.

G If a lower extremity DVT is detected, heparin anticoagulation therapy should be initiated and the patient treated as explained in Chapter 56. If an upper extremity, catheter-induced DVT is detected, the need for anticoagulation is less phlebitis, duplex ultrasound scanning should be has been reported in such patients, and an anticoagulation agent is appropriate if no contraindications exist, especially in patients who would poorly tolerate even a small pulmonary embolus (see Chapter 58).

H When catheter-induced phlebitis is associated with infection (either with or without associated DVT), several weeks of antibiotic therapy may be required for resolution of the process. During this treatment, continued examination of the site of phlebitis must be maintained to ensure that suppurative infection with abscess formation does not develop.

I Uncomplicated superficial phlebitis is common and is managed with symptomatic treatment, including anti-inflammatory medication and local application of warm compresses. This treatment nearly always suffices to bring resolution and relief to the patient, although residual firmness may last for several months until the clot and associated inflammation resolves.[16, 17] In rare cases, symptomatic treatment may be unsuccessful; if so, anticoagulation may be required. Compression stockings and ambulation are encouraged to reduce stasis and prevent DVT formation.

If patients present with several episodes of spontaneous superficial phlebitis, evaluation of a possible hypercoagulable state should be undertaken (see Chapter 3). Recurrent, spontaneous phlebitis in the same lower extremity vein is an indication for vein excision, usually when accompanied by varicose segments (see Chapter 59).

J Suppurative phlebitis, although rare, nearly always requires vein excision, and may produce severe bacteremia and sepsis if not adequately treated. Delayed primary closure of the wound is usually necessary. The most extensive

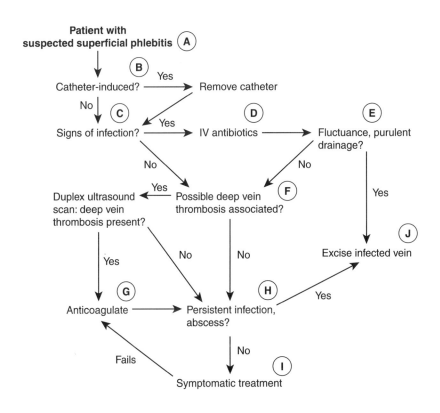

experience with suppurative phlebitis has concerned burn patients, and results have emphasized the need for aggressive resection of the involved peripheral vein.[3-5, 10, 17]

In those rare instances when sepsis associated with a central thrombus exists and is not improved by antibiotic treatment, radical removal of central veins has been employed with a successful outcome.[18] This can be a complex surgical procedure requiring both clavicular and sternal incisions if the subclavian vein is involved.[19, 20]

REFERENCES

1. Maki DG: Infections associated with intravascular lines. Curr Clin Top Infect Dis 1982;3:1229-1233.
2. Wermeling DP, Rapp RP, DeLuca PP, et al: Osmolality of small-volume intravenous admixtures. Am J Hosp Pharm 1985;42:1739-1744.
3. Pruitt BA Jr, Stein JM, Foley FD, et al: Intravenous therapy in burn patients: Suppurative thrombophlebitis and other life-threatening complications. Arch Surg 1970;100:399-404.
4. Stein JM, Pruitt BA Jr: Suppurative thrombophlebitis—a lethal iatrogenic disease. N Engl J Med 1970;282:1452-1455.
5. O'Neill JA, Pruitt BA Jr, Foley FD, Moncrief JA: Suppurative thrombophlebitis—a lethal complication of intravenous therapy. J Trauma 1968;8:256-267.
6. Maki DG, Goldman DA, Rhame FS: Infection control in intravenous therapy. Ann Intern Med 1993;79:867-887.
7. Herrmann M, Vaudaux PE, Pittet D, et al: Fibronectin, fibrinogen and laminin act as mediators of adherence of clinical *Staphylococcus* isolates to foreign material. J Infect Dis 1988;158:693-701.
8. Cheung AL, Fischetti VA: The role of fibrinogen in mediating staphylococcal adherence to fibers. J Surg Res 1991;50:150-155.
9. Costerton JW, Lewandowski Z, Caldwell DE, et al: Microbial biofilms. Ann Rev Microbiol 1995;49:711-745.
10. Pruitt BA Jr, McManus WF, Kim SH, et al: Diagnosis and treatment of cannula-related intravenous sepsis in burn patients. Ann Surg 1980;191:546.
11. Hammond JS, Varas R, Ward CG: Suppurative phlebitis: A new look at a continuing problem. South Med J 1986;81:969-971.
12. Knudson GJ, Wiedmeyer DA, Erickson SJ, et al: Color Doppler sonographic imaging in the assessment of upper extremity deep venous thrombosis. Am J Roentgenol 1990;154:399-403.
13. Bergquist D, Jaroszewski H: Deep vein thrombosis in patients with superficial phlebitis of the leg. Br Med J 1986;292:658-659.
14. Skillman JJ, Kent KC, Porter DH, Kim D: Simultaneous occurrence of superficial and deep thrombophlebitis in the lower extremity. J Vasc Surg 1990;11:818-824.
15. Edwards EA: Thrombophlebitis of varicose veins. Surg Gynecol Obstet 1938;66:236-245.
16. Johnson RA, Zajac RA, Evans ME: Suppurative thrombophlebitis: Correlation between pathogen and underlying disease. Infect Control 1986;7:582-585.
17. Righter J, Bishop LA, Hill B: Infection and peripheral venous catheterization. Diag Microbiol Infect Dis 1983;1:89,93.
18. Munster AM: Septic thrombophlebitis: A surgical disorder. JAMA 1974;230:1010-1011.
19. Winn RE, Tuttle KL, Gilbert DN: Surgical approach to extensive suppurative thrombophlebitis of the central veins of the chest. J Thorac Cardiovasc Surg 1981;81:564-568.
20. Weinberg G, Pasternak BM: Upper extremity suppurative thrombophlebitis and septic pulmonary emboli. JAMA 1978;240:1519-1520.

SUPERFICIAL PHLEBITIS

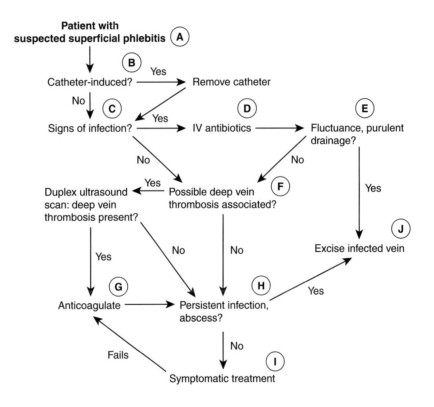

Chapter 56 Lower Extremity Deep Vein Thrombosis

MARK H. MEISSNER, MD

(A) Accurate diagnosis of acute deep venous thrombosis (DVT) is important, since improperly withholding anticoagulation therapy is associated with the risk of pulmonary embolism, whereas inappropriate treatment carries the inconvenience, expense, and hazards of anticoagulation. Unfortunately, the clinical diagnosis of DVT is inaccurate; the classic findings of pain, swelling, and tenderness are equally as common in limbs with and without objectively confirmed thrombosis. The diagnosis of DVT, therefore, requires confirmatory testing.

(B) Despite the inaccuracy of clinical diagnosis alone, an assessment of the probability of thrombosis is necessary prior to diagnostic testing. As none of the noninvasive tests for DVT is 100% accurate, the positive and negative predictive values depend on the pretest probability of DVT in individual patients. A thorough clinical assessment is thus required in defining the need for serial noninvasive studies as well in determining the duration of anticoagulation and the need for further diagnostic studies to exclude underlying conditions (e.g., hypercoagulable states, malignancy).

On the basis of signs and symptoms, associated thrombotic risk factors, and the plausibility of alternative diagnoses, it is possible to stratify patients as having a high, moderate, or low pretest probability of disease.[1,2] Major outpatient risk factors include:

- Active malignancy
- Paralysis or limb immobilization
- More than 3 days of bed rest or surgery within 4 weeks
- A strong family history of DVT

Minor factors include recent limb trauma and hospitalization within the previous 3 months.

Thigh and calf swelling, calf swelling more than 3 cm, and tenderness along the deep veins are considered major clinical signs; unilateral pitting edema, dilated superficial veins, and erythema are considered minor signs.

Outpatients with one or fewer major risk factors or signs have a low pretest probability of thrombosis. Those with more than two major and two minor or more than three major factors or signs in the absence of an alternative diagnosis have a high probability of disease.[2]

More empirical stratification has also been of value,[1] with the prevalence of positive noninvasive studies increasing from 2.1% among outpatients without swelling or thrombotic risk factors to 13% in patients with thrombotic risk factors but no swelling and approximately 50% in patients with acute unilateral swelling.[3] The negative predictive value of the absence of unilateral swelling or an existing thrombotic risk factor in outpatients is greater than 97%.[3] Although the value of clinically screening hospitalized patients is less clear, similar strategies have been validated for inpatients.[4]

(C) Although ascending venography remains the diagnostic reference standard, duplex ultrasonography has largely replaced venography for clinical purposes. More than 80% of symptomatic venous thrombi involve the easily interrogated proximal veins, and uniformly high sensitivities of 93% to 97% and specificities of 94% to 99% have been reported for the ultrasound diagnosis of proximal DVT.

Measurement of D-dimer cross-linked fibrin degradation products (FDPs), formed by the action of plasmin on cross-linked fibrin, has been proposed as an alternative to initial noninvasive testing. A sensitivity of 96.8% and a specificity of 35.2% have been reported for enzyme-linked immunosorbent assay (ELISA),[5] making it theoretically possible to limit noninvasive testing to those with positive D-dimer results. Unfortunately, the ELISA test is time-consuming and impractical as a screening test, while most rapid latex agglutination assays have had insufficient sensitivity. More rapid ELISA assays, returning results within 1 hour, have now become available and appear promising.[6] However, prospective evaluation of the safety of withholding anticoagulation therapy in patients with negative D-dimer tests has been limited. The number of false-positive results may also limit the utility of this approach in hospitalized patients with a high prevalence of malignancy, infection, or recent surgery. It is likely that these tests may become useful in the management of patients in the future.

(D) Strategies for withholding anticoagulation based on duplex ultrasound examination alone require serial testing, since 3% to 7% of documented thromboses show initial findings that are negative for proximal thrombosis. Initial diagnostic failure rates may be higher among inpatients and those with persistent symptoms. However, the incidence of thromboembolism within 6 months of serially negative ultrasound scans is less than 2%, and withholding anticoagulation in symptomatic patients with two negative ultrasound scans 5 to 7 days apart has proved safe.[7,8]

Unfortunately, serial testing is expensive, inefficient, and inconvenient. Approximately 95% of follow-up studies are found to be negative, and several alternatives to serial testing have been proposed. A single, technically adequate examination that includes the calf veins potentially eliminates the need for serial studies in many patients, although the safety of this approach has not been prospectively evaluated.

D-Dimer testing also theoretically can identify patients requiring serial studies. With this strategy, only patients with an initially normal ultrasound scan and an abnormal D-dimer level would be referred for serial testing. Although such an approach may permit definitive management on the day of presentation in 42% to 69% of patients, it may not be significantly more cost-effective than serial venous ultrasound surveillance alone.[9]

Strategies combining clinical assessment with duplex ultrasonography have been the most extensively evaluated. Using distinct inpatient and outpatient criteria, groups with low, moderate, and

LOWER EXTREMITY DEEP VEIN THROMBOSIS

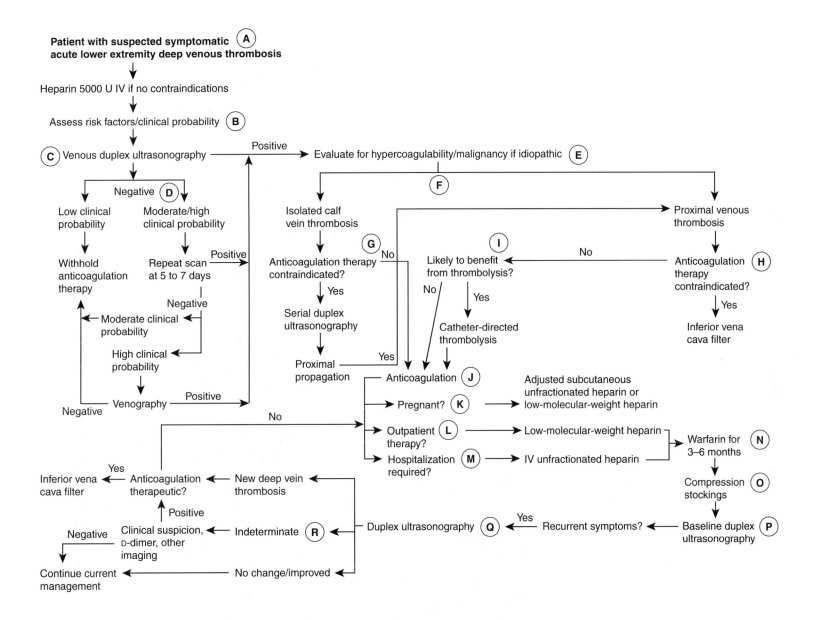

high pretest probabilities can be defined as having respective DVT prevalences of 10%, 20%, and 76% for inpatients and 5%, 33%, and 85% for outpatients.[2,4] Because the negative predictive value of a normal ultrasound scan in the low-probability group is high, serial scanning may be unnecessary in these patients. However, duplex ultrasonography has clear limitations in imaging the iliac and calf veins, and further testing is appropriate for patients with a moderate or high probability of thrombosis.

Anticoagulation may be safely withheld in moderate probability patients with two negative scans, whereas venography should be considered either before or after a second negative scan in patients with high clinical suspicion of venous thrombosis. The role of alternative modalities, such as magnetic resonance venography and nuclear medicine imaging, has not yet been fully defined in these patients.

(E) Most patients with an acute DVT associated with identifiable risk factors require no further evaluation; however, patients with no apparent precipitating events or risk factors (i.e., idiopathic DVT) need to be considered for underlying hypercoagulability or malignancy. Investigation of a *congenital* (factor V Leiden, prothrombin 20210 A mutations; protein C, protein S, antithrombin deficiency; hyperhomocyst(e)inemia) or an *acquired* (particularly antiphospholipid antibodies) thrombophilic state is appropriate when the patient has had:

- Idiopathic DVT and is younger than age 50 years
- A family history of thrombosis
- Thrombosis in an unusual site
- Recurrent DVT
- Recurrent fetal loss

DVT may also herald a previously undetected malignancy in 3% to 23% of patients with idiopathic thrombosis, with the incidence of occult malignancy diagnosed within 6 to 12 months being 2.2 to 5.3 times higher than that expected in the general population.[10,11] Although the value of an intensive search for occult malignancy has not been demonstrated, screening based on the history, a complete physical examination, standard laboratory tests, and chest x-ray is warranted. Further evaluation should be guided by any abnormalities detected and recommended screening guidelines.

(F) The primary goal in the treatment of DVT is prevention of the two major complications: pulmonary embolism and the post-thrombotic syndrome. On the basis of perceived differences in the risk of these complications, acute DVT is often defined as involving either the proximal veins, encompassing segments from the popliteal vein to the inferior vena cava, or isolated to the calf veins. Without treatment, pulmonary embolism may complicate up to 50% of proximal thrombi, whereas as many as two thirds of patients may experience long-term manifestations of pain, edema, hyperpigmentation, or ulceration.

Although the incidence of complications is lower after isolated calf vein thrombosis, it is not trivial, and these thrombi should not be ignored. Approximately 20% of such thrombi will propagate proximally, with a theoretical 2% risk of fatal pulmonary embolism and 5% to 10% risk of symptomatic pulmonary embolism.[12] Furthermore, approximately 25% of patients with isolated calf vein thrombosis will have persistent symptoms of pain and edema during follow-up.[13]

(G) Options for the management of symptomatic, isolated calf vein thrombosis include anticoagulation versus serial noninvasive follow-up with anticoagulation only in the event of proximal extension. Based on the risk of proximal propagation and the associated risks of pulmonary embolism and the post-thrombotic syndrome, many have concluded that the benefits of treatment exceed the risk and inconvenience of anticoagulation in most patients.[12,14] Anticoagulation may be particularly warranted in patients with a previous history of DVT, in whom recurrence rates of 50% have been documented, as well as in those with malignancy or multiple thrombotic risk factors, in whom the risk of proximal thrombosis is higher.[13]

Serial duplex ultrasonography may be a reasonable alternative in patients with contraindications to anticoagulation who can be reliably monitored. Current recommendations include follow-up testing at 2- to 3-day intervals for 10 to 14 days after presentation.[12,14]

(H) Randomized clinical trials have established anticoagulation therapy as the standard of care for patients with proximal DVT. However, placement of an inferior vena cava (IVC) filter is appropriate in patients with contraindications to anticoagulation. Other conventional indications for IVC filter placement include recurrent thrombosis despite adequate anticoagulation and complications of anticoagulation.[14] A significant rate of recurrent DVT has been associated with IVC filters,[15] and anticoagulation should be considered if any contraindication resolves.

(I) Despite the absence of randomized clinical trials demonstrating long-term efficacy, thrombolytic therapy may have a role in the treatment of patients at substantial risk for post-thrombotic disability. This would include otherwise healthy patients with proximal thrombosis and a good life expectancy. Furthermore, limited evidence suggests that the best results are obtained with a catheter-directed approach in patients with iliofemoral DVT having symptoms of less than 10 days' duration and without a prior history of DVT. In this selected population, complete thrombolysis can be achieved in 65% of patients and close to 85% show complete or major clot resolution, with a 1-year patency of 96%.[16]

More information is needed prior to similar recommendations for femoropopliteal DVT. A standard course of anticoagulation should be instituted after completion of thrombolytic treatment.

(J) Anticoagulation with heparin, followed by warfarin, remains standard therapy for acute DVT. Although the availability of low-molecular-

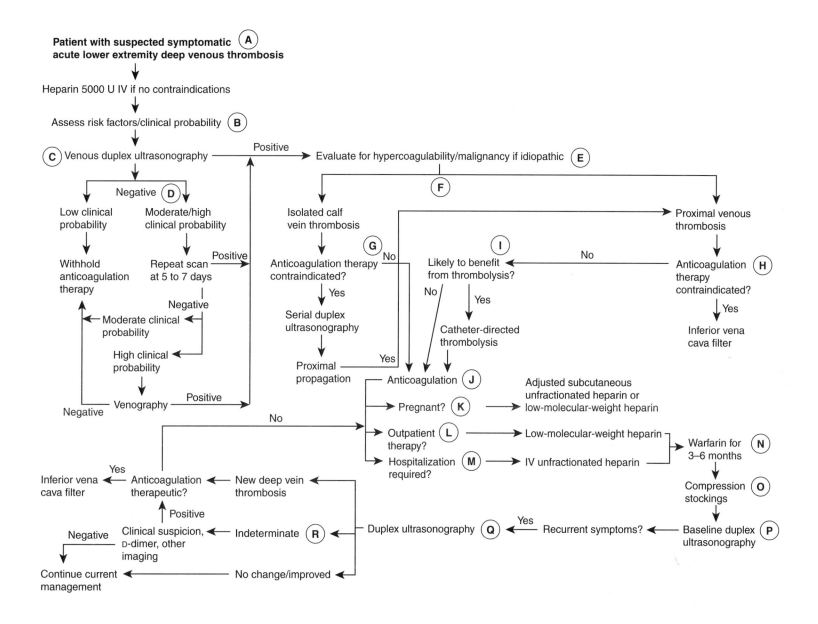

weight (LMW) heparins and other anticoagulants has expanded treatment options, these drugs remain expensive and incompletely evaluated in some patient populations. Appropriate anticoagulation must therefore be tailored for the individual patient.

(K) Thromboembolism during pregnancy is associated with higher rates of preterm delivery and perinatal mortality, whereas pulmonary embolism is second only to abortion as a cause of maternal mortality. It is thus generally conceded that the benefits of anticoagulation for DVT during pregnancy exceed the potential risks.

Unfortunately, warfarin readily crosses the placenta and has both teratogenic and fetal effects. Exposure between the 6th and 12th weeks is associated with the fetal warfarin syndrome, consisting of nasal hypoplasia, stippled epiphyses, and growth retardation, whereas exposure during the second and third trimesters may lead to central nervous system abnormalities.[17, 18] Warfarin is thus contraindicated in pregnancy, although its use does not appear to be associated with adverse effects in the breast-fed infant.

In contrast, neither unfractionated heparin nor the LMW heparins cross the placenta. Unfractionated heparin administered intravenously (IV) for 5 to 10 days, followed by adjusted-dose subcutaneous (SC) unfractionated heparin every 12 hours to maintain the activated partial thromboplastin time (aPTT) in the therapeutic range, is recommended for the treatment of DVT during pregnancy.[17] IV heparin is again used immediately before delivery, discontinued once the active phase of labor is reached, and resumed within 6 hours of vaginal delivery.[18] Anticoagulation with warfarin should be continued for 4 to 6 weeks post partum.

Unfractionated heparin administered over prolonged periods, however, is associated with osteopenia in one third of patients and vertebral fractures in approximately 2% of patients.[17] The LMW heparins appear to be associated with less osteopenia, which together with their more predictable dose-response relationship, lack of a requirement for laboratory monitoring, and lower incidence of thrombocytopenia theoretically makes them better suited for the long-term treatment of venous thromboembolism during pregnancy. Unfortunately, LMW heparins are expensive, and information to guide dosing in pregnancy is limited. However, LMW heparins have been recognized as safe and effective during pregnancy, with several small case series suggesting an expanded role for these drugs.[19]

(L) The availability of LMW heparins, together with evidence that early ambulation does not increase the incidence of pulmonary embolism, now makes the outpatient treatment of DVT feasible.[20] Potential advantages of LMW heparins include:

1. Increased bioavailability, allowing once-daily or twice-daily SC injection.
2. Dosing without the need for laboratory monitoring.
3. A longer half-life.
4. Less risk of heparin-induced thrombocytopenia.
5. Possibly a reduced risk of bleeding.[14, 21]
6. Proof that they are at least as safe and effective as unfractionated heparin in the treatment of proximal venous thrombosis.

Although individual studies have not consistently shown a clear benefit associated with the LMW heparins, a meta-analysis of published studies suggests a lower rate of recurrent thromboembolic and bleeding complications.[21] However, despite their potential superiority and the likelihood that these drugs will become the standard of care for DVT, they are substantially more expensive than unfractionated heparin. Although limited data suggest that some of these drugs may be more cost-effective in inpatients as well as outpatients, their use currently requires some justification based on the decreased costs associated with hospitalization and the need for laboratory monitoring. Not all patients are candidates for outpatient treatment, and the optimal dosing of these agents in some situation, such as in obese patients and patients with renal failure, remains poorly defined.

Various criteria have been suggested as absolute or relative contraindications to outpatient management, including:

- Residence remote from medical care
- Other indications for hospital admission
- Pregnancy
- Advanced age (>75 years)
- The potential for bleeding complications
- Symptomatic pulmonary embolism
- Limited cardiopulmonary reserve
- Abnormal vital signs and arterial blood gas analyses
- Abnormal electrocardiogram[22]

Absence of these criteria has been found, retrospectively, to have a negative predictive value of 100% for the occurrence of serious complications during outpatient treatment. Using these criteria, which are conservative, 9% of patients with proximal thrombosis have been noted to be eligible for outpatient treatment, with an additional 9% possibly eligible and 82% ineligible. In contrast, Wells and coauthors,[23] using more liberal exclusion criteria including only massive pulmonary embolism, active bleeding, high risk for major bleeding, phlegmasia, and co-morbid conditions requiring hospitalization, have noted that up to 83% of outpatients may be eligible for home treatment with risks of recurrent thromboembolism and major hemorrhage as low as 3.6% and 2.0%, respectively. Also, some patients, although not candidates for the initiation of treatment as outpatients, may be able to complete therapy at home by using LMW heparin.

(M) For patients requiring hospitalization, treatment guidelines for initial anticoagulation with unfractionated heparin have been developed.[14] Failure to achieve early therapeutic anticoagulation, which is critically important in preventing recurrent venous thromboembolism, is perhaps the most common error in the treatment of acute DVT.

LOWER EXTREMITY DEEP VEIN THROMBOSIS

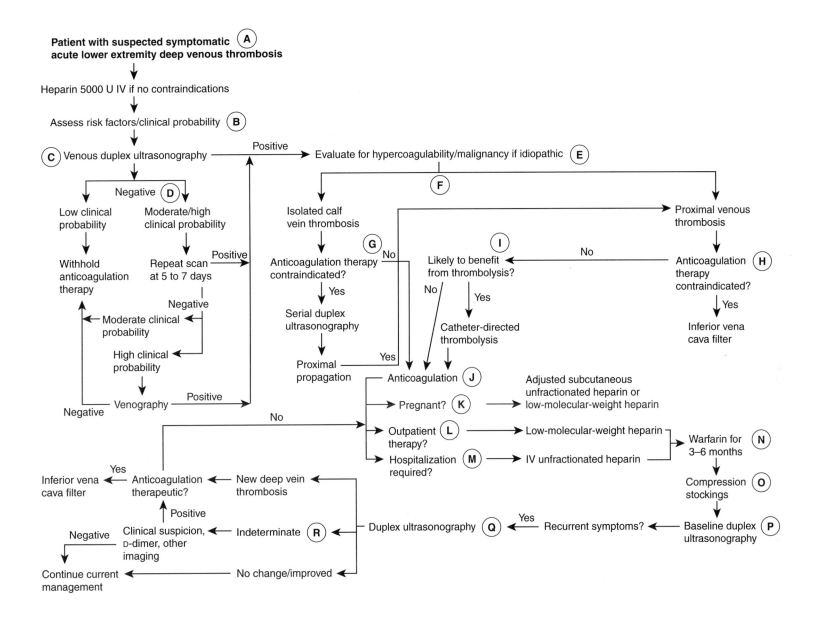

Several clinical trials have now demonstrated that failure to achieve an aPTT above 1.5 times the control value within 24 hours is associated with a significantly higher risk of recurrent thrombotic events. According to these considerations, an initial bolus of 80 IU/kg of heparin IV should be followed by a maintenance infusion of 18 IU/kg per hour, with subsequent dosage adjustment to maintain the aPTT within the *therapeutic range*, defined as the range of the aPTT in seconds corresponding to plasma heparin levels of 0.2 to 0.4 IU/mL by protamine titration.[14]

The importance of rapidly attaining a therapeutic aPTT has made it clear that subsequent dose adjustments should be nomogram-driven rather than empirically driven. Weight-based nomograms outperform nonindividualized standard nomograms, increasing the aPTT above the therapeutic threshold more rapidly, better estimating eventual heparin requirements, and requiring fewer dosage adjustments.[24]

Platelet counts should be monitored daily to check for the presence of heparin-induced thrombocytopenia. Heparin should be discontinued, and anticoagulation with danaparoid or recombinant hirudin should be considered if the platelet count falls precipitously or to below 100,000/μL.[14]

(N) The inconvenience of adjusted-dose SC heparin and the risk of osteopenia make heparin inappropriate for long-term anticoagulation of most patients, and warfarin is most often used following an initial course of unfractionated or LMW heparin. Warfarin at a dose of 5 mg can be started on the first day of treatment, with subsequent dosage adjustments to achieve an International Normalized Ratio (INR) of 2.0 to 3.0. Combined therapy with heparin and warfarin should be continued for 5 to 7 days until the INR is therapeutic for 2 consecutive days.[14]

Determining the appropriate duration of anticoagulation after an episode of acute DVT is based on balancing the risks of hemorrhage with those of recurrent thromboembolism and should be tailored to the individual patient. Patients with idiopathic DVT, recurrent DVT, inherited thrombophilic states, and malignancy are particularly susceptible to recurrent thrombosis and need long-term anticoagulation.[25] In contrast, patients with reversible risk factors, such as surgery and trauma, are at substantially lower risk for recurrent thromboembolism.

Although the optimal duration of anticoagulation therapy remains unresolved in many patients, general guidelines include:

1. Anticoagulation for 3 months in patients with isolated calf vein thrombosis.
2. Three to 6 months in patients with a first episode of DVT and either heterozygous activated protein C resistance or reversible risk factors.
3. At least 6 months in patients with idiopathic DVT.
4. Twelve months to lifelong anticoagulation in patients with recurrent DVT or a first DVT in association with malignancy, congenital anticoagulant deficiencies, persistent antiphospholipid antibodies, or homozygous activated protein C resistance.[14]

Some authors, however, have suggested that a shorter 6-week to 3-month course of anticoagulation therapy be considered for postoperative DVT.[25, 26]

(O) Prevention of the post-thrombotic syndrome is the second objective in the treatment of acute DVT. Although anticoagulation sufficient to prevent recurrent thrombosis is important, randomized trials have also shown that the use of graded elastic compression stockings (40 mmHg at the ankle) reduces the incidence of objectively documented post-thrombotic syndrome by approximately 50%.[27]

(P) One third of patients with an acute DVT present with recurrent symptoms within 1 year, although a new thrombotic episode can be objectively documented in only one third of these. Unfortunately, a diagnosis of recurrent DVT may be difficult to establish with most imaging modalities. Variable degrees of residual occlusion, partial recanalization, intimal thickening, and collateral formation may mask new intraluminal filling defects on venography and limit the utility of venous ultrasonography in this setting. Since compression ultrasound studies may remain abnormal in 27% to 70% of patients after 1 year, a baseline examination obtained 3 to 6 months after an acute event may be useful in defining future thrombotic events.

(Q) Despite limitations, duplex ultrasonography is often the most appropriate initial study for the evaluation of recurrent symptoms. A newly incompressible venous segment or a free-floating tail is diagnostic of recurrent thrombosis, whereas the presence of multiple collateral vessels, several flow channels, and brightly echogenic thrombus may suggest chronic thrombosis. An examination that reveals no alterations from baseline values requires no change in treatment, but clear evidence of new thrombus requires an evaluation of the adequacy of anticoagulation.

If the patient has completed treatment or anticoagulation is subtherapeutic, appropriate anticoagulation is necessary. However, if recurrent thrombosis has developed despite adequate anticoagulation, placement of an IVC filter is appropriate.

(R) Unfortunately, ultrasonography may be indeterminate in many patients with recurrent symptoms. Venography may have a limited role in this setting, whereas strategies demonstrating active thrombus formation may also be effective adjuncts. Theoretically, D-dimer levels may be useful in this regard but have not been extensively evaluated in the setting of recurrent DVT. Short-term studies have demonstrated that although D-dimer levels decline early after treatment, they remain significantly elevated at 10 days. Absolute elevations of D-dimer levels may therefore have

LOWER EXTREMITY DEEP VEIN THROMBOSIS

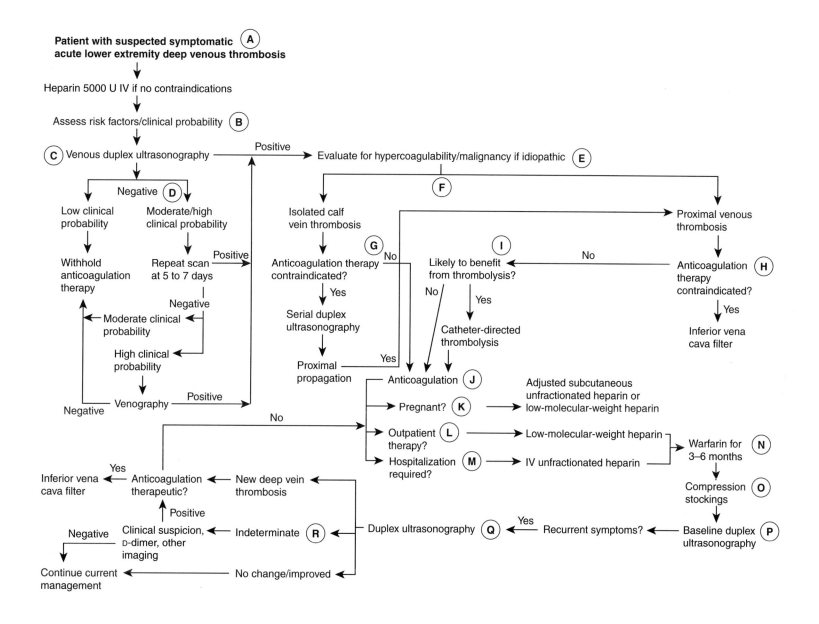

limited utility. Small series have inconsistently related secondary D-dimer increases to recurrent thromboembolism.

Perhaps more useful are the use of radiopharmaceuticals specific for components of actively forming thrombus. Those containing synthetic peptides specific for the surface integrin glycoprotein IIb/IIIa expressed on activated platelets are the most promising and have undergone early feasibility testing in humans. One such agent, technetium 99m apcitide (AcuTect, Diatide, Inc., Nycomed Amersham), is now commercially available.

Unfortunately, prospective studies of these adjunct approaches are lacking, and firm guidelines are difficult to establish. Optimal management of the patient with noninvasive results indeterminate for recurrent thrombosis requires appreciation of the limitations of the available tests and integration of clinical suspicion with the results of venous duplex ultrasonography supplemented by these adjunctive strategies.

REFERENCES

1. Perrier A, Desmarais S, Miron MJ, et al: Non-invasive diagnosis of venous thromboembolism in outpatients. Lancet 1999;353(9148):190.
2. Wells PS, Hirsh J, Anderson DR, et al: Accuracy of clinical assessment of deep-vein thrombosis. Lancet 1995;345(8961):1326.
3. Glover JL, Bendick PJ: Appropriate indications for venous duplex ultrasonic examinations. Surgery 1996;120(4):725.
4. Wells PS, Anderson DR, Bormanis J, et al: Application of a diagnostic clinical model for the management of hospitalized patients with suspected deep-vein thrombosis. Thromb Haemost 1999;81(4):493.
5. Bounameaux H, de Moerloose P, Perrier A, et al: Plasma measurement of D-dimer as a diagnostic aid in suspected venous thromboembolism: An overview. Thromb Haemost 1994;71(1):1.
6. Janssen MC, Wollersheim H, Verbruggen B, et al: Rapid D-dimer assays to exclude deep venous thrombosis and pulmonary embolism: Current status and new developments. Semin Thromb Hemost 1998;24(4):393.
7. Birdwell B, Raskob G, Whitsett T, et al: The clinical validity of normal compression ultrasonography in outpatients suspected of having deep venous thrombosis. Ann Intern Med 1998;128(1):1.
8. Cogo A, Lensing AWA, Koopman MMW, et al: Compression ultrasonography for diagnostic management of patients with clinically suspected deep vein thrombosis: Prospective cohort study. BMJ 1998;316(7124):617.
9. Heijboer H, Ginsberg JS, Buller HR, et al: The use of the D-dimer test in combination with non-invasive testing versus serial non-invasive testing alone for the diagnosis of deep-vein thrombosis. Thromb Haemost 1992;67(5):510.
10. Nordstrom M, Lindblad B, Anderson H, et al: Deep venous thrombosis and occult malignancy: An epidemiological study. BMJ 1994;308(6933):891.
11. Sorensen HT, Mellemkjaer L, Steffensen FH, et al: The risk of a diagnosis of cancer after primary deep venous thrombosis or pulmonary embolism. N Engl J Med 1998;338(17):1169.
12. Raskob G: Calf-vein thrombosis. In Hull R, Raskob G, Pineo G (eds): Venous Thromboembolism: An Evidence-Based Atlas. Armonk, NY, Futura Publishing Company, 1996, p 307.
13. Meissner M, Caps M, Bergelin R, et al: Early outcome after isolated calf vein thrombosis. J Vasc Surg 1997;26(5):749.
14. Hyers TM, Agnelli G, Hull RD, et al: Antithrombotic therapy for venous thromboembolic disease. Chest 1998;114(5 Suppl):561S.
15. Decousus H, Leizorovicz A, Parent F, et al: A clinical trial of vena caval filters in the prevention of pulmonary embolism in patients with proximal deep-vein thrombosis. N Engl J Med 1998;338(7):409.
16. Mewissen MW, Seabrook GR, Meissner MH, et al: Catheter-directed thrombolysis of lower extremity deep venous thrombosis: Report of a national multicenter registry. Radiology 1999;211(1):39.
17. Ginsberg JS, Hirsh J: Use of antithrombotic agents during pregnancy. Chest 1998;114(5):524S.
18. Ramin SM, Ramin KD, Gilstrap LC: Anticoagulants and thrombolytics during pregnancy. Semin Perinatol 1997;21(2):149.
19. Sanson B-J, Lensing AWA, Prins MH, et al: Safety of low-molecular weight heparin in pregnancy: A systematic review. Thromb Haemost 1999;81(5):668.
20. Koopman MMW, Prandoni P, Piovella F, et al: Treatment of venous thrombosis with intravenous unfractionated heparin administered in the hospital as compared with subcutaneous low-molecular-weight heparin administered at home. N Engl J Med 1996;334(11):682.
21. Siragusa S, Cosmi B, Piovella F, et al: Low-molecular-weight heparins and unfractionated heparin in the treatment of patients with acute venous thromboembolism: Results of a meta-analysis. Am J Med 1996;100(3):269.
22. Yusen RD, Haraden BM, Gage BF, et al: Criteria for outpatient management of proximal lower extremity deep venous thrombosis. Chest 1999;115(4):972.
23. Wells PS, Kovacs MJ, Bormanis J, et al: Expanding eligibility for outpatient treatment of deep venous thrombosis and pulmonary embolism with low-molecular-weight heparin: A comparison of patient self-injection with homecare injection. Arch Intern Med 1998;158(16):1809.
24. Raschke R, Reilly B, Guidry J, et al: The weight-based heparin dosing nomogram compared with a "standard care" nomogram: A randomized controlled trial. Ann Intern Med 1993;119(9):874.
25. Hirsh J: The optimal duration of anticoagulant therapy for venous thrombosis. N Engl J Med 1995;332(25):1710.
26. Diuguid DL: Oral anticoagulant therapy for venous thromboembolism. N Engl J Med 1997;336(6):433.
27. Brandjes D, Buller H, Heijboer H, et al: Randomised trial of effect of compression stockings in patients with symptomatic proximal-vein thrombosis. Lancet 1997;349(9054):759.

LOWER EXTREMITY DEEP VEIN THROMBOSIS

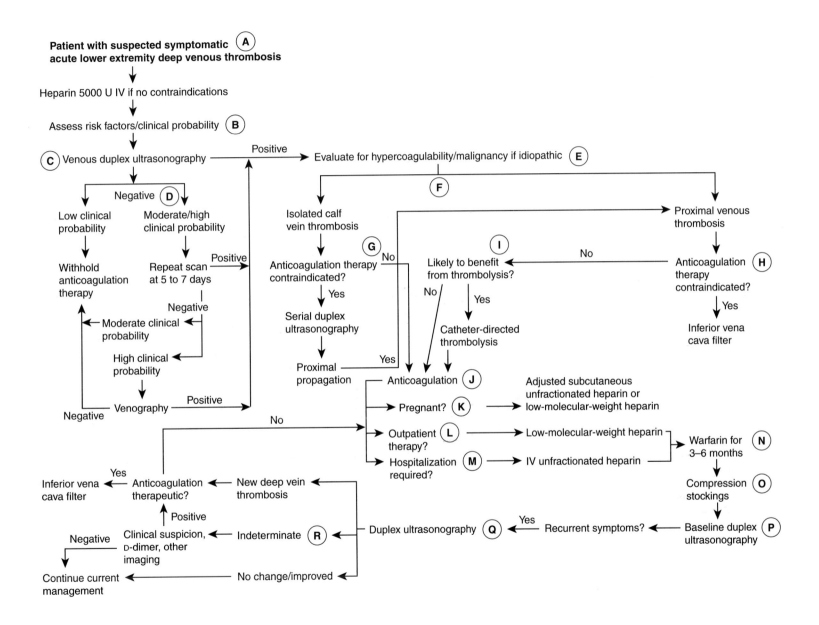

Chapter 57 *Iliofemoral Deep Vein Thrombosis*

ANTHONY J. COMEROTA, MD

A The diagnosis of iliofemoral deep venous thrombosis (DVT) often is suspected on a clinical basis and confirmed with venous duplex ultrasound imaging. The distribution of clot in the infrainguinal venous system is well detailed by the venous duplex examination. The proximal extent of thrombus is evaluated in patients who are to undergo venous thrombectomy or catheter-directed lysis. If anticoagulation therapy is chosen as the preferred treatment, details about the proximal extent of clot are of interest but will not alter treatment.

B After the diagnosis of iliofemoral DVT is established, patients are evaluated for their risk of treatment (lytic therapy or thrombectomy), their level of activity prior to DVT, and their life expectancy. If the patient is not active and not ambulatory, has a high risk for intervention, or has short life expectancy, anticoagulation therapy is recommended.

C When treating patients with anticoagulation for acute DVT, my colleagues and I administer large doses of heparin initially to achieve "supratherapeutic" partial thromboplastin time (PTT > 100 seconds). This is not associated with increased bleeding risk in the absence of co-morbidities for bleeding.[1,2] Supratherapeutic anticoagulation with heparin ensures full anticoagulation and reduces the number of blood tests required to monitor therapy. In addition to anticoagulation, the patient's leg is elevated to reduce swelling.

D If anticoagulation and elevation control symptoms, this treatment is continued. If patients demonstrate progressive edema, pain, cyanosis or particularly, skin blistering, however, reconsideration must be given to therapy that removes the clot and reduces venous hypertension. Because the last two signs of progression are often followed by venous gangrene if obstruction is not promptly relieved, thrombectomy rather than catheter-directed thrombolysis may be indicated for more rapid clot removal.

E Current data support anticoagulation for a minimum of 1 year or more after the initial episode of DVT.[3] In patients with extensive iliofemoral DVT, however, anticoagulation extending beyond 1 year may be necessary. If the patient has an underlying inherited hypercoagulable disorder or a history of recurrent DVT, indefinite anticoagulation is recommended. Leg elevation and compression are recommended during the remainder of the hospitalization to speed resolution of symptoms and to relieve persistent edema. Long-term support with a well-fitting elastic stocking, with a minimum of 30 to 40 mmHg pressure applied at the ankle, is important in control of post-thrombotic leg edema.

F All patients considered for venous thrombectomy and catheter-directed thrombolysis undergo full iliocavagraphy via the opposite groin. Knowledge of the proximal extent of thrombus and its configuration is important to properly plan both catheter directed thrombolysis and venous thrombectomy. The principles behind these interventions are:

1. Removing the clot.
2. Restoring unobstructed venous drainage to the vena cava (at least from profunda femoris vein).
3. Correcting any underlying iliac vein lesion.
4. Avoiding rethrombosis.

G Catheter-directed thrombolysis is the preferred initial therapeutic approach unless lytic therapy is contraindicated.[4-7] Contraindications include:

1. Intracranial disease.
2. Recent eye operations (within 3 months).
3. A current source of bleeding.
4. Recent major trauma.
5. Severe hypertension.

H If there are no contraindications to lytic therapy, the phlebogram is assessed for the presence of free-floating caval thrombus.

I If free-floating caval thrombus is present, a vena caval filter is placed above the caval clot because of concern that early lysis will dislodge the anchoring thrombus before the bulk of the caval thrombus is dissolved, thereby producing a pulmonary embolus.

J The preferred access for catheter-directed lytic therapy is ultrasound-guided popliteal vein puncture with antegrade advancement of the infusion catheter. Alternatively, ultrasound-guided posterior tibial vein access can be considered. Both techniques allow antegrade advancement of the catheters and infusion of the plasminogen activator directly into the thrombus.

The majority of the experience with catheter-directed thrombolysis is with urokinase, given as a bolus of 250,000 to 500,000 units, followed by a continuous infusion of 250,000 to 400,000 units/hr. We have used recombinant tissue plasminogen activator (rt-PA), infusing a bolus of 4 to 5 mg, followed by a continuous infusion of 2 to 4 mg/hr. The progress of clot lysis is monitored by repeated phlebography at 8- to 12-hour intervals, and the catheters are repositioned, as needed, to maximize intrathrombus infusion.

K After successful catheter-directed thrombolysis or venous thrombectomy, completion iliofemoral phlebography is performed to evaluate the iliac veins for an underlying stenosis. Common iliac vein stenotic lesions are frequently found, particularly on the left. If one exists, it must be corrected to maintain long-term patency. Generally, balloon angioplasty is performed. If recoil of the lesion is observed, a venous stent is inserted. If recoil is not observed and luminal integrity is maintained, a stent is not required.

L Venous thrombectomy is recommended if lytic therapy is contraindicated, if catheter placement within the thrombus has failed, or if lysis has been unsuccessful despite proper catheter positioning. Occasional patients with painfully

ILIOFEMORAL DEEP VEIN THROMBOSIS

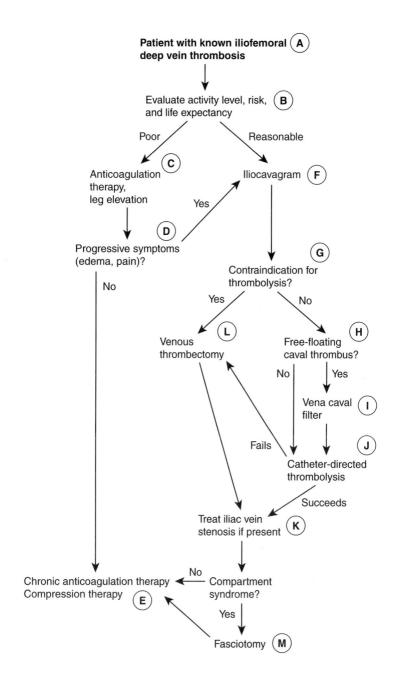

swollen cyanotic legs (phlegmasia cerulea dolens) progress to blistering or blebbing and may need thrombectomy rather than thrombolysis because the latter procedure is much slower, often taking 48 (or more) hours to complete. In rare instances, it may be applied when there is an urgent need for clot removal (e.g., impending venous gangrene), since adequate clot lysis may take days to achieve.

The technical details of venous thrombectomy have been well described.[8-11] The principles are to restore patency and to provide unobstructed venous drainage from the common femoral vein into the vena cava. If inflow to the common femoral vein is compromised because of infrainguinal venous thrombosis, an infrainguinal venous thrombectomy is also required.

Following the thrombectomy, completion iliofemoral phlebography is used to document that the thrombus is removed and to evaluate the status of the iliac venous system. If an underlying stenosis is present, plans are made to correct the iliac lesion. In patients with vena caval clot, retroperitoneal exposure of the vena cava via a right flank incision and concomitant caval thrombectomy are performed.

An arteriovenous fistula (AVF) is constructed by means of either a large proximal branch of the saphenous vein or the saphenous vein itself via anastomosis (end to side) to the superficial femoral artery. A thrombectomy may be required to restore patency to the saphenous vein. The anastomosis should be no larger than 3.5 to 4 mm. Femoral venous pressures are measured before and after the AVF is opened. If the venous pressure rises, the patient must be evaluated for iliac vein obstruction or excessive flow through the fistula.

(M) In patients with massive lower extremity swelling due to venous thrombosis, compartment syndrome may develop, compromising arterial inflow. In such a case, the patient may require fasciotomy, although after successful thrombus removal, fasciotomy is rarely required. Compartment pressures can be measured in these cases as a guide to performing fasciotomy, but this procedure often requires a decision based on clinical assessment.

REFERENCES

1. Conti S, Daschbach M, Blaisdell FW: A comparison of high dose versus conventional dose heparin therapy for deep vein thrombosis. Surgery 1982;92:972.
2. Hull RD, Raskob GE, Rosenbloom D, et al: Optimal therapeutic level of heparin therapy in patients with venous thrombosis. Arch Intern Med 1992;152:1589.
3. Kearon C, Gent M, Hirsh J, et al: A comparison of three months of anticoagulation with extended anticoagulation for a first episode of idiopathic venous thromboembolism. N Engl J Med 1999; 342:955–960.
4. Comerota AJ, Aldridge SC, Cohen G, et al: A strategy of aggressive regional therapy for acute iliofemoral venous thrombosis with contemporary venous thrombectomy or catheter-directed thrombolysis. J Vasc Surg 1994; 20:244–254.
5. Comerota AJ (ed): Thrombolytic therapy for acute deep vein thrombosis. In Thrombolytic Therapy for Peripheral Vascular Disease. Philadelphia, JB Lippincott, 1995.
6. Bjarnason H, Kruse JR, Asinger DA, et al: Iliofemoral deep venous thrombosis: Safety and efficacy outcome during 5 years of catheter-directed thrombolytic therapy. J Vasc Interv Radiol 1997;8:405–418.
7. Mewissen MW, Seabrook GR, Meissner MH, et al: Catheter-directed thrombolysis for lower extremity deep venous thrombosis: Report of a national multicenter registry. Radiology 1999; 211:39–49.
8. Comerota AJ: Venous thrombectomy. In Ginsberg J, Kearon C, Hirsh J (eds): Critical Decisions in Thrombosis and Hemostasis. Hamilton, Ontario, BC Decker, 1998.
9. Comerota AJ: Venous thromboembolism. In Rutherford RB (ed). Vascular Surgery, 4th ed. Philadelphia. W.B. Saunders, 1995.
10. Plate G, Einarsson E, Ohlin P, et al: Thrombectomy with temporary arteriovenous fistula: The treatment of choice in acute iliofemoral venous thrombosis. J Vasc Surg 1984;1:867–876.
11. Plate G, Eklof B, Norgren L, et al: Venous thrombectomy for iliofemoral vein thrombosis: 10-year results of a prospective randomized study. Eur J Vasc Endovasc Surg 1997;14:367.

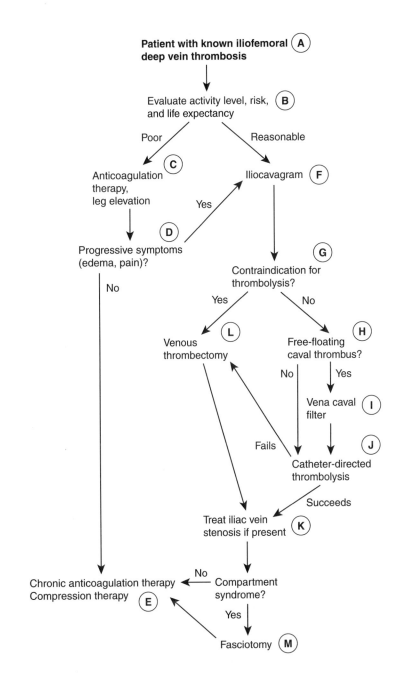

Chapter 58 Pulmonary Embolism

LAZAR J. GREENFIELD, MD • MARY C. PROCTOR, MS

(A) Clinical diagnosis of pulmonary embolism (PE) is highly unreliable, but the presence of *dyspnea, tachypnea,* or *pleuritic chest pain,* which are frequently associated with PE, should lead to objective diagnostic evaluation. If *none* of these features is present, the chance of missing a PE is less than 3%. Among patients with PE, 80% to 90% have at least one recognized risk factor for thromboembolism. As identified in a 1998 report on thromboembolic prophylaxis, the clinical suspicion for PE should be based on a combination of clinical signs and symptoms in addition to risk factors.[1]

Heparin should usually be given immediately to patients in whom PE is suspected; this therapy can be discontinued if the diagnosis proves incorrect (see H and I).

(B) For patients in unexplained shock, immediate evaluation and treatment, including aggressive resuscitation, may prove life-saving. The diagnosis must be confirmed as quickly as possible with a definitive imaging study. Transesophageal echocardiography (TEE) is an accurate, noninvasive method for bedside evaluation of large emboli. The finding of an abnormal intraluminal structure with different echogenicity relative to the blood or vessel wall is diagnostic. In one small series of patients, a positive TEE diagnosis of PE was followed by thrombolytic therapy, which resulted in a decrease in mean pulmonary artery pressure and pulmonary resistance within 24 hours. Surface echocardiography findings of an increase in right ventricular end-diastolic diameter or right ventricular filling pressure or both were associated with PE, as was tricuspid valve regurgitation and right ventricular dysfunction.[2]

Pulmonary angiography remains the standard for diagnosis of PE. When used, it results in low morbidity and mortality, overall cost of treatment is reduced by 40%, and fewer than 5% of patients are treated unnecessarily. This procedure is safe, but the volume of contrast medium should be minimized in the presence of severe pulmonary hypertension.[3] The choice of imaging study often depends on availability of diagnostic methods and the stability and portability of the patient.

(C) A chest x-ray, electrocardiogram, arterial blood gas analysis, and echocardiogram should be obtained in hemodynamically stable patients because all these tests are useful in ruling out other causes of the clinical symptoms or further supporting the diagnosis of PE.[4] They are supportive tests but are not diagnostic in themselves.

(D) A radionuclide ventilation-perfusion ratio ($\dot{V}/\dot{Q}$) scan is next obtained in stable patients through the use of a gamma camera, with relative levels of ventilation and perfusion of the lung mass signifying different levels of suspicion for PE (e.g., normal/low, intermediate/indeterminate, and high suspicion).[5]

(E) Three tests are used to further delineate the diagnosis of PE in those with intermediate or indeterminate $\dot{V}/\dot{Q}$ scan results. The D-dimer test can be used, but the time required to obtain the result makes it impractical in patients with hemodynamic instability.[6] Two methods are available, but the enzyme-linked immunosorbent assay (ELISA) should be used because it has greater predictive value. Using a cutoff ELISA value of 500 µg/L effectively rules out thromboembolism in patients with nondiagnostic $\dot{V}/\dot{Q}$ scan results.

Helical computed tomography (CT) is an alternative diagnostic method receiving much attention. It has reported sensitivities of 60% to 100% and specificities ranging from 81% to 96%. The diagnostic CT criterion for acute PE is an area of low attenuation that completely or partially fills the lumen of a vessel. The sensitivity increases to 86% when subsegmental emboli are excluded. On the basis of available evidence, helical CT is not suitable as a definitive screening test for PE but may clarify nondiagnostic $\dot{V}/\dot{Q}$ findings.[7,8]

The sensitivity and specificity of magnetic resonance imaging (MRI), another noninvasive imaging study for diagnosis of PE, are comparable to those of helical CT (73% and 97%, respectively). The limitations of MRI include poor sensitivity in subsegmental branches and the usual patient contraindications to the procedure (e.g., the need to continue close monitoring and resuscitation, claustrophobia, morbid obesity). The costs of MRI falls between those of $\dot{V}/\dot{Q}$ scanning and pulmonary angiography. Its major advantage is the ability to scan the lungs, inferior vena cava, and lower extremities at the same time.

The choice of an adjunctive test depends on several factors. If the $\dot{V}/\dot{Q}$ results are indeterminate and the clinical suspicion for PE is low, the most appropriate choice may be a D-dimer test, which can effectively rule out PE. If, however, the clinical suspicion for PE remains high, CT or MRI may prove more useful. These imaging methods are fairly comparable with respect to costs and their limitations in viewing PE in the subsegmental branches, where they both lack sensitivity. For patients with renal failure or sensitivity to contrast medium, MRI is preferable to helical CT. When other factors are equal, the decision should be based on availability of testing and the experience and preference of the local radiologists.[9]

(F) When the patient with a major or massive PE is unable to maintain adequate blood pressure and oxygenation without the use of vasopressor agents, fluid resuscitation, and mechanical ventilation and when the diagnosis of PE has been made, rapid intervention is required.

(G) Patients with a diagnosis of PE requiring hemodynamic and ventilatory support must be treated promptly with some form of clot removal technique. The basic options are embolectomy and thrombolysis.

Use of the Greenfield embolectomy catheter offers rapid treatment without the risks associated with thrombolytic therapy or surgical embolectomy with cardiac bypass. Immediately following pulmonary angiography, the embolectomy catheter can be advanced through the right heart to the pulmonary arteries under fluoroscopic guidance. The tip is advanced to the thrombus, which is drawn into the cup by syringe suction. The catheter is then withdrawn while the suction is maintained. The procedure is continued until enough clot is removed to render the patient hemodynamically stable or until no further thrombus can be retrieved.[10, 11]

Thrombolytic therapy should be considered for patients who have major PE with syncope, hypotension, hypoxemia, or heart failure. It may also be used in patients with massive PE who are hemodynamically stable enough to survive the time required for lysis. Streptokinase, urokinase, and tissue plasminogen activator (t-PA) are able to restore lung perfusion, reduce pulmonary hypertension, and lyse residual thrombus. The risks of serious hemorrhagic complications preclude the use of thrombolytic therapy in patients with a recent (2 weeks) history of surgery, pregnancy, gastrointestinal bleeding, hemorrhagic stroke, or trauma.

Thrombolytic therapy has life-saving potential for patients with major or massive PE. It can improve flow dynamics, normalize gas exchange, relieve right ventricle failure, and increase both short-term and long-term exercise capacity. Because the cost of thrombolytic therapy is high, however, it should *not* be used in all hemodynamically stable patients with major PE but instead should be reserved for patients who do not do well with heparin therapy. Furthermore, trials have not been able to demonstrate statistically significant improvement in survival with thrombolytic therapy compared with heparin.[12-14]

The choice between catheter embolectomy and thrombolytic therapy should be based primarily on:

1. The patient's hemodynamic status and resuscitative requirements.
2. The patient's ability to tolerate thrombolytic therapy, in terms of contraindications and the time required.
3. The relative costs of the procedures.

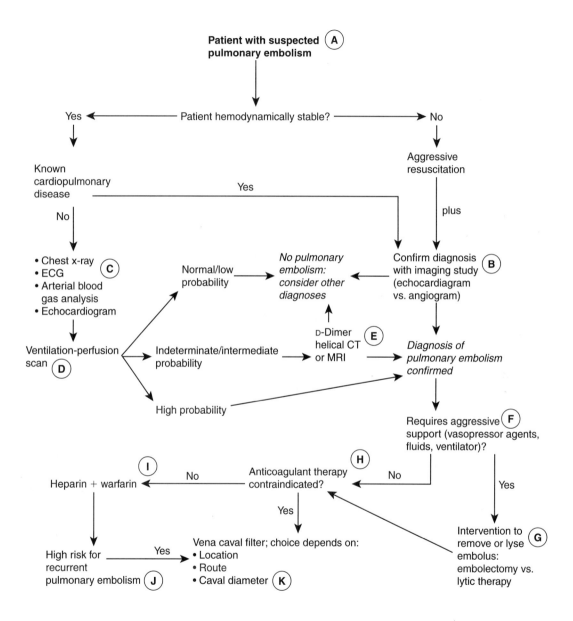

When time is the overriding issue, pulmonary embolectomy is the treatment of choice because it can be performed in any institution with an angiography suite. The procedure does not require cardiopulmonary bypass and can be performed in virtually all patients. When thrombolytic therapy is not contraindicated and the patient is stable enough that time for lysis is not a factor, PE may be treated with thrombolytic agents. Open surgical embolectomy for acute PE is reserved for those rare occasions in which the patient has experienced a cardiac arrest requiring chest compression, making catheter embolectomy impossible, or in which catheter embolectomy has been unsuccessful.

(H) Patients in whom anticoagulation therapy is unsuccessful or who have recurrence of thromboembolism despite adequate anticoagulation are candidates for vena caval interruption with a vena caval filter.

(I) In patients with PE who are initially stable or whose hemodynamic status has been stabilized by clot removal or lysis, anticoagulation with heparin and warfarin is the accepted standard of care. It is given to all patients who do not have a contraindication to anticoagulant therapy.

Unfractionated heparin, given intravenously in doses adjusted to maintain the activated partial thromboplastin time at 1.5 to 2 times the control value, is effective, and this value should be attained within the first 24 hours. Low-molecular-weight heparins administered subcutaneously, with doses adjusted according to body weight, have proved comparable to unfractionated heparin with respect to efficacy and safety. They are also suitable for home administration in patients without massive PE. Oral anticoagulation with warfarin can be initiated concomitantly until the International Normalized Ratio value reaches 2.0 to 3.0, at which time the heparin can be discontinued. Warfarin should be continued up to 6 months after the first episode of major PE.[15]

(J) In addition to patients in whom anticoagulants are contraindicated, some patients may benefit from placement of a vena caval filter even though they are also being given anticoagulants. Placement of such a filter is indicated for patients who undergo pulmonary embolectomy or who are at high risk for an additional PEs because of significant underlying cardiac or respiratory compromise.[12, 16]

A second group of patients who remain at risk for additional PEs are those with an underlying coagulopathy, ongoing immobility, or fresh thrombus in the lower extremities. In such patients, placement of a vena caval filter may be performed in addition to anticoagulation.

(K) The choice of vena caval filter should be based on its demonstrated efficacy and safety. Four types of vena caval filters are currently approved for marketing by the U.S. Food and Drug Administration: (1) Simon Nitinol, (2) VenaTech, (3) Bird's Nest, and (4) Greenfield. Although all the devices appear to be roughly comparable with respect to efficacy in prevention of PE, each has advantages and liabilities of variable significance that may influence its choice. Material integrity, vena caval patency, and mechanical stability should be considered.

Beyond that, the choice of filter may be affected by vena caval diameter, desired filter position, and available access sites. In the rare instance in which the vena caval diameter exceeds 28 mm, the Bird's Nest filter can be used, or one of the other devices can be placed in each of the iliac veins. The most common route for placement is the right femoral vein, followed by the left femoral or right internal jugular vein. All the devices mentioned can be placed via these access sites. When none of these routes is available, a Simon Nitinol filter may be placed via the antecubital vein, but this is an extremely rare circumstance.[17, 18]

When the patient is a female of childbearing potential or if thrombus is filling the vena cava, the filter may need to be positioned above the renal veins. In this case, a titanium Greenfield filter is preferred because it remains patent in this position in 96% to 98% of cases.

REFERENCES

1. Ryu JH, Olson EJ, Pellikka PA: Clinical recognition of pulmonary embolism: Problem of unrecognized and asymptomatic cases. Mayo Clin Proc 1998;73:873–879.
2. Krivec B, Voga G, Zuran I, et al: Diagnosis and treatment of shock due to massive pulmonary embolism. Chest 1997;112:1310–1316.
3. Oudkerk M, Van Beek EJR, Van Putten WLJ, Buller HR: Cost-effectiveness analysis of various strategies in the diagnostic management of pulmonary embolism. Arch Intern Med 1993;153:947–954.
4. Stein PD, Terrin ML, Hales CA, et al: Clinical, laboratory, roentgenographic, and electrocardiographic findings in patients with acute pulmonary embolism and no pre-existing cardiac or pulmonary disease. Chest 1991; 100:598–603.
5. Value of the ventilation/perfusion scan in acute pulmonary embolism: Results of the Prospective Investigation of Pulmonary Embolism Diagnosis (PIOPED). JAMA 1990;268:2753–2759.
6. Perrier A, Bounameaux H, Morabia A, et al: Diagnosis of pulmonary embolism by a decision analysis-based strategy including clinical probability, D-dimer levels, and ultrasonography: A management study. Arch Intern Med 1996;156:531–536.
7. Drucker EA, Rivitz SM, Shepard JO, et al: Acute pulmonary embolism assessment of helical CT for diagnosis. Radiology 1998;209:235–241.
8. Garg K, Welsh CH, Feyerabend AJ, et al: Pulmonary embolism: Diagnosis with spiral CT and ventilation-perfusion scanning—correlation with pulmonary angiographic results or clinical outcome. Radiology 1998;208:201–208.
9. Tapson VF: Pulmonary embolism—new diagnostic approaches. N Engl J Med 1997;336:1449–1451.
10. Greenfield LJ, Proctor MC, Williams D, Wakefield T: Long-term experience with transvenous catheter pulmonary embolectomy. J Vasc Surg 1993;18:450–458.
11. Greenfield LJ, Proctor MC: Long-term experience with transvenous catheter pulmonary embolectomy: Why we should be doing it. In Veith FJ (ed): Current Critical Problems in Vascular Surgery, 6th ed. St. Louis, Quality Medical Publishing, 1994, pp 92–98.
12. Hirsh J, Hoak J: Management of deep vein thrombosis and pulmonary embolism: A statement for healthcare professionals. Circulation 1996;93:2212–2245.
13. Turkstra F, Koopman MMW, Buller HR: The treatment of deep vein thrombosis and pulmonary embolism. Thromb Haemost 1997;78:489–496.
14. Pini M: The role of thrombolytic therapy in the treatment of pulmonary embolism. Haematologica 1997;82:258–261.
15. Haas SK: Treatment of deep venous thrombosis and pul-

monary embolism. Med Clin North Am 1998;82:495–511.
16. Handler JA, Feied CF: Acute pulmonary embolism: Aggressive therapy with anticoagulants and thrombolytics. Postgrad Med 1995;97:61–72.
17. Cho KJ, Proctor MC, Greenfield LJ: Efficacy and problems associated with inferior vena cava filters. In Cope C (ed): Current Techniques in Interventional Radiology. Philadelphia, Current Medicine, 1994, pp 8.1–8.17.
18. Greenfield LJ, Cho KJ, Proctor MC, et al: Late results of suprarenal Greenfield vena cava filter placement. Arch Surg 1992;127:969–973.

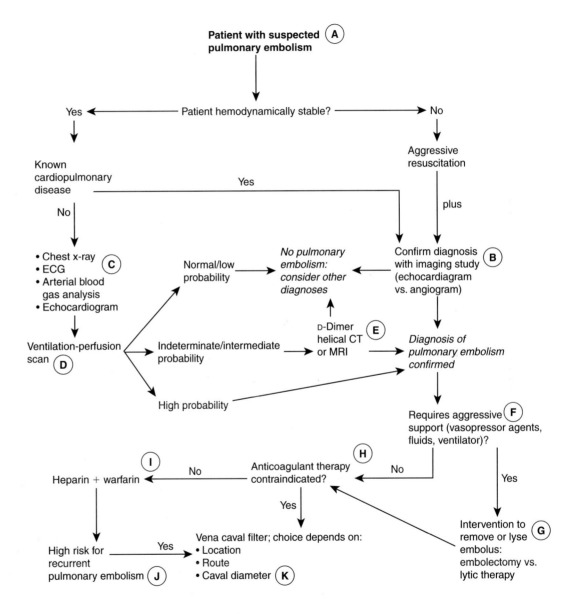

Chapter 59 Varicose Veins

ROBERT B. RUTHERFORD, MD

(A) Clinical evaluation of a patient with varicose veins (VVs) should focus on (1) the patient's symptoms and cosmetic concerns (to establish indications for intervention), (2) the extent and distribution of the varicosities themselves, (3) the severity and location of any associated venous insufficiency in terms of edema and secondary changes in the skin and subcutaneous tissue, and (4) separation of primary varicose veins from varicose veins secondary to prior deep vein thrombosis (DVT) or congenital venous malformations (CVMs) or arteriovenous malformations (AVMs).

Of historical importance are (1) family history of varicose veins or clotting tendency, (2) time of onset and rate of progression, (3) past and anticipated future pregnancies or occupational or medical causes of increased intra-abdominal pressure, and (4) history of venous thrombosis, either deep (DVT) or in the varicosities themselves.

Most patients with primary varicose veins have inherited a predisposition to them, and their family history is frequently positive for the disease. Doppler ultrasound studies have shown a significantly higher incidence of saphenofemoral incompetence in the children of patients with varicose veins.[1] Primary varicose veins may appear in the first years after puberty in such an individual but often not until a first pregnancy. They commonly first appear on the medial calf, if of greater saphenous vein origin (GSV), or the posterior calf, if of lesser saphenous vein (LSV) origin. A localized cluster of varicose veins in the calf may suggest an incompetent perforating vein as the origin. Earlier onset or atypical distribution should suggest that the varicose veins may be a part of a CVM, and a pathognomonic "birthmark" should be sought (see Chapter 71).

The appearance of patients with primary varicose veins who present late with secondary skin changes (pigmentation, cutaneous atrophy, subcutaneous fibrosis, ulceration) may be quite similar to that of patients with late sequelae from DVT. For diagnosis, the sequence is important. Patients with primary varicose veins describe having the varicose veins for years before the secondary changes. Patients with secondary varicose veins, however, may not recall a DVT but do at least describe having normal legs before a certain time when swelling began, with the appearance of varicose veins some time later. Physical examination should determine the extent and distribution of varicose veins and any associated edema and secondary skin changes.

(B) *Significant edema, secondary skin changes*, or *ulceration* is a clear indication for intervention, but each may require additional procedures beyond those for dealing with the varicose veins themselves (e.g., perforating vein interruption). The additional treatment can be planned only after venous duplex scanning, which is therefore the next step for such patients.

(C) For patients without edema or skin changes, the decision concerning varicose vein treatment is more involved. *Pain* is an accepted indication for surgery, but is not an absolute one, and must be considered in relation to the varicose veins. If the pain is significant and is clearly associated with the varicose veins (i.e., localized to the varicose veins, exacerbated by standing, and relieved by elevation), the decision is straightforward. The patient with more diffuse discomfort or atypical pain, particularly when it is out of proportion to the apparent varicose veins, is better given a trial of elastic stockings to see whether they relieve the symptoms.

Some patients with long-standing painless varicose veins who experience leg pain may assume that the pain is due to the varicosities, as may their primary care physician, but it may be due to arthritis or some other cause. Compression therapy with periodic leg elevation is optimal advice not only for patients with diffuse symptoms and minor varicose veins but also for elderly patients, poor-risk patients, and patients with secondary varicose veins that are a relatively small part of their venous insufficiency (i.e., those with major deep venous insufficiency; see Chapters 60 and 61).

In patients with primary varicose veins, there is often controversy about the treatment of essentially asymptomatic veins for cosmetic reasons. Health care agencies often do not reimburse for treatment of this indication, further complicating the issue. Because cosmetic concerns may have a major psychological impact, I believe that healthy patients with *unsightly varicosities* deserve treatment.

There is also some prophylactic benefit to this approach; varicose veins progress with time to become larger, with potentially complicating involvement of perforating veins. Women presenting late after multiple pregnancies with long-standing varicose veins that have led to secondary skin changes and ulceration are not uncommon. Surgery for the extensive varicosities and incompetent perforating veins in such patients is much more difficult than treatment of isolated saphenofemoral incompetence in young women.

(D) Patients with varicosities of typical greater saphenous vein distribution and no significant edema or secondary skin changes (CEAP category C2 [see Chapter 60]) *may* be treated without formal vascular laboratory studies *if* the physical examination, along with the findings of a Trendelenburg test, hand-held Doppler ultrasound probe examination, or both are clear.

In many patients, particularly those with straightforward primary varicose veins, the Trendelenburg test can confirm saphenofemoral incompetence and exclude incompetent perforating veins. It is performed either (1) by first collapsing the varicose veins with leg elevation and then showing a delay (>20 seconds) of varicose vein filling after the patient resumes an upright position or (2) by using digital or tourniquet compression at or just below the saphenofemoral junction and observing rapid refilling when the compression is removed.

A hand-held Doppler ultrasound transducer can be used to evaluate the saphenofemoral and saphenopopliteal junctions and even common perforating vein locations. In most vascular practices located in close proximity to a vascular laboratory, it is customary to send all patients with varicose veins to the laboratory for noninvasive testing, although this practice is not worldwide.

(E) All but the simplest cases (see D) are best studied in the vascular diagnostic laboratory. This statement applies to any patient in whom the results of examination and simpler tests are not clear, because proper treatment depends on stratifying disease according to the underlying venous abnormalities. Any patient with significant edema (category C3), secondary skin changes (category C4), or venous ulceration (category C6) deserves vascular laboratory study because these findings indicate that the varicose veins are likely associated with more than saphenofemoral incompetence.

In the past, plethysmographic studies—which involved timing the venous return (VRT) after a series of ankle flexions and then monitoring the effect of a tourniquet placed successively at the upper thigh, lower thigh, upper calf, and lower calf levels on the VRT—were used to distinguish patients with pure greater saphenous vein incompetence from those with associated perforating vein incompetence or lesser saphenous vein incompetence. However, duplex ultrasound scanning now provides more accurate physiologic and anatomic information about venous insufficiency. It can easily distinguish patients with greater saphenous vein incompetence alone from those with perforating venous insufficiency or deep venous insufficiency or both, and can be used to localize incompetent perforating veins. Venography is rarely used unless venous reconstruction is contemplated (see Chapter 61).

(F) Isolated greater saphenous vein incompetence is the most common underlying abnormality associated with primary varicose veins. It

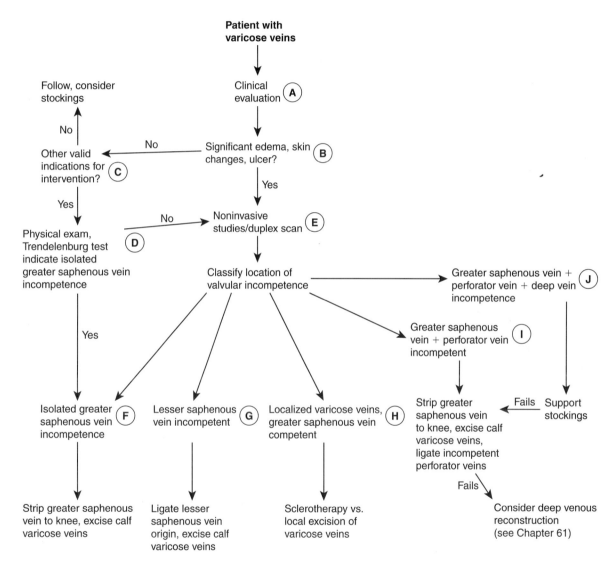

Varicose Veins (continued)

may be treated in a number of ways, but high ligation (usually with stripping) is the standard. Sclerotherapy does not reliably control incompetence,[2] and there is not yet sufficient follow-up of radiofrequency obliteration to prove its efficacy.[3] Management of the greater saphenous vein after high ligation has varied from complete stripping to the ankle (associated with annoying saphenous nerve trauma) to preservation of the vein for future use by sclerosis or excision of varices after high ligation. High ligation without stripping has led to a high recurrence rate, however,[4, 5] so that greater saphenous vein stripping to just below the knee (near the confluence with the posterior arch and anterior branch) is most commonly performed today.

Varicose veins that cannot be reached through the lower incision are usually treated by stab avulsion, although smaller varicose veins can be controlled by sclerotherapy. Very large varicose veins, especially so-called medusa head clusters, should be directly excised.

The word "stripping" here is used in a generic sense. It is still the most common way of excising the greater saphenous vein, but video-assisted techniques, developed for vein harvest, are also being used, as is an inversion technique that turns the greater saphenous vein inside out as it is removed. Chandler and associates[3] have described advancing a radiofrequency-heated catheter up the greater saphenous vein to near its termination and using the catheter to obliterate the vein lumen. A significant incidence of nerve complications associated with this procedure is said to have been reduced with greater experience. Until these alternative approaches show a significant reduction in morbidity and long-term control of the greater saphenous vein, stripping will remain the standard treatment.

(G) Isolated lesser saphenous incompetence as the cause of calf varicose veins is also relatively uncommon. When calf varicosities are associated with greater saphenous vein varicosities, a communicating vein of Giacomini should be sought. The location of the saphenopopliteal junction is variable and may be quite high.[6] It should be determined by duplex scanning to allow the necessary high ligation to be performed with ease. The varicose veins can be treated as described in D.

(H) After thorough study, localized clusters of varicose veins may occasionally be seen that are found not associated with incompetence of a communicating vein.[7] They may be treated with local excision (commonly, avulsion through small stab incisions[6]) or sclerotherapy. The latter procedure is effective, in carefully selected cases, for small to medium-sized varicosities.

(I) When there are also *significant* incompetent perforating veins, they should undergo interruption in addition to the greater saphenous vein stripping and high ligation. The method of perforating vein interruption has evolved from the open techniques of Cockett and Linton, to the multiple incisions of DePalma, to clipping of the perforating veins through a strategically placed lower incision for stripping, to opening of the fascia and use of long instruments developed for laparoscopic procedures (subfascial endoscopic perforating vein surgery [SEPS]).[8, 9]

The choice between performing all these maneuvers at one operation and first performing greater saphenous vein stripping and later perforating vein interruption in those who need it is a matter of debate. Stripping the greater saphenous vein does not interrupt and correct perforating vein incompetence.[10] The most commonly involved perforating veins communicate with the posterior arch tributary, not with the greater saphenous vein itself, and are therefore missed even if stripping is carried down to the ankle. Stripping of the greater saphenous varicosities may obviate the need for perforator interruption. However, in patients with advanced secondary changes and multiple incompetent perforating veins, a case can be made for concomitant procedures.

(J) In a patient with varicose veins plus perforating vein and deep vein incompetence, conservative treatment with support stockings is used initially, because by itself this treatment may control symptoms and because support stockings would probably be necessary even if the varicose veins are removed. In patients with venous ulcers or other advanced disease, however, support stockings may be insufficient. (see Chapters 60 and 61). In these cases, it is usually recommended to excise the incompetent greater saphenous vein and ligate incompetent perforating veins before considering deep vein reconstruction.

A number of studies have shown that interruption of superficial or perforating veins, or both, has significantly benefited such patients and that the deep venous insufficiency has actually improved or disappeared.[11, 12] If this approach fails, deep vein reconstruction is appropriate for selected patients (see Chapter 61).

REFERENCES

1. Regan B, Folse R: Lower limb venous hemodynamics in normal patients and children of patients with varicose veins. Surg Gynecol Obstet 1971;132:15–18.
2. Bishop CC, Fronek HS, Fronek A, et al: Real-time color duplex scanning after sclerotherapy of the greater saphenous vein. J Vasc Surg 1991;14:505–508.
3. Chandler JG, Pichot O, Sessa C, et al: Results of radiofrequency ablation of the greater saphenous. J Vasc Surg (in press).
4. McMullin, GM, Colleridge Smith PD, Scurr JH: Objective assessment of high ligation without stripping the long saphenous vein. Br J Surg 1991;78:1139–1141.
5. Munn SR, Morton JB, MacBeth WAAG, McLeisch AR: To strip or not to strip the long saphenous vein? A varicose vein trial. Br J Surg 1981;68:426–428.
6. Ricci S, Giogiev M, Goldman MP: Ambulatory Phlebectomy. St. Louis, CV Mosby, 1995.
7. Labropolous N, Kang SS, Mansour MA, et al: Primary superficial vein reflux with competent saphenous trunk. Eur J Vasc Endovasc Surg 1999;18:201–206.
8. Pierek EGJM, van Urk H, Hop WCJ, Wittens CHA: Endoscopic vs. open subfascial division of incompetent perforator veins in the treatment of venous leg ulceration: A randomized trial. J Vasc Surg 1997;26:1049–1054.
9. Gloviczki P, Bergan JJ, Rhodes JM, and the North American Study Group: Mid-term results of endoscopic perfora-

tor vein interruption for chronic venous insufficiency: Lessons learned from the North American Subfascial Endoscopic Perforator Surgery (NASEPS) registry. J Vasc Surg 1999;29:489–499.
10. Stuart WP, Adam DJ, Allan PL, et al: Saphenous surgery does not correct perforator incompetence in the presence of deep venous reflux. J Vasc Surg 1998;28:834–838.
11. Sales CM, Bilof ML, Petrillo KA, Luka NL: Correction of lower extremity deep venous incompetence by ablation of superficial venous reflux. Ann Vasc Surg 1996;10:186–189.
12. Walsh JC, Bergan JJ, Beeman S, Comer TP: Femoral venous reflux abolished by greater saphenous stripping. Ann Vasc Surg 1994;8:566–570.

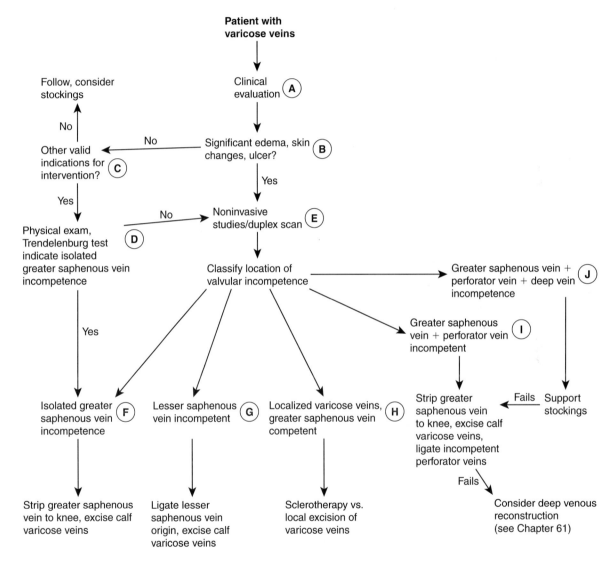

Chapter 60 Deep Vein Insufficiency: Evaluation and Conservative Management

AHMED M. ABOU-ZAMZAM, MD • GREGORY L. MONETA, MD

(A) Twenty-seven percent of people in the United States have some degree of chronic venous disease (CVD) of the lower extremity. In Europe, 1.5% of adults have venous stasis ulcers. Venous ulceration leads to severe physical impairment and diminished quality of life with limitation of earning capacity and leisure activities.[1] Severe CVD, primarily venous valvular insufficiency, may manifest as leg swelling, heaviness, aching pains associated with and worsened by prolonged standing or sitting, chronic edema, stasis dermatitis, or ulceration.

Multivariate analysis has identified greater age, previous deep vein thrombosis (DVT), lower extremity trauma, male sex, and obesity as independent risk factors for venous stasis ulcers. Any previous episodes in the patient history of venous thromboembolism are important, as is any family history of venous disease or hypercoagulable states. Most patients have a history of these risk factors. Other causes of edema, such as congestive heart failure and renal failure, should also be excluded.

(B) Physical examination should be directed toward identifying and characterizing the severity of the signs of CVD:

- Lower extremity telangiectases
- Reticular veins
- Varicose veins
- Edema
- Skin changes (brawny induration, stasis dermatitis, hemosiderin deposition)
- Evidence of healed ulcers
- Any active ulcers

A thorough pulse examination should be performed to rule out concomitant arterial insufficiency, which can be associated with CVD and can contribute to nonhealing of venous ulcers. A bedside Trendelenburg test (elevating the leg, applying a tourniquet, then observing varicose vein filling with standing alone and then with early release of the tourniquet) may be performed as a gross estimate of the presence of superficial and deep venous insufficiency. The presence of Homans' sign is not a worthwhile indicator because it lacks accuracy.

(C) The CEAP system is a means of characterizing patients with CVD.[2]

Clinical (C) signs are graded as 0 through 6:

0   No disease
1   Telangiectases
2   Varicose veins
3   Edema without skin changes
4   Skin changes due to venous disease
5   Healed ulceration
6   Active ulceration

Etiologic (E) classification is defined as congenital, primary, or secondary (i.e., due to DVT).

Anatomic (A) distribution is listed as superficial, deep, perforating, or any combination.

Pathophysiologic (P) dysfunction is described as reflux, obstruction, or combined.

The CEAP classification system allows more accurate comparisons of patient groups and should provide more reliable assessment of the results of therapeutic interventions.

(D) Lymphedema can usually be distinguished from CVD on the basis of the history and physical examination. Young patients who present with unilateral leg edema near or soon after puberty are very likely to have lymphedema. The quality of the edema is typically "brawny and pitting" in venous disease, whereas it is "soft and spongy" in early lymphedema. Venous edema often markedly diminishes with overnight elevation, but lymphedema does not respond promptly to limb elevation. Involvement of the dorsum of the feet and base of the toes is classic for lymphedema; venous edema generally spares the feet and centers on the ankle and lower leg. Chronic venous swelling is associated with stasis pigmentation of the lower leg and cutaneous atrophy; lymphedema is associated with cutaneous thickening, and pigmentation is usually limited or absent.

If doubt persists about the differential diagnosis, noninvasive venous testing may be performed. The presence of unilateral edema and normal results of venous studies strongly suggest lymphedema.

(E) Patients with grossly infected venous ulcers may require hospitalization. In all patients, bed rest to control edema and local wound care with soap-and-water scrubs are used. Intravenous antibiotics may be required. For long-neglected wounds, whirlpool therapy may be of some aid. DVT prophylaxis is important in this patient group. Surgical débridement is occasionally necessary.

(F) Noninvasive vascular laboratory studies can characterize the location, extent, and pathophysiology of CVD. The following tests are employed:

1. *Photoplethysmography:* Provides a noninvasive measure of venous recovery time and an assessment of overall lower extremity venous function. Occlusion of the superficial system with a tourniquet is routinely performed to document the pattern of disease—isolated superficial disease or combined superficial and deep disease.
2. *Air plethysmography:* Provides several measurements helpful in the assessment of venous disease. The venous filling index is a measure of venous reflux. The venous ejection fraction reflects reflux and calf muscle pump function. The residual volume fraction indicates overall venous function.

3. *Venous duplex scan:* Has several advantages. Any obstruction due to venous thrombosis (acute or chronic) can be accurately identified. Reflux can also be reliably localized to specific venous segments (e.g., greater saphenous vein, femoral vein, profunda femoris vein).

G Some patients may have normal or mildly abnormal noninvasive test results yet may show signs and symptoms entirely consistent with CVD. These patients are best treated with long-term compression therapy.

H Compression therapy may involve the use of graded-compression stockings (knee-high, 30 to 40 mmHg), elastic wraps, layered bandages, or Unna boots. In patients with oddly shaped legs, a legging orthosis is available. Called a CircAid, this device consists of multiple pliable, adjustable compression bands that wrap around the leg from the ankle to the knee and are held in place with hook-and-loop tape (Velcro).

The goals of compression therapy are to:

1. Control the leg swelling with counterpressure to offset the ambulatory venous hypertension that is present in all patients with significant CVD.
2. Promote healing of venous ulcers, if present.
3. Prevent future ulcer formation.

Compression therapy devices are worn from the time the patient arises from bed in the morning until the patient goes to bed in the evening. In patients with severe CVD, leg elevation for short periods during the day (e.g., 10 minutes every 2 hours, during coffee and lunch breaks) is helpful, especially in those with jobs requiring long periods of standing.

I Patients with venous ulcers can usually be successfully treated with compression therapy. All that is required for the ulcer is placement of a dry gauze over the wound and, occasionally, a small foam insert directly over the bandage, under the compression garment or bandage. Soap-and-water scrubs of the ulcer are carried out

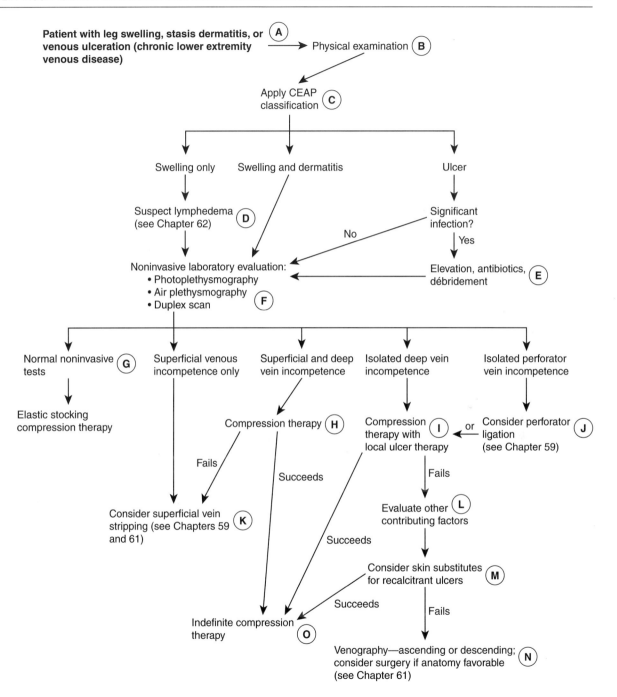

twice daily. Topical steroids can be applied to the areas of surrounding dermatitis but never to the ulcer itself. We have utilized Unna boots or multi-layered wraps in patients who are debilitated, noncompliant, or otherwise unable to perform dressing changes. We avoid gels and other topical agents because of their high cost and unconvincing efficacy.

(J) Patients with isolated perforating vein incompetence directly underlying an ulcer may be considered for ligation or interruption of perforating veins. This procedure may be performed via the subfascial endoscopic approach.[3]

(K) Patients with isolated superficial venous incompetence are candidates for surgical ablation of the involved superficial veins. In the setting of combined superficial and deep venous insufficiency, treatment of the superficial disease alone appears to bring about significant improvement.[4] The patient with this pattern of disease whose symptoms remain incompletely resolved after compression therapy may be considered for superficial venous procedures.

(L) Although we have found that noncompliance is the most common reason for nonhealing of ulcers, other causes must be excluded. Underlying arterial insufficiency must always be ruled out. Fungal or bacterial infection must be controlled and eradicated. In rare instances, malignancy may arise in the area of chronic ulceration; this possibility can be evaluated with a biopsy.

(M) Apligraf, a bioengineered skin substitute, has proved beneficial in speeding the healing of venous ulcers. This agent consists of a keratinocyte-containing epidermis and a dermal layer of fibroblasts separated by a basement membrane. The cells are derived from cultured human neonatal foreskin. Apligraf appears most beneficial in large ulcers (area >10 cm^2), deep ulcers, and chronic ulcers (present > 6 months).[5] The application of an Apligraf is very similar to that of split-thickness skin grafting. All applications are accompanied by rigorous compression therapy.

(N) Venography has been reserved, in our hands, for patients considered for surgical repair or reconstruction. Ascending phlebography defines obstruction accurately, whereas descending phlebography identifies areas of valvular incompetence. These tests are no more helpful than duplex scanning with valve closure times in evaluating the severity of deep venous reflux[6] but are useful for specific surgical planning (see Chapter 61).

(O) We have reviewed the results in 113 patients with venous ulcers who were treated in our institution over a 15-year period.[7] All patients received local wound care and compression therapy. Overall, 93% experienced complete ulcer healing at a mean time of 5.3 months. In patients who were compliant with the compression therapy, a 97% rate of ulcer healing was seen, whereas noncompliant patients experienced a rate of only 55%. Ulcers recurred in 16% of patients who were compliant with compression therapy and in 100% of patients who were noncompliant with the use of elastic stockings. This experience underscores the value of compression therapy and compliance in managing CVD.

REFERENCES

1. Moneta GL, Nehler MR, Porter JM: Pathophysiology of chronic venous insufficiency. In Rutherford RB (ed): Vascular Surgery, 5th ed. Philadelphia, WB Saunders, 2000, pp 1982–1989.
2. Porter JM, Moneta GL, and an International Consensus Committee on Chronic Venous Disease: Reporting standards in venous disease: An update. J Vasc Surg 1995;21:635–645.
3. Gloviczki P, Bergan JJ, Menawat SS, et al: Safety, feasibility, and early efficacy of subfascial endoscopic perforator surgery: A preliminary report from the North American registry. J Vasc Surg 1997;25:94–105.
4. Padberg FT, Pappas PJ, Araki CT, et al: Hemodynamic and clinical improvement after superficial vein ablation in primary combined venous insufficiency with ulceration. J Vasc Surg 1996;24:711–718.
5. Falanga V, Margolis D, Alvarez O, et al: Rapid healing of venous ulcers and lack of clinical rejection with an allogenic cultured human skin equivalent. Arch Dermatol 1998;134:344–349.
6. Welch HJ, Faliakou EC, McLaughlin RL, et al: Comparison of descending phlebography with quantitative photoplethysmography, air plethysmography, and duplex quantitative valve closure time in assessing deep venous reflux. J Vasc Surg 1992;16:913–920.
7. Mayberry JC, Moneta GL, Taylor LM, Porter JM: Fifteen-year results of ambulatory compression therapy for chronic venous ulcers. Surgery 1991;109:575–581.

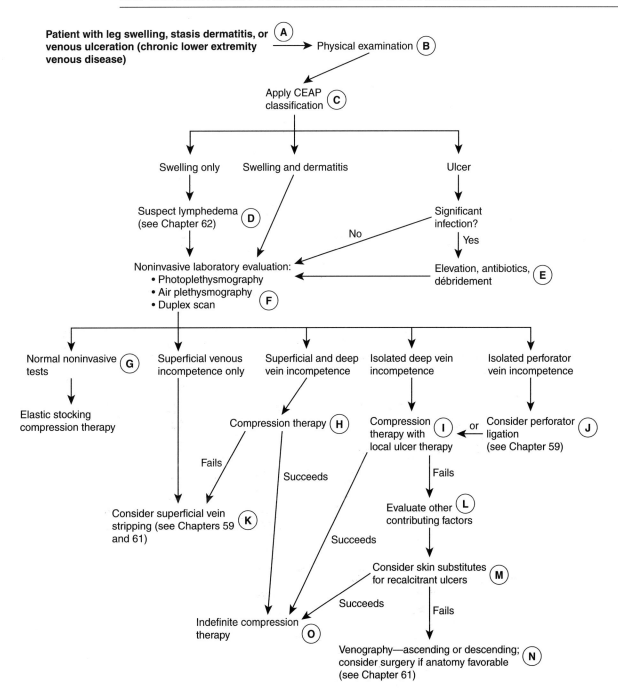

Chapter 61 Deep Vein Insufficiency: Surgical Treatment

ROBERT L. KISTNER, MD • BO EKLOF, MD, PhD

A The candidate for deep venous reconstruction is usually selected because of disabling symptoms that have not responded to more conservative measures (compression therapy) (see Chapter 60) or to surgery of the superficial and perforator veins (see Chapter 59). They have been previously evaluated in the vascular laboratory by tests (duplex scanning, plethysmography) that identify the nature of the venous disease causing the patient's problem (also see Chapter 60).

The primary determinants of surgical treatment of deep venous insufficiency are (1) disabling symptoms and signs that significantly interfere with the individual's way of life and (2) reasonable prospects for relieving them with the contemplated procedure. Surgery offers the opportunity to adapt the venous disease to the patient's way of life rather than making the patient adapt or modify his or her life to the limitations imposed by the disease, as occurs in all nonsurgical therapy. This decision requires consideration of the individual's age, overall health, occupation, and important activities.

The overall strategy of deep venous reconstruction is to provide patency *above* the common femoral vein (CFV), because valve function plays no role proximally, and to provide competence as well as patency in the venous tree *below* the CFV, where reflux is the usual dominant physiologic problem.[1,2]

B Ascending and descending phlebography is usually required for patients with disease *below* the CFV. When the ascending venogram shows a patent venous system and the duplex scan shows severe reflux, descending venography is needed to search for a repairable valve and to classify the extent of reflux. Whereas the duplex scan defines the presence and the segmental location of reflux and obstruction below the CFV, venography demonstrates the exact sites of the valves and provides the best anatomic information about all the major veins draining the extremity. Venography also provides the ultimate preoperative differentiation between primary and secondary disease[3] and identifies the anatomy of congenital venous disease.

C The differentiation between primary and secondary disease and congenital venous disease and their characterization are essential to the development of an appropriate surgical strategy, for the following reasons.

In primary venous insufficiency (PVI), the lumina of the veins and their anatomic course in the extremity are normal. Primary disease is anatomically and physiologically pure reflux disease and involves only veins below the CFV.[4,5] Secondary disease (usually *post-thrombotic syndrome* [PTS]) typically includes an obstructive pattern, which may vary from totally obstructed segments to subtle striae or wall thickening that represents the residue of prior obstruction.[6] The hallmark of significant obstruction is development of abnormally prominent collateral vessels. Both ascending venography and descending venography demonstrate changes that are diagnostic of secondary disease; in addition, descending venography may show abnormal valve sinuses. Secondary obstructive disease, in contrast to primary disease, involves veins both above and below the CFV.

When primary disease is the sole problem in the deep veins, there is frequently a repairable valve in the refluxing veins, the reconstruction of which by direct valvuloplasty offers the best opportunity for a successful long-term correction.[7] When secondary disease is the sole problem, there is rarely the opportunity for valvuloplasty and some form of valve substitution procedure (transplantation or transposition) is necessary.

Congenital venous disease is marked by atypical venous anatomy and variable valvular defects, and in each case venography is necessary to identify its individual characteristics.

Finally, a significant number of cases demonstrate both distal secondary (post-thrombotic) and proximal primary disease, in which a repairable valve is still available in the proximal segment even though the more distal veins are obstructed. After successful valvuloplasty of the proximal valve, these cases of mixed PVI and post-thrombotic syndrome have a superior long-term outcome compared with cases of pure post-thrombotic syndrome, which require a valve substitution procedure.[8]

D Reflux and obstruction may coexist in both secondary and congenital venous disease, presenting the dilemma whether to perform an antireflux operation to treat the valvular incompetence or a bypass or endovascular disobliteration to treat the obstructive problem. In such cases, it is important to determine whether the obstruction or the reflux is dominant. The determination requires consideration of the location and severity of the obstructive lesion. In extreme cases, these features may be obvious from imaging studies, but physiologic tests may be required to solve the dilemma. The following guidelines are offered:

1. Obstruction *above* the CFV is relatively more important and is poorly tolerated in the presence of reflux below the CFV and should be corrected. Subsequently, restoring competence to the axial divisions below the CFV may nevertheless be required to adequately relieve symptoms.
2. If venous pressure is normal immediately below an anatomic obstruction (because of extensive collateral circulation), the obstruction can be ignored and attention devoted to correction of reflux.[9]
3. Because gauging the physiologic significance of an obstruction is the weakest part of venous evaluation, plethysmographic studies, such as air plethysmography (APG), may be combined with venous pressure recordings to solidify the diagnosis. For example, when APG shows severe reflux (venous filling index [VFI] $>$ 8 to 10 mL/sec) and mild obstruction (outflow fraction

[OF] < 40 ± 3 mL/sec), reflux is the dominant problem.

4. When a clear determination cannot be made whether reflux or obstruction is dominant, surgical treatment should be directed first toward the most likely correctable defect, such as repair of a primary valve or endovascular disobliteration of a partially occluded iliac vein. Then a determination should be made as to whether the treatment would suffice.

(E) The important finding on descending venography that helps identify the candidate for a reflux corrective operation is the presence of axial reflux involving both thigh and calf, presenting a continuous column of blood from the heart to the leg below the knee. When a competent valve in either the popliteal vein or superficial femoral vein (SFV) interrupts the axial reflux, deep venous repair or reconstruction is seldom indicated.

(F) In patients with primary reflux or with secondary disease but dominant reflux, the first consideration is that saphenous vein and perforating vein reflux be controlled.[10] In many cases, this control will have already been achieved.[8] In most others, the usual recommendation is to treat the saphenous and large perforating veins before the deep veins, in the hope that persisting symptoms and signs of the deep venous reflux may not require a second operation. A valid exception may be the young patient who performs heavy work, who has severe reflux in all systems, and whose work capacity is limited by advanced venous disease. In this situation, a case can be made for early repair of reflux in all systems, including the deep veins.[11] Patients who have disabling symptoms after superficial and perforator vein surgery deserve consideration for deep venous repair or reconstruction and careful evaluation to determine the most appropriate operation.

(G) The choice of operation for deep venous reflux depends on whether or not there are repairable valves in each of the refluxing axial segments. Control of all continuous axial reflux from groin level to the calf by at least one competent valve per axial division is usually needed to

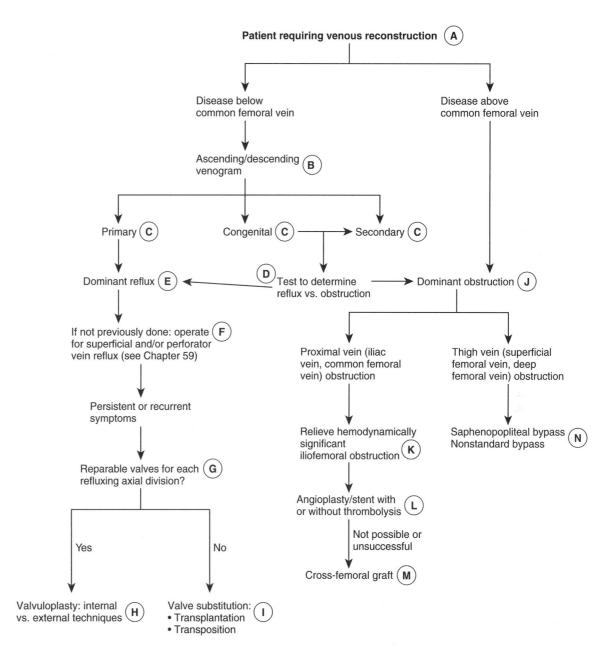

control the venous insufficiency. Therefore, it is important to define valve sites in each of the three axial divisions:

- Greater saphenous vein (GSV)
- Superficial femoral vein (SFV)/popliteotibial vein
- Profunda femoris (deep femoral) vein (PFV)/popliteotibial vein

The option to ligate the incompetent SFV may be useful when other axial segments are competent.[12]

Potentially repairable valves are identified with descending venography. Venographic technique is critical if reliable information is to be gleaned.[13-15] Valve locations in the SFV, GSV, and PFV must be identified separately.

The determination as to operability of the valve is based on the specific findings at the valve site. When the contrast agent refluxes freely down the vein without identifying any valve stations and if there is no sign of diseased intima that would indicate secondary disease, the valves may have been lost to atrophy or there may be aplasia in the vein. The absence of a repairable valve requires a valve substitution procedure, such as transplantation or transposition.

(H) For patients with reflux due to primary disease who have a repairable valve, valvuloplasty is the procedure of choice. One form or another (internal or external) of valve repair can be used for reflux of the SFV, PFV, and GSV. The important point is to achieve at least one site of competence in each axial system. In the case of the PFV, repair is necessary when there is a large, incompetent communication between the distal PFV and the popliteal vein or distal SFV that causes this pathway to become a continuous source of axial reflux from the thigh to the calf.[16] When reflux is limited to the PFV in the thigh, correction of reflux in the PFV valve is usually not warranted.

When the decision to perform valve repair is made, the choice between internal and external repair involves the following considerations:

1. The advantage of an internal over an external valve repair is that the internal repair has been reported in several large series to have consistently good long-term results at more than 5 years,[14, 17-20] and in one series at more than 10 years.[8] This repair is thus a reproducible standard that can be used to judge other approaches. The results of external repair have not been reported in a definitive manner, but there is reason to believe that long-term follow-up will show this repair to be less favorable than the internal approach (S. Raju, 2000, and V.S. Sottiurai, 2001, personal data).
2. The advantages of an external repair, whether by a suture[17, 21] or cuffing[22] technique, over the internal approach are that it is much simpler, is less invasive, does not require heparin, and can more readily be performed on several valves in a single operation. An interesting approach to external repair is the angioscopically guided method that is under investigation in several centers.[23, 24]

(I) When there is no valve to be repaired, a valve substitution procedure is needed, and such procedures confer a less favorable prognosis.[8] The most commonly performed valve substitution procedure is the axillary vein valve transplant to either the SFV or the popliteal vein.[25-27] This procedure has been widely reported, but the results have not been uniform. Some studies[26, 27] have reported very favorable results at 4 years (80% to 90%); other studies with similar or shorter follow-up periods[8, 10, 18] have reported discouraging rates (35% to 45%).

The discrepancy between these reported outcomes is not fully explained but may relate to (1) the placement of the valves in the popliteal vein rather than the superficial vein, (2) repairs of the incompetent valves at the time of transfer, or (3) other technical differences. At harvest, many of the arm valves are found to be incompetent and they require repair at the time of transplant.[11]

Another substitution operation is the transposition procedure. An incompetent axial segment is divided proximally, and its distal end is anastomosed to an adjacent segment that has a competent proximal valve.[28] This procedure has generated a number of reports of inferior long-term results but has continued to have appeal in well-selected cases reported by a few investigators.[8, 18] The discrepancy between the favorable and unfavorable reports is so far unexplained, but the possibilities include the selection of patients and the techniques of dissection and repair.

A later technique is the use of cryopreserved homologous vein valve segments.[29] The advantage of this approach is its availability for patients in whom no valved segments are available, especially those with aplasia or post-thrombotic syndrome who also have incompetent axillary vein valves. This technique carries a high failure rate at 12 months, perhaps largely due to late rejection (M. Dalsing, personal communication, 2000).

A nonreconstructive approach to restore competence to the popliteal vein was reported by Psathakis,[30] who developed a "sling" operation to occlude the popliteal vein during exercise and thereby mimic the valve effect. This procedure has not been widely accepted in the United States, but there are anecdotal cases with favorable results.

(J) When the evaluation reveals obstruction to be the dominant problem (see D), phlebographic study is needed if operation is contemplated. When the problem is limited to obstruction in the iliofemoral segment and the duplex scan shows the veins below the CFV to be patent and competent, descending venography is not performed. In the case of unilateral iliac vein obstruction or stenosis, iliocaval venography is needed to study the proximal inferior vena cava (IVC) for patency and the contralateral iliac vein for extension of the occlusion. In the case of SFV obstruction, other sources of drainage of the calf and popliteal veins need to be found.

(K) Demonstrating the presence of obstruction in the iliac vein by an imaging technique does not in itself constitute an indication for treatment because it may be physiologically insignificant. When the collateral veins are well developed, compensation for the anatomic obstruction is often sufficient for the patient's activity and bypass is superfluous. An important clinical symptom of severe obstruction is venous claudication, which occurs when the extremity becomes congested and may require long periods of elevation to decompress. In the absence of claudication, it is important to perform physiologic studies to confirm that the obstruction is hemodynamically significant. This step establishes not only the need for intervention but also the likelihood of its success.

With the techniques of bypass or disobliteration used to relieve the obstruction, thrombosis tends to occur in the bypassed or disobliterated segment unless there are elevated pressure gradients to generate high flows across the segment.[9, 31] Therefore, it is important to demonstrate elevated femoral vein pressures distal to the obstruction, and plethysmographic confirmation of reduced outflow is supportive.[31]

(L) Treatment of iliac vein obstruction can be achieved with disobliteration of the occlusion using the endovascular techniques of thrombolysis, balloon angioplasty, and stenting[32, 33] or using the surgical techniques of endovenectomy (unpublished data) or bypass of the iliac occlusion using synthetic (ringed) prosthetics[34] or autogenous vein.[35-37] An adjunctive femoral arteriovenous (A-V) fistula can be employed to increase flow and reduce the likelihood of thrombosis of the bypass.[38]

The recent development of endovascular disobliteration of the iliac vein has provided good early results when the occlusion can be crossed with a wire and balloon dilatation achieved. Stenting of the dilated vein appears successful in the first year or two of follow-up.[32, 33] Because this is an endovascular procedure, it is readily tolerated by the patient. A femoral A-V fistula has not been used in the majority of these disobliteration procedures, and there is no present evidence that it is needed. There is some fear that an A-V fistula would create more turbulence, leading to earlier endothelial hyperplasia and thereby creating an unfavorable environment over the long term.

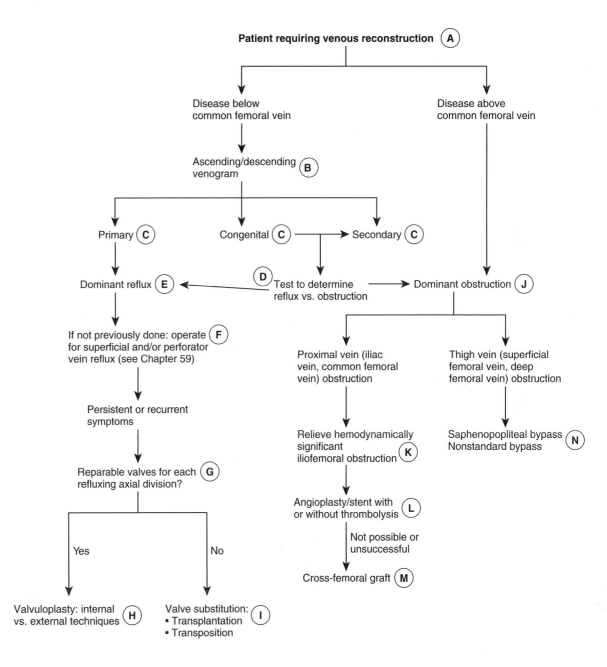

Deep Vein Insufficiency: Surgical Treatment (continued)

(M) When the iliac vein cannot be disobliterated, the only way to provide outflow from the extremity is to use a bypass. The contralateral saphenous vein has been used for many years in the form of the Palma-Dale transfemoral bypass.[35-37] An important limitation to this bypass is its small size, which has led to the use of a ringed polytetrafluoroethylene (PTFE) synthetic bypass from the ipsilateral femoral vein to the contralateral iliac or femoral vein[34] or, in some cases, to the IVC.[39] These synthetic bypasses are always performed with an adjunctive femoral A-V fistula. Results of these bypasses are mixed.[31]

(N) A few patients are very symptomatic from obstruction of the SFV and may benefit from bypass of the SFV by means of a saphenopopliteal anastomosis.[40] This situation occurs in the post-thrombotic state and occasionally after traumatic occlusion, when either the SFV and its collateral vessels are occluded or when the SFV lacks effective collateral vessels and communications via the GSV and the PFV are deficient. The selection of such cases is based on the presence of venous claudication and confirmation by duplex scan and venography of extremely poor outflow from the popliteal vein. Because the popliteal vein is partially occluded in many of these cases, the candidate for bypass must still have an adequate popliteal vein for anastomosis and, of course, a patent GSV.

The venous pressure measured in the foot is not very helpful because elevated foot pressure can be due to many causes. It is possible, however, that evaluation of the popliteal pressure in this particular group of patients would show local hypertension due to outlet obstruction at this level.[41] In some of these bypasses, the GSV will have remained competent; in others, the dilated GSV becomes incompetent but a retained valve in the vein may be present that can be repaired to provide a competent outflow from the congested calf.

In patients qualifying for bypass of the SFV, the anatomy may not be suitable for a popliteosaphenous bypass. However, with thorough imaging, it may be possible to find anatomic variants that permit bypass decompression of the congested calf. We have used a Giacomini vein and a lateral branch of the CFV for this purpose.

REFERENCES

1. Labropoulos N, Delis K, Nicolaides AN, et al: The role of the distribution and anatomic extent of reflux in the development of signs and symptoms in chronic venous insufficiency. J Vasc Surg 1996;23:504–510.
2. Ackroyd JS, Browse NL: The investigation and surgery of the post-thrombotic syndrome. J Cardiovasc Surg 1986;27:5–15.
3. Masuda EM, Kistner RL: Prospective comparison of duplex scanning and descending venography in the assessment of venous insufficiency. Am J Surg 1992;164:254–258.
4. Kistner RL: Primary venous valve incompetence of the leg. Am J Surg 1980;140:218–224.
5. Browse NL, Burnand KG, Thomas ML: Varicose veins: Pathology. In Diseases of the Veins: Pathology, Diagnosis and Treatment. London, Edward Arnold, 1988, pp 151–165.
6. Browse NL, Burnand KG, Thomas ML: Pathologic features of a deep vein thrombosis. In Diseases of the Veins: Pathology, Diagnosis and Treatment. London, Edward Arnold, 1988, pp 460–463.
7. Kistner RL, Eklof B, Yang D, Masuda EM: Venous reconstruction: Evidence-based analysis of results. In Ballard JL, Bergan JJ (eds): Chronic Venous Insufficiency: Diagnosis and Treatment. London, Springer, 2000, pp 139–150.
8. Masuda EM, Kistner RL: Long-term results of venous valve reconstruction: A 4- to 21-year follow-up. J Vasc Surg 1994;19:391–403.
9. Raju S, Fredericks R: Venous obstruction: An analysis of 137 cases with hemodynamic, venographic and clinical correlations. J Vasc Surg 1991;13:91–100.
10. Ericksson I, Almgren B, Nordgren L: Late results after venous valve repair. Int Angiol 1985;4:413–417.
11. Sottiurai VS: Surgical correction of recurrent venous ulcer. J Cardiovasc Surg 1991;32:104–109.
12. Masuda EM, Kistner RL, Ferris EB: Long-term effects of superficial femoral vein ligation: Thirteen-year follow-up. J Vasc Surg 1992;16:741–749.
13. Kamida CB, Kistner RL: Descending phlebology: The Straub technique. In Bergan JJ, Kistner RL (eds): Atlas of Venous Surgery. Philadelphia, WB Saunders, 1992, pp 105–109.
14. Herman RJ, Neiman HL, Yao JST, et al: Descending venography: A method of evaluating lower extremity venous valvular function. Radiology 1980;137:63–69.
15. Morano JU, Raju S: Chronic venous insufficiency: Assessment with descending venography. Radiology 1990;174:441–444.
16. Eriksson I, Almgren B: Influence of the profunda femoris vein on venous hemodynamics of the limb. J Vasc Surg 1986;4:390–395.
17. Raju S, Fredericks RK, Neglen PN, Bass JD: Durability of venous valve reconstruction techniques for "primary" and postthrombotic reflux. J Vasc Surg 1996;23:357–367.
18. Cheatle TR, Perrin M: Venous valve repair: Early results in fifty-two cases. J Vasc Surg 1994;19:404–413.
19. Perrin MR: Reconstructive surgery for deep venous reflux: A report on 144 cases. Cardiovasc Surg 2000;8:246–255.
20. Sottiurai VS: Results of deep vein reconstruction. Vasc Surg 1997;31:276–278.
21. Kistner RL: Surgical technique of external venous valve repair. The Straub Foundation Proceedings 1990;55:15–16.
22. Schanzer H, Skladany M, Peirce EC: The role of external banding valvuloplasty in the surgical management of chronic deep venous disease. Phlebology 1994;9:8–12.
23. Gloviczki P, Merrell SW, Bower TC: Femoral vein valve repair under direct vision without venotomy: A modified technique using angioscopy. J Vasc Surg 1991;14:645–648.
24. Welch HJ, McLaughlin RL, O'Donnell TF: Femoral vein valvuloplasty: Intraoperative angioscopic evaluation and hemodynamic improvement. J Vasc Surg 1992;16:694–700.
25. Taheri SA, Lazar L, Elias SM, et al: Surgical treatment of postphlebitic syndrome with vein valve transplant. Am J Surg 1982;144:221–224.
26. Bry JDL, Muto PA, O'Donnell TF, Isaacson LA: The clinical and hemodynamic results after axillary-to-popliteal vein valve transplantation. J Vasc Surg 1995;21:110–119.
27. Nash T: Long-term results of vein valve transplants placed in the popliteal vein for intractable post-phlebitic venous ulcers and pre-ulcer skin changes. J Cardiovasc Surg 1988;29:712–716.
28. Kistner RL: Deep venous reconstruction. Int Angiol 1985;4:429–433.
29. Dalsing MC, Raju S, Wakefield TW, Taheri SA: A multicenter, phase 1 evaluation of cryopreserved venous valve allografts for the treatment of chronic deep venous insufficiency (CDVI). Presented at the American Venous Forum Eleventh Annual Meeting, Dana Point, Calif, February 21, 1999.
30. Psathakis ND: The substitute "valve" operation by technique II in patients with post-thrombotic syndrome. Surgery 1984;95:542–548.
31. Abu Rahma AF, Robinson PA, Boland JP: Clinical, hemodynamic and anatomic predictors of long-term outcome

of lower extremity venovenous bypasses. J Vasc Surg 1991;14:635–644.
32. Motarjeme A, Gordon GI, Bodenhagen K: Thombolysis and angioplasty of chronic iliac artery occlusions. J Vasc Interv Radiol 1995;6(Suppl):66S–72S.
33. Neglen P, Berry MA, Raju S: Endovascular surgery in the treatment of chronic primary and post-thrombotic iliac vein obstruction. Eur J Vasc Endovasc Surg 2000;20:560–571.
34. Gruss JD: Venous bypass for chronic venous insufficiency. In Bergan JJ, Yao JST (eds): Venous Disorders. Philadelphia, WB Saunders, 1991, pp 316–330.
35. Palma EC, Esperon R: Vein transplants and grafts in surgical treatment of the postphlebitic syndrome. J Cardiovasc Surg 1960;1:94–107.
36. Dale WA: Crossover grafts for iliofemoral venous occlusion. In Bergan JJ, Yao JST (eds): Venous Problems. Chicago, Year Book Medical Publishers, 1978, pp 411–429.
37. Halliday P, Harris J, May J: Femoro-femoral crossover grafts (Palma operation): A long-term follow-up study. In Bergan JJ, Yao JST (eds): Surgery of the Veins. Orlando, Fla, Grune & Stratton, 1985, pp 241–254.
38. Eklof B: Temporary arteriovenous fistula in reconstruction of iliac vein obstruction using PTFE grafts. In Eklof B, Gjores JE, Thulesius O, Bergqvist D (eds): Controversies in the Management of Venous Disorders. London, Butterworth, 1989, pp 280–290.
39. Gloviczki P, Pairolero PC, Toomey BJ, et al: Reconstruction of large veins for nonmalignant venous occlusive disease. J Vasc Surg 1992;16:750–761.
40. Husni EA: Venous reconstruction in postphlebitic disease. Circulation 1971;43(Suppl 1):147–150.
41. Neglen P, Raju S: Ambulatory venous pressure revisited. J Vasc Surg 2000;31:1206–1213.

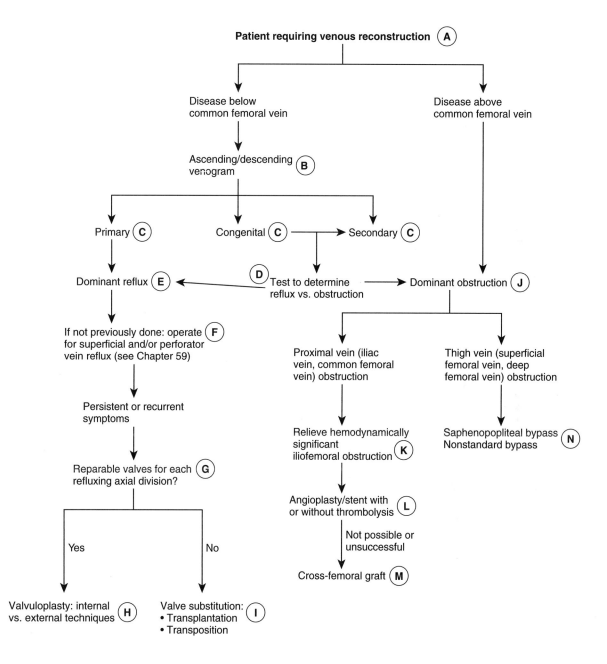

MISCELLANEOUS TOPICS

Chapter 62 Portal Hypertension

KAJ H. JOHANSEN, MD, PhD

A Most patients requiring intervention because of complications of portal hypertension have gastrointestinal (GI) tract bleeding. The majority of such patients suffer massive, painless hematemesis—vomiting large volumes of dark blood or clots. A much smaller percentage of patients (10% to 15% of those bleeding from portal hypertension) do not have hematemesis but instead pass large amounts of blood per rectum. No matter how it presents, bleeding may be become massive, leading to hypovolemic shock.

A very small percentage of patients who undergo operation for portal hypertension (<5%) do not have GI hemorrhage but instead require intervention because of another complication of portal hypertension—usually ascites (especially when patients have the Budd-Chiari syndrome) or hypersplenism.

B Both for diagnostic reasons and for acute therapy, fiberoptic esophagogastroduodenoscopy (EGD) should be performed as soon as possible in all patients with significant upper GI hemorrhage. These diagnostic efforts can and should occur simultaneously with volume resuscitation, including transfusion. The source of the upper digestive tract hemorrhage (esophagogastric varices, gastritis or esophagitis, peptic ulcer disease, Mallory-Weiss tear, or tumor) usually can be detected by EGD. Among patients with portal hypertension and varices complicated by GI bleeding, up to 20% may be bleeding from a source not related to the portal hypertension.

Although initial upper endoscopy was traditionally performed with the patient under general anesthesia with rigid gastroscopes, the advantages of flexible fiberoptic scopes for the diagnosis and management of upper digestive tract hemorrhage are now established.

C The majority (80%) of portal hypertensive bleeding is from esophageal varices, usually in the lowest 5 to 10 cm of the esophagus; 10% of portal hypertensive bleeding is from the stomach, divided equally between proximal gastric (fundal) varices and portal hypertensive gastropathy. Other sites of occasional bleeding resulting from portal hypertension include (1) hemorrhoidal varices (resulting in rectal bleeding), (2) duodenal or other small intestinal or colonic varices, or (3) varices forming at the site of various portosystemic venous communications (e.g., abdominal wall stomata, scars, or adhesions).

D Endoscopic therapy has been very effective treatment for bleeding from esophageal varices. Although initial therapy included injection sclerotherapy with a variety of sclerosant materials (hypertonic saline, sodium morrhuate, alcohol, sodium tetradecyl sulfate), prospective randomized trials by Stiegmann and colleagues comparing injection sclerotherapy and variceal banding clearly demonstrated that the latter technique is both more effective (in controlling bleeding) and safer (in minimizing late complications).[1] Endoscopic therapy should be performed by operators skilled in the technique. Because both sclerotherapy and banding result in intense fibrosis, repeated endoscopic therapy is often much more difficult if early rebleeding occurs.

E The means by which endoscopic therapy actually halts bleeding is disputed. Intravariceal sclerosant injection obviously results in thrombosis of the bleeding varices; however, paravariceal sclerosant injection, as promoted by Paquet and others,[2] appears to work by causing fibrotic thickening of the esophageal mucosa, thereby diminishing the likelihood of rebleeding because the varices are less superficial. Esophageal variceal banding works by causing necrosis of the varix with surrounding inflammation, fibrosis, and variceal thrombosis. Both techniques may fail, resulting in early rebleeding; even if the technique is successful, esophageal perforation and mediastinitis or late esophageal stricture formation or dysmotility may occur as a consequence of endoscopic variceal therapy.

Endoscopic therapy is not useful for the management of bleeding from gastric varices, although experimental trials of injection of methyl methacrylate have been attempted. Endoscopic therapy also has no role to play in bleeding from portal hypertensive gastropathy.

F Approximately 90% of esophageal variceal bleeding can be controlled by aggressive endoscopic therapy (injection sclerotherapy or banding). In about 10% of patients, endoscopic therapy cannot be performed (e.g., because endoscopic expertise may not be available), or esophageal variceal bleeding cannot be controlled or rapidly recurs. In these patients, as well as in those with bleeding from gastric fundal varices, one of several devices used for esophagogastric variceal balloon tamponade should be inserted. Use of these devices requires an understanding of the goal of balloon tamponade and avoidance of serious and even lethal complications (esophageal rupture, pulmonary aspiration). Balloon tamponade must be halted within 48 to 72 hours, by which time further efforts to provide definitive control of bleeding, such as endoscopic therapy, transjugular intrahepatic portosystemic shunt (TIPS), or operative portal decompression, should be applied.

G Although balloon tamponade does halt portal hypertensive bleeding in approximately 90% of patients, control is not possible for some patients with this method; for patients in this circumstance, a more aggressive intervention is required. TIPS may be highly effective, especially in a patient who is otherwise severely compromised or is in the process of resuscitation following massive sustained variceal hemorrhage. It is not prudent to attempt TIPS in unstable patients (i.e., those who are actively bleeding, who are hypotensive, or who are being actively resuscitated).[3]

Emergency esophageal transection may be

highly effective in controlling persistent bleeding refractory to less invasive treatments.[4] Such esophageal devascularization, usually performed by means of the EEA stapling device after midline laparotomy and high gastrotomy, is obviously ineffective for variceal or mucosal bleeding from the stomach; furthermore, whereas esophageal variceal hemorrhage can be acutely controlled in this fashion, rebleeding may occur within months. This therapy should not be considered to be definitive.

Orloff has, for 30 years, championed the concept of emergency portacaval shunt in patients with bleeding esophageal varices.[5] In his practice, now in excess of 500 patients treated in this fashion, patients are transferred directly to the operating room following endoscopic proof of portal hypertensive bleeding. His results, which show a 75% survival rate after emergency portacaval shunt, independent of hepatocellular function, are unequalled at any other centers, but his approach has not been widely adopted.

(H) Once acute portal hypertensive bleeding has been controlled, consideration of one or another form of definitive therapy to prevent recurrent hemorrhage is obligatory. This is because untreated variceal bleeding has a 50% to 90% likelihood of recurring within the next 12 months. Absent definitive therapy, mortality from recurrent bleeding or progressive liver failure is 90% within 5 years of the index bleeding episode. Multiple treatment options—pharmacologic, endoscopic, interventional radiologic, surgical (by shunt, devascularization, or transplantation)—are available. The proper choice depends upon the patient's hepatocellular and general medical status, the urgency of treatment, and available expertise. The first question to be answered is whether the patient is a near-term candidate for liver transplantation.

(I) Orthotopic liver transplantation (OLT), which involves substituting a healthy liver for the cirrhotic one, completely resolves the problem of recurrent portal hypertensive bleeding as well as the hepatic structural and metabolic abnormalities that are the underlying cause of the problem. Patients whose end-stage liver disease is compli-

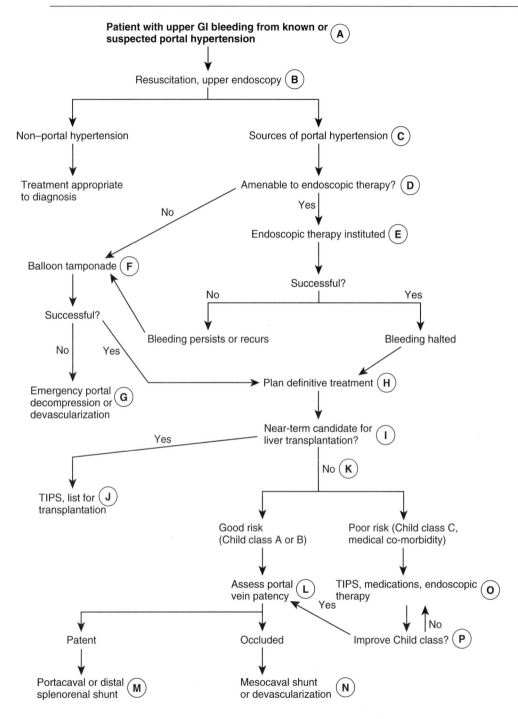

cated by portal hypertensive bleeding have outcomes equivalent to those undergoing hepatic transplantation for other causes.[6] For patients undergoing transplantation because of the late consequences of alcoholic liver disease, rates of return to alcohol consumption are acceptably low.

These favorable findings regarding OLT in patients with portal hypertensive bleeding notwithstanding, most patients with portal hypertensive bleeding should not or cannot be considered for OLT. On the one hand, a significant proportion of such patients are *not* in end-stage hepatocellular decompensation; they have compensated hepatic disease and need to have variceal bleeding controlled, not replacement of the liver. Numerous other patients with portal hypertensive bleeding are not candidates for OLT because of significant medical co-morbidities, because they are too old, or because they are still actively consuming alcohol (most hepatic transplantation programs require 6 months of demonstrated alcohol abstinence before transplantation in patients with alcoholic cirrhosis can be considered). Furthermore, the ethical dilemma inherent in offering a precious societal resource—a donor liver—to treat what is 90% of the time the self-inflicted consequences of a disease of substance abuse is self-evident.[7]

(J) Patients with portal hypertensive bleeding who might be considered legitimate candidates for near-term OLT are characterized by the following:

- Decompensated hepatocellular status
- If alcoholic, abstinent for at least 6 months
- Age younger than 70 years
- Relatively free of advanced cardiac, pulmonary, renal, pancreatic, or other medical co-morbidities
- Well insured
- Predictably compliant with follow-up and lifelong immunosuppression.

Portal hypertensive bleeding for these patients can be rapidly and effectively controlled by TIPS[8]; operative portosystemic shunting of any variety is relatively contraindicated and should be avoided.

(K) The majority of patients with portal hypertensive bleeding who do not fit criteria for near-term OLT require definitive nontransplant management of their bleeding. The Child-Pugh classification,[9] tempered by available expertise and the exigency of definitive bleeding control, remains the most effective means for discriminating accurately among treatment alternatives. In general, Child class A and "good" Child class B patients with variceal bleeding are best managed by operative portal decompression. Less-favorable Child class B and all Child class C patients, as well as those of any Child class who are unfavorable operative candidates for other reasons (irreversible coagulopathy, acute hepatitis), are better managed by nonsurgical therapies, including medication, repeated endoscopic therapy, or TIPS.

(L) Among good-risk cirrhotic patients in whom an operative portosystemic shunt is planned, assessment of portal vein patency plays an important role in the choice of operative shunt. Portal vein thrombosis, partial or complete, is present in approximately 10% of patients with bleeding from portal hypertension. Causes include an underlying hypercoagulable state (usually secondary to a congenital clotting protein deficiency), stagnant portal vein flow secondary to far-advanced cirrhosis, and hepatocellular carcinoma. Portal vein patency can be determined by duplex ultrasonography, computed tomographic portography, or late-phase visceral arteriography.

(M) With a demonstration of portal vein patency, all forms of operative portosystemic decompression are possible: The choice of which one to perform is based primarily on surgeon experience and preference. Direct side-to-side portacaval shunt has the highest likelihood of protection against variceal rebleeding (permanent control of recurrent bleeding 95% to 99% in all large series).

This procedure may be technically somewhat challenging, especially when the portal vein and inferior vena cava are difficult to appose for anastomosis. The introduction of the short polytetrafluoroethylene (PTFE) interposition graft by Sarfeh and coworkers[10] has significantly facilitated management of this technical dilemma.

The major long-term complication of standard portacaval shunt is a significantly increased likelihood of late portosystemic encephalopathy (PSE). Experimental and clinical validation of the concept of "partial portal decompression" by Sarfeh[11] and Johansen and colleagues[12] has suggested that limiting the degree of portal decompression can significantly diminish the risk of late PSE without increasing the likelihood of recurrent variceal hemorrhage.

The other commonly accepted portosystemic shunt that is used electively in good-risk cirrhotic patients with variceal hemorrhage is the distal splenorenal shunt. It provides good protection against variceal rebleeding; whether the distal splenorenal shunt's ability to prevent PSE is less than that of the standard portacaval shunt is disputed.[13, 14] This procedure is extremely challenging and is relatively contraindicated in a number of relatively common clinical settings such as refractory ascites, need for emergency portal decompression, thrombosed portal vein, and "unfavorable" venous anatomy.

(N) Good-risk patients requiring portal decompression who have been found on preoperative imaging to have portal vein thrombosis are generally best managed by mesocaval shunting utilizing externally-supported PTFE interposition grafts.[15] Recently or focally occluded portal veins may occasionally be thrombectomized, permitting portacaval shunting. Patients with diffuse splanchnic venous thrombosis and refractory portal hypertensive bleeding are best managed by esophagogastric devascularization (usually including splenectomy).[16]

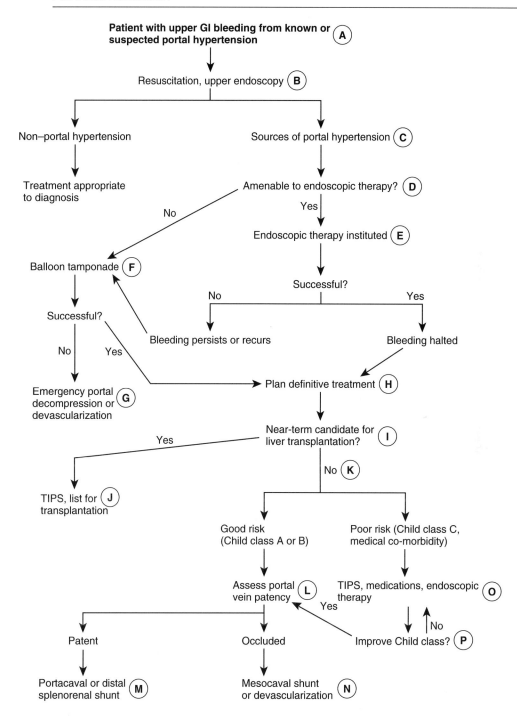

O "Poor-risk" patients (1) are in Child-Pugh class C or "unfavorable" class B; (2) have another medical problem (advanced cardiopulmonary or renal failure, acute hepatitis, or irreversible coagulopathy) which makes them poor candidates for a general anesthetic or a major operation; or (3) cannot be managed operatively because of a lack of available surgical expertise. The propensity of such patients toward variceal rebleeding may be greatly reduced by one or more therapeutic approaches, including various medications, repeated endoscopic therapy, or TIPS. As for operative portal decompression, each approach has advantages and disadvantages, and local expertise and experience must be taken into consideration.

Pharmacologic therapy to lower portal pressure, primarily by means of administration of β-antagonist medications, results in a lower risk of first variceal hemorrhage when administered *prophylactically* (i.e., in cirrhotic patients with no previous variceal bleeding).[17] Whether β blockade offers equivalent protection when administered *therapeutically* (i.e., in patients with previous variceal bleeding) is unclear. While the concept of lowering portal pressure by chronic orally administered medication is attractive, a potential risk of β blockade is, of course, a blunting of the patient's ability to increase heart rate and cardiac output in compensatory fashion if a significant variceal hemorrhage *were* to occur.

In patients compliant with long-term follow-up and repeated endoscopic examinations, chronic endoscopic therapy—either by sclerosant injection or by banding—may be reasonably effective at limiting future rebleeding from varices. As noted in E, this approach is ineffective for patients with prior bleeding from gastric fundal varices or from portal hypertensive gastropathy. Following complete eradication of esophageal varices, protection against variceal rebleeding exceeds 50% at 5 years.[18] Whether effective obliteration of esophageal varices results in increasing likelihood of bleeding from sources in the stomach is unclear.

TIPS is technically relatively straightforward in centers where it is routinely practiced, and initial technical success rates exceed 95%. TIPS provides immediate, complete portal decompression without the risks inherent in general anesthesia and a major operation. Used as a "bridge" to OLT in severely decompensated cirrhotic patients with variceal bleeding, TIPS has been lifesaving.[18] Unfortunately, the durability of TIPS is low, with up to 50% of patients demonstrating TIPS stenosis or thrombosis or variceal rebleeding within 6 months.[19] Stenotic or occluded TIPS channels can be identified by ultrasonographic surveillance protocols, permitting restoration of portal decompression by revision TIPS. This requires that patients treated with TIPS be compliant with such surveillance programs and that they remain willing to undergo multiple subsequent angiographic studies. Also, TIPS is associated with a 30% risk of new cases of PSE, probably a result of this procedure's complete decompression of the portal system and the fact that it is commonly utilized in patients with marginal hepatocellular function. A sudden improvement in encephalopathy in a TIPS patient frequently signifies that the TIPS channel has become stenotic or is occluded.

(P) The primary determinant of a cirrhotic patient's clinical status is the degree of hepatocellular decompensation, as indicated by their calculated Child-Pugh score.[9] With improved nutrition, cessation of alcohol intake, and protection against recurrent variceal hemorrhage, some patients may show improvement in Child classification status and even may become candidates for a shunt procedure.[20]

REFERENCES

1. Stiegmann GV, Goff JS, Michaletz-Onody PA, et al: Endoscopic sclerotherapy as compared with endoscopic ligation for bleeding esophageal varices. N Engl J Med 1992;326:1527–1532.
2. Paquet K-J: Endoscopic paravariceal injection sclerotherapy of the esophagus—indications, techniques, complications: Results of a period of 14 years. Gastrointest Endosc 1983;29:310–315.
3. Helton WS, Belshaw A, Althaus S, et al: Critical appraisal of the angiographic portacaval shunt (TIPS). Am J Surg 1993;165:566.
4. Burroughs AK, Hamilton G, Phillips A, et al: A comparison of sclerotherapy with staple transection of the esophagus for the emergency control of bleeding from esophageal varices. N Engl J Med 1979;321:857.
5. Orloff MJ, Bell RH Jr: Long-term survival after emergency portacaval shunting for bleeding varices in patients with alcoholic cirrhosis. Am J Surg 1986;151:176.
6. Iwatsuki S, Starzl TE, Todo S, et al: Liver transplantation in the treatment of bleeding esophageal varices. Surgery 1988;104:697–705.
7. Moss AH, Siegler M: Should alcoholics compete equally for liver transplantation? JAMA 1991;262:1295.
8. Ring EJ, Lake JR, Roberts JP, et al: Using transjugular intrahepatic shunts to control variceal bleeding before liver transplantation. Ann Intern Med 1992;116:304–309.
9. Conn HO: A peek at the Child-Turcotte classification. Hepatology 1981;1:673.
10. Sarfeh IJ, Rypins EB, Fardi M, et al: Clinical implications of portal hemodynamics after small-diameter portacaval H graft. Surgery 1984;96:223.
11. Collins JC, Ong MS, Rypins EB, Sarfeh IJ: Partial portacaval shunt for variceal hemorrhage: Longitudinal analysis of effectiveness. Arch Surg 1998;133:590–592.
12. Johansen KH: Prospective comparison of partial versus portal decompression for bleeding esophageal varices. Surg Gynecol Obstet 1992;175:528.
13. Millikan WJ, Warren WD, Henderson JM, et al: The Emory prospective randomized trial: Selective vs. nonselective shunt to control variceal bleeding. Ten-year follow-up. Ann Surg 1985;201:712.
14. Grace ND, Conn HO, Resnick RH, et al: Distal splenorenal vs. portal systemic shunts after hemorrhage from varices: A randomized controlled trial. Hepatology 1988;8:1475.
15. Paquet K-J, Mercado MA, Gad HA: Surgical procedures for bleeding esophagogastric varices when sclerotherapy fails: A prospective study. Am J Surg 1990;160:43.
16. Caps MT, Helton WS, Johansen K: Left upper quadrant devascularization for "unshuntable" portal hypertension. Arch Surg 1996;131:834.
17. Conn HO, Grace ND, Bosch J, et al: Propranolol in the prevention of the first hemorrhage from esophagogastric varices: A multicenter randomized clinical trial. Hepatology 1991;13:902–912.
18. Westaby D, MacDougall BR, Williams R: Improved survival following injection sclerotherapy for esophageal varices: Final analysis of a controlled trial. Hepatology 1985;5:827–830.
19. Sanyal AJ, Freedman AM, Luketic VA, et al: The natural history of portal hypertension after transjugular intrahepatic portosystemic shunts. Gastroenterology 1997;112:1040.
20. Holman JM, Rikkers LF: Success of medical and surgical management of acute variceal hemorrhage. Am J Surg 1980;140:816.

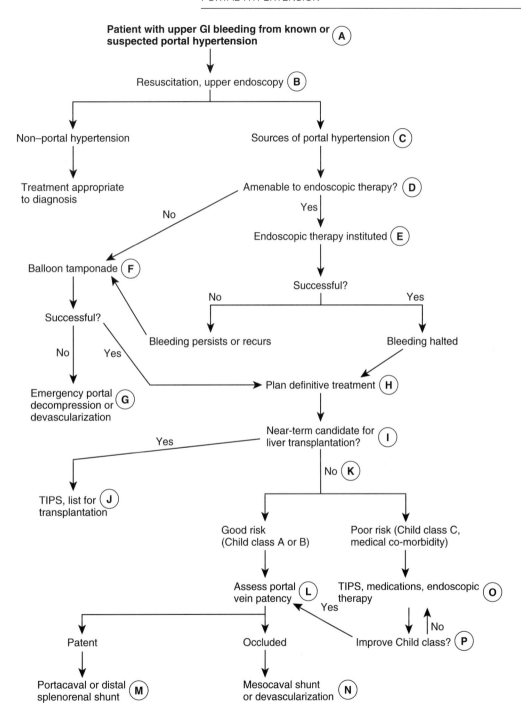

Chapter 63 Lymphedema

AUDRA A. NOEL, MD • PETER GLOVICZKI, MD

(A) The patient's history and physical examination are the keys to the diagnosis of lymphedema. A family history of congenital lymphedema (Milroy's disease) and a patient history of malignancy, radiation therapy, previous surgery, infections, deep venous thrombosis, or vascular malformations should be sought. A history of cardiac, renal, or hepatic disease is important in the differential diagnosis of a swollen limb.

Edema of systemic origin is characteristically bilateral. The most common systemic form, cardiac edema, is pitting. Skin changes of chronic venous disease (pigmentation, varicosities, ulcers) and swelling that diminishes overnight are clues to edema of venous origin. In contrast, lymphedema frequently is unilateral and progresses proximally, although it originates in the dorsum of the foot and the toes, with "squaring" of the toes and inverted Y–shaped interdigital creases. The toes are spared with other edemas. Although early lymphedema may be spongy or pitting in nature, it soon becomes firm as a result of subcutaneous fibrosis, hyperkeratosis, and the development of small vesicles that may drain lymph.

Time of onset of edema is important in differentiating primary from secondary lymphedema. Primary lymphedema typically occurs at birth or during puberty, although a subtype, lymphedema tarda, may occur in patients older than 35 years. Secondary lymphedema, however, is associated temporally with its cause (e.g., infection, malignancy, trauma). Bacterial or fungal infections occur frequently with both primary and secondary lymphedemas, and the latter may be caused by parasitic infection.

(B) Venous noninvasive studies are useful in differentiating venous edema from lymphedema. Duplex ultrasound scanning may identify deep vein or perforating vein incompetence to account for a swollen limb. In addition, plethysmography (air or strain-gauge) may facilitate the diagnosis of venous outflow obstruction or reflux. One should consider the diagnosis of lymphedema in a patient with a mildly swollen limb and normal results of venous studies.

(C) Computed tomography (CT) may demonstrate pelvic masses causing unilateral, or possibly bilateral, venous or lymphatic obstruction. In addition to ruling out obstructing masses, CT confirms the presence of a nonenhancing tubular reticular pattern in the subcutaneous tissues in patients with primary lymphedema. Unfortunately, CT cannot distinguish whether the pattern is of lymphatic channels or fluid-filled spaces.

Magnetic resonance imaging (MRI), however, has been found to be useful in distinguishing between different types of limb swelling (lymphedema, lipedema, venous edema), showing the honeycomb pattern seen on CT in patients with lymphedema.[1] In patients with lymphatic obstruction, MRI may show nodal anatomy and dilated lymphatics proximal to an obstruction that are not visualized by lymphoscintigraphy.

Finally, MRI is valuable in determining the extent of congenital vascular malformations. Many of the venous and even some of the microfistulous congenital vascular malformations have a significant lymphatic component, and some manifest as a swollen leg (see Chapter 71).

Clearly, neither CT nor MRI is routinely used, but both of these methods are applied when the diagnosis of lymphedema is unclear clinically or to investigate cases of lymphedema suspected of being obstructive in nature.

(D) Lymphoscintigraphy is performed by injecting technetium 99m–labeled antimony trisulfide colloid or labeled human albumin into the interdigital space of the foot or hand and then scanning the limb with a gamma camera. Accumulation of the radiolabeled isotope can be observed in lymph vessels or nodes, and delayed transport or obstruction may be identified. This study provides functional information rather than anatomic detail (see contrast lymphangiography in N). A semiquantitative transport index is derived from five components: (1) transport kinetics, (2) distribution pattern, (3) time of appearance of isotope in lymph nodes, (4) lymph nodes, and (5) lymph vessels. The transport index is 92% sensitive and nearly 100% specific in demonstrating lymphedema.[2]

Lymphoscintigraphy cannot differentiate primary from secondary lymphedema, but this examination is ideal for identifying lymphedema as the cause of extremity swelling. Because lymphoscintigraphy is minimally invasive, it is the examination of choice for diagnosis of lymphedema and for serial monitoring of the progression of disease.

(E) Primary lymphedema may be classified as *congenital* when it appears at birth, *praecox* when onset occurs between the ages 1 and 35 years, and *tarda* if onset occurs later in life. Primary lymphedema is most commonly due to fibrosis or hypoplastic disorders of the lymphatics, although 8% to 10% of patients may present with hyperplastic lymphatics.

Of patients with primary lymphedema, 80% experience bilateral swelling at the time of puberty; the swelling begins at the ankles and progresses slowly. This type is attributed to distal lymphatic obliteration. Another 10% of patients may have rapid progression of unilateral leg and thigh edema associated with proximal lymphatic obliteration. A final 10% have whole-limb congenital swelling due to lymphatic hyperplasia.

Familial congenital lymphedema (Milroy's disease) is an autosomal dominant disorder with incomplete penetrance that has been linked to specific genotypic markers in an investigation of several generations of North American and British families.[3, 4]

(F) In the United States, the most common causes of secondary lymphedema are malignant metastases to lymph nodes and surgical exci-

LYMPHEDEMA

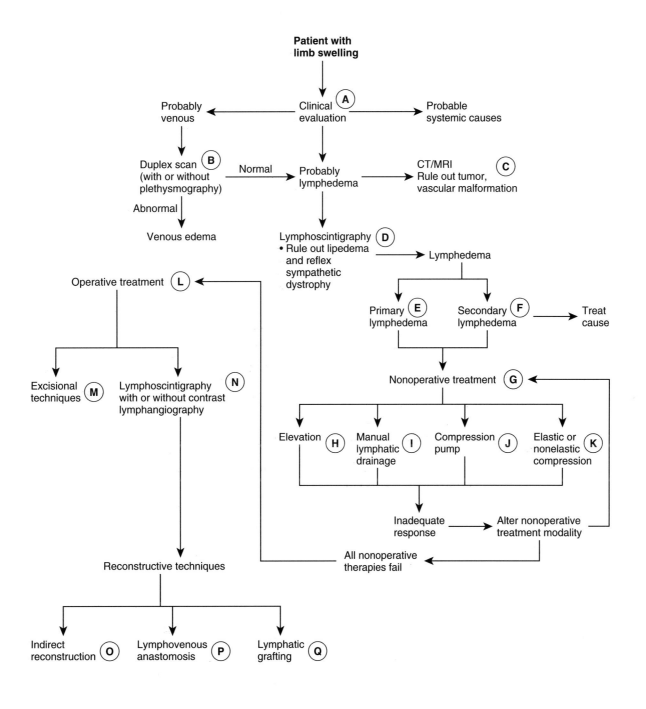

sion of lymph nodes with or without concomitant radiation therapy. In tropical countries, filariasis is a common cause of lymphedema. Other secondary causes are infection, chemical agents, and trauma.

(G) The components of nonoperative treatment, which is the mainstay of therapy in most cases of lymphedema, are discussed separately in *H* through *K*, but they are used together in varying combinations.

In general, all patients with primary lymphedema are advised to elevate their legs and to wear elastic stockings and are given a thorough trial of compression pump therapy. In patients with positive responses to compression pump therapy, these "gains" are consolidated by elastic compression and, eventually, newly fitted stockings. Manual massage has proved effective in Europe and is becoming more popular in North America, being applied by physiotherapists as part of lymphedema treatment programs.

(H) Limb elevation often is used in conjunction with other nonoperative methods to reduce lymphedema. The use of slings or arm boards, 3 to 5 days of elevation, and bed rest may diminish edema significantly. However, elevation may produce little reduction in lymphedema, unlike the response with venous and systemic edemas. If elevation does improve lymphedema, it should be considered a temporary solution and should be used in conjunction with manual lymphatic drainage or with pneumatic pump compression rather than as primary treatment alone.

(I) Manual lymphatic drainage, initially popularized in Europe, is being employed increasingly in the United States, particularly in the management of postmastectomy lymphedema. Specific regimens, described by various researchers, combine skin care, massage therapy, exercise, and compression garments with or without compression pumps.[5-7] The underlying theory of massage therapy is to manually move lymph fluid through the limb from distal to proximal lymphatics until the fluid can ultimately drain into normal lymph channels. Manual treatment can be effective but should be performed by a trained therapist and may be time-consuming, with daily therapy necessary initially.[5] Sessions are subsequently reduced to once a week for 4 to 6 weeks, but the entire series of therapeutic sessions must be repeated two or three times a year.

(J) Intermittent compression pump therapy has been effective in reducing lymphedema. Sequential-compression devices with multiple chambers per boot or sleeve appear more effective than single-chamber devices. The pneumatic compression reaches 90 to 100 mmHg of pressure and sequentially utilizes segmental compartments to mechanically propel lymph from the distal extremity to the proximal, normal lymphatics. In one study, sequential external pneumatic compression, in conjunction with elastic compression stockings and daily skin care, produced long-term reduction in limb girth in 90% of patients ($n = 49$) monitored for a mean time of 25 months.[8]

(K) Elastic garments, stockings, elastic bandages, or nonelastic external garments with hook-and-loop tape (Velcro) reinforcement are critical components of the nonoperative management of lymphedema. Once manual or mechanical compression therapy is instituted, external compression is employed in an attempt to maintain the reduced volume of the limb. Graduated compression stockings for patients with lymphedema frequently have a pressure of 40 to 50 mmHg at the ankle.

(L) Surgical intervention is considered in a small subgroup of patients whose lymphedema is refractory to medical treatment and who have considerable extremity dysfunction because of the extreme size and weight of the limb. This subgroup includes patients with impaired extremity movement, recurrent superimposed cellulitis, or, on occasion, severe pain. Another subset of patients may request intervention for primarily cosmetic reasons. Such patients occasionally may be considered for surgery but only after they have been counseled regarding the experimental nature and the limitations of lymphatic surgery (see *M, O, P,* and *Q*). In addition, the presence of lymphangiosarcoma necessitates operative treatment.

The surgical approaches described here are selectively applied in terms not only of their infrequent use, but also of the patients selected for each. Excisional techniques are mainly used for debulking of massive soft tissue enlargement to achieve better limb function and appearance. Reconstructive techniques, and even the indirect bridging techniques, are of value only in patients with lymphatic channels below a point of obstruction. Direct reconstructive techniques can be applied only to join sizable lymphatic pathways in continuity above and below a point of obstruction.

(M) Classic "*radical*" circumferential excisional procedures (e.g., the Charles procedure) have been abandoned as a result of poor healing and the need for large-surface skin grafting. Instead, several staged excisional procedures have been developed with the basic goal of creating adequate flap closure over the excised subcutaneous tissue.[9-11] After excision of excess skin, the flaps are approximated over closed-system drains. Excisional procedures, even if accomplished in stages, must be considered palliative and, as such, continue to require the use of compression garments. In addition, complications of excisional procedures include wound infection, poor healing, persistent edema, and sensory nerve injury.

(N) Prior to consideration of lymphatic reconstruction in a patient with lymphedema, lymphoscintigraphy is required for documentation of dilated lymphatics, proximal obstruction, and the characteristic pattern of lymphatic transport (see *D*).[2]

In addition, direct contrast lymphangiography, in rare instances, may be indicated to identify specific anatomic details of the lymphatics prior to lymphovenous anastomoses or lymphatic grafting. In such patients, if contrast lymphangiography is

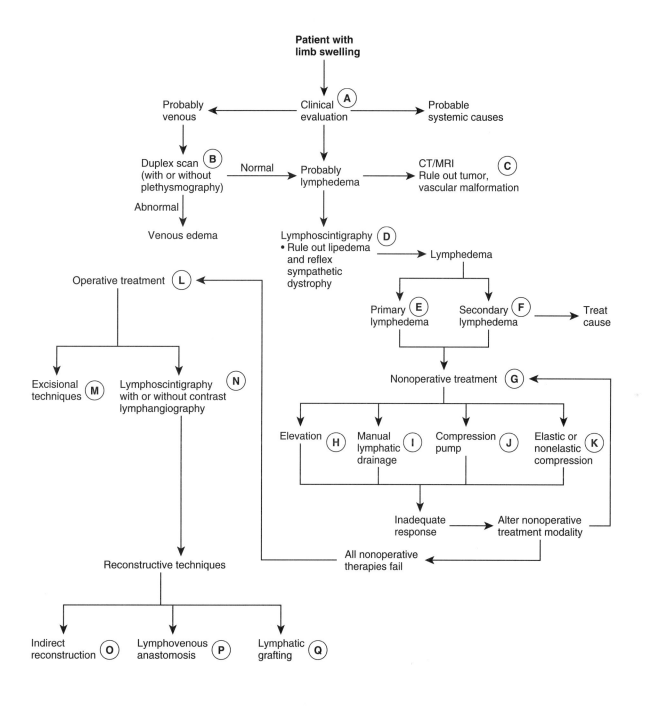

performed within 24 hours before surgery, the lymphatics may be visualized with fluoroscopic guidance during surgery.

O The concept of indirect lymphatic reconstruction relies on the theory that lymphatics spontaneously form collateral drainage. Patients with intact inguinal lymph nodes but who have obstruction proximal to the nodes may be candidates for the mesenteric bridge procedure. A segment of ileum is opened longitudinally with mucosa removed. The segment is anastomosed to fibrotic transected inguinal nodes. This procedure, with careful patient selection, has been reported to provide reduction of lymphedema with normal lymphatic clearance at 5 years in five of eight patients.[12,13]

Although the use of omental free flaps has been performed successfully in dogs,[14] previous patient experience with the procedure was fraught with complications and the procedure is not currently recommended.[15] Autotransplantation of free lymphatic node flaps has been a promising technique, especially in postmastectomy patients treated with axillary node transplants.[16]

P Lymphatic reconstruction with lymphovenous anastomoses can be achieved through the use of high-power microscopy, microsurgical instruments, and fine (9–0 or 10–0) monofilament suture.[17] Despite a considerable learning curve for this approach, the overall patency rate in 34 dogs was 50% at 8 months in one study.[17]

Patients selected for lymphovenous anastomoses include those who have secondary lymphedema without prior lymphangitis or chronic venous insufficiency. Lymphatics are visualized intraoperatively with the use of isosulfan blue or with contrast angiography. The lymphatic vessels are anastomosed end to end to the veins with interrupted monofilament suture. Postoperatively, the patient must wear an elastic bandage and must keep the operated limb elevated. Although clinical improvement in patients has been well documented,[18] imaging studies to confirm long-term patency of such grafts in humans are not available.[19]

Q Normal lymphatic channels, harvested from a nonedematous leg, have been used as lymphatic grafts for patients with postmastectomy lymphedema. In patients with unilateral leg lymphedema, the contralateral lymphatics are harvested and used as suprapubic lymphatic grafts.

The lymphatics in the normal limb are dissected along the greater saphenous vein; two or three lymphatic channels are transected distally, and they are passed through a suprapubic tunnel to be anastomosed to lymphatics in the groin of the affected limb. Postoperative imaging with lymphoscintigraphy is performed to confirm patency and improved drainage.

The experience of Baumeister and colleagues,[20] from Munich, Germany, with this approach has been most promising. In their series of 55 patients with at least 3 years of follow-up, reduced extremity volume was achieved in 80% of patients. Patency, however, was not consistently documented in the grafts of patients who showed clinical improvement.

A later report by Campisi and associates[21] describes the utilization of autologous vein to create a lymphatic-venous-lymphatic bypass with invagination of several lymphatic vessels into the vein graft. Further experience in both lymphatic grafting and lymphatic-venous-lymphatic bypass may confirm the efficacy of these interventions.

REFERENCES

1. Duewell S, Hagspiel KD, Zuber K, et al: Swollen lower extremity: Role of MR imaging. Radiology 1992;184:227–231.
2. Cambria RA, Gloviczki P, Naessens JM, Wahner HW: Noninvasive evaluation of the lymphatic system with lymphoscintigraphy: A prospective, semiquantitative analysis in 386 extremities. J Vasc Surg 1993;18:773–782.
3. Evans AL, Brice G, Sotirova V, et al: Mapping of primary congenital lymphedema to the 5q35.3 region. Am J Hum Genet 1999;64:547–555.
4. Witte MH, Erickson R, Bernas M, et al: Phenotypic and genotypic heterogeneity in familial Milroy lymphedema. Lymphology 1998;31:145–155.
5. Kasseroller RG: The Vodder School: The Vodder method. Cancer 1998;83:2840–2842.
6. Leduc O, Leduc A, Bourgeois P, Belgrado JP: The physical treatment of upper limb edema. Cancer 1998;83:2835–2839.
7. Casley-Smith JR, Boris M, Weindorf S, Lasinski B: Treatment for lymphedema of the arm—the Casley-Smith method: A noninvasive method produces continued reduction. Cancer 1998;83:2843–2860.
8. Pappas CJ, O'Donnell TF Jr: Long-term results of compression treatment for lymphedema. J Vasc Surg 1992;16:555–628.
9. Kim DI, Huh S, Lee SJ, et al: Excision of subcutaneous tissue and deep muscle fascia for advanced lymphedema. Lymphology 1998;31:190–194.
10. Miller TA, Wyatt LE, Rudkin GH: Staged skin and subcutaneous excision for lymphedema: A favorable report of long-term results. Plast Reconstr Surg 1998;102:1486–1498.
11. Mavili ME, Naldoken S, Safak T: Modified Charles operation for primary fibrosclerotic lymphedema. Lymphology 1994;27:14-20.
12. Hurst PA, Stewart G, Kinmonth JB, Browse NL: Long term results of the enteromesenteric bridge operation in the treatment of primary lymphoedema. Br J Surg 1985;72:272–274.
13. Browse NL: The diagnosis and management of primary lymphedema. J Vasc Surg 1986;3:181–184.
14. O'Brien BM, Hickey MJ, Hurley JV, et al: Microsurgical transfer of the greater omentum in the treatment of canine obstructive lymphoedema. Br J Plast Surg 1990;43:440–446.
15. Goldsmith HS: Long term evaluation of omental transposition for chronic lymphedema. Ann Surg 1974;180:847–849.
16. Trevedic PCJ: Free axillary lymph node transfer. In Cluzan RV (ed): Progress in Lymphology. Amsterdam, Elsevier Science, 1992, pp 415–420.
17. Gloviczki P, Hollier LH, Nora FE, Kaye MP: The natural history of microsurgical lymphovenous anastomoses: An experimental study. J Vasc Surg 1986;4:148–156.
18. O'Brien BM, Mellow CG, Khazanchi RK, et al: Long-term results after microlymphaticovenous anastomoses for the treatment of obstructive lymphedema. Plast Reconstr Surg 1990;85:562–572.
19. Gloviczki P, Fisher J, Hollier LH, et al: Microsurgical lymphovenous anastomosis for treatment of lymphedema: A critical review. J Vasc Surg 1988;7:647–652.
20. Baumeister RG, Siuda S: Treatment of lymphedemas by microsurgical lymphatic grafting: What is proved? Plast Reconstr Surg 1990;85:64–74.
21. Campisi C, Boccardo F, Tacchella M: Reconstructive microsurgery of lymph vessels: The personal method of lymphatic-venous-lymphatic (LVL) interpositioned grafted shunt. Microsurgery 1995;16:161–166.

LYMPHEDEMA

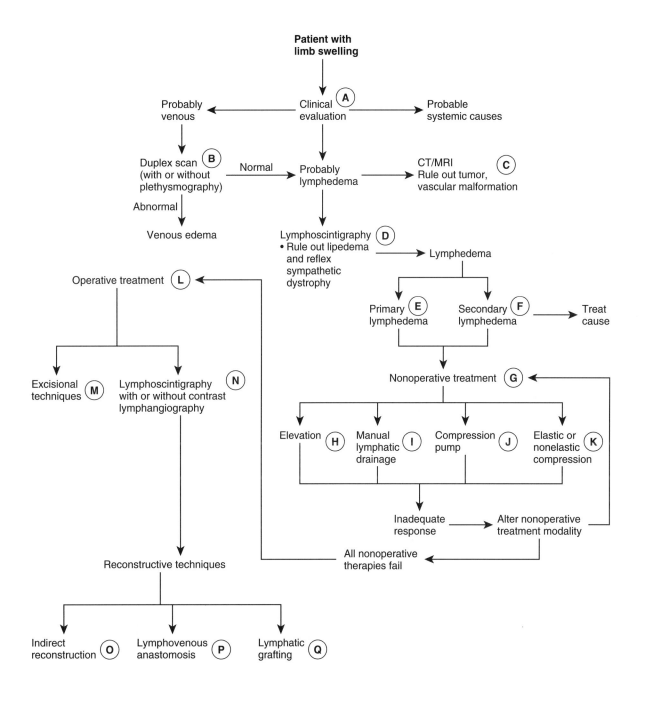

Chapter 64 Brachiocephalic Vascular Trauma

MALCOLM O. PERRY, MD • KENNETH E. McINTYRE, JR, MD

(A) For the patient with brachiocephalic trauma, the ABCs of initial trauma resuscitation must be first applied: The airway must be secured, adequate breathing ensured, and the circulation supported, as needed. Flint and associates[2] reported that 40% of 146 patients with major vascular injuries in the base of the neck were in shock when first seen. Reul and colleagues[4] observed that almost 50% of their patients with injuries to the great vessels were hypotensive and more than 40% had other serious wounds.[1-4]

Two large-bore intravenous (IV) lines are inserted, and usually the line opposite the neck or chest wound is advanced to a central position. If an innominate vein or superior vena cava wound is suspected, a lower extremity IV line may be needed. An infusion of a balanced salt solution is begun while blood is obtained for transfusion.

If chest tubes are required, they should be placed *before* pressure-assisted respiration is started to avoid tension pneumothorax. If breath sounds are absent and if dullness to percussion, tracheal shift, or other clinical signs of a hemopneumothorax are present, closed-chest tube thoracostomy must be performed. Thoracotomy is needed if more than 1500 mL of blood is found or if bleeding continues at a rate greater than 200 mL per hour.[3]

A Foley catheter is inserted into the bladder, and often a radial arterial line is inserted into an uninjured extremity. Nasogastric tubes should *not* be inserted in the patient with potential vascular injuries in the base of the neck because this may cause gagging, which can dislodge a clot or disrupt tamponade. The wounds should not be probed digitally or locally explored, and foreign bodies should not be removed until control of bleeding is possible.

(B) Most penetrating neck and chest wounds are caused by knives or gunshots. Associated injuries are present in up to one third of the patients.[1] Wounds of the aerodigestive tract and damage to major nerves are common. Patients who have been in motor vehicle collisions at speeds greater than 30 miles per hour or who have fallen from a level of two stories or higher are more likely to have blunt trauma to the aortic arch and great vessels. In hemodynamically stable patients, a long delay between the injury and admission to the hospital suggests that a life-threatening wound is not present. The patient and any observer should be questioned about symptoms, including transient neurologic deficits, difficulty in breathing or speaking, and vomiting or coughing of blood.

(C) Many patients initially have no clinical signs of vascular injury, as was the case in 30% of the patients in the series reported by Flint and associates.[2] Small wounds of the upper chest can be associated with serious vascular injuries of the aortic arch and great vessels, and bleeding may initially cease but can recur at any time. Reduction or absence of pulses in the arms strongly suggests an arterial injury, but this is not always the case. The pulse wave can be transmitted through soft clot or beyond intimal flaps. The rich collateral circulation about the shoulder can lead to a palpable distal pulse, even with a significant proximal injury.[1,3] Calhoon and associates[3] reported that 64% of their patients with proven proximal thoracic arterial injuries had palpable pulses when initially seen.

The location and nature of all wounds are recorded, and priorities of treatment established. It is helpful to separate the neck wounds according to zones, as follows[5]:

Zone I: Below 1 cm above the clavicle.
Zone II: Between 1 cm above the clavicle and the angle of the mandible.
Zone III: Between the angle of the mandible and the base of the skull.

Associated injuries of important nerves are common in vascular wounds, and a paralyzed vocal cord or the presence of Horner's syndrome suggests that nearby vessels may also be injured. Many patients with serious vascular injuries in this area have hematoma at the base of the neck, a wide mediastinum, continued bleeding, or hemothorax. Persistent bleeding in the chest may not be apparent until after a period of observation and more blood loss.

(D) A hemodynamically unstable patient is taken immediately to the operating room. Control of bleeding is essential, and delay for time-consuming diagnostic tests is not recommended. If additional studies are needed, they can be performed in the operating room while preparations for operation are under way.[6] The neck and chest should be prepared for surgery; control of bleeding may necessitate wide exposure and more than one incision. The patient is anesthetized, and an endotracheal tube is inserted carefully to avoid dislodging clots. At the same time, the position of the vocal cords is recorded and the aerodigestive tract examined for accumulations of air or blood.

(E) An upright posteroanterior chest x-ray film is an important study that can usually be obtained even in patients with relatively unstable hemodynamic status. Blood in the chest cavities or mediastinum may be visible, and other injuries occasionally can be detected. Ultrasound studies can be employed to detect the presence of blood in the tissues. In some patients, duplex ultrasound studies of the vessels of the neck may reveal the presence or absence of an arterial injury. These tests are useful mainly when their results are positive. In most patients with trauma to the neck and chest, an electrocardiogram is needed, and arterial blood gas tensions are measured. It is often wise to analyze the blood for alcohol and drugs.

In stable patients, biplane arteriography can be of help in defining the location and extent of the injuries. Arteriograms are generally obtained for one of these three reasons[7]:

1. To expose injuries that are not detectable by other means.

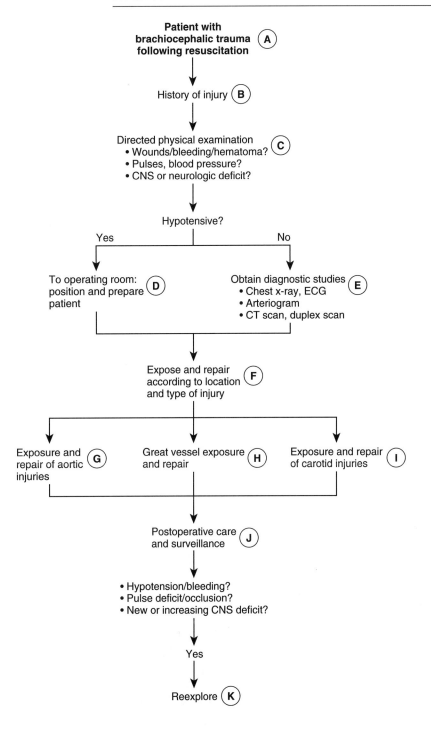

Brachiocephalic Vascular Trauma (continued)

2. To exclude the need for an operation in patients who have no other indication for surgery.
3. To plan an operation when special maneuvers or techniques may be needed.

Arteriograms are often needed in treating the patient who has penetrating or blunt trauma to the great vessels and the carotid and vertebral arteries. They are recommended in all hemodynamically stable patients with zone I or zone III injuries (see C). Pulse deficits and reduced arterial pressures in the upper extremities may dictate arteriography to locate the site of injury. Continued bleeding in the chest, a wide mediastinum, obscuration of the aortic knob, an apical cap, and tracheal or esophageal deviation are signs suggesting vascular injuries in the thorax, and arteriography is usually required.

In addition to the standard chest x-ray and electrocardiogram, echocardiography of the heart may be helpful in some instances to detect fluid in the pericardium or abnormalities of the heart. Studies by Fabian and associates[8] have shown that helical computed tomography (CT) is a highly sensitive method for the diagnosis of blunt aortic injuries.

(F) Although determining the location and type of vascular injury is not always possible in hemodynamically unstable patients, an attempt to do so is important in directing the most appropriate exposure and repair. The decision regarding surgical exposure of arterial injuries in zone I of the neck or in the chest can be difficult (e.g., whether to approach the wound through a lateral thoracotomy or a median sternotomy) (see G and H).

(G) A midline sternum-splitting incision affords access to the heart, aortic arch, and the great vessels except for the origin of the left subclavian artery. This incision can be extended into the supraclavicular area to expose the subclavian vessels, or into the anterior triangles of the neck along the sternomastoid muscle to reach the common carotid artery. The incision can be extended laterally into the intercostal space if necessary, but most surgeons prefer a separate third or fourth interspace thoracotomy to control the origin of the left subclavian artery

Wounds of the aortic arch pose a difficult and dangerous problem. Small lacerations can be repaired with partial occlusion and lateral suture techniques using pledgets. If the blood pressure is not low, compression of the proximal aorta while the sutures are placed may be helpful in reducing the pressure. It is particularly important to remember the fragility of the great vessels, especially the subclavian artery, during repair of these injuries.[3]

Whenever possible, repair of the aorta and great vessels *without* the use of cardiopulmonary bypass is probably safer. Systemic heparinization, trauma to the elements of the blood, and the technical problems of bypass increase the risk. The use of total bypass can usually be limited to specific problems in which extensive repairs of the aortic arch are needed. Experience with the Biomedicus centrifugal pump suggests that this device may simplify such operations because less priming solution is needed, no heparin is necessary, and no oxygenator is used.[9] The bypass is usually performed from the left atrium or the left pulmonary vein to the aorta; multiple catheters attached to the system add the possibility of separate perfusion of some of the great vessels.

(H) If the presence and location of a brachiocephalic arterial injury have been established, exposure and repair of the arterial injury are usually straightforward. A hematoma in the arterial sheath or in the adventitia is an indication for more extensive exposure. Direct control of bleeding usually can be accomplished with digital pressure. In some cases, lateral wounds of the large vessels can be controlled with partial-occlusion clamps.

Preliminary anterior third interspace thoracotomy may be required to achieve control of bleeding from subclavian arteries into the chest. Packing may be helpful while incisions are being widened or additional ones opened. If control cannot be obtained by encircling the vessels proximally and distally or by applying vascular clamps and if bleeding is profuse, balloon catheters can be inserted into the wounds and gently retracted to control bleeding.[1] In some cases, balloon occlusion catheters can be inserted from a remote site and advanced to the wound to assist in control of bleeding.

Once vascular clamps are in place and bleeding is controlled, standard vascular techniques are used to repair the vessels. Lateral repair may be possible in larger vessels. Resection and anastomosis of medium-sized vessels are recommended if the injury is not tangential and limited. If the repair cannot be accomplished without tension, an interposition graft is needed; most surgeons use prosthetic grafts for repair of the larger brachiocephalic vessels. If a hematoma obscures the origin of the innominate artery, it is often prudent to insert a prosthetic graft before it is disturbed. An 8-mm or 10-mm tube graft is first sewn end to side to the ascending aorta with a partial occlusion clamp and then end to end to the artery distally. The origin of the innominate artery can then be safely exposed and oversewn.[6]

Marin and associates[10] have shown that, in hemodynamically stable patients, endovascular techniques can be useful in managing large arteriovenous fistulae and false aneurysms in the chest. The devices are inserted from remote sites in the extremities. Although endovascular methods have mainly been used to treat large chronic lesions, they may be helpful in managing acute wounds of the great vessels. The long-term outcome obtained with the devices is as yet unknown, but early results are promising.

(I) For most carotid injuries, standard exposure with an incision along the anterior border of the sternocleidomastoid muscle is all that is required. If injuries of the internal carotid artery in zone III are suspected, exposure can be difficult. Exposure can usually be accomplished with nasotracheal intubation, section of the digastric muscle,

BRACHIOCEPHALIC VASCULAR TRAUMA

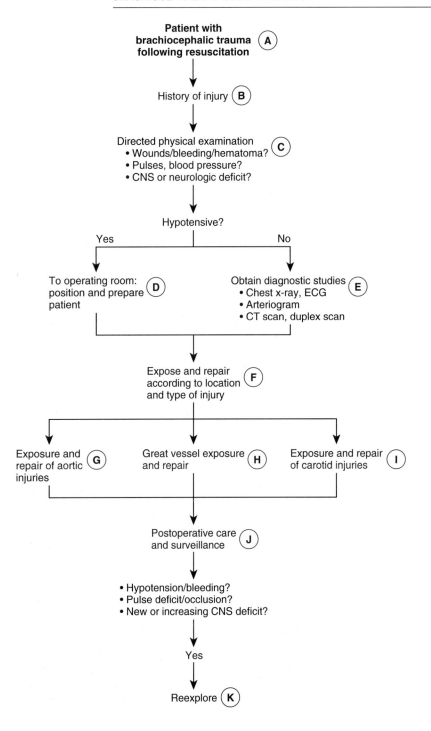

excision of the styloid process, and insertion of a bite block to open the jaw. In some patients, it may be necessary to subluxate the mandible anteriorly to reach the base of the skull. This maneuver requires preoperative planning and the insertion of dental appliances by oral surgery colleagues.

When one is deciding on repair, it is helpful to consider the presence and degree of neurologic deficit and whether the vessel is occluded or still has prograde flow. The final outcome in most patients with carotid artery wounds is usually determined by the extent of the neurologic deficit prior to repair.[1, 7] Whether the injury has caused occlusion or not also plays a role.

It is our practice to repair all injuries of carotid arteries in patients who have prograde flow. The results of repair are less favorable in patients with complete occlusion of the internal carotid artery and a profound stroke with altered consciousness,[11] but if the clots can be completely removed and there is good back-flow, repair in such cases is indicated.[7, 12] Thus, the only injuries we do not repair are those in patients with profound neurologic deficit with altered state of consciousness and those with complete occlusions without prospects for restoration of flow.

Carotid artery wounds are repaired by direct suture, patch graft angioplasty, or, more commonly, resection and end-to-end anastomosis. More extensive injuries may require a replacement graft, and usually the saphenous vein from the groin is chosen. For the larger arteries, prosthetic grafts are used. Completion arteriography is recommended.

Injured veins are usually ligated; however, if both internal jugular veins are injured, the larger vein is repaired if feasible. Direct suture or patch venoplasty can be chosen. Grafts are rarely employed.

Wounds of the trachea and esophagus are repaired and drained. Cranial nerves may be repaired in clean wounds, and the repairs are marked with metallic clips. If delayed nerve reconstruction is planned, the nerve ends are tagged for identification.

J Postoperatively, patients are observed in the intensive care unit. Frequent evaluations of the airway, chest tube drainage, vital signs, and neurologic status are indicated. Blood pressure is controlled in a normal range. The patency of the vascular repairs is followed by means of physical examination, Doppler or duplex ultrasound studies, and arteriography, if required.

K Significant bleeding from the chest tube or neck wound or unexplained hypotension may signal breakdown of the repair or anastomosis and requires reexploration. If a patient demonstrates a new neurologic deficit or if there is extension of a mild preoperative deficit after carotid artery repair, immediate reoperation is indicated. Often an acute occlusion of an arterial repair or reconstruction can be successfully treated, and a delay for confirmatory arteriograms may compromise the results, especially if the common or internal carotid arteries are involved. A limited change in the neurologic status thought to be the result of distal embolism rather than occlusion of the carotid arteries is, however, an indication for arteriography.

A fall in limb blood pressures or a pulse deficit also suggests a problem with the arterial repair. Arteriography may be needed to plan the operation. If the immediate operation is successful, the outcome is likely to be good.

REFERENCES

1. Perry MO: Management of Acute Vascular Injuries. Baltimore, William & Wilkins, 1981, pp 55–65.
2. Flint LM, Snyder WH, Perry MO, Shires GT: Management of major vascular injuries in the base of the neck: An 11-year experience with 146 cases. Arch Surg 1973;106:407–413.
3. Calhoon JH, Grover FL, Trinkle JT: Chest trauma: Approach and management. Clin Chest Med 1992;13:55–67.
4. Reul GJ, Beall AC, Jordon GL, Mattox KL: The early operative management of injuries to the great vessels. Surgery 1973;74:862–868.
5. Monson DO, Saletta JD, Freeark RJ: Carotid-vertebral trauma. J Trauma 1969;9:987–999.
6. Perry MO: Penetrating injuries of the aortic arch, innominate, and subclavian arteries. In Ernst CB, Stanley JC (eds): Current Therapy in Vascular Surgery, 4th ed. Philadelphia, Mosby, in press.
7. Perry MO: Injuries in the neck. In Chant ADB, Barros D'Sa AAB (eds): Emergency Vascular Practice. London, Edward Arnold, 1997, pp 214–222.
8. Fabian TC, Davis KA, Gavant ML, et al: Prospective study of blunt aortic injury: Helical CT is diagnostic and antihypertensive therapy reduces rupture. Ann Surg 1998;227:666–677.
9. Hess PJ, Howe HR, Robiesek R, et al: Traumatic tears of the thoracic aorta: Improved results using the Biomedicus pump. Ann Thorac Surg 1989;48:6–9.
10. Marin ML, Veith FJ, Panetta TF, et al: Transluminally placed endovascular stented graft repair for arterial trauma. J Vasc Surg 1994;20:466–473.
11. Liekweg WG, Greenfield LJ: Management of penetrating carotid injuries. Surgery 1974;76:955–962.
12. Teehan EP, Padberg FT, Thompson PN, et al: Carotid arterial trauma: Assessment with the Glasgow Coma Scale (GCS) as a guide to surgical management. Cardiovasc Surg 1997;5:196–203.

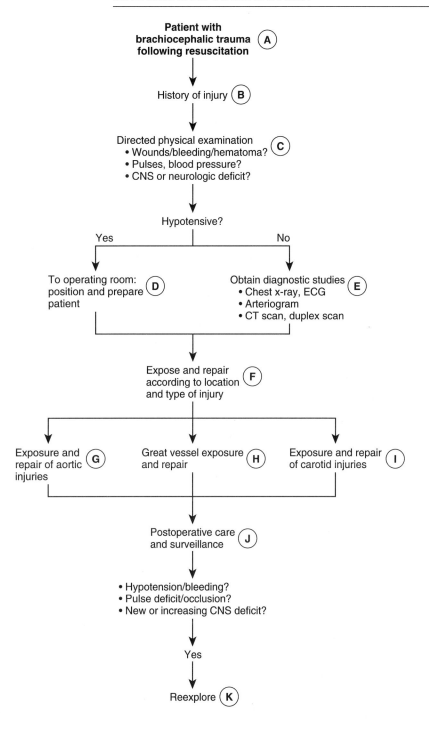

Chapter 65 Abdominal Vascular Trauma

JAMES T. LEE, MD • FRED S. BONGARD, MD

(A) Abdominal vascular injuries result from blunt and penetrating trauma and remain one of the more challenging scenarios in today's trauma centers. Injury to the abdominal vessels is seen in 12% of patients with penetrating abdominal trauma and in 2% to 3% of patients with blunt trauma.[1]

(B) The clinical diagnosis in a patient with a penetrating abdominal wound who is hypotensive is fairly straightforward. In contrast, blunt vascular injury in a normotensive patient can manifest as clinical evidence that is often ambiguous. Conscious patients may give a history of the nature of the trauma. If not, an understanding of the mechanism of vascular injury from blunt trauma can be facilitated by a report from someone on the scene, such as an emergency medical services (EMS) technician.

Body position and speed on impact, the object with which the patient had impact, the nature of wounds, visible bleeding and vital signs at the scene, and similar information all provide the treating physicians with a better perspective of the nature of the trauma. Sudden deceleration or compression of the torso can result in avulsion or thrombosis of major intra-abdominal vessels. Avulsion from fixed mesenteric attachments is particularly likely for branches or tributaries connected with the superior mesenteric artery (SMA) and portal vein as well as hepatic veins that empty into the retrohepatic vena cava. In other instances, an intimal tear can result from the sheer stress of overstretching of a vessel. Occlusion by an intimal flap is thought to be responsible for the "seat belt aorta" and for thrombosis of the renal arteries.[2]

Physical examination includes checking the vital signs (especially for hypotension, which is likely to be associated with a major vascular injury); inspecting for wounds and abdominal wall contusions (e.g., seat belt marks); and noting abdominal distention, tenderness, and guarding, and ileus.

(C) Certain studies are routine for most patients with major injuries. A chest x-ray is obtained to evaluate associated injuries, including hemothorax, pneumothorax, and bony fractures. Plain films of the abdomen and pelvis, with markers placed at entrance and exit sites in patients with penetrating trauma, can direct and focus attention to likely areas of injury. Displaced viscera, obscured muscle contours, excessive intraperitoneal fluid, and an elevated diaphragm may all signal a source of bleeding. Laboratory studies commonly include serial hematocrit measurements, typing and crossmatching of blood, and urinalysis.

The utility of urinalysis to demonstrate the presence of microscopic hematuria continues to be a topic of controversy. The presence of shock with microscopic hematuria has been reported to be more characteristic of renovascular injury than microscopic hematuria alone.[3-5] In the past, a "one-shot" intravenous pyelogram (IVP) was often used in hemodynamically stable patients with microscopic hematuria and transient hypotension after flank or abdominal trauma. Because of the 30% rate of false-negative results associated with an IVP, however, computed tomography (CT) has become the study of choice for the diagnosis of renal parenchymal injury in a stable patient.[6]

(D) Most patients with abdominal vascular injuries arrive in shock, and many are in extremis. Standard resuscitation protocols, such as Advanced Trauma Life Support (ATLS), should be instituted. Warm physiologic fluid resuscitation through bilateral upper extremity intravenous (IV) lines is needed to obtain an adequate arterial pressure. It may be necessary to place additional IV lines. Caution is warranted in the use of lower extremity venous access. In the patient with a major iliocaval *venous* injury, crystalloid infusion given through lower extremity venous access will spill into the peritoneal cavity or retroperitoneum and will not reach the central circulation.[5, 7]

(E) Physiologic derangements from injury to other organ systems are almost invariably associated with abdominal vascular trauma.[8] The hemodynamic status is pivotal in the decision whether to pursue further diagnostic studies or to proceed directly with surgical exploration.

(F) If hemodynamic stability can be achieved, diagnostic peritoneal lavage (DPL) is worthwhile in patients with *blunt* trauma because negative results may obviate laparotomy. In contrast, there is *no* role for DPL in a patient who is hypotensive or who has a penetrating injury to the abdomen.

(G) In patients with abdominal vascular injuries, hemodynamic instability often precludes extensive preoperative studies. In hemodynamically stable patients, however, a CT scan of the abdomen and pelvis is extremely valuable. It is sensitive in defining solid organ injuries after blunt trauma.[9] CT characterization of retroperitoneal hematomas secondary to abdominal vascular disruption—more specifically to the renal arteries, aorta, and mesenteric branches—has been well described.[9, 10] Thus, CT may indicate that the source of bleeding is partly or temporarily contained or slow enough that the patient remains hemodynamically stable. This finding may provide an opportunity for arteriography and even for angiographic control of the bleeding.

(H) Advances in interventional radiology have provided opportunities beyond angiographic localization of the bleeding source in the form of adjunctive techniques for controlling hemorrhage. The utility of angiographically controlled embolization of bleeding pelvic vessels is well documented.[11-13]

Asymptomatic deceleration injury to the renal vasculature may be suspected when the kidney does not opacify on IVP or CT scan. It is perhaps the only abdominal vascular injury to require angiographic proof for diagnosis.[8] Placement of stents to correct intimal dissection of the renal arteries from sudden deceleration has been performed successfully.[14, 15] Blunt intimal disruption usually occurs 2 cm from the origin of the renal artery. This disruption more often involves the left renal artery, which is shorter and less fixed than the right and thus has a shorter surface area to absorb sheer stress from stretching.[16, 17]

When an initial CT scan demonstrates fractures of the liver or spleen, angiographically controlled embolization of the associated arteries can be therapeutic. This procedure can also be accomplished in selected patients in whom surgery has been unsuccessful and reoperation is undesirable.[18]

Aortography should be performed in all hemodynamically stable patients with suspected aortic injury.[19] Once an injury to the aorta or its major branches is diagnosed, a balloon catheter may be placed under real-time fluoroscopic guidance into the abdominal aorta preoperatively to assist in obtaining proximal control of bleeding.[20] Failure to achieve satisfactory, permanent control of hemorrhage by means of these techniques is an indication for laparotomy.

(I) Anterolateral thoracotomy in the emergency department is associated with a dismal prognosis (6% to 8% survival).[9, 21] However, it may be the only option available to the surgeon when a patient demonstrates progressive hemodynamic instability and increased abdominal distention.[20]

(J) Once the need for laparotomy has been established, certain objectives should be met in an organized fashion. Adequate blood products should be present and body warming measures instituted. The patient, and the surgeon, must be prepared for entry into either the thorax or the abdominal cavity.[22] The source of hemorrhage must be exposed and identified. Operative principles include four-quadrant packing of the abdomen to obtain temporary hemostasis, with supraceliac

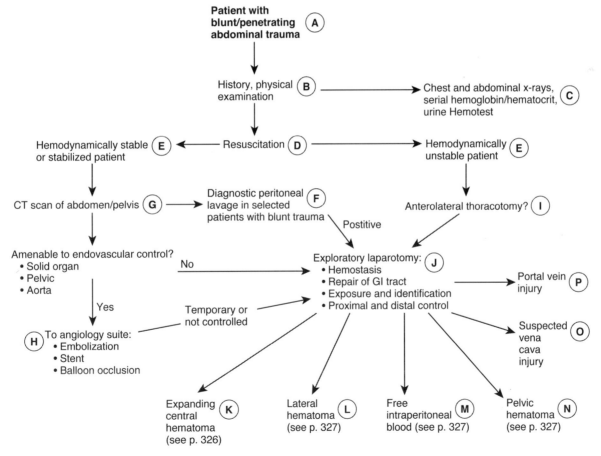

Illustration continued on following page

Abdominal Vascular Trauma (continued)

aortic control if necessary. The retroperitoneum, base of mesentery, lateral pelvic area, and portal triad must not be overlooked.[9] Control of enteric defects and removal of soilage should be accomplished before definitive vascular repair is undertaken.

(K) An expanding central hematoma usually indicates aortic disruption. The abdominal aorta is divided into three surgical regions[23]:

- Diaphragmatic (supraceliac)
- Suprarenal
- Infrarenal

Penetrating injuries to the *supraceliac* aorta have a high mortality rate owing to exsanguination. The major challenges in its treatment are exposure and control.[20] Direct pressure controls the bleeding while exposure is obtained. Proximal control is established by blunt dissection through the lesser omentum, with mobilization of the esophagus to the left and application of a clamp at the diaphragmatic hiatus.[24] Left-to-right rotation of medial viscera exposes the aorta and its branches from T9 to the bifurcation.

The aorta is repaired primarily with a lateral suture. If a large defect is present, an autogenous patch styled from an opened hypogastric artery is preferred, although polytetrafluoroethylene (PTFE) or polyester (Dacron) can be used if necessary.[23] The celiac axis arteries can be individually ligated without sequelae if the SMA and cephalad collateral vessels remain patent. The common hepatic artery should be ligated proximal to the origin of the gastroduodenal artery, which serves as the major collateral from the SMA. Splenic infarction necessitating subsequent splenectomy can occur after ligation of the splenic artery if collateral flow from the short gastric arteries proves insufficient.

Suprarenal aortic injuries are associated with a mortality rate of 28% to 46%.[25] Concomitant injury to the inferior vena cava (IVC) has a reported mortality rate of 100%.[26] SMA injuries may manifest as hemorrhage, intestinal ischemia, or arteriovenous fistula.[27] Chronic atherosclerotic occlusion of the SMA may be tolerated because of collateral flow. In acute SMA occlusion, however, this established collateralization is not sufficient to prevent bowel ischemia in patients with previously normal mesenteric circulation.[28]

Proximal control of the supraceliac aorta is established either at the diaphragm (by means of entry into the lesser sac through the gastrohepatic omentum and blunt division of the left crus) or through the left chest. Mobilization of all left-sided intra-abdominal viscera, including the left colon, pancreas, spleen, left kidney, and fundus of the stomach, is a valuable maneuver in dealing with major vascular injuries to the aorta and the origin of its major visceral branches.[10] When injury to the IVC is suspected, however, medial rotation of the right viscera is preferred. Access to the SMA is best achieved through an incision at the base of the mesentery. In some instances, when the SMA is approached anteriorly, division of the pancreas with distal pancreatectomy may be necessary.[27]

Lateral repair of the suprarenal aorta is preferred. Adjacent defects should be connected and either closed primarily or by patch aortoplasty using PTFE or polyester (Dacron).[29] Injuries at or near the origin of the SMA can be oversewn or ligated if the pancreaticoduodenal arteries as well as the collateral vessels from the celiac and inferior mesenteric artery remain intact. More distal injuries (1 to 2 cm) must be repaired with lateral arteriorrhaphy or reconstructed with use of a bypass graft. Saphenous vein is the preferred conduit, but success with PTFE has also been reported.[30] The proximal anastomosis is performed below the inferior edge of the pancreas to avoid a potential

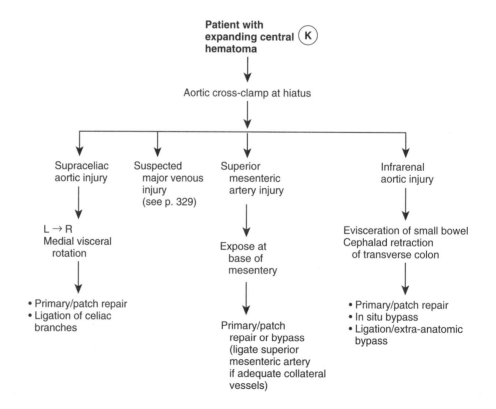

fistula. Fluorescein dye and Doppler ultrasound examination can determine the adequacy of mesenteric blood flow.[31]

Finally, a low threshold for a second-look laparotomy is advocated.[9, 22, 28, 32] A 58% survival after SMA injury has been reported; however, if more than lateral repair is required, the survival rate is only 22%.[27] Concomitant injuries to the superior mesenteric vein (SMV) occur in 50% of patients with SMA injuries.[27, 28] Exposure is often difficult, especially in the segment that lies just beneath the pancreas. Primary repair, interposition of a saphenous vein graft, or splenic vein anastomosis is favored over ligation.[8, 9, 22, 28]

Infrarenal aortic injuries are associated with a survival rate of 48% to 55%.[23] Commonly, a large midline retroperitoneal hematoma with flank extension is seen intraoperatively. Coexistent laceration of the vena cava and an acute aortocaval fistula in the setting of penetrating trauma must be anticipated.[33]

After blunt trauma, avulsion of posterior lumbar branches of the aorta or IVC account for major blood loss.[10] Exposure requires cephalad retraction of the transverse colon and evisceration of the small bowel. The proximal clamp is applied below the left renal vein. Distally, an obliquely applied vascular clamp affords control of the posterior lumbar arteries. Repair of the infrarenal aorta is performed in the same manner as described previously for suprarenal aortic injuries. Primary repair is accomplished in arterial tears or lacerations smaller than 1 cm.[23, 33] When a large segment is involved, either in situ bypass or ligation with extra-anatomic bypass is required.

For penetrating wounds, examination of the posterior wall of the aorta can exclude a potential missed injury to the back wall.[29] If an in situ graft is placed, the retroperitoneum is carefully closed with a pedicle of omentum interposed between the duodenum and prostheses. Consideration of four-compartment fasciotomies of the lower extremities is warranted after prolonged clamp time in patients undergoing extra-anatomic bypass.[34]

(L) Lateral retroperitoneal hematomas often develop following injuries to the renal vasculature. These hematomas are routinely explored when caused by penetrating trauma. Stable hematomas secondary to blunt trauma are generally left intact. When necessary, surgical intervention for blunt trauma should be pursued in the most expedient manner after injury.[35–37]

Prior to exploration of a perirenal or paracolic hematoma, proximal control of the renal pedicle is established. The surgeon obtains control of the left renal artery by opening the root of the mesentery once the small bowel is reflected to the right and the colon retracted cephalad. The left renal vein is also mobilized superiorly through ligation of its major branches to provide adequate exposure to the left renal artery. The left renal vein may be ligated and divided in the midline as it crosses the aorta. The same approach is used to achieve control of the right renal artery. In addition, a Kocher maneuver may be necessary to improve exposure of the right renal vessels.[38] This approach is ideal for renal parenchymal wounds, allowing for individual ligation of bleeding vessels and diminishing the incidence of nephrectomy.[39]

Once proximal control is accomplished, revascularization can be achieved with the use of lateral arteriorrhaphy, end-to-end anastomosis, prosthetic or autologous bypass, and (in rare instances) autotransplantation. Transposition of the splenic artery with concomitant splenectomy has also been reported.[20, 29]

Traumatic disruption of the renal veins should be repaired through lateral venorrhaphy. The left renal vein can be ligated proximal to the junction of the adrenal and gonadal veins. Nephrectomy must accompany ligation of the right renal vein.[9, 29] Reports of formation of collateral circulation validate the argument against early nephrec-

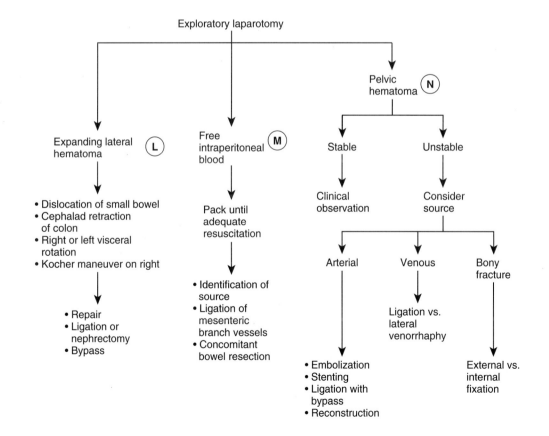

Abdominal Vascular Trauma (continued)

tomy.[17, 37, 40] However, a common sequela of renal trauma is the development of refractory hypertension, which may require future nephrectomy.[35, 37]

(M) When unrecognized, free intraperitoneal blood originating from the aorta and its major branches leads to fatal exsanguination. Once the abdomen is opened, four-quadrant packing and manual compression should be the initial step. Mesenteric bleeding points are controlled by digital compression and individual suture ligatures. Other sources, once identified, are managed as outlined in the algorithms in this chapter. Repair and restoration of bowel continuity are undertaken to prevent further intra-abdominal contamination.

In the event of hemodynamic instability, intractable acidosis, hypothermia, and coagulopathy, "damage control laparotomy" is an acceptable option. The abdomen is packed in all quadrants, and the patient is taken to the intensive care unit for resuscitation, correction of coagulopathy, and rewarming. Once these issues have been addressed, the patient can be brought back to the operating room for definitive management.

(N) During exploratory laparotomy for other injuries, there is no indication for routine exploration of pelvic hematomas secondary to *blunt trauma*, especially if (1) they are associated with pelvic fractures or normal genitourinary study findings or (2) they are expanding slowly.[10, 39, 41] Nonoperative management is discounted in the presence of a ruptured or pulsatile hematoma, a rapidly expanding hematoma, absence of femoral pulses, intraperitoneal transection of the urethra in a male patient, or rupture of the bladder.[10, 39, 42] The cause of continuing hemorrhage is arterial, venous, a result of fracture edges, or a combination of these sources.

Defining the source and obtaining control of pelvic bleeding in a large hematoma are technical challenges. Often the size of the hematoma makes it impossible to define which side is injured. A sound maneuver is to obtain initial control proximal to the hematoma through aortic or vena caval compression concurrent with direct pressure at the site of active bleeding.[8]

Pelvic veins are frequently the cause of continued hemorrhage in the patient with blunt trauma.[22] In such cases, tight packing of the pelvis with subsequent external fixation of the associated pelvic fracture is usually effective.

Therapeutic angiographic embolization of deep pelvic arteries can be performed in the operating suite in the presence of massive exsanguination.[43] The insertion of Fogarty balloon catheters offers an efficacious temporary reprieve prior to proximal ligation.[44, 45]

Rarely seen blunt traumatic injuries to the iliac arteries include intimal disruption and thrombosis. Endovascular stenting of traumatic intimal dissection of the iliac system has been described to be theoretically feasible.[46] Endovascular devices have been placed successfully in the setting of traumatic pseudoaneurysms and arteriovenous fistulas of the common iliac arteries.[47, 48] Crush injuries to the pelvis can result in thrombosis of the iliac arteries.[49, 50] In situ reconstruction with an interposition graft, iliofemoral bypass, and extra-anatomic femorofemoral bypass graft are good limb-sparing options. Major arterial injury occurs in 1% of patients with blunt trauma and carries an 83% mortality rate.[42, 51] Whenever a vascular injury is suspected

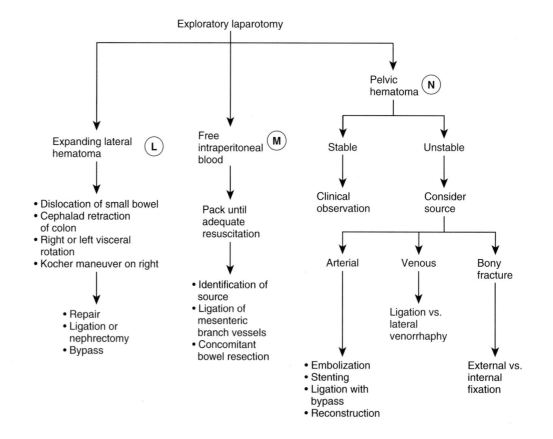

after *penetrating trauma* to the pelvis, surgical intervention is pursued. Iliac artery injuries are frequently associated with colonic violation.[52] When primary repair is unsuccessful, reconstruction with vein or prosthetic graft is used. The ipsilateral hypogastric artery may also be used as a conduit.[29]

In the presence of gross fecal contamination and hemodynamic instability, ligation of the injured common iliac artery is an acceptable alternative, followed by restoration of bowel continuity or diversion ("damage control"). Postoperatively, careful serial neurovascular examinations document limb viability. In the event that ischemia is observed, a femorofemoral crossover with four-compartment fasciotomy is performed.[20, 29, 34, 53, 54] Primary iliac artery ligation without revascularization is associated with an amputation rate of 45% to 55%.[55]

Venous injuries to the iliac system are rare and potentially difficult to control. Surgical options include lateral venorrhaphy and ligation. Occasionally, when access is technically difficult, transection of the right common iliac artery provides the necessary exposure to repair the underlying venous injury. This is followed by repair of the respective iliac artery.[8, 56] A layer of peritoneum, omentum, or mesenteric fat can be placed between the artery and vein if the two suture lines lie in close proximity.[9]

O Injuries to the IVC and portal vein can lead to unexpected catastrophic hemorrhage. Fatal exsanguination is the major cause of early postoperative mortality. Late death is often due to sepsis.[57–59] Infrarenal vena caval injuries occur in one third to one half of patients.[23, 57] Initial control of small lacerations is often achieved through direct pressure applied manually or with sponge sticks. Repair is with lateral venorrhaphy, provided that the vessel's diameter is not compromised by more than 50%.[23, 58, 59]

Patients with complex injuries require more aggressive dissection. Exposure is gained through a right-to-left medial visceral rotation or an extended Kocher maneuver. The infrarenal vena cava can also be approached in the same manner as the infrarenal aorta (see previously). Significant defects have been repaired with the use of thin-walled PTFE or autogenous vein in the form of a panel graft or a spiral vein graft.[60, 61] When an extensive section of the infrarenal vena cava is disrupted and hemodynamic stability is tenuous, ligation is an acceptable intervention. Should this occur, aggressive administration of fluids is necessary to maintain an adequate circulatory volume.

As with all vascular trauma, especially penetrating trauma, inspection of the posterior surfaces of the vasculature is essential. Repair of posterior wounds to the vena cava can be facilitated through extension of the anterior defect and repair of the posterior venotomy, followed by closure of the entrance site.[20, 29, 58, 62]

Expeditious identification and management of a suprarenal or retrohepatic vena caval injury are challenging endeavors. Delay in diagnosis is often associated with massive hepatic and visceral trauma, which may mask the source of bleeding. The overall mortality rate is 33% to 67%.[2]

A right-to-left rotation of the medial viscera with an extended Kocher maneuver exposes the extrahepatic suprarenal vena cava. Hemostasis is achieved through digital compression, use of sponge sticks, or intraluminal balloon occlusion. Owing to the fragile nature of the vein wall, caution must be exercised with balloon inflation. Restorative techniques include repair with prosthetic or autogenous materials similar to those used in infrarenal vena caval injuries. Ligation at this location has largely been abandoned because of the associated high mortality rate.[57–62]

The retrohepatic vena cava is the most difficult to expose and control. Preparation for a median sternotomy should be anticipated in case more proximal control is necessary. Mobilization of the liver is attained by division of the coronary and triangular ligaments. In the event of massive liver trauma, extension of the hepatic laceration along the injury tract can adequately expose the confluence of the hepatic veins and vena cava.[63] Several

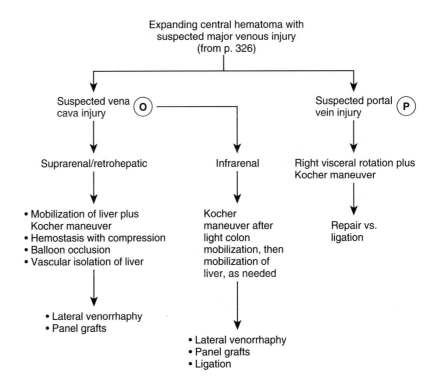

techniques, including atrial–vena cava shunting and venovenous bypass, have been reported for vascular isolation.[59, 64, 65] The more popular approach is placement of an endotracheal tube through a right atrial cardiotomy to lie just above the renal veins.[2, 66] Once the shunt is in place, vessel repair or hepatic resection can be attempted.

Perioperative care involves meticulous fluid balance and the use of sequential venous compression devices, elastic bandage (Ace) wraps, and limb elevation to minimize venous pooling.[2, 23, 62] Long-term anticoagulation in the late postoperative period is suggested because the incidence of pulmonary embolism in such cases approaches 25%.[58]

(P) Because of the frequent association of other morbid injuries and the difficulty with anatomic accessibility, portal vein injuries often manifest as exsanguinating hemorrhage.[57] The mortality rate is 41% to 71%.[67]

An extended Kocher maneuver provides access to the porta hepatis. The portal vein is then isolated from the common bile duct and hepatic artery. Application of a noncrushing clamp across all three structures (Pringle's maneuver) may be required. Further exposure may necessitate division of the pancreatic head. Lateral venorrhaphy or end-to-end anastomosis should be performed, although panel grafts may be required when significant disruption has occurred.[2, 23] Other surgical options are interposition grafting and direct anastomosis of the proximal splenic vein to the SMV.[29, 57, 68] Postoperative surveillance guides the use of anticoagulation therapy.[69]

In the setting of multiple intra-abdominal or extra-abdominal injuries, particularly with onset of coagulopathy, acidosis, or hypothermia, it may be necessary to ligate the portal vein.[60, 70, 71] This maneuver may lead to frank hepatic necrosis, especially in the hypotensive patient. It is therefore important to ensure preservation of the hepatic artery if portal vein ligation is considered. Mesocaval shunting can be performed but is associated with multiple complications.[57, 60, 61, 67, 72] The development of severe intestinal edema following ligation necessitates aggressive replacement of intravascular volume.[23, 39, 60, 70] A "second-look" laparotomy is recommended to remove any necrotic bowel resulting from venous hypertension.[57]

ACKNOWLEDGMENT

The authors would like to thank Colleen L. Brayack for her timely assistance in preparing the decision tree for this chapter.

REFERENCES

1. Mattox KL, Feliciano DV: Visceral vascular trauma. In Moore EE, Eiseman B, Van Way CW III (eds): Critical Decisions in Trauma. St. Louis, CV Mosby, 1984, p 222.
2. Bongard FS: Thoracic and abdominal vascular trauma. In Rutherford RB (ed): Vascular Surgery, 5th ed. Philadelphia, WB Saunders, 2000, p 871.
3. Mee SL, McAninch, JW, Robinson, AL, et al: Radiographic assessment of renal trauma: A ten-year prospective study of patient selection. J Urol 1989;141:1095.
4. Mee SL, McAninch JW: Indications for radiographic assessment in suspected renal trauma. Urol Clin North Am 1989;16:187.
5. Perry MO, Bongard FS: Vascular trauma. In Moore WS (ed): Vascular Surgery: A Comprehensive Review, 5th ed. Philadelphia, WB Saunders, 1998, p 648.
6. Wilson RF, Zeigler DW: Diagnostic and treatment problems in renal injuries. Am Surg 1987;53:399.
7. Mattox KL, Hirshberg A, Wall M: Alternate approaches to resuscitation. In Ivatury RR, Cayten CG (eds): The Textbook of Penetrating Trauma. Baltimore, Williams & Wilkins, 1996, p 196.
8. Mattox KL, Hirshberg A: Vascular trauma. In Haimovici H, Ascer E, Hollier LH, et al (eds): Vascular Surgery. Cambridge, Mass, Blackwell Scientific, 1996, p 480.
9. Carrillo EH, Bergamini TM, Miller FB, et al: Abdominal vascular injuries. J Trauma 1997;43:164.
10. Feliciano DV: Management of traumatic retroperitoneal hematoma. Ann Surg 1990;211:109.
11. Ben-Menachem Y, Handel SF, Thaggard A, et al: Thera-

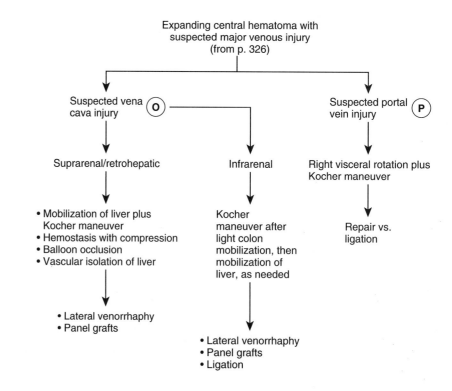

peutic arterial embolization in trauma. J Trauma 1979; 19:944.
12. Yellin AE, Lundell CJ, Finck EJ: Diagnosis and control of post-traumatic pelvic hemorrhage: Transcatheter angiographic embolization techniques. Arch Surg 1983; 118:1378.
13. Panetta T, Sclafani SJ, Goldstein, AS, et al: Percutaneous transcatheter embolization for massive bleeding from pelvic fractures. J Trauma 1985;25:1021.
14. Whigham CJ Jr, Bodenhamer JR, Miller JK: Use of the Palmaz stent in primary treatment of renal artery intimal injury secondary to blunt trauma. J Vasc Interv Radiol 1995;6:175.
15. Goodman DNF, Saibil EA, Kodama RT: Traumatic intimal tear of the renal artery treated by insertion of a Palmaz stent. Cardiovasc Intervent Radiol 1998;21:69.
16. Barlow B, Gandi R: Renal artery thrombosis following blunt trauma. J Trauma 1980;20:614.
17. Carrol PR, McAninch JW, Klosterman P, et al: Renovascular trauma: Risk, assessment, surgical management, and outcome. J Trauma 1990;30:547.
18. Velmahos GC, Demetriades D, Chahwan S, et al: Angiographic embolization for arrest of bleeding after penetrating trauma to the abdomen. Am J Surg 1999;178:367.
19. Brathwaite CEM, Rodriguez A: Injuries of the abdominal aorta from blunt trauma. Am Surg 1992;58:350.
20. Mattox KL, Burch JM, Richardson R, et al: Retroperitoneal vascular injury. Surg Clin North Am 1990;70:635.
21. Ivatury RR, Kazigo J, Rohman M, et al: Directed emergency room thoracotomy: A prognostic prerequisite for survival. J Trauma 1991;31:1076.
22. Mullins RJ, Huckfeldt R, Trunkey DD: Abdominal vascular injuries. Surg Clin North Am 1996;76:813.
23. Bongard FS: Vascular injury. In Cameron JL (ed): Current Surgical Therapy. St. Louis, CV Mosby, 1995, p 843.
24. Veith FJ, Gupta S, Daly V: Technique for occluding the supraceliac aorta through the abdomen. Surg Gynecol Obstet 1980;151:427.
25. Bongard FS, Dubrow T, Klein SR: Vascular injuries in the urban battleground: Experience at a metropolitan trauma center. Ann Vasc Surg 1990;4:415.
26. Accola KD, Feliciano DV, Mattox KL, et al: Management of injuries to the suprarenal aorta. Am J Surg 1987; 154:613.
27. Accola KD, Feliciano DV, Mattox KL, et al: Management of injuries to the superior mesenteric artery. J Trauma 1986;26:313.
28. Bourland WA, Kispert JF, Hyde GL, et al: Trauma to the proximal superior mesenteric artery: A case report and review of the literature. J Vasc Surg 1992;15:669.
29. Feliciano DV: Abdominal vascular injuries. Surg Clin North Am 1988;68:741.
30. Lucas AE, Richardson JD, Flint LM, et al: Traumatic injury of the proximal superior mesenteric artery. Ann Surg 1981;193:30.
31. Marfuggi RA, Greenspan M: Reliable intraoperative prediction of intestinal viability using a fluorescent indicator. Surg Gynecol Obstet 1981;152:33.
32. Courcy PA, Brotman S, Oster-Granite ML, et al: Superior mesenteric artery and vein injuries from blunt abdominal trauma. J Trauma 1984;24:843.
33. Talhouk AK, Lim RC, Bongard FS: Abdominal aortic injuries. In Bongard FS, Wilson SE, Perry MO (eds): Vascular Injuries in Surgical Practice. Norwalk, Conn, Appleton & Lange, 1991, p 165.
34. Padberg FT Jr, Hobson RW II: Fasciotomy in acute limb ischemia. Semin Vasc Surg 1992;5:52.
35. Dinchman KH, Spirnak JP: Traumatic renal artery thrombosis: Evaluation and treatment. Semin Urol 1995; 13:90.
36. Wein AJ, Arger PH, Murphy JJ: Controversial aspects of blunt renal trauma. J Trauma 1997;17:662.
37. Maggio AJ, Brosnan S: Renal artery trauma. Urology 1987;11:125.
38. McAninch JW, Carroll PR: Renal trauma: Kidney preservation through improved vascular control. J Trauma 1982;22:285.
39. Canizaro PC, Pessa ME: Management of massive hemorrhage associated with abdominal trauma. Surg Clin North Am 1990;70:621.
40. Feliciano DV, Burch JM, Graham JM: Abdominal vascular injury. In Feliciano DV, Moore WS, Mattox KL (eds): Trauma. Norwalk, Conn, Appleton & Lange, 1996, p 615.
41. Klein SR, Bongard FS, Mehringer CM: Management strategy of vascular injuries associated with pelvic fractures. J Cardiovasc Surg (Torino) 1992;33:349.
42. Rothenberger DA, Fischer RP, Perry JF Jr: Major vascular injuries secondary to pelvic fractures: An unsolved clinical problem. Am J Surg 1978;136:660.
43. Saueracker AJ, McCroskey BL, Moore EE, et al: Intraoperative hypogastric artery embolization for life-threatening pelvic hemorrhage: A preliminary report. J Trauma 1987;27:1127.
44. Paster SB, VanHouten FX, Adams DF: Percutaneous balloon catheterization, a technique for the control of arterial hemorrhage caused by pelvic trauma. JAMA 1974; 230:573.
45. Sheldon GF, Winestock DP: Hemorrhage from open pelvic fracture controlled intraoperatively with balloon catheter. J Trauma 1987;18:68.
46. Landreneau RJ, Lewis DM: Complex iliac arterial trauma: Autologous or prosthetic vascular repair? Surgery 1993;114:9.
47. Moore WS, Marin ML: Endovascular grafting. In Moore WS (ed): Vascular Surgery: A Comprehensive Review, 5th ed. Philadelphia, WB Saunders, 1998, p 330.
48. White RA, Donayre CE, Walot I, et al: Preliminary clinical outcome and imaging criterion for endovascular prosthesis development in high risk patients with aortoiliac and traumatic arterial lesions. J Vasc Surg 1996;24:556.
49. Smejkal R, Izant T, Born C, et al: Pelvic crush injuries with occlusion of the iliac artery. J Trauma 1988;28:1479.
50. Brown JJ, Greene FL, Mcmillin RD: Vascular injuries associated with pelvic fractures. Am Surg 1984;50:150.
51. Rothenberger D, Fischer R, Strate R, et al: The mortality associated with pelvic fractures. Surgery 1978;84:356.
52. Mattox KL, Rea J, Ennix CL, et al: Penetrating injuries to the iliac arteries. Am J Surg 1978;136:663.
53. Burch JM, Richardson RJ, Martin RR, et al: Penetrating iliac vascular injuries: Recent experience with 233 consecutive patients. J Trauma 1990;30:1450.
54. Rutherford RB: Acute limb ischemia: Clinical assessment and standards for reporting. Semin Vasc Surg 1992;5:4.
55. DeBakey ME, Simeone FA: Battle injuries of the arteries in World War II: An analysis of 2,471 cases. Ann Surg 1946;123:534.
56. Salam AA, Stewart MT: New approach to wounds of the aortic bifurcation and inferior vena cava. Surgery 1985;98:105.
57. State DL, Bongard FS: Abdominal venous injuries. In Bongard FS, Wilson SE, Perry MO (eds): Vascular Injuries in Surgical Practice. Norwalk, Conn, Appleton & Lange, 1991, p 185.
58. Burch JM, Feliciano DV, Mattox KL: Injuries to the inferior vena cava. Am J Surg 1988;156:548.
59. Wiencek RG, Wilson RF: Inferior vena cava injuries—the challenge continues. Am Surg 1988;54:423.
60. Mattox KL: Abdominal venous injuries. Surgery 1982;91:497.
61. Conti S: Abdominal venous trauma. In Blaisdell FW, Trunkey DD (eds): Trauma Management, Vol I. Abdominal Trauma. New York, Thieme-Stratton, 1982, p 253.
62. Ward RE, Blaisdell FW: Abdominal aorta and vena cava injuries. In Moore EE, Eiseman B, Van Way CW III (eds): Critical Decisions in Trauma. St. Louis, CV Mosby, 1984, p 218.
63. Pachter HL, Spencer FC, Hofstetter S, et al: The management of juxtahepatic venous injuries without an atriocaval shunt: Preliminary clinical observations. Surgery 1986;99:569.
64. Beall SL, Wards RE: Successful atrial caval shunting in the management of retrohepatic venous injuries. Am J Surg 1988;158:409.
65. Baumgartner F, Scudamore C, Nair C: Veno-veno bypass for major hepatic and caval trauma. J Trauma 1995; 39:671.
66. Rovito PF: Atrial caval shunting in blunt hepatic vascular injury. Ann Surg 1987;205:318.
67. Weil PH: Management of retroperitoneal trauma. Curr Probl Surg 1982;20:545.
68. Sheldon GF, Lim RC, Yee ES, et al: Management of injuries to the porta hepatis. Ann Surg 1985;202:539.
69. Ivatury RR, Nallathambi M, Lankin DH, et al: Portal vein injuries: Noninvasive follow-up of venorrhaphy. Ann Surg 1987;206:733.
70. Stone HH, Fabian TC, Turkleson ML: Wounds of the portal venous system. World J Surg 1982;6:355.
71. Pachter HL, Drager S, Godfrey N, et al: Traumatic injuries to the portal vein. Ann Surg 1979;189:383.
72. Peterson SR, Sheldon GF, Lim RC: Management of portal venous injuries. J Trauma 1979;19:616.

Chapter 66 Extremity Vascular Trauma

S. RAM KUMAR, MD • DOUGLAS B. HOOD, MD • FRED A. WEAVER, MD

(A) Approximately 90% of all peripheral arterial injuries are located in the extremities, and more than 50% are caused by penetrating trauma. The following recommendations are valid only for injuries distal to the deltopectoral groove or inguinal ligament. For more proximal iliac or axillary injuries, diagnostic arteriography is required in the stable patient.

(B) Fewer than 5% of patients with peripheral vascular injuries arrive at the emergency department with active hemorrhage, an expanding hematoma, or an acutely ischemic extremity.[1] Patients with any or all of these findings have a high likelihood of major vascular injury and should proceed to the operating room without delay. Intraoperative arteriography may be required for precise localization and characterization of the injury.

(C) In a prospective analysis of 514 patients with penetrating extremity trauma,[1] a pulse deficit or a minimum ankle-brachial or wrist-brachial index (MABI) below 1.00 was present in all major arterial injuries requiring repair. Pulse deficit alone was significantly correlated with arterial injury but was present in only 25% of documented arterial injuries. Doppler indices have a significant and complementary role to the physical examination in detecting clinically occult injuries. Systolic pressure is measured by Doppler studies in the involved extremity and then compared with a normal extremity to obtain the pressure index. Use of a lower index threshold (i.e., <0.90 or 0.95) improves specificity but is significantly less sensitive.

(D) Several studies have investigated the accuracy of duplex ultrasound examination for detecting arterial injuries in patients with extremity trauma.[2,3] However, this modality is technically demanding and dependent on the skill of the technologist and the ability of a surgeon or radiologist to interpret the findings. Only institutions with significant technical expertise should use duplex ultrasonography as the first diagnostic test. When duplex ultrasonography is not available or if it provides inconclusive results, an arteriogram should be obtained; however, arteriograms are less than perfect, with about a 5% incidence of false-positive and false-negative results.[4]

(E) Some low-velocity penetrating ("minimal") injuries do not impair distal circulation or cause active hemorrhage. Arteriographically, these lesions are intimal defects, pseudoaneurysms smaller than 5 mm in diameter, and adherent or downstream intimal flaps.[5] Minimal injuries do not require immediate repair.

(F) Patients with a normal pulse and a Doppler index at or above 1.00 may be observed for 24 hours or even a briefer period and discharged.[1,5] Patients with negative duplex ultrasound or arteriographic findings may also be discharged after a brief period of observation.

(G) Over 90% of minimal injuries heal spontaneously or remain stable. Nonoperative management of these injuries is safe in both the short and the long term.[6] Evidence of vessel healing should be obtained by serial arteriography or duplex evaluation. Should these suggest a change (e.g., enlargement of a pseudoaneurysm), repair should be considered.

(H) Transcatheter embolization with particles, coils, or detachable balloons is indicated for low-flow arteriovenous fistulae, small pseudoaneurysms of noncritical arteries, and actively bleeding noncritical arteries, such as branches of the distal profunda femoris or muscular branches of major arteries.[7] Embolization can be done at the time of diagnostic arteriography. For selected proximal extremity large-vessel injuries (pseudoaneurysms or arteriovenous fistulae), stent-graft repair has also been successfully employed.[8]

(I) The injured extremity should be prepared and draped in its entirety. The contralateral lower extremity should also be draped for harvest of the saphenous vein if autogenous conduit is required. For upper extremity injuries, the contralateral arm or either lower extremity should be part of the operative field.

(J) Intraoperative arteriograms are required for multiple penetrating injuries or extensive blunt injuries when a preoperative study has not been obtained. Percutaneous or open cannulation of the common femoral artery or any arterial segment proximal to the injury, hand injection of contrast medium, and C-arm fluoroscopy can localize injuries requiring surgical repair.

(K) Assessment of all associated injuries plays a critical role in deciding the timing and nature of vascular intervention. The management of life-threatening head and neck, thoracic, or abdominal injuries takes precedence over restoration of extremity perfusion. On occasion, extremity vessel ligation may be necessary to arrest hemorrhage so that other, more life-threatening injuries can be addressed. The adage "life before limb" continues to be operational.

(L) The type of arterial repair depends on the site and magnitude of injury. Tension-free lateral repair or resection with end-to-end anastomosis or interposition grafting is commonly used to repair focal injuries. Bypass grafts are sometimes required for more extensive trauma with associated soft tissue and bone injury. If a vein graft is required, the vein should be harvested from an uninjured leg or arm. For more proximal repairs, especially in an unstable patient or in a patient with inadequate vein, prosthetic grafts may be used with satisfactory results. Polytetrafluoroethylene (PTFE) is currently the prosthetic material of choice. Any popliteal or infrapopliteal repair requires an autogenous conduit. At the time of repair, systemic use of heparin has been shown to improve limb salvage for popliteal injuries.[9] Intravenous administration of antioxidants (e.g., mannitol) prior to revascularization may be helpful in minimizing reperfusion injury.

M All arterial repairs require a routine completion study to document technical perfection and to assess the distal arterial tree for emboli or unsuspected injuries. Either intraoperative arteriography or duplex ultrasonography may be used.

N After all arterial repairs, the need for fasciotomy should be considered. Extremities with combined arterial and venous injuries, significant blunt soft tissue injury, more than 6 hours of limb ischemia, or occlusive popliteal injuries are susceptible to compartment syndrome. Compartments that are tense after reperfusion or with measured pressures in excess of 30 mmHg require a complete fasciotomy and dermotomy. Decompression of the four compartments of the lower leg require both medial and lateral incisions. A single volar incision is used to decompress the forearm.[10] If all soft tissue is viable, immediate coverage of fasciotomy sites with tension-free reapproximation of skin edges or split-thickness skin grafts decreases the risk of wound sepsis.[10] All patients who do not undergo fasciotomy should be carefully monitored postoperatively. The appearance of pain, especially to passive movements, diminished distal sensation, or a tense compartment should prompt fasciotomy. Loss of a distal pulse is a late finding in compartment syndrome and should not be relied upon to make this diagnosis.

O Orthopedic and arterial injuries commonly occur in the same extremity. If the limb is stable, arterial repair should be completed first and distal perfusion restored prior to orthopedic repair. Following the orthopedic procedure, it is incumbent on the surgeon to confirm the integrity of the vascular reconstruction before the patient leaves the operating room.

P When severe musculoskeletal injury renders the limb unstable, an external fixator can be placed rapidly, followed by the vascular repair. More definitive orthopedic repair may follow if needed. The use of an intravascular shunt across the injured portion of the artery to immediately reestablish distal perfusion before orthopedic stabilization has been suggested.[11] If external fixation

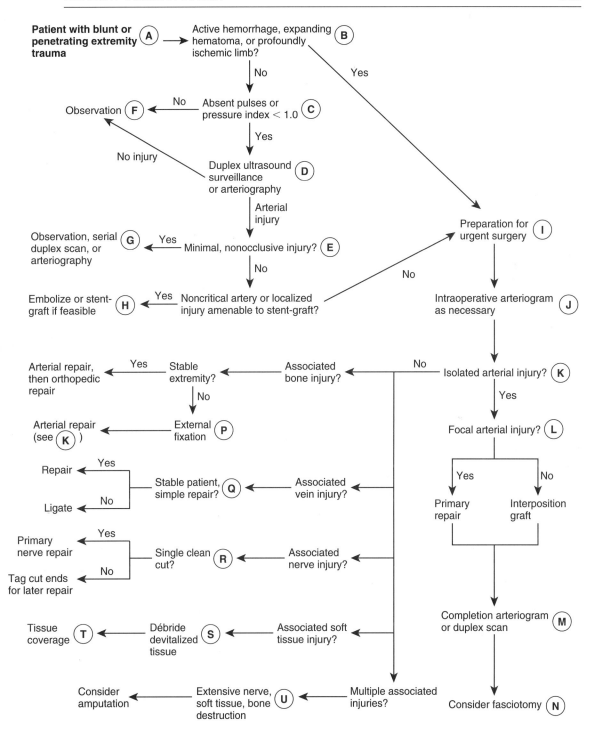

(Q) Major venous injuries should be managed according to location, associated injuries, and the patient's condition. Popliteal venous injuries carry the greatest potential for acute and chronic morbidity.[12] Simple lateral or end-to-end repair of venous injuries may be undertaken in the stable patient. When injured veins are repaired, meticulous attention to technique is essential because thrombosis ensues with the slightest anastomotic imperfection. For more extensive injuries, complex repairs using panel or spiral vein grafts have not proved durable. Most complex venous repairs thrombose within 14 days.[13] Following venous repair or ligation, the extremity should be elevated and wrapped with a compressive dressing.

(R) Neurologic injury occurs in association with 50% of upper and 25% of lower extremity vascular injuries and is a critical determinant of ultimate extremity function. In-continuity nerve injuries usually recover spontaneously and should be left intact. A nerve cleanly transected by a sharp instrument can be primarily repaired at the time of initial vascular repair, but this type of injury is uncommon. Most injured nerves should be tagged with nonabsorbable suture at the time of initial operation to facilitate easier identification at the time of subsequent repair 2 to 3 months later.[14]

(S) Peripheral vascular injuries are associated with varying degrees of damage to the surrounding soft tissues. More severe soft tissue injuries occur with blunt trauma, high-velocity gunshot wounds, and shotgun blasts. Effective management of major soft tissue injury requires débridement of all clearly nonviable tissues at the initial operation. Removal of devitalized tissue reduces the incidence of wound sepsis, an important cause of limb loss following successful arterial repair. Soft tissue wounds should be inspected frequently, in the operating room if necessary. For extensive complex wounds, return to the operating room may be necessary for inspection every 48 to 72 hours until all devitalized tissue is removed.

to stabilize the limb cannot be accomplished rapidly, an intravascular shunt can be considered but in our experience is seldom required.

(T) Soft tissue coverage of exposed bone, vessels, and nerves is important. In most penetrating extremity injuries, except for shotgun injuries, this is possible. For injuries with extensive soft tissue destruction, coverage may require mobilization and rotation of adjacent uninjured muscle or, rarely, the use of free flaps using the rectus abdominis or latissimus dorsi muscle.[15]

(U) Associated nerve, musculoskeletal, and venous injuries are factors that may affect the long-term functional status of the injured extremity. Several indices, such as the Mangled Extremity Severity Score (MESS) and the Limb Salvage Index (LSI), have been proposed in an attempt to identify those injured limbs that will be functionally useless.[16] However, we have found none of them sufficiently accurate to be relied upon in practice. Patients with extensive soft tissue, bone, nerve, and vascular injuries should be considered for primary amputation. The decision to amputate should involve, whenever possible, the patient and his or her family.

REFERENCES

1. Schwartz MR, Weaver FA, Bauer M, et al: Refining the indications for arteriography in penetrating extremity trauma: A prospective analysis. J Vasc Surg 1993; 17:116–124.
2. Fry WR, Smith RS, Sayers DV, et al: The success of duplex ultrasonographic scanning in diagnosis of extremity vascular proximity trauma. Arch Surg 1993;128: 1368–1372.
3. Bynoe RP, Miles JW, Bell RM, et al: Noninvasive diagnosis of vascular trauma by duplex ultrasonography. J Vasc Surg 1991;14:346–352.
4. Weaver FA, Yellin AE, Bauer M, et al: Is arterial proximity a valid indication for arteriography in penetrating extremity trauma? Arch Surg 1990;125:1256–1260.
5. Stain SC, Yellin AE, Weaver FA, Pentecost MJ: Selective management of nonocclusive arterial injuries. Arch Surg 1989;124:1136–1141.
6. Dennis JW, Fryberg ER, Veldenz HC, et al: Validation of nonoperative management of occult vascular injuries and accuracy of physical examination alone in penetrating extremity trauma: 5- to 10-year follow-up. J Trauma 1998;44:243–252; discussion, 242–243.
7. Yellin AE, Lundell CJ, Finck EJ: Diagnosis and control of posttraumatic pelvic hemorrhage: Transcatheter angiographic embolization techniques. Arch Surg 1983; 118:1378–1383.
8. Parodi JC, Schonholz C, Ferreira LM, Bergan J: Endovascular stent-graft treatment of traumatic arterial lesions. Ann Vasc Surg 1999;13:121–129.
9. Wagner WH, Calkins ER, Weaver FA, et al: Blunt popliteal artery trauma: One hundred consecutive injuries. J Vasc Surg 1988;7:736–743.
10. Johnson SB, Weaver FA, Yellin AE, et al: Clinical results of decompressive dermotomy-fasciotomy. Am J Surg 1992;164:286–290.
11. Johansen K, Bandyk D, Thiele B, Hansen ST Jr: Temporary intraluminal shunts: Resolution of a management dilemma in complex vascular injuries. J Trauma 1982; 22:395–402.
12. Rich NM: Principles and indications for primary venous repair. Surgery 1982;91:492–496.
13. Meyer J, Walsch J, Schuler J, et al: The early fate of venous repair after civilian vascular trauma. Ann Surg 1987;206:458–464.
14. Visser PA, Hermreck AS, Pierce GE, et al: Prognosis of nerve injuries incurred during acute trauma to peripheral arteries. Am J Surg 1980;140:596–599.
15. Levin LS: The reconstructive ladder: An orthoplastic approach. Orthop Clin North Am 1993;24:393–409.
16. O'Sullivan ST, O'Sullivan M, Pasha N, et al: Is it possible to predict limb viability in complex Gustilo IIIB and IIIC tibial fractures? A comparison of two predictive indices. Injury 1997;28:639–642.

EXTREMITY VASCULAR TRAUMA

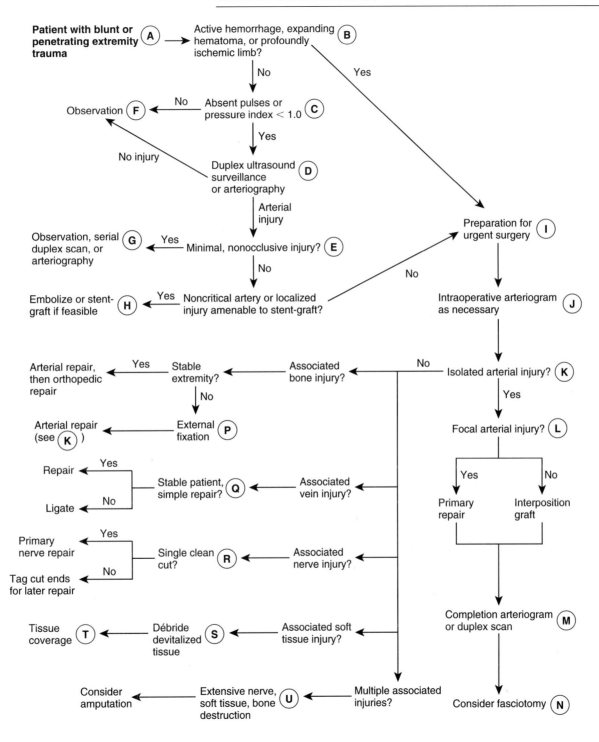

Chapter 67 Post-traumatic Pain Syndrome

ALI F. ABURAHMA, MD

A Post-traumatic pain syndromes (PTPSs), often called *causalgia* or *reflex sympathetic dystrophy*, remain one of the most poorly understood and frequently misdiagnosed entities encountered in clinical practice. Recently, the terminology "complex regional pain syndrome" (CRPS) has been suggested to encompass these terms.[1-3] PTPS can develop following irritation or damage to peripheral nerves in various settings. The initiating event may be relatively insignificant, even obscure. One form is caused by ischemic damage to nerves following delayed revascularization.

B The classic triad of PTPS is burning pain, hyperesthesia, and vasomotor abnormalities in the affected part of the limb. Unfortunately, it does not always present in classic form, so that clinical diagnosis can be challenging. The pain of PTPS is characteristically disproportionate to that expected following the initial event; it may be spontaneous or evoked and is usually reported as "burning" or at least an intense, diffuse aching. In the absence of penetrating nerve trauma, it is not consistent with the distribution of a peripheral nerve. This distinguishes PTPS from other more specific neuropathic pain disorders. The pain may be reported as intermittent or continuous and is often exacerbated by physical or emotional stresses. The patient often adopts a "guarding" posture to protect the affected extremity.

Sensory changes are usually reported at some stage, usually hyperesthesia in the region of the pain. This may occur in response to thermal stimulation (cold or warm), deep pressure, light touch, or joint movement. Sympathetic dysfunction is reported as a sudomotor or vasomotor instability in the affected extremity compared with the unaffected extremity. This dysfunction may vary from time to time and with different stages of the condition; thus, the patient may report that the extremity is warm and red or cold and blue, purple, or mottled. Skin temperature is altered in 92% of patients.[4] Sweating, particularly of the palms or soles, may be reported as increased, decreased, or unchanged. Normal sympathetic function may occasionally be present.

Swelling or the sensation of swelling may be reported at any stage of this syndrome. The swelling is typically peripheral, may be intermittent or permanent and may be exacerbated in the dependent position of the extremity. Motor dysfunction is uncommon but may include dystonia, tremor, and loss of strength of the affected muscle groups. Joint swelling and stiffness may also be reported, particularly of the digits and particularly in advanced stages.

Trophic changes of the skin may be reported later in the course of the syndrome. The nails may be atrophic or hypertrophic. Hair growth and texture may be decreased or increased, and the skin may become atrophic and shiny.

C Radiologic findings of CRPS may take several weeks to develop. Osteoporosis and abnormal bone scans can be found in the majority of patients with PTPS.[5-7] Asymmetric blood flow is usually seen, with most patients showing increased flow and uptake, whereas few patients at later stages may show diminished flow and uptake. These tests, although helpful if results are positive, cannot exclude the diagnosis if there is a strong clinical suspicion.

D The clinical diagnosis of PTPS is greatly strengthened by a positive response to sympathetic blockade. Patients should be encouraged to quantitate the degree of relief obtained using a numeric scale. The degree of pain relief is an excellent predictor of the likely benefit that can be expected should sympathectomy be undertaken.[8] Some caution should be exercised here, however, because sympathetic block can give some degree of nonspecific relief of almost any pain, including ischemic pain.[9,10] Causalgic pain is usually dramatically relieved by sympathetic blockade (e.g., 75% to 100% relief), whereas other pain is usually relieved only mildly to moderately (e.g. 25% to 50% relief). A positive response to sympathetic block not only provides good pain relief but persists beyond the duration of the anesthetic agent used.

E Drucker and colleagues have divided the natural history of causalgia into three clinical stages.[11] Although these stages may be oversimplified, they provide a framework for diagnosis, treatment, and prognosis in patients with PTPS.

1. *Acute (stage I)*. At this stage, the clinical course is reversible and is characterized by warmth, erythema, burning, edema, hyperalgesia, hyperhidrosis, and, after a few months, patchy osteoporosis. At stage I, a good result can be expected with a Bier block or chemical sympathectomy, often lasting beyond the normal duration of the block. Spontaneous resolution may occur, particularly with therapeutic support.
2. *Dystrophic (stage II)*. The clinical course is marked by a longer, fixed duration, but there is still a good response to sympathetic block. Patients rarely experience spontaneous resolution. Characteristics include coolness; mottling of the skin; cyanosis; brawny edema; dry, brittle nails; continuous pain; and diffuse osteoporosis. At this stage, bone scan finding are positive and changes in the bone structure are seen on plain films.
3. *Atrophic (stage III)*. Pain beyond the area of injury is common, and fixed, trophic changes occur, including atrophy of the skin and its appendages and fixed joint contractures. Radiographs show severe demineralization and ankylosis.

F In the differential diagnosis of PTPS, one of the most important diagnoses to consider is that of nerve entrapment. Causalgia-like pain may also occur if a nerve is caught in a suture, entrapped by a scar, or compressed by surrounding structures. Obviously, the former must be considered in causalgic pain appearing immediately postoperatively, but since nerve irritation or injury can occur by any compressing or pinching mechanism, there may be a causalgic component to the pain associated with any nerve compression. This is important because relief of the compression may only partially relieve the pain, and the causalgic component may persist. If peripheral nerve entrapment is suspected, there will often be a "trigger point" where the focal application of pressure causes sharp pain. The pain is relieved by the infiltration of a small amount of local anesthetic at this point.

Patients presenting with signs and symptoms characteristic of Drucker's stage II may be thought to have Raynaud's syndrome. In the latter syndrome, however symptoms are intermittent, related primarily to cold exposure, and relieved by warmth. Furthermore, hyperesthesia is rare and pain is not usually severe or burning in character.

The pain of peripheral neuritis is often burning and associated with hyperesthesia and vasomotor phenomena. In fact, the pathogenetic mechanisms for the two may be quite similar. However, the process here is more diffuse in location and gradual in onset, without a history of trauma or some other discrete precipitating event.

G. Medical treatment consists of drug therapy, intermittent sympathetic blocks, and physiotherapy. In stage I patients, in whom sympathetic blocks provide relief for days or weeks beyond the duration of the block itself, intermittent blocks are useful in providing relief during which physiotherapy can be actively pursued. In others, these intervals may be too short to justify repeated blocks, so that drugs must be used to control pain while physiotherapy is pursued. Drug therapy may require nonspecific analgesics, but these should be superimposed, only if necessary, on a background of medication designed to attenuate the symptoms by direct effect. Of these, phenytoin, amitriptyline, carbamazepine, and baclofen may be used effectively, usually in that order, because of increasing side effects. Nonsteroidal anti-inflammatory agents may be useful not only in relieving joint swelling but also—in combination with the agents just

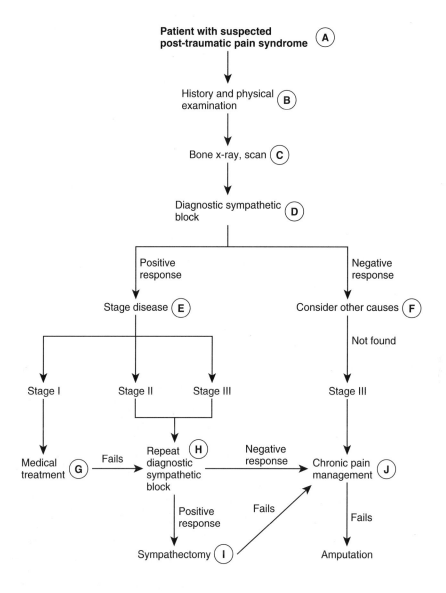

Post-traumatic Pain Syndrome (continued)

listed—in allowing reduced dosage and fewer side effects.

A short course of high-dose steroids may be helpful as well.[7,12] Amitriptyline (Elavil) is recommended in a dose of 50 to 75 mg nightly or divided during the day with 150 mg maximum.[13] A phenothiazine such as fluphenazine (Prolixin) is also recommended because it potentiates any narcotic, possesses an analgesic property of its own, and depresses the response to peripheral stimuli. A sympatholytic drug such as phenoxybenzamine (Dibenzyline) should be begun at 10 mg daily and increased to 40 mg daily as tolerated.

Intensive physical therapy should be initiated for patients with an inadequate response to the above measures. This regimen should include full range-of-motion exercises and whirlpool bath exercises. Timely physical therapy can be helpful in most patients with PTPS.[16]

Transcutaneous electrical nerve stimulation (TENS) has been used in patients with PTPS.[14] Results have been mixed; however, since this method is rapid and safe, it may be tried before a more aggressive treatment is used. Success or failure of the TENS device in the hands of an experienced examiner will be apparent by the third to fifth treatment.[15] A course of steroids should be tried in patients with a poor response to physical therapy or TENS.[16]

A serious mistake in medical management is to persist too long if the method is unsuccessful. This not only subjects nonresponders to additional time, expense, and suffering but may also compromise their opportunity to obtain complete and lasting relief by sympathectomy.

(H) Patients who do not respond to medical treatment or who present with advanced stage II PTPS are considered for sympathectomy if their response to sympathetic block has been positive. In most cases, since some time will have elapsed after the initial diagnostic block, this should be repeated at this time. At this point, a subsequent block may show a more limited response to sympathectomy, still positive, but now lasting for only the duration of the anesthetic agent used. A positive response, combined with failure of medical therapy, is an indication for sympathectomy in most patients. Without a positive response to sympathetic block at this point, however, chronic pain management without sympathectomy is more appropriate.

(I) Sympathectomy may be performed by open surgery, minimally invasive surgery (laparoscopic or thoracoscopic), or percutaneous techniques. In the past, phenol and alcohol blocks were performed in the hope of producing a lasting sympathectomy. Although up to 70% success rates were claimed, repeated blocks were often required and follow-up was short. Also, a significant incidence of neuritic pain complicated this approach.

Radiofrequency ablation has been advocated as a precise method of achieving percutaneous sympathetic denervation.[17] Although it may represent an advance over phenol or alcohol blocks, its effect is still not as complete or durable as surgical sympathectomy, and its local inflammatory reaction, as with repeated alcohol or phenol blocks, seriously interferes with the safety of subsequent sympathectomy. For this reason, surgical sympathectomy is preferred in most patients.

Cervical sympathectomy should include removal of T2 and T3 ganglia and division of the rami to the lower part of the stellate ganglion. This can be performed with precision and safety with the thoracoscopic approach.[18-20] For PTPS of the lower extremity, excision of the L2 and L3 ganglia is performed, including all encountered rami and interganglionic fibers. More complete resection has been advocated[21] to reduce the possibility of incomplete denervation. Inclusion of the L4 ganglion is necessary to remove possible crossover fibers; however, except for proximally localized causalgic pain, L1 ganglionectomy seems to add little benefit and increases the risk of retrograde ejaculation, particularly if done bilaterally. Lumbar sympathectomy is usually performed through retroperitoneal incisions, but laparoscopic techniques are also being developed.[22] If sympathectomy is limited to patients obtaining excellent relief from a sympathetic block produced by local anesthesia, it produces long-term relief in nearly 90% of patients.[8,23-24]

(J) Treatment of stage III PTPS consists of chronic pain management, often aided by referral to a specialized pain clinic. If the initial diagnostic sympathetic block yields a moderate response (e.g., 25% to 60% pain relief), sympathectomy can be considered. In severe cases that cannot be controlled by advanced pain management, amputation is occasionally necessary.

REFERENCES

1. Stanton-Hicks M, Janig W, Hassenbusch S, et al: Reflex sympathetic dystrophy: Changing concepts and taxonomy. Pain 1995;63:127–133.
2. Haddox JD: A call for clarity. Pain 1996: An updated review. International Association for Pain Refresher Courses on Pain Management held in conjunction with the 8th World Congress on Pain. Seattle, IASP Press, 1996, pp 97–99.
3. Merskey H, Bogduk N: Classification of Chronic Pain, 2nd ed. Seattle, IASP Press, 1994.
4. Veldman PHJM, Reynen HM, Arntz IE, et al: Signs and symptoms of reflex sympathetic dystrophy: Prospective study of 829 patients. Lancet 1993;342:1012–1016.
5. Davidoff G, Werner R, Cremer S, et al: Predictive value of the three-phase technetium bone scan in diagnosis of reflex sympathetic dystrophy syndrome. Arch Phys Med Rehabil 1989;70:135–137.
6. Kozin R, Genant HK, Bekerman C, et al: The reflex sympathetic dystrophy syndrome: II. Roentgenographic and scintigraphic evidence of bilaterally and of periarticular accentuation. Am J Med 1976;60:332–338.
7. Kozin F, Ryan LM, Carerra GF, et al: The reflex sympathetic dystrophy syndrome: III. Scintigraphic studies, further evidence for the therapeutic efficacy of systemic corticosteroids and proposed diagnostic criteria. Am J Med 1981;70:23–30.
8. AbuRahma AF, Robinson PA, Powell M, et al: Sympathectomy for reflex sympathetic dystrophy: Factors affecting outcome. Ann Vasc Surg 1994;8:372–379.
9. Bobin A, Anderson WP: Influence of sympathectomy in α-2 adrenoreceptor binding sites in canine blood vessels. Life Sci 1983;33:331.
10. Lon L, Nathan PW: Painful peripheral states and sympathetic blocks. J Neurol Neurosurg Psychiatr 1978;41:664.

11. Drucker WR, Hubay CA, Holden WD, et al: Pathogenesis of posttraumatic sympathetic dystrophy. Am J Surg 1959;97:454.
12. Kozin F. The painful shoulder and reflex sympathetic dystrophy syndrome. In McCarty DJ (ed.): Arthritis and Allied Conditions, 10th ed. Philadelphia, Lea & Febiger, 1985.
13. Benson WF: Discussion of Chuinard RG, Annual Meeting, American Society for Surgery of the Hand, 1980, Atlanta.
14. Meyer GA, Fields HL: Causalgia treated by selective large fibre stimulation of peripheral nerve. Brain 1972;95:163–168.
15. Wilson RL: Management of pain following peripheral nerve injuries. Orthop Clin North Am 1981;12:343–359.
16. Trudel J, DeWolfe VG, Young JR, et al: Disuse phenomenon of the lower extremity: Diagnosis and treatment. JAMA 1963;186:1129–1131.
17. Noe CE, Haynsworth RF Jr: Lumbar radiofrequency sympatholysis. J Vasc Surg 1993;17:801.
18. Appleby TC, Edwards WH Jr: Thoracoscopic dorsal sympathectomy for hyperhidrosis: Technique of choice. J Vasc Surg 1992;16:121.
19. Horgan K, O'Flanagan S, Duignan PJ, et al: Palmar and axillary hyperhidrosis treated by sympathectomy by transthoracic endoscopic electrocoagulation. Br J Surg 1984;71:1002.
20. Malone PS, Cameron ALP, Rennie JA: Endoscopic thoracoscopic sympathectomy in the treatment of upper limb hyperhidrosis. Ann Coll Surg Engl 1986;68:93.
21. Kim GE, Ibraheim IM, Imparato AM: Lumbar sympathectomy in end stage arterial occlusive disease. Ann Surg 1976;183:157–160.
22. Kathouda N, Wattanasirichaigoon S, Tang E, et al: Laparoscopic lumbar sympathectomy. Surg Endosc 1997;11:257–260.
23. Mockus MB, Rutherford RB, Rosales C, et al: Sympathectomy for causalgia: Patient selection and long-term results. Arch Surg 1987;122:668.
24. Olcott C, Eltherington LG, Wilcosky BR, et al. Reflex sympathetic dystrophy: The surgeon's role in management. J Vasc Surg 1991;14:488–492.

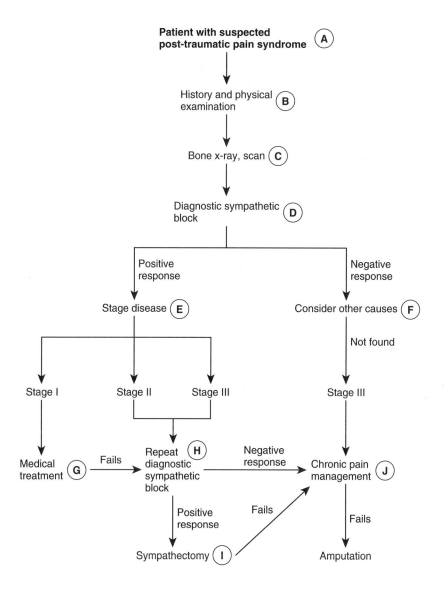

Chapter 68 Neurogenic Thoracic Outlet Syndrome

RICHARD J. SANDERS, MD • SHARON L. HAMMOND, MD

(A) Most patients with neurogenic thoracic outlet syndrome (TOS) have a history of some type of neck trauma, with whiplash injuries being the most common. Patients may not always remember the event without appropriate questioning by the examiner. Repetitive stress injuries at work are the next most common cause. The mechanism is probably repeated small traumata to the scalene muscles caused by repeated hyperextension of the neck. In 10% to 15% of patients, no history of trauma is found.

(B) Paresthesia most often involves all five fingers, but is worse in the fourth and fifth fingers. In some patients, paresthesia involves the whole arm. Pain may be constant or intermittent and may involve the neck, trapezius, anterior chest wall, shoulder, arm, elbow, and forearm. Pain and paresthesia occur in more than 90% of patients with TOS, although this combination of symptoms is not required to make the diagnosis.

Occipital headaches are present in about 70% and sometimes are the biggest complaint. In rare instances, headache and neck pain are the only symptoms. Another common point in the history is that symptoms are often elicited by arm elevation to perform such tasks as combing one's hair, driving a car, and sleeping with the arms overhead. Frequently, paresthesia occurs at night and interferes with sleeping.

(C) Scalene muscle tenderness is present in more than 90% of patients. Spurling's sign (direct pressure over the brachial plexus) and Tinel's sign (tapping over the brachial plexus) are each positive in about 67%. Ninety-degree abduction in external rotation (90° AER) is held for 3 minutes. This position reproduces symptoms within 30 to 60 seconds in more than 90% of patients, whereas this position reduces the radial pulse in fewer than 30%. We use the 90° AER position in place of the Adson maneuver that we abandoned many years ago because of its inconsistencies.

Other common findings on examination include pain and paresthesia in the contralateral neck, arm, and hand on full neck rotation and head tilt and reduction of the sensation of light touch in the fingers of the hand. These findings are more impressive in unilateral disease. The minimal requirements to establish a diagnosis of neurogenic TOS are tenderness over the scalene muscles and duplication of symptoms on 90° AER. We usually require both of these findings but do accept just one if there are at least one or two other corroborative findings. The more additional positive physical findings, the stronger the reinforcement of the presumptive diagnosis of TOS.

(D) Neuroelectric diagnostic studies, such as electromyography (EMG), nerve conduction velocity (NCV), somatosensory evoked potentials (SSEP), and F-wave latency measurements are primarily of help in diagnosing or excluding more peripheral entrapments. In almost all patients with TOS, results of these studies are normal or show nonspecific changes.[1,2]

(E) Radiographs are obtained to exclude skeletal abnormalities. Cervical ribs are associated with arterial TOS, but only 5% to 10% of patients operated upon for neurogenic TOS have cervical ribs, and in most of these patients a history of trauma precedes the onset of symptoms. Magnetic resonance imaging of the cervical spine is indicated when there is a clinical question of cervical spine disease. It is not routinely ordered for all patients with TOS. Our indications include symptoms in the upper brachial plexus distribution (paresthesia in the first 3 fingers) and degenerative disc disease noted on neck radiographs.

(F) Scalene muscle block is performed by injecting 1% lidocaine into the belly of the anterior scalene muscle.[3] We perform this without EMG control, but it can be done with such control.[4] The rationale for this test is that we presume scalene muscle spasm or fibrosis to be the root of neurogenic TOS in most patients. Lidocaine relaxes the muscle or breaks the spasm. Fibrosis is supported by histologic studies that have demonstrated increased connective tissue in the scalene muscles of all patients with TOS studied.[5]

A positive response is noted by improvement in physical findings for several minutes after the block. A negative response means that TOS is less likely, and we look harder for another diagnosis. The block is a diagnostic test only, although a patient may rarely derive prolonged symptomatic relief.

(G) Perhaps 1% of TOS patients demonstrate objective findings, such as hand atrophy and EMG changes typical of ulnar neuropathy.[6] In such patients, when radiography reveals a cervical rib, surgical therapy may be indicated without trying conservative therapy.

(H) Lack of response to a scalene block may be due to an inadequate block or to the fact that TOS is not the diagnosis. After searching for and not finding other treatable diagnoses and if the patient has the clinical diagnostic criteria for TOS, we treat the patient for TOS.

(I) Conservative therapy includes a variety of modalities of physical therapy and exercises.[7,8] We advocate a home program of neck stretching, abdominal breathing, posture awareness, and behavior modification to avoid positions and activities that produce symptoms. Physical therapy to manage associated diagnoses, such as fibromyalgia, is included.

(J) Surgical decompression includes anterior and middle scalenectomy, first rib resection,[9] or combined scalenectomy and first rib resection.[10-12] Statistically, the supraclavicular and transaxillary approaches have been equally effective. Differences in results between scalenectomy with and without first rib resection are small and not statistically significant.

K Disabling symptoms are those that interfere with work, sleep, recreation, or activities of daily living.

REFERENCES

1. MacLeader HI, Moll F, Nuwer M, Jordan S: Somatosensory evoked potentials in the assessment of thoracic outlet compression syndrome. J Vasc Surg 1987;6:177–184.
2. Komanetsky RM, Novak CB, Mackinnon SE, et al: Somatosensory evoked potentials fail to diagnose thoracic outlet syndrome. J Hand Surg (Am) 1996;21:662–666.
3. Sanders RJ, Haug CE: Thoracic outlet syndrome: A common sequela of neck injuries. Philadelphia, JB Lipppincott, 1991, pp 91–93.
4. Jordan SE, Machleder HI: Diagnosis of thoracic outlet syndrome using electrophysiologically guided anterior scalene muscle blocks. Ann Vasc Surg 1998;12:260–264.
5. Sanders RJ, Jackson CGR, Banchero N, Pearce WH: Scalene muscle abnormalities in traumatic thoracic outlet syndrome. Am J Surg 1990;159:231–236.
6. Passero S, Paradiso C, Giannini F, et al: Diagnosis of thoracic outlet syndrome: Relative value of electrophysiological studies. Acta Neurol Scand 1994;90:179–185.
7. Novak CB: Conservative management of thoracic outlet syndrome. Semin Thorac Cardiovasc Surg 1996;8:201–207.
8. Walsh MT: Therapist management of thoracic outlet syndrome. J Hand Ther 1994;11:131–144.
9. Roos DB: The place for scalenectomy and first rib resection in thoracic outlet syndrome. Surgery 1982;92:1077–1085.
10. Cheng SWK, Reilly LM, Nelken NA, et al: Neurogenic thoracic outlet decompression: Rationale for sparing the first rib. Cardiovasc Surg 1995;3:617–623.
11. Thomas GI: Diagnosis and treatment of thoracic outlet syndrome. Perspect Vasc Surg 1995;8:1–28.
12. Sanders RJ, Pearce WH: The treatment of thoracic outlet syndrome: A comparison of different operations. J Vasc Surg 1989;10:626–634.

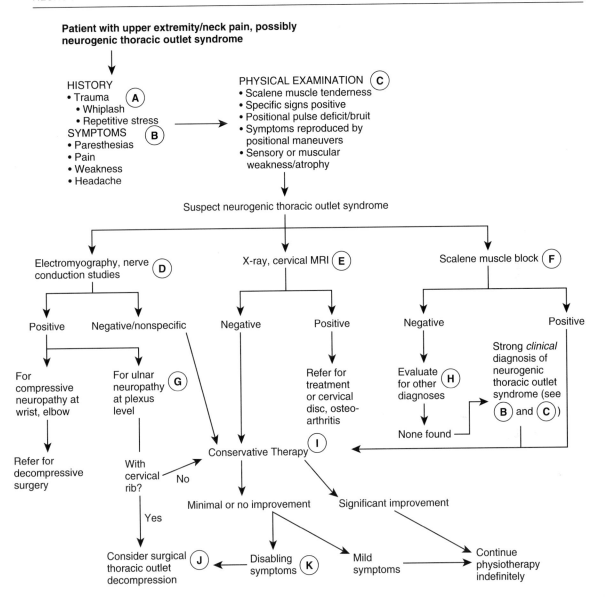

Chapter 69 Raynaud's Syndrome

GREGORY J. LANDRY, MD • JOHN M. PORTER, MD

(A) The skin color changes of Raynaud's syndrome (RS) consist of initial pallor caused by spasm of digital arteries and arterioles. When arteriolar spasm relaxes, the initial blood flow into the dilated capillaries rapidly desaturates, causing cyanosis. As blood flow increases in the dilated capillary beds, rubor occurs. This classic tricolor skin change is, in fact, rarely seen, and patients with any combination of these skin color changes may qualify for a diagnosis of RS. Pain associated with skin color changes is frequently noted but is an inconsistent finding and, therefore, not essential for diagnosis.

(B) All patients presenting for evaluation of RS or digital ischemia should be carefully questioned and examined for signs and symptoms of connective tissue diseases (CTD), specifically arthralgia, myalgia, skin rash, alopecia, sclerodactyly, dysphagia, xerostomia, xerophthalmia, telangiectasia, and hand swelling. Connective tissue diseases are the most frequently detected diseases noted in association with RS, and include scleroderma, systemic lupus erythematosus (SLE), Sjögren's syndrome, rheumatoid arthritis, and mixed connective tissue diseases. The diagnosis of individual connective tissue diseases is based on a combination of serologic abnormalities and associated multisystem symptoms.

A history of angina pectoris, transient ischemic attacks, or findings of diminished peripheral pulses or bruits should be carefully sought as an indication of generalized atherosclerosis. Symptoms of carpal tunnel syndrome should be sought, as this syndrome is present in up to 15% of patients with RS. Other causes of digital artery occlusion should be sought, such as a history of frostbite, repetitive trauma (hypothenar hammer syndrome), accidental intra-arterial drug injection, proximal embolic source, and drug ingestion (ergotism). The physical examination should include palpation for cervical rib and clavicular anomalies.

(C) Laboratory evaluation is performed to identify disease processes that may be associated with digital ischemic symptoms. In our experience, at least 70% of patients with RS have associated diseases.[1] Our initial routine screen includes a complete blood count including platelet count, urinalysis, erythrocyte sedimentation rate, automated multichemistry, and immunologic screening consisting initially of rheumatoid factor and antinuclear antibody. More detailed immunologic evaluation is performed for specific connective tissue diseases if initial screening tests indicate positive serologic findings.

(D) Digital photoplethysmography (PPG) along with finger pneumatic cuffs is used to obtain digital pressures and waveforms, which permits both the detection and quantification of obstructive digital artery disease.[2] The digital hypothermic challenge (Nielsen) test indicates the absence or presence of digital artery vasospasm. In our experience, this has been the most accurate (92%) test for RS.[3]

(E) Division of patients into categories according to their initial vascular laboratory and serologic findings is of great prognostic significance. It is generally believed that primary vasospastic RS is a benign disease constituting little more than a nuisance condition. Patients with vasospastic RS and positive serologic findings are at increased long-term risk for the subsequent development of connective tissue diseases and thus should be monitored with increased vigilance. Patients with obstructive RS, regardless of initial serologic profiles, are at highest risk for subsequent development of digital ulcers, gangrene, and the need for digital or phalangeal amputation.[1]

(F) The mainstay of treatment for RS remains medical management. Most patients with RS achieve acceptable relief of symptoms through avoidance of cold and tobacco and through hand warming. Moving to a warmer climate region may be considered in patients with severe symptoms if they live in colder regions.

Numerous medical therapies have been used in the treatment of RS. Among such therapies, the calcium channel blockers are the first line of therapy. Nifedipine is the most potent vasodilator among the calcium channel blockers. Multiple clinical trials have indicated that as many as two thirds of patients demonstrate some improvement,[4] and these tend to be people with vasospastic RS. Numerous other medications have been used and have shown variable benefit. These include prostaglandins, angiotensin-converting enzyme (ACE) inhibitors, serotonin antagonists, α-adrenergic antagonists, and platelet inhibitors. To date, none of these have proved as effective as the calcium channel blockers.

Behavioral therapy, or biofeedback, has shown some promise, with reduction in symptoms noted in 66% of patients.[5] Investigators theorize that biofeedback works by increasing β-adrenergic stimulation.

(G) Digital photoplethysmography with digital blood pressure determination is as accurate as arteriography in the detection of significant digital obstruction, and the finding of a digital blood pressure 10 mmHg below brachial pressure establishes the diagnosis.[6] Although the use of the noninvasive vascular laboratory allows the objective evaluation of digital ischemia, it does not eliminate the need for upper extremity arteriography in certain patients. Digital gangrene always implies digital artery occlusion, since this does not result from vasospasm alone.

The purpose of arteriography is not to confirm distal arterial obstruction, obviously present in these patients, but to rule out a proximal disease process, such as subclavian artery stenosis or aneurysm, which may be serving as a source of emboli and which may be amenable to surgical repair. If no diagnosis of connective tissue disease can be made on the basis of laboratory data, and

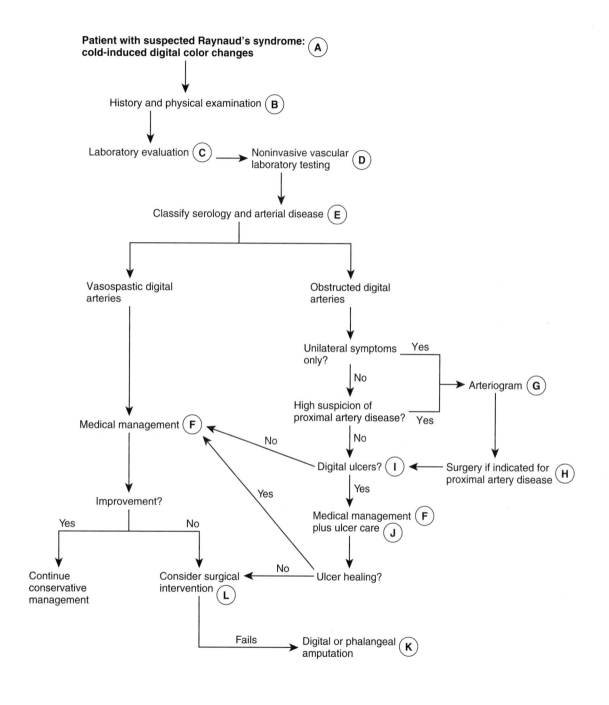

Raynaud's Syndrome (continued)

particularly if the signs and symptoms are unilateral, the diagnosis of isolated distal small artery occlusive disease can be established with certainty only after proximal arterial disease has been arteriographically eliminated. In recent years, we have been increasingly willing to forgo arteriography in patients with bilateral finger ischemia and normal upper extremity arterial findings to the wrist. The probability of finding bilateral proximal arterial disease in such patients is remote.

(H) Patients with an obstructive pattern of disease with demonstrable subclavian, axillary, brachial, radial, or ulnar artery aneurysms, stenoses, or occlusions may benefit from autogenous reconstruction. Resection of associated bony abnormalities in patients with arterial thoracic outlet syndrome (e.g., cervical ribs) is also indicated.[7]

(I) In our clinical experience, ischemic digital ulcerations occurred at some time in 52% of patients with obstructive RS and is often the initial presenting symptom of associated connective tissue disease. Digital ulcers do not occur in patients with only vasospastic RS. In approximately 50% of patients with digital ulcerations, ulcer recurrence develops over time. The incidence of digital ulceration in patients with obstructive RS does not increase with increasing lengths of follow-up. If patients have had RS for more than 10 years and have not had problems with digital ulceration, it is unlikely that this will develop subsequently.[1]

(J) In addition to standard medical management (see F), patients with ulcers require specific, local treatment. A healing rate of at least 85% can be achieved with soap and water scrubs, antibiotics as indicated by bacterial culture, and selective, minimal débridement.[8] These results are equal to the healing rate achieved after thoracic sympathectomy, underscoring the lack of critical data in support of more extensive surgical intervention.

(K) In one study, digital or phalangeal amputations were required in approximately 15% of patients with obstructive RS.[1] Given that most patients with digital ulcerations improve with conservative management, it is important to avoid premature amputation in these patients. Digital amputation is virtually never required for patients with vasospastic disease for pain control alone.

(L) Cervicothoracic sympathectomy has been employed as a treatment of RS for many years, and the most consistent result has been only short-term improvement in symptoms of vasospastic RS. Patients typically experience improvement for about 6 months, then a return to baseline values is seen. The same cycle is observed when repeated sympathectomy is tried, and the exact cause of this treatment failure remains unclear.[9] Endoscopic transthoracic dorsal sympathectomy has met with a similar outcome.

Given these poor results, we do not recommend upper extremity sympathectomy for RS.[10] However, this negative view of sympathectomy is not universal. Most investigators admit that overall results are poor; however, some think that carefully selected patients can benefit, and they will try this before amputation. However, the selection of those patients who might benefit from sympathectomy is difficult. In contrast, lumbar sympathectomy has proved to have durable beneficial effects in 90% of patients with lower extremity vasospastic arterial disease.[11]

The technique of periarterial sympathectomy involves disruption of neural input to the arterial wall. This is done by stripping 4 to 5 cm of arterial adventitia just past the bifurcation of the common digital artery.[12] Results of this procedure have been uniformly poor, and it is not recommended.

Attempted digital revascularization with microvascular bypasses and arteriovenous reversal at the wrist has also been attempted, but results have been poor. An occasional patient with radial or ulnar artery obstruction at the wrist, however, may benefit from a palmar artery bypass.[13]

REFERENCES

1. Landry GJ, Edwards JM, McLafferty RB, et al: Long-term outcome of Raynaud's syndrome in a prospectively analyzed patient cohort. J Vasc Surg 1996;23:76–86.
2. Gates KN, Tyburczy JA, Zupan T, et al: The non-invasive quantification of digital vasospasm. Bruit 1984;8:34–37.
3. Nielsen SL, Lassen NA: Measurement of digital blood pressure after local cooling. J Appl Physiol 1977;43:907–910.
4. Smith CD, McKendry RJ: Controlled trial of nifedipine in the treatment of Raynaud's phenomenon. Lancet 1982;2:1299.
5. Freedman RR: Physiological mechanisms of temperature biofeedback. Biofeedback Self-Regulation 1991;16:65–115.
6. McLafferty RB, Edwards JM, Taylor LM, et al: Diagnosis and long-term outcome in patients diagnosed with hand ischemia. J Vasc Surg 1995;22:361–369.
7. Nehler MR, Taylor LM, Moneta GM, et al: Upper extremity ischemia from subclavian artery aneurysms caused by bony abnormalities of the thoracic outlet. Arch Surg 1997;132:527–532.
8. Mills JL, Friedman EI, Taylor LM, et al: Upper extremity ischemia caused by small artery disease. Ann Surg 1987;206:521.
9. Machleder HI, Wheeler E, Barber WF: Treatment of upper extremity ischemia by cervico-dorsal sympathectomy. Vasc Surg 1979;13:399–404.
10. Lowell RC, Gloviczki P, Cherry KJ, et al: Cervicothoracic sympathectomy for Raynaud's syndrome. Int Angiol 1993;12:168.
11. Janoff KA, Phinney ES, Porter JM: Lumbar sympathectomy for lower extremity vasospasm. Am J Surg 1985;150:147–152.
12. Flatt AE: Digital artery sympathectomy. J Hand Surg 1980;5:550.
13. Nehler MR, Dalman RL, Harris EJ, et al: Upper extremity arterial bypass distal to the wrist. J Vasc Surg 1992;16:633–640.

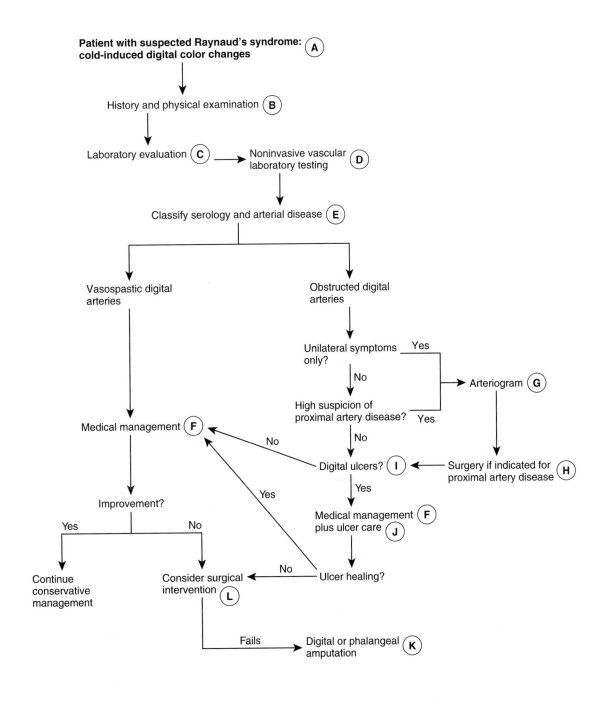

Chapter 70 Erectile Dysfunction

RALPH G. DePALMA, MD

(A) Erectile dysfunction (impotence) is defined as the persistent or repeated inability, for at least 3 months' duration, to attain or maintain an erection sufficient for satisfactory performance in the absence of an ejaculatory disorder such as premature ejaculation.[1] Impotence is a symptom, not a disease. Although it is a dramatic vascular failure, it may have a variety of causes. Therefore, no single treatment algorithm exists for diagnosis and therapy. With the availability of effective oral drugs[2] and the knowledge that a minority of men require vascular surgery,[3] the algorithm in this chapter outlines my preferences for decision making. Diagnosis and treatment are interrelated. The approach begins with responsiveness or unresponsiveness to initial therapy; if oral medications are unsuccessful, more elaborate investigations are advised.[4]

(B) A comprehensive medical, sexual, and psychosocial history is an essential step, followed by careful physical examination. Normal nocturnal erections may indicate psychological rather than physiologic causes. Leg pulse deficits or femoral bruits suggest macroarterial disease. The genitalia are carefully examined, including prostatic palpation rectally. Sensory testing of the extremities, perineum, and glans may detect neuropathy, which is particularly relevant in diabetic patients.[4] The bulbocavernosus reflex is also tested. When neuropathy is associated with erectile dysfunction, with the exception of overt spinal injury, gross neurologic examination is unrewarding in the usual case.

(C) Risk factors for vascular disease, such as hyperlipidemia, diabetes, cigarette smoking, and hypertension, are often present. Efforts are made to control risk factors not only for treatment of erectile dysfunction but also for avoiding, as possible, later progression of vascular disease.

(D) I continue to use a noninvasive vascular screening along with initial office examination. The screening consists of penile pressures and pulse volume recording,[5] which for the vascular specialist can define the presence of aortoiliac and pelvic occlusive disease.[6] Plethysmographic testing, however, does not detect venous leakage or small vessel or cavernous muscle dysfunction, common causes of erectile dysfunction.

I no longer recommend neurologic screening (pudendal and peripheral sensory evoked potentials, bulbocavernous latency, and cortical evoked potentials)[4] initially. Vascular and neurologic dysfunction often overlap,[7] usually in diabetic patients. Often diabetic men can respond to oral therapy or intracavernous injection (ICI) of vasoactive agents. Neurologic testing is expensive and time-consuming. When severe or combined neurologic disorders are unresponsive to initial therapy, prostheses can be considered as treatment. Neurologic abnormality probably contraindicates microvascular reconstruction. Sleep studies are mainly useful when medicolegal issues complicate presentation; a normal erection during formal sleep study observation rules out organicity.[4]

(E) For diabetes and rare cases of prolactinemia, specific therapy should be initiated. When hypogonadism is suspected, based on shrunken testes, and confirmed by laboratory studies, hormonal therapy can also be initiated, provided that older men are observed carefully for prostate malignancy. Unfortunately, treatment of thyroid disorders has had little effect on erectile dysfunction.[4]

I have observed that high levels of blood glucose, in excess of 300 mg/dL, are common in men presenting with a complaint of erectile dysfunction. These men, typically, have been treated as "borderline diabetics" and are unaware of the seriousness of their metabolic disorder. Impotence is often the presenting complaint. Further, the corpus cavernosal smooth muscle is refractory to ICI at high levels of blood glucose as well as in cases of hyperprolactinemia (personal observation). With treatment, the cavernosal smooth muscle again becomes capable of relaxation in response to vasoactive agents.

(F) Because cavernous smooth muscle dysfunction is the most frequent cause of erectile dysfunction, treatment will probably be medical for most men presenting with this complaint. Initial oral therapy currently uses sildenafil (Viagra), a selective inhibitor of cyclic guanosine monophosphate (cGMP)–specific phosphodiesterase type 5 (PDE_5), available in oral form. Overall, this drug was initially effective in 40% of attempts at sexual intercourse compared with 20% of attempts in a placebo group receiving a fixed dosage. With titration of dosage, the drug was effective in 59% of attempts compared with 20% in groups receiving placebo.[8, 9] One study has shown that sildenafil is an effective drug in diabetic men.[10]

The use of *nitrates* or *terazosin* is a specific contraindication to sildenafil therapy. In the initial study, eight deaths were reported in the study groups (n = 861) from cardiovascular causes and the popular press has reported several scores of deaths as well among a large but unknown denominator. Caution is mandated in warnings for sildenafil for men who have had a heart attack, stroke, or life-threatening arrhythmia within the previous 6 months; resting hypotension or hypertension; cardiac failure; unstable angina; or retinitis pigmentosa.

Other oral drugs are currently being developed. Additional oral agents prescribed for impotence include pentoxifylline, phentolamine, apomorphine, and an α blocker, isoxsuprine. The last has been useful and safe in my experience.

(G) If oral drugs fail, ICI therapy using either prostaglandin E_1 (PGE_1) or mixtures of PGE_1, phentolamine, and papaverine is employed.[3, 4] Inability to become erect with increasing doses of a vasoactive agent suggests a need for more invasive testing and possible vascular intervention. In my clinic, intraurethral installation of alprostadil

ERECTILE DYSFUNCTION

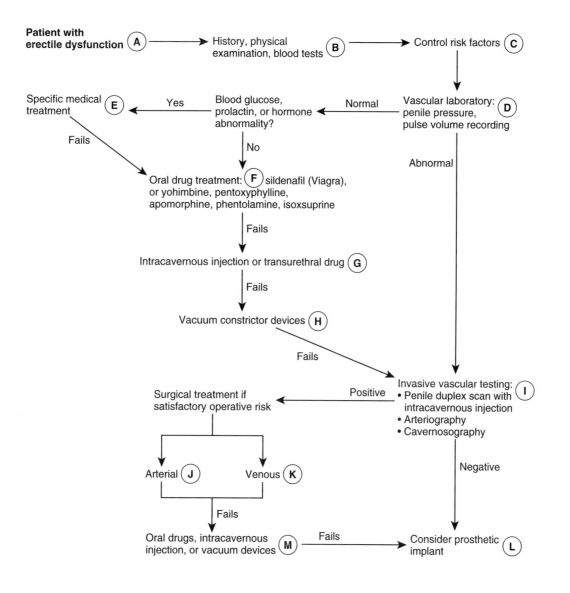

(PGE$_1$) has proved highly effective when time for teaching is taken. Among 84 patients, average age 61 years, 93% continued effective intercourse at 6 months of follow-up, with three patients dropping out because of pain or transient urethral irritation.

(H) If ICI or transurethral therapy is unsuccessful or is not tolerated, we suggest vacuum constrictor devices. With these modalities, most men respond, although 6% to 7% require further testing and treatment.[4]

(I) Some authorities proceed directly to ICI therapy and study of cavernous artery Doppler wave forms using duplex ultrasound scanning while an erection develops from use of ICI.[11] ICI is a useful screening test for arteriogenic impotence. Systolic cavernosal peak flow velocities above 30 cm/sec have been described as normal. In comparing the results of duplex scanning with arteriography, Valji and Bookstein[12] concluded that duplex scanning during ICI-induced erection is a successful screening tool, but its sensitivity and specificity, compared with those in angiography, are limited. The use of duplex scanning for detection of venous insufficiency is even less secure. I prefer this test for documenting vascular abnormalities and lesion extent in Peyronie's disease.

Abdominal ultrasonography and conventional arteriography are used in men with large vessel disease. Occult aneurysms can cause sudden onset of impotence,[3] probably as a result of embolism into the hypogastric and pudendal arteries. Small vessel disease involving pudendal and penile arteries is defined by ICI to achieve tumescence and highly selective pharmacoarteriography. Dynamic infusion cavernosometry and cavernosography are used to quantify and to detect venous leakage or traumatic penile injuries.[4] The results of invasive testing determine surgical approaches.[13]

(J) For aortoiliac occlusive disease or aneurysms, direct reconstruction or angioplasty is used. Overall results in these older men have been quite favorable.[3] Such causes, however, occur in only a minority of men with erectile dysfunction. For small vessel occlusive disease (i.e., pudendal or penile) in young patients, epigastric to dorsal penile artery microvascular bypass is used when the disease is highly localized. Dorsal vein arterialization is offered when diffuse penile arterial disease does not permit bypass, again in young subjects. Favorable results with vascular surgery are seen in older men with large vessel disease and in younger men with trauma.[13, 14]

(K) Venous procedures include interruption of the deep dorsal vein, ligation and suture of demonstrable leakage, or transcatheter occlusion. The choice is determined by documentation of magnitude and sites of leakage and by absence of arterial disease demonstrated by selective pharmacoangiography.[4] These procedures are useful in young men with post-traumatic leakage. It must be reemphasized that, according to a meta-analysis by a Clinical Guidelines Panel,[15] the chances of success with venous and arterial surgery do not justify their routine use. The problems of diagnosis and classification make procedure choice critical, as emphasized in my review.[13]

(L) Prosthetic implantation is considered either after revascularization when oral or injection therapy remains ineffective or as a primary procedure in the presence of severe spinal or neurologic dysfunction or in nonresponsive diabetic patients.

(M) After vascular reconstruction, erectile function can be enhanced by supplemental oral, intracavernosal, or intraurethral drug therapy when the patient had been previously unresponsive. In older men with large vessel disease, approximately 70% respond spontaneously after reconstruction, in contrast to younger men with small vessel or arterial dysfunction, who commonly require additional therapy.[3] After unsuccessful revascularization, a prosthesis can also be offered; however, once a prosthesis is inserted, vascular reconstruction is not possible.

REFERENCES

1. The Process of Care Consensus Panel: Position paper. The process of care model for evaluation and treatment of erectile dysfunction. Int J Impot Res 1999;11:59–74.
2. DePalma RG: The best treatment for impotence. Vasc Surg 1998;32:519–521.
3. DePalma RG, Olding M, Yu GE, et al: Vascular interventions for impotence: Lessons learned. J Vasc Surg 1995;21:576–585.
4. DePalma RG: New developments in the diagnosis and treatment of impotence. West J Med 1996;164:54–61.
5. DePalma RG, Emsellem HA, Edward CM, et al: A screening sequence for vasculogenic impotence. J Vasc Surg 1987;5:228–236.
6. DePalma RG, Michal V: Point of view: Déjà vu—again: Advantages and limitations of methods for assessing penile arterial flow. Urology 1990;36:199–200.
7. Fabra M, Porst H: Bulbocavernous-reflex latencies and pudendal nerve SSEP compared to penile vascular testing in 609 patients with erectile failure and other sexual dysfunctions. Int J Impot Res 1999;11:167–175.
8. Center for Drug Evaluations and Research/Viagra (Sildenafil) "Joint Clinical Review" for New Drug Application 20-895.
9. Goldstein I, Lue TF, Padma-Nathan H, et al: Oral sildenafil in the treatment of erectile dysfunction. N Engl J Med 1998;338:1397–1404.
10. Kendell MS, Rajfer J, Wicker PA, et al: Sildenafil for treatment of erectile dysfunction in men with diabetes. JAMA 1999;281:421–426.
11. Lue TF, Hricak H, Marich KW, Tanago EA: Vasculogenic impotence evaluated by high resolution ultrasonography and pulsed Doppler spectrum analysis. Radiology 1985;155:777–781.
12. Vaji K, Bookstein JJ: Diagnosis of arteriogenic impotence: Efficacy of duplex sonography as a screening tool. AJR Am J Roentgenol 1993;160:65–69.
13. DePalma RG: Vascular surgery for impotence: A review. Int J Impot Res 1997;9:61–67.
14. Hatzichristou DG: Current treatment and future perspectives for erectile dysfunction. Int J Impot Res 1998;10 (Suppl F):S3–S11.
15. Montague DK: Clinical Guidelines Panel on erectile dysfunction: Summary report on the treatment of erectile dysfunction. J Urol 1996;156:2007–2011.

ERECTILE DYSFUNCTION

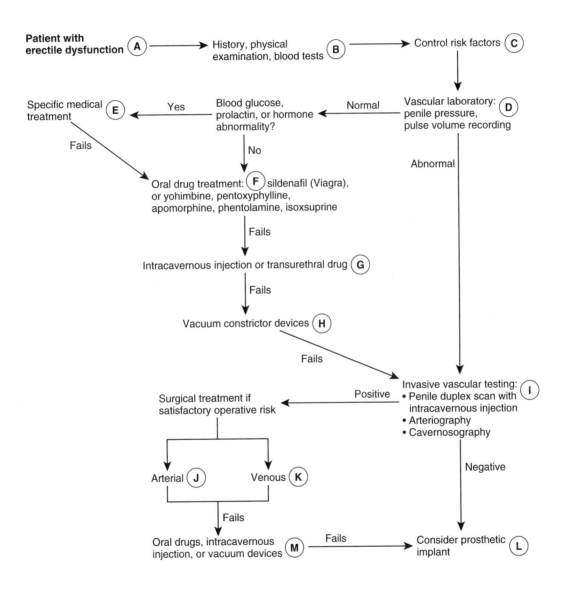

Chapter 71 Congenital Vascular Malformations

ROBERT B. RUTHERFORD, MD

A Congenital vascular malformations (CVMs) are uncommon, occurring in approximately 1% of births,[1] with many of these not presenting for treatment. This rarity, combined with variable severity and clinical presentation, makes clinical diagnosis difficult. The triad of birthmark, varicosities, and changes in limb girth or length is helpful, but all three are present in a bare majority of arteriovenous malformations (AVMs).[2]

Predominantly venous malformations account for approximately 50% of CVMs presenting for treatment, whereas about a third are malformations containing arteriovenous fistulae (AVFs), called AVMs. Isolated arterial defects represent only 1% of CVMs.[1] The remainder are capillary CVMs (most of which do not present for treatment), and lymphatic and mixed element defects. Some present as a mass lesion, others with diffuse changes involving all or most of the extremity, and still others with no more obvious abnormality than a "birthmark."

Although none of these features is pathognomonic for a given type, the presence of one or more of these features should lead one to at least suspect a CVM. Noting whether there is a "birthmark" or colored skin lesion, atypical (onset or distribution) varicosities, a mass lesion, or changes in limb dimension can help direct the diagnostic evaluation.

B One of the first steps in clinical diagnosis in children is to distinguish CVM skin lesions (e.g., capillary or cavernous malformations) from true hemangiomas.[3] Hemangiomas are truly neoplastic, with accelerated growth and endothelial turnover rates; CVMs (often misnamed hemangiomas) are non-neoplastic, with a normal endothelial turnover and a growth rate which is commensurate with the growth of the child.

CVMs are present at birth, but hemangiomas appear shortly after birth, although this occurrence may be missed. It is important to differentiate because juvenile hemangiomas usually involute spontaneously and can be treated expectantly unless they (1) are in a critical location and encroach upon important anatomy (e.g., eyes, mouth, airway), (2) become ulcerated and produce significant bleeding or infection, or (3) cause disseminated intravascular coagulation (DIC).

C The first diagnostic step is to detect or rule out AVFs. Birthmarks or varicosities may be the only extrinsic signs of deeper AVFs. Segmental limb systolic pressures (SLPs), segmental plethysmography or pulse volume recordings (PVRs), and arterial velocity waveforms (VWFs) can detect most congenital AVFs of the extremities. SLPs and PVRs are increased above an AVF and, depending on degree of steal, are normal or decreased below it.

The arterial VWF over a major inflow artery loses it sharp triphasic or biphasic shape in the presence of an AVF where continuous flow during diastole occurs.[4] Although this can be demonstrated with a continuous wave Doppler study, a duplex ultrasound scan using color flow imaging demonstrates AVFs more definitively.

In superficially placed lesions, duplex scans can visualize macro-AVFs, venous "lakes" (clusters), or cystic components. When there is no significant arteriovenous (A-V) shunting, particularly in a patient presenting with varicose veins, limb swelling or sequelae of chronic venous hypertension, a duplex venous scan is indicated to investigate the possibility of a predominantly venous defect, such as an anomaly of the deep system (see L) and venous angiomata (see J).

A nuclear medicine A-V shunt study may be used to quantitate A-V shunting. Pulmonary counts on a gamma camera following the injection of ^{99m}Tc-labeled albumen microsphere into the major inflow artery of the involved extremity are compared as a ratio to any venous injection, 100% of which are trapped in the lungs.[5] Normally, no more than 3% physiologic shunting is present. The degree of shunting has a prognostic value for AVMs and is thus helpful in counseling parents and in deciding which AVMs will likely need treatment and for monitoring the success of such treatment. It is also extremely valuable in separating Klippel-Trenaunay syndrome from Parkes Weber syndrome. Both present with this triad, but by convention the former is purely venous and the latter is characterized by AVFs, although in the microfistulous variety, the distinction cannot be made clinically.

The screening tests for AVMs just mentioned share the weakness that they cannot precisely localize the anatomic extent of the AVMs and are not applicable to very proximal (aortoiliac, pelvic, shoulder girdle) AVMs.

D For significant CVMs, and particularly in CVMs with high A-V shunting, magnetic resonance imaging (MRI) offers sufficient advantages to be used in the initial diagnostic evaluation.[6] MRI demonstrates the lesions, their flow characteristics (e.g., distinguishing venous malformations from AVMs), and their anatomic extent, particularly the involvement of surrounding muscle, bone, and subcutaneous tissues, which in turn determines operability. MRI has supplanted computed tomography (CT) because it provides better soft tissue definition and avoids the need for an intravenous (IV) contrast agent.

E A number of classification systems have been suggested, but none has become universally adopted. The most logical and useful is the Hamburg clinicopathologic classification system.[7] It contains no eponyms.

CVMs are divided into predominantly arteriovenous, venous, arterial, lymphatic, and mixed types of *defects*, with each of these divided into *truncular* (involving main or axial vessels) and *extratruncular* (involving peripheral branches) forms. The truncular forms are then divided into *dilating* versus *aplastic/obstructive* subgroups for all but A-V defects, which are divided into *superficial* and *deep* groups. The extratruncular forms are separated into *limited (localized)* and *diffuse* groups.

Although not all of the resultant 20 groups are represented clinically and are too cumbersome for this algorithm, the Hamburg system provides a better framework for stratifying CVMs for treatment and reporting purposes than any other system. Only the relatively common clinical types are featured here. Lymphatic defects include a dilating type (lymphocele) and an aplastic/obstructive type (lymphedema). For simplicity, and because they present differently, lymphatic defects are not considered here. Lymphocele presents as a painless mass, usually in the neck or retroperitoneum. Lymphedema presents as typical (onset and distribution) painless leg swelling (see Chapter 63).

(F) Congenital AVFs that are localized enough for complete surgical excision are rare, representing fewer than 10% of those presenting to a vascular surgery center.[2] In the past, many patients have been subjected to extensive surgery in the misguided hope that AVFs could be excised or controlled. In addition to MRI, an arteriogram is necessary in identifying appropriate cases for surgical treatment. Essentially all of such AVFs are macrofistulae.

(G) Because embolotherapy, including ethanol sclerotherapy, is not curative for the most part, *localized* AVFs should be excised, although preoperative embolotherapy may facilitate this in selected cases. Isolated use of embolotherapy might be considered for high-risk patients (but most are young and otherwise healthy) and small fistulae in critical locations where surgery would be difficult or disfiguring.

(H) Multiple, extensive, high-flow macrofistulae are associated with the worst prognosis and are the most difficult to treat effectively. As a rule, they should *not* be treated surgically, and attempts to "control" them by partial excision or ligation are fruitless and subject the patient to unnecessary risk. Ligation of inflow arteries precludes subsequent embolotherapy, the patient's best chance for control.

Embolotherapy,[8] including ethanol injections,[9]

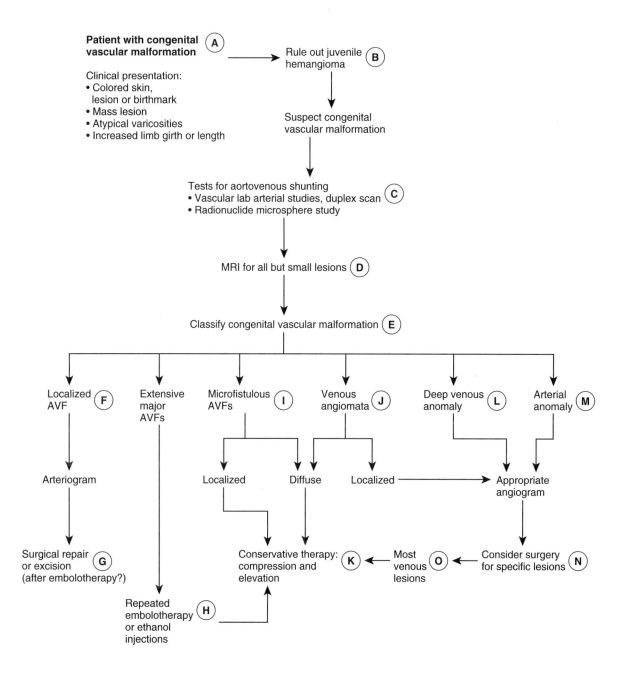

Congenital Vascular Malformations (continued)

has now become the primary method of treatment in this setting, that is, macrofistulous AVMs too extensive for complete (curative) surgical excision. For the method to be effective, the AVF must have a visible "nidus" and the injection must be made there. Cures have been accomplished with absolute ethanol injections following this dictum, but this necrosant is potentially dangerous if the dose and localization of each injection are not precise. Nerve injury is the most bothersome complication. In addition, multiple sessions with the patient under general anesthesia to avoid severe pain, as well as expensive imaging (MRI plus duplex ultrasound scanning), are required at each step of the way. This fact, along with the uncertainty of "cure," suggests that absolute ethanol injections be used only for symptomatic macrofistulous AVFs with specific mandatory indications for intervention, such as chronic critical ischemia from distal steal, bleeding or infected ulcerated lesions, systemic hemodynamic effects (rare), local mass with pressure effects in critical locations, intolerable disfigurement, and DIC.

Intervention to control limb overgrowth has been an accepted indication for embolotherapy in the past, but epiphyseal closure, timed on the basis of bone age film monitoring, is effective and safer.

(I) Microfistulous AVMs are almost always diffuse, are not well visualized by arteriography, have no nidus to inject, produce only a minor hemodynamic effect (mainly increased venous pressure), and do not pose a threat of critical ischemia or limb loss. There is negligible risk of a microfistulous AVM transforming into a hemodynamically significant macrofistulous AVM.

Parental assurance, in pediatric cases, and conservative treatment of any associated venous hypertension are the keys to proper management. Limb length can be controlled by timed epiphyseal closure. Varicose veins may be treated by stab avulsion or sclerotherapy as appropriate (see Chapter 59) but it must be understood that, unlike primary varicose veins, the underlying cause is not being controlled and recurrences are likely. Therefore, this method should be undertaken only for pressing indications.

(J) Venous angiomata are peripherally located (small tributary) venous lesions that form grape-like clusters (lakes), which may be relatively well localized and superficially located or diffuse and disseminated through deeper tissues, like muscle. They are not ordinarily associated with dysfunction of the deep veins and do not result in venous hypertension. The diffuse form is usually best treated conservatively (see K). The localized form may be excised if it is cosmetically unacceptable. Sclerotherapy with ethanol or another sclerosant has been used to treat venous angiomata, but it is seldom indicated because:

1. Angiomata, for the most part, are cosmetic problems.
2. Sclerosing very large veins usually produces painful masses and discoloration, which are very slow to resolve.
3. Multiple sessions, general anesthesia, and expensive imaging are required.

(K) Compression therapy with elastic support stockings, combined with intermittent elevation, is effective in controlling venous hypertension. It is not only the mainstay of management of otherwise untreatable lesions (diffuse microfistulous AVMs and venous angiomata) but serves as interval treatment between interventions for extensive macrofistulous AVFs and for other venous lesions in which surgery is inappropriate or incomplete (see N).

(L) Truncal venous lesions are rare. Obstructive lesions (aplastic or hypoplastic segments, localized membranes, webs, stenoses) may justify surgery. The more extensive deep venous obstructions, with associated embryonal and marginal veins, may be appropriately treated by bypass of the involved deep veins. Excision of huge but dysfunctional collaterals (marginal or embryonal veins) may be indicated if the remaining system is not functionally obstructed. The most common dilating form is a popliteal venous aneurysm, which may present with venous thromboembolism and require intervention. The procedures employed for these diverse lesions must be individualized after careful functional and anatomic characterization of each.[10]

(M) Isolated arterial defects are the rarest of all CVMs. The only one provoking general awareness is persistent primitive sciatic artery. Most of the others are localized dilations or strictures (coarctations), but detailed elaboration on these is beyond the scope of this chapter.

(N) The following CVMs may justify surgery, depending on the severity of their symptoms, their predicted natural history, and the likelihood that surgery can produce lasting benefit: (1) localized AVMs, (2) localized venous angiomata, (3) localized venous truncal defects and deep segment aplasia or hypoplasia, (4) venous aneurysms, and (5) mature arterial defects, be they aneurysm or obstructing lesion (persistent sciatic artery aneurysm, coarctation). In each case, preoperative angiography is needed to demonstrate exact anatomy.

(O) Because most venous lesions do not require surgical intervention and since some that do cannot be made entirely normal functionally, compression therapy with periodic leg elevation remains an important part of management.

REFERENCES

1. Tasnadi G: Epidemiology and etiology of congenital vascular malformations. Semin Vasc Surg 1993;6:200–203.
2. Szilagyi DE, Smith RF, Elliot JP, et al: Congenital arteriovenous anomalies of the limbs. Arch Surg 1976;111:423–429.
3. Mulliken JB: Cutaneous vascular anomalies. Semin Vasc Surg 1993;6:204–218.
4. Rutherford RB: Noninvasive testing in the diagnosis and assessment of arteriovenous fistula. In Bernstein E (ed): Noninvasive Diagnostic Techniques in Vascular Disease, 3rd ed. St. Louis, CV Mosby, 1985, pp 666–679.

5. Rhodes BA, Rutherford RB, Lopez-Majano V, et al: Arteriovenous shunt measurements in extremities. J Nucl Med 1972;13:357–362.
6. Pearce WH, Rutherford RB, Whitehill TA, et al: Nuclear magnetic resonance imaging: Its diagnostic value in patients with congenital vascular malformations of the limbs. J Vasc Surg 1988;8:64–70.
7. Belov S: Anatomopathological classification of congenital vascular defects. Semin Vasc Surg 1993;6:219–224.
8. Gomes AS, Mali WP, Oppenheim WL: Embolization therapy in the management of congenital vascular malformations. Radiology 1982;144:41.
9. Yakes WF, Leuthke JM, Merland JJ, et al: Ethanol embolization of arteriovenous fistulas: A primary mode of therapy. J Vasc Interv Radiol 1990;1:89.
10. Loose DA: Surgical treatment of predominantly venous defects. Semin Vasc Surg 1993;6:252–259.

BIBLIOGRAPHY

Rutherford RB, Anderson BO, Durham JD: Congenital vascular malformations of the extremities. In Moore WS (ed): Vascular Surgery: A Comprehensive Review, 5th ed. Philadelphia, WB Saunders, 1998, pp 191–202.

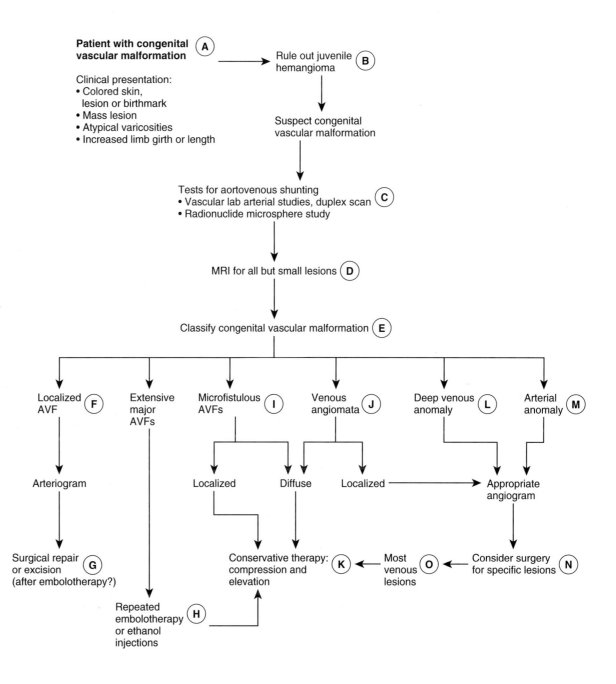

Chapter 72 Vascular Access for Hemodialysis

MICHAEL B. SILVA, JR., MD • BRAJESH K. LAL, MD

Patients Requiring New Hemodialysis Access

(A) Three types of procedures are commonly performed for hemodialysis access: (1) an autogenous fistula (AF), (2) a prosthetic bridging graft (BG), and (3) an indwelling central venous catheter. The ideal access delivers a flow rate sufficient for effective dialysis, is easily cannulated, has a long life, and has a low complication rate.

Autogenous fistulas come closest to fulfilling these criteria,[1] but their use is dependent on identification of a suitable artery and vein, which in patients presenting for access today is frequently not evident on simple physical examination. Past reliance on physical examination alone to select arteries and veins suitable for formation of an AF contributed to high early failure rates and disenchantment with routine selection of the single-incision radiocephalic fistula for initial access. This and other factors (poor planning, desire for early access) contributed to a reduction in AF use and a concomitant increase in the placement of prosthetic bridging grafts.

The U.S. Renal Data System (USRDS), which accumulates and reviews data from the nation's dialysis centers, reported in 1995 that the frequency of native AF construction in the United States was less than 30% of total access procedures performed, with some regions having AF placement rates in fewer than 10%.[2] In 1996, the Dialysis Outcomes Quality Initiative (DOQI) Vascular Access Work Group met at the behest of the National Kidney Foundation to address all aspects of current medical and surgical issues associated with hemodialysis and to publish a set of practice guidelines that could be adopted.[3] These recommendations, based on both evidential data and opinion, have received widespread attention among nephrologists, who are primarily responsible for the ongoing management of dialysis patients in the nation. Of significance for the vascular surgeon is that the recommendations designate an AF as preferential to a BG and set a minimum standard of 50% AF placement.

In order to meet these goals, surgeons must develop strategies to increase placement of an AF and to reduce the characteristically high failure to mature rates associated with usage of suboptimal arteries and veins. We have used upper extremity noninvasive duplex ultrasound evaluation of all prospective access candidates to enhance our ability to identify arteries and veins suitable for AF formation.[4] This is the starting point for our algorithm for patients requiring a new access as well as for patients with a failing or failed access.

(B) The first step in establishing hemodialysis access is to select the best available site, based on optimal arterial inflow and venous outflow, observing the preference of an AF over a BG, forearm over upper arm, and nondominant upper extremity over dominant upper extremity. Visual inspection and physical examination of the upper extremity are performed but may be inadequate to assess certain aspects, especially vein size, quality, and adequacy of central venous outflow. For this reason, we use duplex ultrasound scanning in all patients.

The examination is initiated at the wrist of the nondominant upper extremity, and a tourniquet is placed at the mid-forearm. After dilatation of the superficial veins by gentle tapping and stroking, the veins are insonated with a 5- or 7-MHz scanning probe. They are evaluated for diameter, compressibility, and continuity with upper arm veins. Patency of the deep system and continuity with patent axillary and subclavian veins are also verified. Central venous stenosis or thrombosis precludes use of that arm.

The largest-diameter superficial vein of good quality is mapped with skin markings. Suitability criteria for access include:

1. Target vein diameter above 2.5 mm for an AF and above 4.0 mm for a BG.
2. Continuity with the deep and central system.
3. Absence of stenoses.

When favorable venous anatomy is found, the arterial system is then evaluated for target artery diameter and patency of the palmar arch. Reduced pressure measurements, compared with the other arm or abnormal Doppler waveforms, indicate proximal arterial stenosis and preclude use of that arm for access unless the problem is successfully addressed. The basic requirements are:

1. An arterial luminal diameter greater than 2.0 mm.
2. Absence of obliterating calcification.
3. Palmar arch patency.

(C) Evaluation of central venous outflow stenosis or occlusion is an integral part of the duplex ultrasound examination. Central venous stenosis usually results from previous use of central catheters, especially in the subclavian vein.[5]

If a unilateral central vein problem is found, the contralateral extremity becomes the preferred choice regardless of the issue of extremity dominance. If bilateral central vein problems exist but are amenable to endovascular treatment, this should be attempted on the least diseased side.

If a subsequent duplex scan confirms effective treatment of the central vein problem, this arm can be selected for access. If not, the patient requires a nonstandard complex access solution (see H).

(D) Anticipated duration of dialysis determines the type of access selected:

1. Patients expected to require dialysis for less than 3 weeks are candidates for noncuffed central venous catheter access for dialysis; these dual-lumen catheters may be placed at the bedside without fluoroscopic guidance.
2. For patients expected to require dialysis longer

than 3 weeks, cuffed, tunneled catheters are placed.

3. For patients undergoing placement of an AF who require immediate dialysis, a cuffed tunneled catheter is placed concurrently, typically in the contralateral internal jugular vein, to provide access while the AF matures.

The internal jugular vein is preferred over the subclavian vein, and the contralateral deep venous system is accessed when possible to avoid catheter obstruction of venous outflow or catheter-induced venous stenosis during the period of AF maturation. We use the duplex scans to aid in the selection of a patent, normal vein for catheter placement. Femoral catheters can also be used on a temporary basis if the deep central venous system of the upper extremity is intractably compromised.

Routine use of upper extremity duplex ultrasound imaging for access planning identifies many patients who have veins suitable for AF formation but that are either too deep for successful cannulation or are remote from the optimal arterial inflow to allow direct anastomosis without tension. We have previously described the technique of superficial venous transposition in the forearm to increase our utilization of AF in these patients.[6] This technique involves extensive dissection of a vein identified by duplex scan as suitable in diameter, with ligation of side branches and transposition to a subcutaneous tunnel along the volar aspect of the forearm, bringing the vein to the inflow artery. This position is optimal for comfortable arm positioning during dialysis.

Preference for the nondominant arm relates to convenience for the patient, allowing the dominant arm to be used for activity during dialysis. When duplex ultrasound surveillance identifies a suitable vein and artery in the nondominant forearm, an AF constructed between them becomes the procedure of choice. We also use duplex ultrasonography to select the optimal anastomotic site. For example, if the radial or ulnar arteries are disadvantaged, a suitable vein in the forearm may be dissected and looped back to the brachial artery

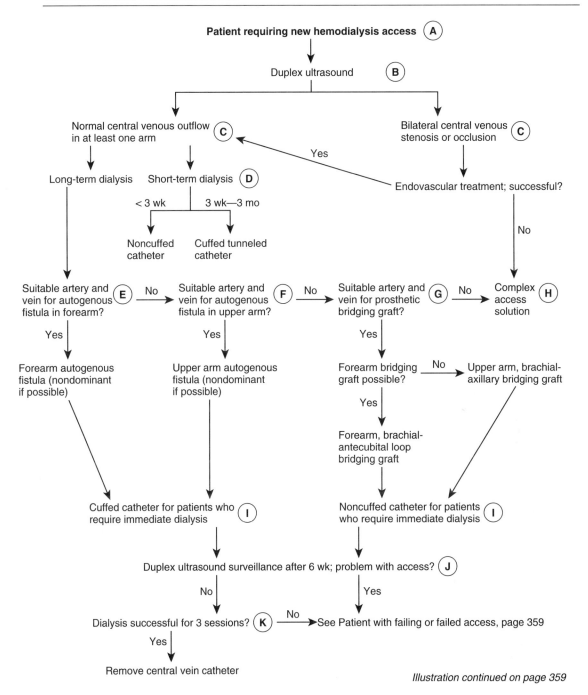

Illustration continued on page 359

Vascular Access for Hemodialysis (continued)

in the antecubital space. We prefer to exhaust all autogenous forearm possibilities before proceeding to autogenous upper arm alternatives, since this maximizes future possible sites.

(F) Absence of suitable veins in both forearms necessitates construction of the access in the upper arm. Again, duplex ultrasonography is valuable in identifying a superficial (preferred) or deep (second-choice) arm vein that can be transposed to a volar subcutaneous location for creation of an AF with the brachial artery. The dominant upper arm is used if arteries and veins in the nondominant upper arm are unsuitable.

(G) If there are no suitable veins for an AF, outflow through the deeper venous system in the arm is examined to identify a possible site of placement of a prosthetic BG. A looped BG configuration is used in the nondominant forearm when an appropriate antecubital vein and brachial artery are present.

The dominant forearm is the next site of choice. If both forearms are unsuitable, the nondominant upper arm, followed by the dominant upper arm, are the next options for curved brachial artery to axillary vein BGs.

Duplex ultrasonography is used to identify and mark the best possible location for the anastomoses and to confirm adequate central venous runoff. In patients who are significantly immunocompromised we avoid, when possible, placing prosthetic BGs because of the significant risk of infection and the complexities involved with removal of the BG and restoration of prograde arterial flow.[7]

(H) Complex access solutions are required when all upper extremity access sites have been exhausted or when extensive central venous obliteration is not responsive to endovascular treatment. If the central venous system is patent, placement of a cuffed catheter is the simplest alternative.

In patients with refractory central subclavian vein occlusion and a patent ipsilateral internal jugular vein, the jugular vein turndown procedure may be performed.[8] The cephalad portion of the jugular vein at the angle of the mandible is divided; after mobilization, the jugular vein is anastomosed to the patent axillary vein segment just proximal to the subclavian occlusion to provide runoff for the upper arm.

Resection of the central portion of the clavicle may be performed to facilitate a favorable anatomic lie of the vein graft. Other nonstandard access configurations, such as axillary artery to axillary vein body wall prosthetic grafts (loop configuration if ipsilateral, crossover or collar graft if contralateral), may be considered.[9] Axillary arterial to right atrial bridging grafts and axillary arterial to arterial prosthetic configurations have been used when extensive central venous obliteration is encountered, but these options are compromised by their potential for increased morbidity.[10,11]

If upper extremity options are unsatisfactory and the superior central venous system is involved, lower extremity access options can be used. Transposition of the saphenous vein in a loop configuration to the superficial femoral artery or common femoral artery has been performed.

Alternatively, a prosthetic BG can be placed in a loop configuration from the common femoral vein to the superficial femoral artery or common femoral artery. A prosthetic BG can also be created from one femoral artery to a contralateral femoral vein and tunneled subcutaneously across the lower anterior abdominal wall. With a percutaneous approach to the femoral vein, a cuffed catheter can be tunneled into the anterior thigh. In patients with lower extremity venous thrombosis, a translumbar approach to the inferior vena cava has been used with a lateral tunnel for the cuffed catheter.

(I) A cuffed central venous catheter is placed in all patients requiring immediate dialysis following AF formation, so that adequate maturation time (6 to 12 weeks) can be provided before cannulation of the AF. Because a BG can usually be used within 3 weeks, temporary noncuffed catheters can be used in this group.

The contralateral internal jugular vein is the preferred site if it is available, since it limits both ipsilateral venous outflow obstruction and would not be associated with development of subclavian vein stenosis. Alternate sites may be as follows:

1. Ipsilateral internal jugular vein; this choice poses some risk of venous outflow obstruction because the catheter physically rests across the confluence of the internal jugular vein, and the now high-flow subclavian vein, but has the benefit of limiting subclavian vein stenosis.
2. Contralateral subclavian vein; perhaps there would be less outflow obstruction but greater potential for negative long-term sequelae if stenosis results.
3. Ipsilateral subclavian vein; this is the least attractive alternative, with potential for both outflow obstruction and stenosis.

(J) We reexamine the AF access by duplex ultrasound scanning approximately 6 weeks following placement to assess maturation and to mark sites most suitable for initial cannulation by the dialysis center personnel. For a new AF, we prefer initial dialysis to be performed through a 16- or 17-gauge needle and for longer periods at minimal rates.

(K) We wait for successful dialysis to be accomplished at least three times before removing the central venous catheter. If flow rates are insufficient for successful dialysis or if follow-up duplex ultrasonography identifies a problem in the access, the access is considered a failure and the patient is referred for evaluation and treatment (see L).

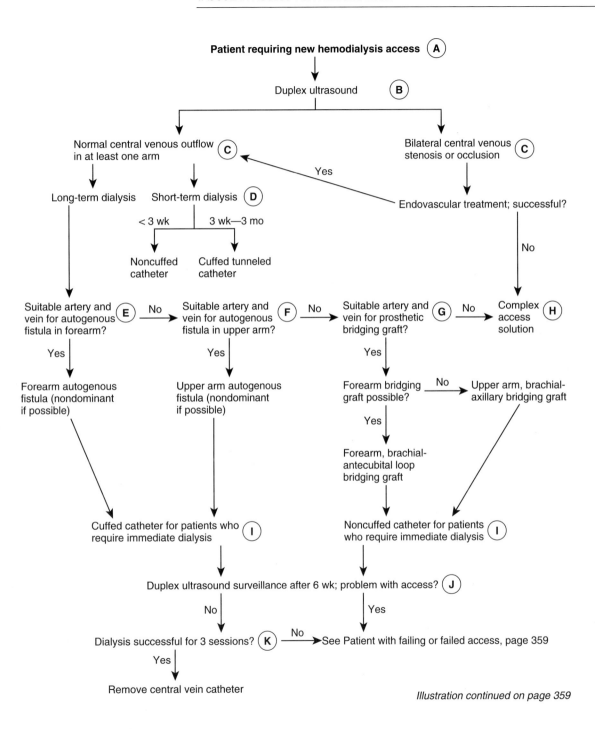

Patients with Failing or Failed Access

(L) For patients with a failing or failed access, the first step is a thorough duplex ultrasound evaluation of both the access and the underlying arterial and venous anatomy to ascertain cause of failure, correctabilty, or salvage and alternative sites. Patients with a prosthetic BG in particular should be evaluated for graft salvage as well as for the identification of a possible site for placement of a new AF, should the BG salvage not be successful.

(M) Patients with a failing dialysis catheter typically present with suboptimal flow on dialysis or, less commonly, upper extremity swelling secondary to pericatheter deep vein thrombosis. A duplex ultrasound scan can easily identify the latter, in which case we consider endovascular treatment to reestablish deep venous outflow following catheter removal. Subsequent imaging is directed at assessing the efficacy of treatment and identifying an alternative insertion site.

(N) In patients with poor catheter flow rates but no evidence of central venous compromise, transcatheter thrombolytic therapy has been effective. Urokinase protocols using 10,000 to 15,000 units, instilled directly through the catheter access port and allowed to dwell for various amounts of time, have been established. As problems of availability persist for this drug, newer protocols that use small doses of alternative thrombolytic agents are under investigation.

Catheters compromised by either malpositioning of the tip or encapsulation in a fibrin sheath can be treated endovascularly.[12] If catheter salvage is unsuccessful, the catheter is exchanged. Over-the-wire techniques may be used for non-cuffed catheters but are more complex with cuffed catheters having exit sites remote from the insertion site. This technique may result in similarly poor flow rates if the problem is a suboptimal subcutaneous tunnel, either acutely angled or compromised by proximity to the clavicle. Most commonly, a new percutaneous placement is performed in the site identified as optimal by duplex ultrasound scans.

(O) Information available from duplex ultrasound examination of a threatened or failed AF or BG is essential for directing treatment. Results with salvaging fistulae or grafts that have thrombosed are significantly worse than with those that are patent but have an identifiable stenosis. Both thrombolytic therapy and surgical thrombectomy have poor 6-month primary efficacy rates.[13] Nonetheless, the value of sustaining each access site in today's dialysis population warrants an attempt at salvage in most cases.

Both thrombolysis and surgical thrombectomy are aimed at removing clot as a prerequisite to identifying the underlying anatomic anomaly. Post-thrombectomy access imaging in the surgical suite is imperative. Appropriate adjunctive management of the offending lesion follows, first with endovascular options, if warranted, and surgical revision if the former prove unsuccessful.

(P) Prospective monitoring of access for hemodynamically significant stenoses, when combined with correction, improves patency and decreases the incidence of thrombosis. A number of techniques have been proposed to monitor for stenoses, including:

1. Intra-access flow.
2. Static or dynamic venous pressure measurements.
3. Measurements of recirculation using urea concentrations or dilution techniques.
4. Observation for changes in characteristics of pulse or thrill in the access.
5. Prolongation of bleeding after needle withdrawal.

Most of these techniques suggest increasing resistance at the venous anastomosis, which is the most common site of myointimal hyperplastic problems.

DOQI guidelines suggest that persistent abnormalities in any of these parameters mandate venography. We prefer a comprehensive duplex scan as the initial examination. The decision to proceed with either endovascular or surgical treatment is determined by the type of lesion identified and the practitioner's local experience.

(Q) Endovascular balloon dilatation of venous outflow stenoses in a BG or segmental stenoses in an AF is our initial choice of treatment. This treatment must result in elimination of the hemodynamically significant stenosis and must restore normal flow for it to be considered a success.

We recommend routine postprocedure evaluation after successful treatment by duplex ultrasound scan at 1 month to assess efficacy. Repeated angioplasty may be performed if indicated. In our practice, two failures of endovascular treatment for the same lesion within a 3-month period prompt surgical intervention.

(R) Surgical revision can be guided by the duplex scan and by subsequent contrast studies obtained during attempted endovascular revision. Surgical revision is focused on eliminating the causative lesion and preserving the maximal usable segment of vein for future use.

Recalcitrant stenoses in an AF can be treated either by patch angioplasty or segmental resection and interposition of a translocated reversed segment of vein or, frequently, by mobilization of the matured vein and primary repair. Arterial or venous stenoses near or involving the anastomosis can be treated with patch angioplasty or, alternatively, with mobilization and formation of a new arteriovenous connection.

For focal defects in a BG, such as midgraft stenosis or pseudoaneurysm, direct excision and interposition of a new segment may be indicated. The BG venous outflow lesion resistant to endovascular treatment may be treated with surgical patch angioplasty or a jump graft to a segment of uninvolved vein with good outflow.

(S) Any failed or failing graft that undergoes successful revision and salvage is reassessed at 1 month by duplex ultrasound examination. To achieve the reported 60% 1-year success rates following either endovascular or surgical intervention, further intervention is typically required.[14]

REFERENCES

1. Kherlakian GM, Roedersheimer LR, Arbaugh JJ, et al: Comparison of autogenous fistula versus expanded polytetrafluoroethylene graft fistula for angioaccess in hemodialysis. Am J Surg 1986;152:238–243.
2. U.S. Renal Data System: USRDS 1995 Annual Data Report. Am J Kidney Dis 1995;26:S12–S166.
3. National Kidney Foundation: Dialysis Outcomes Quality Initiative: Clinical Practice Guidelines. Vascular Access. Am J Kidney Dis 1997;30(4):S152–S191.
4. Silva MB Jr, Hobson RW II, Pappas PJ, et al: A strategy for increasing use of autogenous hemodialysis access procedures: Impact of preoperative noninvasive evaluation. J Vasc Surg 1998;27:302–308.
5. Khanna S, Sniderman K, Simons M, et al: Superior vena cava stenosis associated with hemodialysis catheters. Am J Kidney Dis 1993;21:278–281.
6. Silva MB Jr, Hobson RW II, Jamil Z, et al: Vein transposition in the forearm for autogenous hemoaccess. J Vasc Surg 1997;26:981–988.
7. Curi MA, Pappas PJ, Silva MB Jr, et al: Hemodialysis access: Influence of the human immunodeficiency virus on patency and infection rates. J Vasc Surg 1999;29:608–616.
8. Puskas JD, Gertler JP: Internal jugular to axillary vein bypass for subclavian vein thrombosis in the setting of brachial arteriovenous fistula. J Vasc Surg 1994;19:939–942.
9. McCann RL: Axillary grafts for difficult hemodialysis access. J Vasc Surg 1996;24:457–462.
10. El-Sabrout RA, Duncan JM: Right atrial bypass grafting for central venous obstruction associated with dialysis access: Another treatment option. J Vasc Surg 1999;29:472–478.
11. Scholz H, Zanow J, Petzold M, Petzold K: Arterioarterial interposition as angioaccess for hemodialysis. In Henry ML (ed): Vascular Access for Hemodialysis, vol 6. W. L. Gore & Associates and Precept Press, 1999, pp 255–262.
12. Schwab SJ, Beathard G: The hemodialysis catheter conundrum: Hate living with them, but can't live without them. Kidney Int 1999;56:1–17.
13. Marston WA, Criado E, Jaques PF, et al: Prospective randomized comparison of surgical versus endovascular management of thrombosed dialysis grafts. J Vasc Surg 1997;26:373–381.
14. Valji K, Bookstein J, Roberts A, et al: Pulse-spray pharmacomechanical thrombolysis of thrombosed hemodialysis access grafts: Long term experience and comparison of original and current techniques. AJR Am J Roentgenol 1995;164:1495–1500.

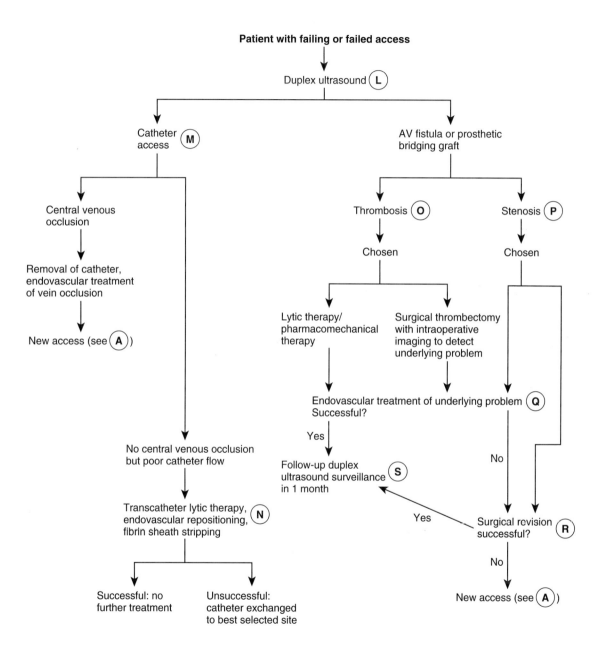

Chapter 73 Takayasu's Disease

JOSEPH M. GIORDANO, MD

(A) Takayasu's disease (TD) occurs most commonly in women during the third to fourth decades of life. Only about 10% of the patients are men. Initially, these patients may present with nonspecific signs and symptoms of systemic inflammatory illness, including fever, myalgia, arthritic complaints, and weight loss. Although the algorithm in this chapter divides TD into *acute* and *chronic* phases, there is considerable overlap.

(B) Often the diagnosis of TD is not made during the acute inflammatory phase. Many young women with systemic inflammatory signs and symptoms would not be thought to have TD. Patients who later present with severe, chronic TD commonly cannot recall a period of time in which they had significant signs and symptoms of systemic inflammatory disease. Either these patients did not have the clinical signs and symptoms of systemic inflammatory disease, or such symptoms were ignored as being nothing more than viral illness in a young patient.

Patients with chronic TD frequently have absent pulses. They may never have gone through an acute phase, or this phase was not recognized by the patient or by the treating physicians. Other patients who are in the "pulselessness" phase of TD are those who had received successful treatment of the acute phase with steroids or cytotoxic drugs and then progressed to a more chronic, inflammatory phase that caused arteries to narrow and, eventually, to occlude.

(C) Some patients have more specific symptoms that lead to the diagnosis of TD during the initial acute phase. A young patient with signs and symptoms of inflammatory disease might present with pain over the involved arteries, in particular the carotid artery or may have bruits on physical examination. The presence of bruits in a young patient is clearly abnormal. These patients may also have absent pulses or differences in brachial arterial pressures between the upper extremities.

The presence of any of these physical findings is an indication for further evaluation. This step often begins with duplex ultrasound scanning but should proceed to arteriography for definitive evaluation.

(D) Arteriography classically shows long, tapered stenoses that most commonly affect the major branches of the aorta, especially the subclavian and carotid arteries. The abdominal aorta below the renal arteries is also commonly involved and again shows a long, tapered narrowing. Aneurysmal dilatations are uncommon but can occur.

Magnetic residence angiography (MRA) can be used as an alternative to conventional arteriography. In the initial evaluation of the patient with potential TD, however, a complete arteriogram involving the thoracic and abdominal aorta and its branches is important to determine the initial presentation of the disease and to determine a baseline value in case newer lesions develop later.[1,2]

(E) The goal of medical treatment of patients with TD is to relieve systemic symptoms, decrease the inflammation of affected arteries, and reduce long-term sequelae from involved major arteries. In one study, 80% of patients required medical treatment but 25% of those treated did not achieve remission. Of those patients who responded with remission, 50% later experienced relapse. Note that current laboratory markers are inadequate to guide clinical management.[3]

Glucocorticoid steroid therapy is the initial treatment modality in controlling clinical manifestations and disease progression in patients with active disease. Patients are maintained on a sufficient dose of daily prednisone to control symptoms for 1 to 3 months. If this therapy is successful, attempts are made to taper and discontinue the prednisone regimen over 6 to 12 months.

(F) Patients who manifest convincing evidence of active disease such as systemic symptoms, progressive angiographic lesions, and elevated sedimentation rate (ESR) despite aggressive therapy, may need to be maintained on daily prednisone at the lowest effective dose. However, long-term steroid therapy is not necessary in patients with only an elevated ESR but no active arterial disease.

Arteriography and perhaps MRA remain the most definitive method of establishing remission or recurrence of disease. These modalities show subtle changes in degree of narrowing and extent of involvement that other, noninvasive studies may miss. It is recommended that arteriography be performed every 6 to 12 months to determine the level of disease activity. If arteriography shows a stable situation, no further treatment is indicated. If the disease remains stable, the frequency of arteriography can be steadily reduced. If the arteriogram shows new lesions, however, further treatment is recommended. In some cases, disease can also be monitored with extremity pressure measurement and duplex ultrasound scanning, reducing the requirement for arteriography, depending on which specific arteries are involved and the duration of a stable interval.

(G) Approximately 25% of patients treated with steroids do not experience a response to therapy. These patients are then treated with cytotoxic therapy. Cyclophosphamide has been effective in the treatment of TD, but it produces important side effects, including infertility, cystitis, bladder carcinoma, and lymphoma. Patients have also been successfully treated with low-dose methotrexate.

(H) As in patients with atherosclerosis, the absence of pulses does not necessitate surgical treatment in asymptomatic patients. Two principles must be considered. These patients are young and therefore may be more disabled by vascular symptoms involving the upper or lower extremities than older patients with atherosclerosis. However,

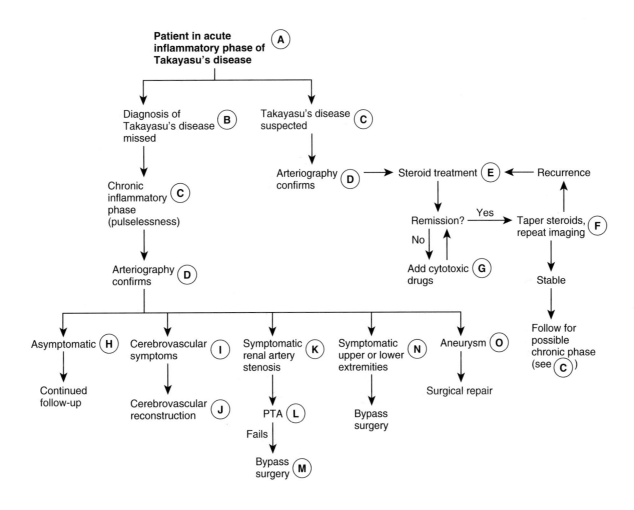

Takayasu's Disease (continued)

young patients with TD may also have had serious medical problems that increase their risk from surgery. They may manifest coronary artery involvement, congestive heart failure, and unrecognized or untreated hypertension.[4] Thus, surgical decision making must include a careful assessment of operative risk.

(I) Branches of the aortic arch are most commonly involved with TD. The subclavian, axillary, common carotid, and even innominate arteries usually develop long, tapered stenoses that extend for most of the length of these arteries.

Involvement of the common carotid artery usually ends just before its bifurcation. Involvement of the innominate artery means that blood flow is limited to the right carotid artery, the right subclavian artery, and therefore the right vertebral artery. Because involvement of the subclavian artery is always distal to the vertebral artery, subclavian steal syndrome never occurs.

I have reported that the incidence of stroke as a presenting symptom is 14%. Although it is difficult to prove, stroke may occur not from emboli but probably from sudden occlusion of one of the narrowed major cerebrovascular arteries.[5]

(J) Bypass is recommended to prevent stroke in symptomatic patients who have hemodynamically significant stenoses of either innominate or carotid arteries as well as in patients who have occlusions that are causing intermittent cerebral or ocular symptoms related to hypoperfusion. The bypass should originate from the ascending aorta because the rate of involvement of this vessel is only 5%, thereby reducing the potential for proximal anastomotic problems. The distal anastomosis can be placed at the carotid bulb, which is usually spared from the long, tapered stenoses that occur in the common carotid artery.

If both carotid arteries are involved, a bifurcation graft can be used. Additional limbs off the bifurcation graft can then also be anastomosed to the axillary or subclavian artery to relieve upper extremity ischemic symptoms.[5]

Good-risk patients with severe asymptomatic cerebrovascular involvement may be candidates for prophylactic surgery, mainly to prevent stroke from sudden occlusion of highly stenotic vessels (see I), but the benefit of this measure has not been clearly established.

(K) The incidence of hypertension in patients with TD is high, ranging from 20% to 72%. In fact, major morbidity and mortality of TD are due to uncontrolled hypertension, sometimes not recognized because artificially low blood pressures are obtained as a result of stenoses in both subclavian arteries. Most cases of hypertension are due to renal artery stenosis, although some may be due to stenosis of the distal descending thoracic aorta, a form of acquired coarctation. Correction of renal artery stenosis is recommended for both renovascular hypertension and kidney salvage.[6]

(L) Percutaneous transluminal angioplasty (PTA) has been used quite successfully for renal artery stenosis resulting from TD. Reports have suggested an initial success rate of 85% to 95%. Recurrence occurs in 15% to 20% of cases and is more likely to occur in renal arteries that have residual stenosis of 20% to 30% after the initial dilatation. Although the use of PTA for other arteries involved with TD has produced mixed results, it is clearly the preferred initial treatment for patients with renal artery stenosis.[7]

(M) Renal artery disease is usually confined to the proximal segment, leaving a considerable amount of renal artery available for surgical bypass. The frequent involvement of the infrarenal aorta may preclude the use of this section of the abdominal aorta for the proximal anastomosis. Therefore, it might be necessary to use the hepatic, splenic, or (when uninvolved) the supraceliac abdominal aorta as the in-flow site. A vein is the preferred conduit for the bypass.

(N) Upper extremity involvement is common, and symptoms can be severe because the involvement of the subclavian and axillary arteries tends to be a long-segment stenosis or occlusion, not the short segment proximal disease that occurs in patients with atherosclerosis. The long-segment involvement of TD restricts the ability of collateral circulation to compensate for proximal obstruction. Since patients with TD tend to be younger and tend to actively use their upper extremities, they become more symptomatic.

Equally important is the inability to obtain accurate blood pressures in patients with TD. If both subclavian arteries are involved, there is no reliable method to measure brachial arterial pressure. Patients can thus have hypertension for many years without being properly treated. In fact, these patients frequently present with congestive heart failure, malignant hypertension, and cardiac decompensation due to unrecognizable hypertension. Bypass of the subclavian or axillary arteries should be considered to treat symptoms from upper extremity involvement and to allow accurate blood pressure measurement.

Claudication of lower extremities occurs less commonly because of the infrequent involvement of the iliac arteries and the low incidence of disease in the femoral circulation. Claudication can be caused by TD of the abdominal aorta, which usually extends from the renal arteries to just proximal to the aortic bifurcation. This problem can be treated with a bypass originating from the lower thoracic aorta to one iliac artery, since this method helps to perfuse both legs.[4]

(O) The incidence of aneurysm formation resulting from TD varies. In the North American experience, aneurysms are relatively uncommon. When they do occur, they tend to be multiple, saccular, and fusiform and are often associated with stenotic lesions.

Aneurysms commonly involve the ascending, thoracic, and abdominal aortas. In the Northern

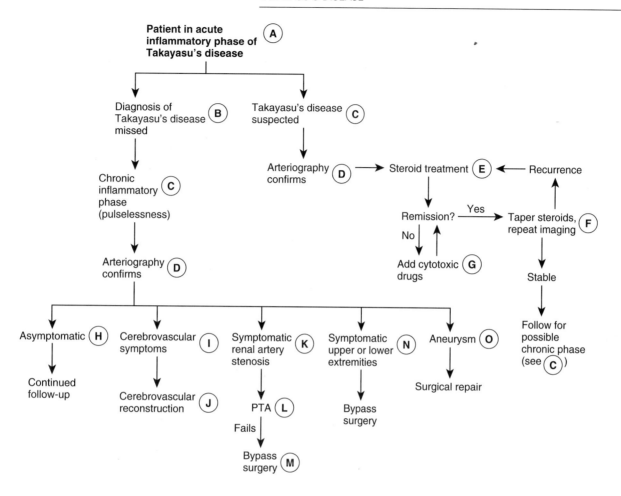

American experience, the incidence of rupture of the aneurysms appears to be quite low. However, large aneurysms of the major arteries probably should be treated with surgical repair in a medically stable patient. These patients are young, and if TD is medically treated, they can anticipate a long life. Therefore, although the frequency of aneurysm rupture is relatively low, if one considers the long life expectancy of young patients with TD, the incidence of rupture over time may actually be high. Resection and aortic valve replacement are recommended for aneurysms of the ascending aorta that are causing clinically significant aortic insufficiency.[6,8]

REFERENCES

1. Lande A, Rossi P: The value of total aortography in the diagnosis of Takayasu's arteritis. Radiology 1975;114:287.
2. Yamada I, Numano F, Suzuki S: Takayasu arteritis: Evaluation with MR imaging. Radiology 1993;188:89.
3. Kerr GS, Hallahan CW, Giordano J, et al: Takayasu arteritis. Ann Intern Med 1994;120:919.
4. Giordano J: Surgical treatment of Takayasu's disease. In Ernst CB, Stanley JC (eds): Current Therapy in Vascular Surgery, 2nd ed. Philadelphia, BC Decker, 1991, p 169.
5. Giordano J, Leavitt RY, Hoffman G, et al: Experience with surgical treatment of Takayasu's disease. Surgery 1991;109:252.
6. Hall S, Barr W, Lie JT, et al: Takayasu arteritis: A study of 32 North American patients. Medicine 1985;64:89.
7. Tyagi S, Singh B, Kaul UA, et al: Balloon angioplasty for renovascular hypertension in Takayasu's arteritis. Am Heart J 1993;125:1386.
8. Matsumura K, Hirano T, Takeda K, et al: Incidence of aneurysms in Takayasu's arteritis. Angiology 1991;42:308.

Chapter 74 Intraoperative Hemorrhage and Bleeding Diathesis

CYNTHIA C. SHORTELL, MD • KENNETH OURIEL, MD

(A) When intraoperative hemorrhage occurs, the most likely cause is an anatomic bleeding source.[1] Before undertaking extensive investigation of a bleeding diathesis, the surgical team must ascertain that no technical problem exists. Bleeding due to a technical problem can be differentiated from bleeding due to a coagulopathy. In the first instance, a single defect in a vascular structure or organ can be identified; with a coagulopathy, a more generalized process is evident. Unfortunately, inability to recognize and promptly correct an anatomic problem may ultimately result in the development of a generalized problem. Therefore, the surgeon should not assume the presence of a coagulopathy without an exhaustive search for a technical error.

(B) The most common causes of intraoperative hypothermia include (1) prolonged operative time (with associated heat loss to the environment), (2) global hypoperfusion due to generalized compromise of the patient, and (3) use of large volumes of unwarmed fluids.[1] Since many laboratories perform tests on samples warmed to 37°C, normal coagulation parameters may be reported in patients who have hypothermia-related coagulopathy.[2] Platelet dysfunction and disseminated intravascular coagulation (DIC) may also be precipitated by hypothermia.[3, 4]

The coagulopathy associated with hypothermia creates a vicious circle in which the above-mentioned factors are exacerbated; increased bleeding leads to longer operative time, greater volume requirements, and worsened tissue perfusion. Once established, therefore, hypothermic coagulopathy is difficult to reverse, and measures aimed at prevention are critical. When the surgeon determines that the operation carries a high risk, prewarming the room, use of warming blankets and prewarmed fluids, and expeditious conduct of the surgery may help to avoid these problems. Acidosis is a particularly common problem for vascular surgeons, as reperfusion of ischemic tissue is often the goal of the procedure. Other causative factors include global hypoperfusion and sepsis.

As with hypothermia, the best treatment is prevention, by administration of appropriate agents, such as bicarbonate prior to restoration of flow. Dilution of coagulation proteins, platelets, and calcium occurs in progressive fashion with increasing administration of fluid and red blood cells to replace shed blood and volume lost to third-space fluid. There is no specific cutoff at which this is known to occur; even in the face of massive blood loss, enough coagulation proteins almost always continue to maintain function.[5, 6] Replacement of platelets and fresh frozen plasma (FFP) should therefore be done in response to documented need, based on laboratory findings consistent with these deficiencies—platelet count, prothrombin time (PT), activated partial thromboplastin time (aPTT), and activated clotting time (ACT).

(C) Although "catastrophic" bleeding is a subjective term, it is one well understood by all surgeons. Most often, it is a result of an anatomic problem, such as a defect in a major vessel or organ, but it can also occur as a result of a severe coagulopathy. Clinically, this is manifested as massive bleeding from virtually all exposed tissue, including previously hemostatic sites.

(D) In the case of catastrophic bleeding due to a coagulopathy, the surgical team is not afforded the luxury of selective therapy (i.e., sending appropriate laboratory tests, waiting for results, and treating the patient accordingly). Instead, a battery of tests designed to screen for all possible problems should be sent immediately, including hematocrit, PT, aPTT, ACT, thrombin time (TT), euglobulin clot lysis time (ECLT), fibrinogen, and fibrin degradation products (FDPs).

(E) Treatment of all reasonable causes using a "shotgun approach" should be instituted prior to return of test results, however, because the patient is at risk for exsanguination in this situation, and replacement of shed blood in addition to correction of the coagulation disorder is crucial for successful resuscitation.

(F) If inadequate heparin reversal is judged to be a problem, administration of protamine sulfate is indicated and is rarely harmful if the patient tolerated the initial protamine dose. If a test dose has not yet been given, care should be taken in administering the protamine, since resultant hypotension may be devastating. Protamine sulfate is a positively charged molecule that works by binding the negatively charged heparin molecule and by restoring antithrombin III to its native state.[7]

(G) Platelets should be administered as the first prophylactic measure in the face of massive hemorrhage.[8] Platelet concentrates replace lost platelets and contain significant amounts of FFP and factor V. Under normal circumstances, a platelet count of 20,000/mL is adequate, but in the setting of severe blood loss, a level of 50,000 to 70,000/mL is advisable.[9] Administration of FFP will treat the majority of dilutional factor deficiencies as well as DIC, unrecognized factor VIII deficiencies, warfarin administration, and liver dysfunction.[10] Empirical use of platelets and FFP is appropriate if there are no obvious clinical causes such as inadequate reversal of anticoagulation or underlying renal disease. The use of desmopressin acetate (DDAVP) may be helpful if platelet function is in question, particularly in patients with renal insufficiency. DDAVP increases levels of factor VIII and von Willebrand factor (VWF) and thereby improves platelet adhesiveness to injured endothelium.[11, 12]

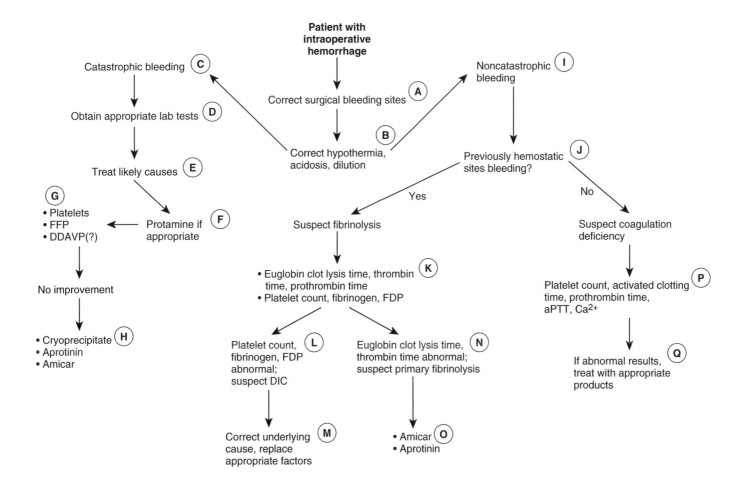

Intraoperative Hemorrhage and Bleeding Diathesis (continued)

(H) When these measures fail to correct the bleeding diathesis, consideration should be given to the use of cryoprecipitate, ϵ-aminocaproic acid (Amicar), and aprotinin. Cryoprecipitate contains large amounts of factor VIII, vWF, and fibrinogen[13, 14] and is indicated in the treatment of consumptive coagulopathy. The use of direct antifibrinolytic agents, such as Amicar, tranexamic acid, and aprotinin, in the situation of undiagnosed bleeding disorder is more problematic. All of these agents block plasminogen directly or block the action of plasmin on fibrin and fibrinogen and are therefore helpful in the treatment of primary fibrinolysis but are contraindicated in the treatment of DIC, since clearance of fibrin from the capillaries is critical in the latter condition.[15–18]

(I) "Noncatastrophic" bleeding due to bleeding diathesis is not qualitatively different from catastrophic bleeding; a generalized "ooze" is noted from all raw surfaces in the absence of a technical problem. In the setting of noncatastrophic bleeding, however, a more considered, selective approach to identification and correction of the underlying disorder is possible.

(J) The first distinction the surgeon should make is based on clinical observation of the bleeding itself: Are previously hemostatic sites bleeding?

(K) If bleeding is shown to be from sites that were previously hemostatic, this suggests active destruction of the hemostatic plug. In this setting, laboratory tests are necessary to help differentiate between the two major causes of this phenomenon—primary fibrinolysis and DIC. These tests include ECLT, TT, platelet count, fibrinogen, and aPTT.

(L) DIC occurs in the presence of severe physiologic insult to the patient, such as sepsis, hypotension, and trauma. In this setting, uncontrolled systemic activation and consumption of all clotting mediators, including thrombin, platelets, and the fibrinolytic system, occur. This leads to the simultaneous and paradoxical development of uncontrolled thrombosis (excess systemic thrombin) and systemic fibrinolysis (excess plasmin).[19–23] The latter process is critical in the clearance of the microvascular thrombi formed as a result of excess thrombin generation and should not be inhibited by administration of antifibrinolytic agents. The laboratory findings suggestive of DIC are elevated TT, PT, and aPTT levels; thrombocytopenia; hypofibrinogenemia; presence of FDPs; and lack of clot formation in the ECLT.

(M) Treatment of the underlying cause of DIC is essential to its management; if the stimulus for excess activation of clotting mediators is not eliminated, all other treatment will fail. In addition, replacement of consumed elements with FFP, cryoprecipitate, and platelets is beneficial. Use of antifibrinolytics is contraindicated, as noted earlier.

(N) Abnormal clotting parameters in the absence of FDPs and thrombocytopenia and an abnormal (shortened) ECLT suggest the diagnosis of primary fibrinolysis, which is distinctly different from DIC. In DIC, fibrinolysis is a secondary event, with the beneficial effect of lysing intravascular thrombi and preventing organ damage, and therefore should not be inhibited. Primary fibrinolysis, in contrast, is not associated with microvascular thrombosis, and reversal can be highly beneficial.[24, 25] The mechanism by which fibrinolysis occurs is by direct plasminogen activation, not indirect activation by high thrombin and fibrin clot levels, as in DIC. Elevation of tissue plasminogen activator (t-PA) is seen in liver failure and in the anhepatic phase of liver transplantation, possibly a result of deficient synthesis of plasminogen activator inhibitor (PAI-1).[26, 27] It may also be seen during supraceliac clamping, particularly if prolonged, probably as a result of hepatic hypoperfusion.[28, 29]

(O) As noted, elimination of ongoing stimulus to fibrinolysis (e.g., release of supraceliac clamp) and reversal of fibrinolytic elements with agents such as Amicar, tranexamic acid, or aprotinin, may result in excellent clinical success.[15–18]

(P) If previously hemostatic sites are not noted to be bleeding, simple deficiencies of procoagulant elements resulting in failure of clot formation, rather than a process in which clot degradation is occurring, should be suspected. The two most likely causes of this problem are dilutional reduction in the elements themselves and failure of the elements to function optimally. Laboratory tests to be performed should include a platelet count, ACT, PT, aPTT, and calcium level.

(Q) Bleeding in the presence of a platelet count below 50 to 70/L should prompt correction with platelet products. If the platelet count is normal but platelet dysfunction is suspected (abnormal bleeding time), DDAVP should be administered.

An isolated elevation of the ACT may represent inadequate reversal of heparin but may also reflect other, more generalized coagulation abnormalities. If inadequate reversal of heparin is suspected, protamine should be given slowly (see F) because of potential hypotension.

The PT can give an assessment of the function of the extrinsic coagulation pathway. An elevated PT may be due to administration of warfarin or liver dysfunction, both of which affect the synthesis of the four vitamin K–dependent clotting factors (II, VII, IX, and X). Administration of FFP is usually sufficient to reverse the bleeding diathesis associated with isolated elevation of PT. Cryoprecipitate contains larger amounts of factor VIII, vWF, and fibrinogen than FFP, and may be used when FFP is ineffective.

An elevated aPTT suggests an abnormality in the intrinsic coagulation pathway. This can be corrected with FFP, protamine, or both. If FFP and

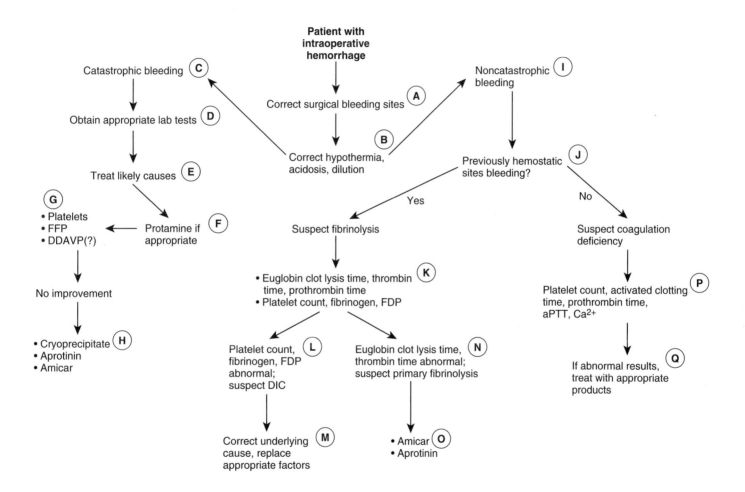

protamine are ineffective, cryoprecipitate may be of value.

Hypocalcemia is usually associated with massive blood loss and transfusion and is rarely seen in isolation. It should be considered when correction of coagulation factor deficiencies has been accomplished and bleeding persists.

REFERENCES

1. Ferrera A, MacArthur JD, Wright HK, et al: Hypothermia and acidosis worsen coagulopathy in the patient requiring massive transfusion. Am J Surg 1990;160:515.
2. Reed RL, Johnston TD, Hudson JD, et al: The disparity between hypothermic coagulopathy and clotting studies. J Trauma 1992;33:465.
3. Yoshihara H, Yamamoto T, Mihara H: Changes in coagulation and fibrinolysis occurring in dogs during hypothermia. Thromb Res 1985;37:503.
4. Valeri CR, Feingold H, Cassidy G, et al: Hypothermia-induced reversible platelet dysfunction. Ann Surg 1987;205:175.
5. Weaver DW: Differential diagnosis and management of unexplained bleeding. Surg Clin North Am 1993;73:353.
6. Lipsett PA, Perler B: The use of blood products for surgical bleeding. Semin Vasc Surg 1996;9:347.
7. National Institutes of Health Consensus Conference: Fresh frozen plasma: Indications and risks. JAMA 1985;253:551.
8. National Institutes of Health Consensus Conference: Platelet transfusion therapy. JAMA 1987;257:1777.
9. Triulzi DJ: Plasma alternatives. Transfusion Medicine Update: Institute for Transfusion Medicine, 1997.
10. Okajima Y, Kanayama S, Maeda Y, et al: Studies on the neutralizing mechanism of antithrombin activity of heparin by protamine. Thromb Res 1981;24:21.
11. Mannucci PM, Ruggeri ZM, Pareti FI, et al: 1-Deamino-8-D-arginine vasopressin: A new pharmacological approach to the management of hemophilia and von Willebrand's disease. Lancet 1987;1:869.
12. Sakariassen S, Catteneo M, vd Berg A, et al: DDAVP enhances platelet adherence and platelet aggregate growth on human artery subendothelium. Blood 1984;64:229.
13. Rutledge R, Sheldon GF, Collins ML: Massive transfusion. Crit Care Clin 1986;2:791.
14. Ratnoff OD: Some therapeutic agents influencing hemostasis. In Colman RW, Hirsh J, Marder VJ, et al (eds): Hemostasis and Thrombosis: Basic Principles and Clinical Practice (3rd ed). Philadelphia, JB Lippincott, 1994, p 1104.
15. Sherry S, Marder VJ: Therapy with antifibrinolytic agents. In Colman RW, Hirsh J, Marder VJ, et al (eds): Hemostasis and Thrombosis: Basic Principles and Clinical Practice (3rd ed). Philadelphia, JB Lippincott, 1994, p 335.
16. Alkjaersig N, Fletcher AP, Sherry S: Epsilon-aminocaproic acid: An inhibitor of plasminogen activation. J Biol Chem 1959;234:832.
17. de Peppo AP, Pierri MD, Scafuri A, et al: Intraoperative antifibrinolysis and blood-saving techniques in cardiac surgery: Prospective trial of 3 antifibrinolytic drugs. Texas Heart Inst J 1995;22:231.
18. Robert S, Wagner BKJ, Boulanger M, et al: Aprotinin. Ann Pharmacother 1996;30:372.
19. Thijs LG, de Boer JP, de Groot MCM, et al: Coagulation disorders in septic shock. Intens Care Med 1993;19(Suppl):S8.
20. White GC, Marder VJ, Colman RW, et al: Approach to the bleeding patient. In Colman RW, Hirsh J, Marder VJ, et al (eds): Hemostasis and Thrombosis: Basic Principles and Clinical Practice (3rd ed). Philadelphia, JB Lippincott, 1994, p 1134.
21. Baglin T: Disseminated intravascular coagulation: Diagnosis and treatment. BMJ 1996;312:683.
22. Feinstein DI: Treatment of disseminated intravascular coagulation. Semin Thromb Hemost 1988;14:351.
23. Levi M, van der Poll T, ten Cate H, et al: The cytokine-mediated imbalance between coagulant and anticoagulant mechanisms in sepsis and endotoxaemia. Eur J Clin Invest 1997;27:3.
24. Lechner K, Niessner H, Thaler E: Coagulation abnormalities in liver disease. Semin Thromb Hemost 1977;4:40.
25. Williams E: Disseminated intravascular coagulation. In Loscalzo J, Schafer A (eds): Thrombosis and Hemorrhage. Boston, Blackwell Science, 1994, p 1023.
26. Francis RB: Clinical disorders of fibrinolysis: A critical review. Blut 1989;59:1.
27. Kang YG, Martin DJ, Marquez J, et al: Intraoperative changes in blood coagulation and thrombelastographic monitoring in liver transplantation. Anesth Analg 1985;64:888.
28. Illig KA, Green RM, Ouriel K, et al: Primary fibrinolysis during supraceliac clamping. J Vasc Surg 1997;25:244.
29. Eagleton M, Illig KA, Riggs PN, et al: Visceral perfusion ameliorates primary fibrinolysis during supraceliac aortic cross-clamping. Surg Forum 1997;4B:419.

INTRAOPERATIVE HEMORRHAGE AND BLEEDING DIATHESIS

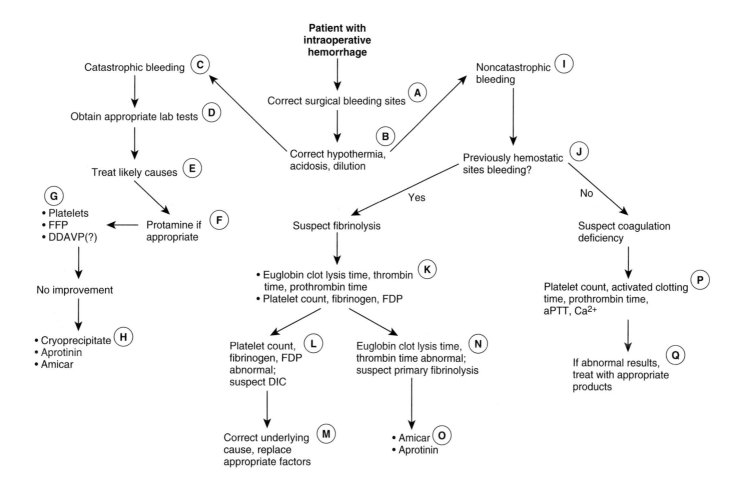

Chapter 75 Heparin-Induced Complications

DONALD SILVER, MD • ANGELA VOUYOUKA, MD

(A) Heparin-induced thrombocytopenia (HIT) occurs in two forms. A nonimmune transient thrombocytopenia, type I, occurs in up to 10% of patients after 3 to 5 days of therapy and remits with no adverse sequelae while heparin is continued. Immune HIT, type II, occurs in 2% to 3% of patients receiving any form of heparin. These patients produce antibodies, usually immunoglobulin G, to a heparin-platelet-protein (usually platelet factor IV) complex, which in the presence of heparin causes platelet aggregation and endothelial damage with thrombocytopenia and less often with arterial or venous thromboses. Bleeding is a rare occurrence. Heparin-associated antiplatelet antibodies (HAAbs) usually appear between the 5th and 8th days of the first exposure to heparin or as early as the first day of reexposure.

Although the mortality and morbidity rates associated with HIT have been as high as 23% and 61%, respectively, with early recognition of the syndrome and prompt cessation of the administration of any form of heparin to which the patient is sensitive these rates can be reduced to 1.1% and 7.4%, respectively.[1]

(B) Once thrombocytopenia (platelet count < 100,000/mm^3, a 30% decrease from initial platelet count or a falling platelet count) occurs, HIT should be excluded by testing for HAAb. The tests include the platelet aggregation assay, serotonin release assay, and enzyme-linked immunosorbent assay (ELISA).

(C) A patient without HAAbs most likely has nonimmune HIT and should do well without discontinuation of heparin. If the thrombocytopenia persists, other causes of the condition should be considered.

(D) If a patient has HAAbs, heparin administration should cease and platelet function should be inhibited (we most often use aspirin).

(E) We have found that HAAbs do not usually cross-react with all the available low-molecular-weight heparins; consequently, we have utilized a nonreactive low-molecular-weight heparin safely in a large number of patients.[2] If another alternative rapid anticoagulant is needed, recombinant lepirudin, which is a direct thrombin inhibitor, is available. For the individual without renal or hepatic impairment, the usual dose of lepirudin is 0.4 mg/kg as a bolus infusion and a continuing infusion of 0.15 mg/kg per hour. Its half-life in individuals with normal renal function is 90 minutes. The activated partial thromboplastin time (aPTT) should be monitored and should be maintained around 2.0 to 2.5 times the control.

(F) Heparin-induced thrombosis is almost always related to the procoagulant activation of platelets and the endothelium by the combination of platelet factor IV/heparin and HAAbs.[3]

(G) The heparin-induced thromboses may occur at or remote from sites of arterial reconstruction. The patient might not become thrombocytopenic; however, a falling platelet count, resistance to heparin anticoagulation therapy, and unexplained thrombosis are the usual manifestations of a heparin-induced thrombosis. All patients who experience a thrombotic event while receiving heparin should be tested for HAAbs.

(H) If the patient has HAAbs, heparin administration should cease and angiograms, thrombolysis, or thrombectomy should be performed with an alternative anticoagulant. Any detected technical errors should be corrected using a nonreactive heparin or an alternative anticoagulant (see E).

(I) A patient who is HAAb-negative can safely receive heparin. If no mechanical or other cause of the thrombosis is apparent, a hypercoagulable condition should be considered.

(J) Insufficient anticoagulation with heparin may contribute to thrombosis in sites of arterial reconstruction. We usually administer heparin intraoperatively, 100 units/kg as a bolus injection and 1000 units/hour thereafter. We do not reverse heparin at the end of the operative procedure. If thrombosis occurs in the patient who is receiving adequate heparin but who has a persistently low aPTT, the antithrombin level may be deficient. In this case, antithrombin can be supplemented with antithrombin concentrates.

(L) We use a low-molecular-weight heparin, usually enoxaparin 30 to 40 mg subcutaneously twice a day, for venous thromboembolism prophylaxis. Venous thromboembolism is a common thrombotic complication of HIT. Therefore, all patients who are receiving or who have recently received heparin who develop venous thromboembolism should be tested for HAAbs.[2]

(M) If HAAbs are present, heparin administration should cease and alternate anticoagulations (see E) should be used for anticoagulation and during times of thrombectomy and thrombolysis.

(N) If the patient is not HAAb-positive, heparin can be continued with the aPTT ranging between 2.5 and 3.5 times the control value. If indicated, thrombolysis or thrombectomy may be offered to resolve the thrombus. Anticoagulation is usually continued with warfarin.

HEPARIN-INDUCED COMPLICATIONS

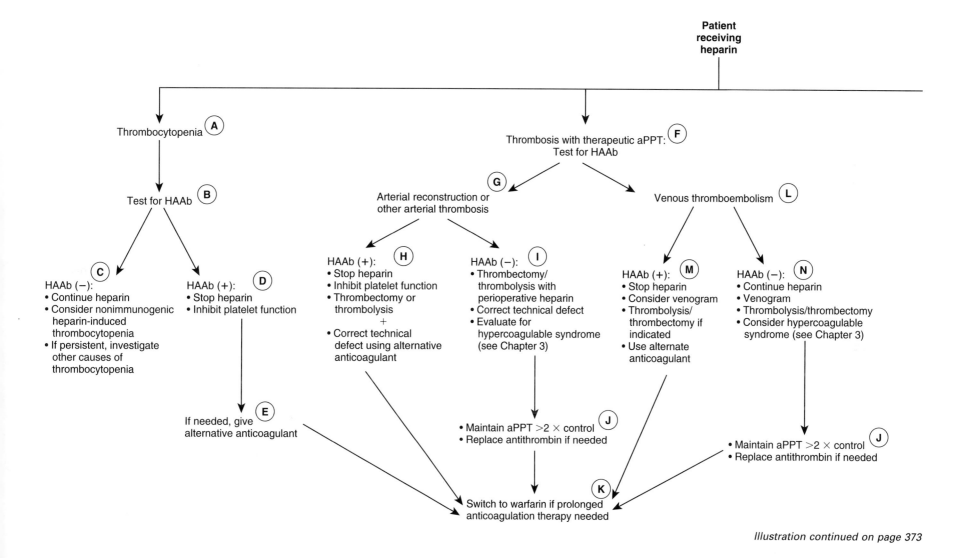

Illustration continued on page 373

Heparin-Induced Complications (continued)

(O) Heparin-induced bleeding is the most common complication of heparin therapy.[4] Approximately 5% of patients (range, 1% to 33%) receiving intravenous or high-dose subcutaneous heparin have major bleeding. If bleeding occurs from the excessive administration of heparin, one should stop administration of heparin for 2 to 3 hours and restart it when bleeding is controlled. The goal should be to achieve an aPTT of 2 to 2.5 times the control value.

(P) Heparin may exacerbate mechanical bleeding. This usually occurs when the aPTT is markedly prolonged (> three times the control value). Few patients experience bleeding from HIT. When the mechanical bleeding is controlled, heparin can be restarted with careful monitoring. A patient with HAAbs should receive alternate anticoagulation (see E) if anticoagulation is needed.

(Q) Nonmechanical heparin-related bleeding usually occurs in patients with one or more risk factors, including advanced age (especially postmenopausal women), renal or hepatic failure, and administration of platelet function inhibitors.

(R) If the patient is HAAb-positive, one should discontinue administration of the sensitizing heparin. If anticoagulation is necessary, carefully controlled anticoagulation with an alternate anticoagulant (see E) is recommended.

(S) If the patient is HAAb-negative, one should discontinue heparin and correct the aPTT. If anticoagulation is necessary, carefully controlled subsequent anticoagulation with heparin and warfarin is recommended.

(T) Heparin-induced skin necrosis usually occurs between the 5th and 6th days of heparin therapy.[5,6]

(U) The lesions may be diffuse, involving the abdominal wall and lower extremities and, less frequently, the hands and the nose. The lesions consist of painful erythematous plaques or necrosis caused by thrombosis of dermal venules and capillaries. If the lesions are diffuse, the patient should be tested for the presence of HAAbs. If the patient has HAAbs, heparin is discontinued and alternative anticoagulation is given when indicated.

(V) If the lesions involve the injection sites, infection should be eliminated as the cause of necrosis. If the culture specimens are negative, the patient should be tested for HAAb (see U). The risk of reinstitution of heparin is not defined and therefore is not recommended for patients with heparin-induced skin necrosis even if HAAbs were not present.

(W) Heparin-induced allergic reactions are rare.[7]

(X) Angioneurotic edema, hypersensitivity reactions, and shock are extremely rare. In these cases, heparin should be discontinued and appropriate cardiovascular support provided.

(Y) The more common forms of allergic heparin reaction are eosinophilia (which occurs in 10% of patients receiving unfractionated heparin; 95% are asymptomatic) and dermal reactions, including urticaria and pruritus. Discontinuation of heparin is not usually required unless symptoms are severe. Antihistamines and different brands of heparin may be helpful.

(Z) Heparin-induced aldosterone suppression with hyperkalemia, hyponatremia, or metabolic acidosis occurs in 7% of patients as a result of heparin's suppressive effect on the adrenal zona glomerulosa. Marked hyperkalemia also requires the evaluation of other conditions affecting renal function. The potassium retention is usually detectable after 1 to 3 days of heparin administration and disappears in 1 to 3 days after heparin discontinuation. Management includes monitoring potassium levels in patients who receive heparin for more than 3 days and, if needed, removing potassium supplements and a saline diuresis. Heparin therapy is usually continued. If symptoms are severe and do not respond to standard management, adrenal hemorrhage should be suspected.[8]

REFERENCES

1. Almeida JI, Coats R, Liem TK, Silver D: Reduced morbidity and mortality rates of the heparin-induced thrombocytopenia syndrome. J Vasc Surg 1998;27:309–316.
2. Slocum MM, Adams JG Jr, Teel R, et al: Use of enoxaparin in patients with heparin-induced thrombocytopenia syndrome. J Vasc Surg 1996;23:839–843.
3. Wallenga J, Bick RL: Heparin-induced thrombocytopenia, paradoxical thromboembolism, and other side effects of heparin therapy. Med Clin North Am 1998;82:635–657.
4. Levine MN, Hirsh J, Salzman EW: Side effects of antithrombotic therapy. In Colman RW, Hirsh J, Mardar VJ, Salzman EW (eds): Hemostasis and Thrombosis: Basic Principles and Clinical Practice, 3rd ed. Philadelphia, JB Lippincott, 1994.
5. Sallah S, Thomas DP, Roberts HR: Warfarin and heparin-induced skin necrosis and the purple toe syndrome: Infrequent complications of anticoagulant treatment. Thromb Haemost 1997;78:785–790.
6. Warkentin TE: Heparin-induced skin lesions. Br J Haemotol 1996;92:494–497.
7. Hirsh J, Raschke R, Warkentin TE, et al: Heparin: Mechanism of action, pharmacokinetics, dosing considerations, monitoring, efficacy and safety. Chest 1995;108(4 Suppl):258S–275S.
8. Oster JR, Singer I, Fishman LM: Heparin-induced aldosterone suppression and hyperkalemia. Am J Med 1995;98:575–586.

HEPARIN-INDUCED COMPLICATIONS

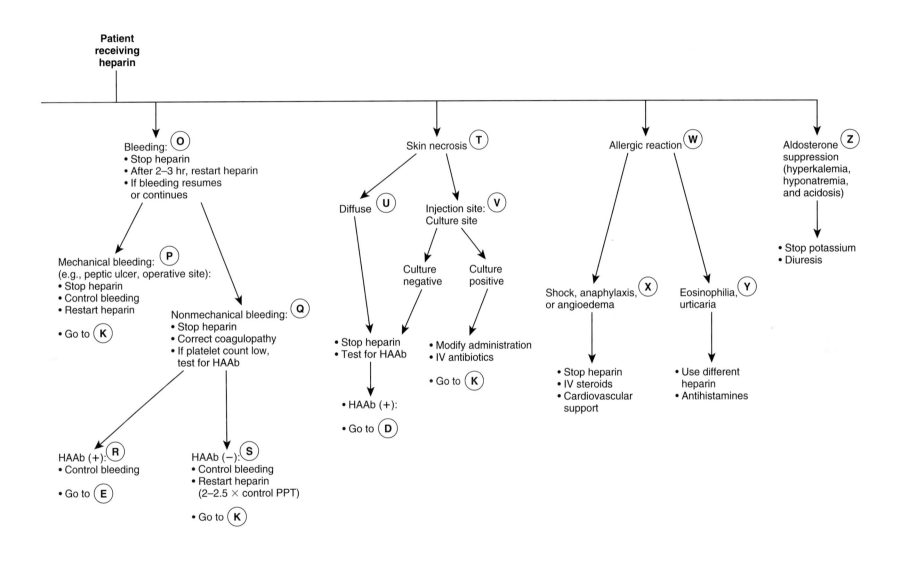

INDEX

Note: Page numbers followed by the letter f refer to figures and those followed by t refer to tables.

Abdominal aortic aneurysm (AAA), 90–96, 91f
  aneurysms associated with, 132, 133f, 136
  endovascular repair of, 120–125, 121f
  fistulas associated with, 108–111, 109f
  life expectancy with, 90, 91f, 92, 92t
  medical management of, 90, 91f, 94
  operative management of, 91f, 92, 94, 96
    mortality risk with, 91f, 92, 92t
    preoperative imaging for, 91f, 94
  renal correlation with, 91f, 94, 246, 247f
  rupture of, 90, 104–106, 105f
    evaluation of, 104–105, 105f
    intraoperative management of, 105–106, 105f
    risk factors for, 90, 91f, 92t
    risk of, estimate related to diameter and, 90, 91f, 91t
  symptomatic vs. asymptomatic, 90, 104
Abdominal compartment syndrome, in ruptured abdominal aortic aneurysm repair, 105f, 106
Abdominal packing, four-quadrant, for abdominal vascular trauma, 327f, 328
Abdominal pain, in mesenteric ischemia, 250, 251f, 256
Abdominal radiographs, for abdominal vascular trauma, 324, 325f
Abdominal vascular trauma, 324–330
  aortic injuries in, 326–327, 326f, 328
  evaluation of, 324–325, 325f
  exploratory laparotomy for, 325–326, 325f
  inferior vena cava injuries in, 329–330, 329f
  pelvic injuries in, 328–329, 328f
  portal vein injuries in, 329–330, 329f
  renal injuries in, 327–328, 327f
  resuscitation of, 324, 325f
ABI. See Ankle-brachial index (ABI).
Ablation therapy
  for pediatric renovascular occlusive disease, 242, 243f
  for post-traumatic pain syndrome, 338
Above-knee amputation (AKA), 218, 219f, 220
Abscess(es)
  with diabetic foot infections, 213f, 214
  with superficial phlebitis, 269, 269f
Acidosis, metabolic
  heparin-induced, 372, 373f
  intraoperative, 364, 365f
Activated clotting time (ACT), intraoperative, 18, 364, 366
Activated partial thromboplastin time (aPTT)
  in heparin therapy complications, 370, 371f, 372

Activated partial thromboplastin time (aPTT) (Continued)
  in hypercoagulable syndrome, 8, 9f
  in intraoperative hemorrhage, 364, 365f, 366
  in lower extremity deep vein thrombosis treatment, 276, 278
Acute limb ischemia (ALI), 168–170, 169f. See also Critical limb ischemia (CLI); specific extremity.
Adenosine thallium stress testing, for preoperative cardiac risk assessment, 3–4
Aerobic exercise, for hyperlipidemia, 6, 7f
AFBP (atriofemoral bypass), in thoracoabdominal aortic aneurysm repair, 99f, 100, 102
Age, advanced
  carotid plus coronary disease and, 84
  perioperative risks with, 2, 3f
  with aneurysms, 90, 92t, 98, 118, 120
Air embolism, in aortovenous fistula repair, 110
AKA (above-knee amputation), 218, 219f, 220
Aldosterone suppression, heparin-induced, 372, 373f
ALI (acute limb ischemia), 168–170, 169f
Alprostadil, for erectile dysfunction, 346, 348
ALRVF (aorta to left renal vein fistula), 108–110, 109f
ε-Aminocaproic acid (Amicar), for intraoperative hemorrhage, 365f, 366
Amitriptyline (Elavil), for post-traumatic pain syndrome, 337, 338
Amputation
  for acute limb ischemia, 169, 169f
  for atheroembolism, 172–173
  for critical limb ischemia, 162, 163f, 164
  for extremity vascular trauma, 333f, 334
  for femoral artery pseudoaneurysm, 143f, 144
  for gangrene, 218, 219f
  for infrainguinal graft thrombosis, 205f, 206
  for infrainguinal occlusive disease, 192, 193f
  for infrainguinal prosthetic graft infection, 208, 209, 209f
  for post-traumatic pain syndrome, 337f, 338
  for Raynaud's syndrome, 343f, 344
  with diabetic foot infections, 212, 213f, 214
Amputation level, determination of, 218, 219f, 220
Anaerobic organisms, in diabetic foot infections, 212
Anastomosis, end-to-end, for vascular trauma
  abdominal, 327, 327f, 330
  brachiocephalic, 322
  extremity, 332, 333f, 334
Anastomotic-neointimal hyperplasia, in acute limb ischemia, 170

Anesthesia, 12–13, 13f
  for abdominal aortic aneurysm
  for carotid endarterectomy, 38, 39f
    with carotid plus coronary disease, 84, 86
  for ruptured abdominal aortic aneurysm repair, 104–105, 105
  with endovascular repair, 124
Aneurysm(s)
  abdominal aortic. See Abdominal aortic aneurysm (AAA).
  as congenital venous malformation, 352
  atheroembolism with, 174
  carotid artery. See Carotid artery aneurysm.
  femoral artery. See Femoral artery aneurysm.
  hepatic artery, 150, 151f
  iliac artery. See Iliac artery aneurysm (IAA).
  in Takayasu's disease, 361f, 362–363
  infectious, 54–56, 55f, 140, 143, 143f
  pelvic artery, 132
  popliteal artery, 146, 147f, 148
    occlusive disease vs., 230, 231f
  renal artery, 152–153, 153f
  thoracoabdominal aortic. See Thoracoabdominal aortic aneurysm (TAA).
  ulnar artery, in upper extremity ischemia, 234
Aneurysmorrhaphy
  of carotid artery, 55f, 56
  of renal artery, 152–153
Angina, unstable, perioperative risks with, 2, 3f
Angiogenesis, gene-induced, for critical limb ischemia, 164
Angiography
  aortic arch, for evaluating cerebrovascular symptoms, 23f, 24
  carotid. See Carotid arteriography.
  cerebral
    for carotid fibromuscular dysplasia, 62
    for ipsilateral stroke, 32
  for aortic dissection, 128
  for aortic graft infection, 186, 187f
  for aortic graft limb thrombosis, 180, 181f, 182, 184
  for aortoenteric fistula, 112, 113f
  for aortoiliac occlusive disease, 176
  for aortovenous fistula, 108, 109f
  for atheroembolism, 173, 173f
  for carotid plus coronary disease, 84, 85f
  for congenital vascular malformations, 351, 351f, 352
  for critical limb ischemia, 162, 163f, 169f
  for diabetic foot infections, 213f, 216

375

Angiography *(Continued)*
    for endovascular abdominal aortic aneurysm repair, 124
    for erectile dysfunction, 347f, 348
    for femoral artery pseudoaneurysm, 143f
    for heparin-induced thrombosis, 370, 371f
    for iliac artery aneurysm, 132, 133f, 134
    for infrainguinal graft surveillance, 198, 199f, 200, 202
    for infrainguinal graft thrombosis, 204, 205f
    for infrainguinal occlusive disease, 192, 193f
    for infrainguinal prosthetic graft infection, 208, 209f
    for lymphedema, 313f, 314, 316
    for mesenteric ischemia
        acute, 250, 251f, 252, 254
        chronic, 256, 257f
    for popliteal artery aneurysm, 146, 147f, 148
    for popliteal artery disease, 228, 229f, 230
    for Raynaud's syndrome, 342, 343f, 344
    for renovascular occlusive disease, 238, 238t, 239f
    for subclavian artery occlusive disease, 76, 77f
    for Takayasu's disease, 360, 361f
    for thoracoabdominal aortic aneurysm, 99f, 100
    for upper extremity ischemia, 232, 233f
    for vascular trauma
        abdominal, 324–325, 325f
        brachiocephalic, 318, 319f, 320, 322
        extremity, 332, 333, 333f
    image-enhanced. *See* Computed tomography angiography; Magnetic resonance angiography.
    pulmonary, for pulmonary embolism, 286, 287f
    renal
        for aneurysm, 152
        for carotid fibromuscular dysplasia, 62
        stenosis correlation with duplex scan, 202
    vertebral, for carotid artery aneurysm, 55, 55f
Angioneurotic edema, heparin-induced, 372, 373f
Angioplasty. *See also specific type.*
    for abdominal vascular trauma, 326, 326f
    for erectile dysfunction, 347f, 348
    for hemodialysis vascular access, 358, 359f
Angioscopy, for aortic graft limb thrombosis, 182
Ankle-brachial index (ABI)
    in asymptomatic carotid artery stenosis, 34
    in critical limb ischemia, 162, 163f
    in extremity vascular trauma, 332, 333f
    in infrainguinal graft surveillance, 199f, 200, 202
    in popliteal artery aneurysm, 146, 147f, 148
Antibiotics
    for aortic graft infection, 186
    for carotid artery aneurysm, 55, 55f
    for deep vein insufficiency, 294, 295f
    for diabetic foot infections, 212, 213f, 214
    for femoral artery aneurysm, 140
    for femoral artery pseudoaneurysm, 143, 143f
    for heparin-induced skin necrosis, 372, 373f
    for infrainguinal prosthetic graft infection, 208, 209f
    for sigmoid ischemia, 118
    for superficial phlebitis, 268, 269, 269f
    for wet gangrene of foot, 218, 219f

Anticoagulation therapy
    alternative, with heparin-induced complications, 370, 371f, 372, 373f
    contraindications to, 18
    for acute limb ischemia, 169f, 170
    for acute mesenteric ischemia, 251f, 252
    for acute stroke, 50–52, 51f
    for carotid artery dissection, 58, 59f, 60
    for carotid artery stenosis, 29f, 32
        recurrent, 45f, 46, 48
    for deep vein thrombosis
        iliofemoral, 282, 283f
        lower extremity, 272, 273f, 274, 276, 278
    for extracranial cerebrovascular disease, 23f, 24
    for hypercoagulable syndrome, 9f, 10
    for infrainguinal graft thrombosis, 204, 205f, 206
    for pulmonary embolism, 286–288, 287f
    for ruptured abdominal aortic aneurysm, 106
    for subclavian-axillary venous thrombosis, 262, 263f, 264, 266
    for superficial phlebitis, 269, 269f
    for vertebral artery disease, 74, 75f
    hematologic disorders with, 14, 370, 371f
    in infrainguinal graft surveillance, 198, 199f, 200
    reversal agents for, 14, 18
    routine intraoperative. *See* Heparin.
Antihistamines, for heparin-induced reactions, 372, 373f
Antihypertensive therapy, for aortic dissection, 128, 129f, 130
Anti-inflammatory agents
    for post-traumatic pain syndrome, 337
    for superficial phlebitis, 269
Antiphospholipid syndrome, 8, 10
Antiplatelet therapy
    for atheroembolism, 172, 173f, 174
    for carotid artery dissection, 58, 59f, 60
    for carotid artery stenosis
        asymptomatic, 34
        recurrent, 45f, 46, 48
        symptomatic, 28, 32
    for carotid fibromuscular dysplasia, 62, 63f
    for carotid plus coronary disease, 84, 85f
    for vertebral artery disease, 74, 75f
    hematologic disorders with, 14
    in infrainguinal graft surveillance, 198, 200
Antithrombin, for heparin-induced thrombosis, 370, 371f
Aorta
    atheroembolism from, 173, 173f, 174
    distal, in aortoiliac occlusive disease, 177f, 178
    in renovascular occlusive disease treatment
        adult fibrodysplastic, 244, 245f
        arteriosclerotic, 246, 247f
    in Takayasu's disease, 362, 363
    infrarenal
        abdominal aneurysm of, 91f, 94
        penetrating injuries of, 326f, 327
    injuries of
        with abdominal vascular trauma, 326–327, 326f, 328

Aorta *(Continued)*
    with brachiocephalic vascular trauma, 319f, 320
    reimplantation of, for pediatric renovascular occlusive disease, 242, 243f
    supraceliac
        in ruptured abdominal aortic aneurysm repair, 105–106
        penetrating injuries of, 326, 326f
    suprarenal
        abdominal aneurysm of, 91f, 94
        atheroemboli of, 174
        penetrating injuries of, 326–327, 326f
Aorta to left renal vein fistula (ALRVF), 108–110, 109f
Aorta–innominate artery bypass, for brachiocephalic artery occlusive disease, 81–82, 81f
Aortic arch
    arteriography of, for evaluating cerebrovascular symptoms, 23f, 24
    in acute stroke, 51, 51f
    in subclavian artery occlusive disease, 78
    in Takayasu's disease, 362
    injuries of, with brachiocephalic vascular trauma, 320
Aortic bypass, multilimb, for brachiocephalic artery occlusive disease, 81f, 82
Aortic clamping
    in chronic mesenteric ischemia repair, 258
    in ruptured abdominal aortic aneurysm repair, 105–106, 105f
    sequential, in thoracoabdominal aortic aneurysm repair, 99f, 100, 102
Aortic dissection, 128, 129f, 130
    subclavian artery occlusive disease *vs.,* 77f
Aortic endarterectomy, for aortoiliac occlusive disease, 177f, 178
Aortic grafts
    for chronic mesenteric ischemia, 258
    infection of, 186, 187f, 188, 190
    limb thrombosis with, 180, 181f, 182, 184
Aortic neck, diameter of, in endovascular abdominal aortic aneurysm repair, 120, 122, 124
Aortic stenosis, perioperative risks with, 2, 3f
Aortic stump blow-out, with graft infection, 190
Aortobifemoral bypass
    for aortoiliac occlusive disease, 177f, 178
    for critical limb ischemia, 163f, 164
Aortocaval fistula, with abdominal aortic aneurysm, 108–111, 109f
Aortoenteric fistula, secondary to aortic reconstruction, 112, 113f, 114, 116
Aortofemoral grafting
    in ruptured abdominal aortic aneurysm repair, 106
    infection of, 186, 188
    limb thrombosis from, 180, 181f, 184
Aortoiliac grafting
    for chronic mesenteric ischemia, 257, 257f, 258
    in ruptured abdominal aortic aneurysm repair, 106
Aortoiliac occlusive disease, 176, 177f, 178
    in critical limb ischemia, 164
    in erectile dysfunction, 348

Aortoiliac occlusive disease *(Continued)*
  in leg pain while walking, 157f, 158
  in renovascular occlusive disease, 246, 247f
Aortorenal bypass, for renovascular occlusive disease
  adult fibrodysplastic, 244, 254f
  arteriosclerotic, 246, 247
  pediatric, 242, 243f
Aortorenal endarterectomy, for renovascular occlusive disease, 246, 247f, 248
Aortovenous fistula, with abdominal aortic aneurysm, 108–110, 109f
Apligraf, for deep vein insufficiency, 296
Aprotinin, for intraoperative hemorrhage, 365f, 366
aPTT. *See* Activated partial thromboplastin time (aPTT).
Arm. *See* Upper extremity.
Arrhythmia, atrial, with acute stroke, 50–51, 52
Arterial occlusive disease
  brachiocephalic, 24, 80–82, 81f
  carotid. *See* Carotid artery occlusive disease.
  distal *vs.* proximal, in upper extremity ischemia, 232, 233f, 234
  in critical limb ischemia, 162, 163f, 164
  in endovascular abdominal aortic aneurysm repair, 122
  in leg pain while walking, 156, 157f, 158
  infrainguinal, 192–194, 193f
    in leg pain while walking, 157f, 158
  peripheral, amputation level in, 218
  popliteal artery, with entrapment syndrome, 230, 231f
  renal. *See* Renovascular occlusive disease.
  small vessel, in erectile dysfunction, 348
  subclavian, 76–78, 77f
Arteriography. *See* Angiography.
Arteriovenous fistula (AVF)
  as hemodialysis vascular access, 354, 355–356, 355f
    failed, 354, 355–356, 355f
  congenital venous malformation as, 350–352, 351f
  in femoral artery pseudoaneurysm, 142, 143f
  in iliac vein obstruction, 299f, 301, 302
  in iliofemoral deep vein thrombosis, 284
  in infrainguinal graft surveillance, 194, 198, 200
  in infrainguinal graft thrombosis, 205f, 206
Arteriovenous malformations (AVM)
  congenital, 350, 351f, 352
  screening tests for, 350
Artery(ies). *See also* named artery, e.g., Carotid artery(ies).
  anomalies of, 351f, 352
Aspirin
  for acute stroke, 50, 51f
  for atheroembolism, 172
  for carotid artery dissection, 58, 59f, 60
  for carotid artery stenosis, 28, 29f, 34, 46
  for carotid fibromuscular dysplasia, 62
  in infrainguinal graft surveillance, 198, 200
Atheroembolism, 172–174, 173f
  in aneurysm repair, 96, 174
  in brachiocephalic artery occlusive disease, 80, 81f
  with carotid artery stenosis, 28, 29f, 32

Atherosclerosis
  in critical limb ischemia, 162, 163f
  in popliteal artery disease, 228, 229f, 230, 231f
  in renovascular occlusive disease, 246, 247f, 248
  leg pain while walking from, 156, 157f, 158
Atrial fibrillation, acute stroke from, 50–52
Atriofemoral bypass (AFBP), in thoracoabdominal aortic aneurysm repair, 99f, 100, 102
Autogenous fistula, as hemodialysis vascular access, 354, 355–356, 355f
  failed, 354, 355–356, 355f
Autoimmune disorders
  carotid artery stenosis with, 28
  transfusions and, 14
Autologous blood transfusions, preoperative *vs.* intraoperative, 15f, 16
Autotransfusion, with abdominal aortic aneurysm repair, 91f, 96
  ruptured, 104
AVF. *See* Arteriovenous fistula (AVF).
AVM (arteriovenous malformations), congenital, 350, 351f, 352
Axillary vein valve transplant, for deep vein insufficiency, 300
Axilloaxillary artery bypass
  for brachiocephalic artery occlusive disease, 82
  for subclavian artery occlusive disease, 77–78, 77f
Axillobifemoral bypass
  for aortic dissection, 130
  for aortic graft infection, 190
  for aortoenteric fistula, 114, 116
  for aortoiliac occlusive disease, 177f, 178
  for atheroembolism, 174

Baclofen, for post-traumatic pain syndrome, 337
Bacterial infections
  carotid artery aneurysm from, 54–55
  femoral artery aneurysm from, 140, 143
  in diabetic foot infections, 216
  in superficial phlebitis, 268
  of aortic grafts, 186, 187f, 188
  of infrainguinal prosthetic graft, 208, 209, 209f, 210
Balloon angioplasty
  open, for carotid fibromuscular dysplasia, 63, 63f
  percutaneous. *See* Percutaneous transluminal angioplasty (PTA).
Balloon dilatation, of hemodialysis vascular access, 358, 359f
Balloon tamponade
  for esophageal varices, from portal hypertension, 306, 307f
  for vascular trauma
    abdominal, 325, 325f, 328, 329, 329f
    brachiocephalic, 320
Behavioral therapy, for Raynaud's syndrome, 342
Below-knee amputation (BKA), 218, 219f, 220
Beta-blockers
  for aortic dissection, 128, 130

Beta-blockers *(Continued)*
  for portal hypertension, 309
Bile resin-binding agents, for hyperlipidemia, 6, 7f
Biopsy(ies), staging, of carotid body tumors, 66, 67f
Birthmark, as congenital venous malformation, 350, 351f
BKA (below-knee amputation), 218, 219f, 220
Bleeding. *See* Hemorrhage.
Blood glucose control
  in diabetic foot infections, 212
  in erectile dysfunction, 346, 347f
  with wet gangrene, 218
Blood pressure
  elevated. *See* Hypertension.
  in Takayasu's disease, 362
  segmental. *See* Segmental limb pressures.
  unequal arm, in subclavian arterial occlusive disease, 76, 77f
Blood transfusions. *See also* Autotransfusion.
  allogeneic, risks with, 16
  autologous, preoperative *vs.* intraoperative, 15f, 16
  strategies for, 14, 15f, 16, 18
Blood type and screen, 15f, 16
Blue toe syndrome, 136, 172
Blunt trauma
  abdominal vascular, 324–325, 325f, 327
  extremity vascular, 333, 333f, 334
Bone injuries
  with abdominal vascular trauma, 328f
  with extremity vascular trauma, 332, 333, 333f, 334
Bone scans
  for diabetic foot infections, 213f, 214
  for post-traumatic pain syndrome, 336, 337f
Bowel evisceration, with abdominal vascular trauma, 326, 326f, 327f, 328, 329
Bowel resection, for acute mesenteric ischemia, 250, 251f, 254
Bowel viability
  in acute mesenteric ischemia, 251f, 252, 254
  in ruptured abdominal aortic aneurysm repair, 105f, 106, 118, 119f
Brachiocephalic artery occlusive disease, 80–82, 81f
  cerebrovascular symptoms of, 24, 80
Brachiocephalic artery reconstruction, in occlusive disease, 80, 81f
Brachiocephalic vascular trauma, 318, 319f, 320, 322
Bridging graft, prosthetic, for hemodialysis vascular access, 354, 355f, 356
  failed, 358, 359f

Calcium channel blockers, 240, 342
Calcium levels, with intraoperative hemorrhage, 365f, 366, 368
Calf vein thrombosis, isolated, 273f, 274, 278
Captopril renography, for renovascular occlusive disease, 239f, 240, 240t
Carbamazepine, for post-traumatic pain syndrome, 337

Carbon dioxide angiography, for renovascular occlusive disease, 238, 238t
Cardiac catheterization
  for preoperative cardiac risk assessment, 2, 3f, 4
  in perioperative care, 12, 13f
Cardiac rhythm, disturbances of, with acute stroke, 50–51, 52
Cardiac risk assessment
  in diabetic foot infections, 212
  preoperative, 2–4, 3f, 12
    for abdominal aortic aneurysm, 92, 92f, 92t
    for thoracoabdominal aortic aneurysm, 98, 99f, 102
    with carotid plus coronary disease, 84, 85f
Cardiology consultation
  for evaluating cerebrovascular symptoms, 23f, 24
  for preoperative risk assessment, 3f, 4
Carotid arteriography
  for carotid artery aneurysm, 55, 55f
  for carotid artery dissection, 58, 59f
  for carotid body tumors, 66, 67f, 68
  for carotid fibromuscular dysplasia, 62, 63f
  for evaluating cerebrovascular symptoms, 23f, 24
  for stenosis diagnosis, 28, 29f
    asymptomatic, 34–36, 35f
    recurrent after endarterectomy, 44, 45f, 46, 48
    symptomatic, 28, 29f
  for stroke following carotid endarterectomy, 70, 71f, 72
  risks of, 23f, 24
Carotid artery(ies)
  bifurcation disease of
    angioplasty risks with, 30
    carotid artery aneurysms as, 56
    evaluating symptoms of, 22, 23f, 24, 74
  common. See Common carotid artery.
  external. See External carotid artery.
  fibromuscular dysplasia of, 62–64, 63f
    dissections with, 58
  in Takayasu's disease, 362
  injuries of, with brachiocephalic vascular trauma, 319f, 320, 322
  internal. See Internal carotid artery.
  ultrasonography of
    advantages of, 22, 23f, 24
    for acute stroke, 50–52, 51f
    for aneurysm, 54, 55f
    for asymptomatic stenosis diagnosis, 34–36, 35f
    for carotid body tumors, 66, 67f, 68
    for dissection, 58, 59f
    for fibromuscular dysplasia, 62, 63f
    for postoperative surveillance, 44, 45f, 48
    for stroke following carotid endarterectomy, 70, 71f
    for symptomatic stenosis diagnosis, 28, 29f, 30
Carotid artery aneurysm, 54–56, 55f
  extracranial, 54–56, 55f, 64
  intracranial, 63f, 64
  with dissections, 59f, 60
  with fibromuscular dysplasia, 63f, 64
Carotid artery dissection, 58, 59f, 60

Carotid artery occlusive disease
  acute, stroke vs., 51f, 52
  plus coronary disease, 84, 85f, 86
  progressive, from stenosis, 29f, 30, 32
  vertebral artery disease with, 74, 75f
Carotid artery reconstruction
  for brachiocephalic artery occlusive disease, 80, 81f, 82
  for carotid artery dissection, 59f, 60
  with carotid body tumors, 67–69, 67f
  with endarterectomy, 39f, 40, 42
Carotid artery stenosis
  acute stroke from, 50–52, 51f
  asymptomatic, 34–36, 35f
    after endarterectomy, 44, 45f
  plus coronary disease, 84, 85f, 86
  progression to occlusion, 29f, 30, 32
  recurrent, 44, 45f, 46, 48
    after endarterectomy, 38, 40, 44, 45f
  symptomatic, 28, 29f, 30, 32
Carotid body tumors, 66–69, 67f
Carotid endarterectomy
  eversion vs. inversion, 38, 39f, 40
  for acute stroke, 51–52, 51f
  for carotid artery stenosis, 38, 39f, 40, 42
    asymptomatic, 34–36, 35f
    recurrent, 44, 45f, 46, 48
    symptomatic, 28, 29f, 30
  for carotid plus coronary disease, 84, 85f, 86
  for subclavian artery occlusive disease, 77, 77f
  stroke following, 70, 71f, 72
  without arteriography, guidelines for, 23f, 24
Carotid shunting, for carotid endarterectomy, 38, 39f
Carotid territory symptoms
  of extracranial cerebrovascular disease, 22, 23f, 24
  with acute stroke, 50–52, 51f
Carotid-carotid bypass, for brachiocephalic artery occlusive disease, 81f, 82
Carotid-subclavian bypass
  for brachiocephalic artery occlusive disease, 81f, 82
  for subclavian artery occlusive disease, 76, 77f, 78
Catheter-induced phlebitis, 268, 269f
Catheter-induced thrombosis, of subclavian-axillary vein, 262, 263f
Causalgia, 336, 337f
Caval thrombus, free-floating, in iliofemoral deep vein thrombosis, 282, 283f
Cavernosography, for erectile dysfunction, 347f, 348
CEAP classification system, for deep vein insufficiency, 294, 295f
Celiac artery(ies)
  in abdominal vascular trauma, 326
  in mesenteric ischemia, 250, 256, 258
Celiac vein, in subclavian-axillary vein thrombosis, 266
Celiotomy, for aortoenteric fistula, 113f, 114
Cellular scanning. See Radioactive cellular scanning.
Cellulitis, with diabetic foot infections, 212, 213f, 214
Central venous catheter, indwelling
  as hemodialysis vascular access, 354–355, 355f, 356

Central venous catheter (Continued)
  occlusion of, 358, 359f
  complications with, 262, 263f, 268, 269f
Central venous stenosis, in hemodialysis vascular access, 354, 355f
  treatment of, 358, 359f
Cerebral arteriography
  for carotid fibromuscular dysplasia, 62
  for ipsilateral stroke, 32
Cerebral ischemia. See Stroke, acute ischemic; Transient ischemic attack (TIA).
Cerebrovascular disease. See also Neurologic deficits.
  carotid artery stenosis in, 28, 29f, 30
  evaluating symptoms of, 22, 23f, 24
  in Takayasu's disease, 361f, 362
  with carotid fibromuscular dysplasia, 62, 63f
Cervical rib
  in neurogenic thoracic outlet syndrome, 340, 341f
  in Raynaud's syndrome, 342, 344
Charles procedure, for lymphedema, 314
Chest radiographs, for vascular trauma
  abdominal, 324, 325f
  brachiocephalic, 318, 319f
Chest tubes, for brachiocephalic vascular trauma, 319f, 320, 322
Chest wounds, brachiocephalic vascular trauma with, 318, 319f
Child-Pugh classification, of portal hypertension, 307f, 308, 310
Cholesterol, management of, 6, 7f
Cilostazol, for leg pain while walking, 158
Circulation
  in compartment syndromes, 222, 223f, 224
  in diabetic foot infections, 213f, 216
"Clamp and sew" techniques, for thoracoabdominal aortic aneurysm, 99f, 100, 102, 130
Claudication
  arteriogenic
    diagnosis of, 156, 157f, 158
    management of, 157f, 158
    neurogenic vs., 156
    Rose criteria for, 156, 157f
    with infrainguinal disease, 192, 204, 205f
  with compartment syndrome, 222, 224, 226
  with iliac vein obstruction, 302
  with popliteal artery entrapment syndrome, 228, 229f
  with Takayasu's disease, 361f, 362
CLI. See Critical limb ischemia (CLI).
Clindamycin, for diabetic foot infections, 212
Clopidogrel
  for atheroembolism, 172
  for carotid artery stenosis, 28, 34, 46
Coagulation studies
  for hypercoagulable syndrome, 8, 9f
  for transfusion strategies, 14, 15f, 18
Coagulopathy, intraoperative, 364, 365f, 366, 368
Collateral circulation, cerebral, with internal carotid artery occlusion, 32

Colon, in ruptured abdominal aortic aneurysm, 105f, 106, 118, 119f
Colonoscopy, for sigmoid ischemia, 118–119, 119f
Colostomy, for sigmoid ischemia, 118
Common carotid artery
  in brachiocephalic occlusive disease, 80–82, 81f
  in carotid body tumor resection, 67f, 68
  in carotid endarterectomy, 39f, 40, 42
  ultrasound surveillance of, 22, 23f, 24
  vertebral artery transposition to, 74
Compartment syndromes
  acute vs. chronic, 222, 223f
  management of, 223f, 224, 226
  pressure measurements in, 222, 223f, 224, 226
  with extremity vascular trauma, 333
  with iliofemoral deep vein thrombosis, 283f, 284
Complete blood count, for hypercoagulable syndrome, 8, 9f
Completion iliofemoral phlebography, for iliofemoral deep vein thrombosis, 282, 284
Complex regional pain syndrome (CRPS), 336, 337f
Composite vein grafts, for infrainguinal occlusive disease, 193f, 194
Compression pump therapy, intermittent, for lymphedema, 313f, 314
Compression stockings
  for congenital venous malformation, 351f, 352
  for deep vein insufficiency, 295, 295f
  for deep vein thrombosis
    iliofemoral, 282, 283f
    lower extremity, 273f, 278
  for lymphedema, 313f, 314
  for varicose veins, 290, 291f, 292
Compression syndromes
  with femoral artery aneurysm, 136, 138
  with iliac artery aneurysm, 133
Compression therapy
  for abdominal vascular trauma, 328, 329f, 330
  for congenital venous malformation, 351f, 352
  for deep vein insufficiency, 295, 295f, 296
  for iliofemoral deep vein thrombosis, 282, 283f
  ultrasound-guided
    for femoral artery aneurysm, 138
    for femoral artery pseudoaneurysm, 142–143, 143f
Computed tomography
  for evaluating cerebrovascular symptoms, 22, 23f, 24, 28
  of abdominal aortic aneurysm, 90, 91f, 94, 96
    in endovascular repair, 120, 121f, 122–123, 124, 125
    ruptured, 104, 105f
  of acute mesenteric ischemia, 250, 251f, 252
  of acute stroke, 50, 51f
  of aortic dissection, 128
  of aortic graft infection, 186, 187f
  of aortoenteric fistula, 112, 113f
  of aortovenous fistula, 108, 109, 109f
  of atheroembolism, 173–174, 173f
  of carotid artery aneurysm, 54, 55f
  of carotid artery dissection, 58, 59f
  of carotid artery stenosis, asymptomatic, 36

Computed tomography (Continued)
  of carotid body tumors, 66, 67, 67f, 68
  of compartment syndromes, 224
  of femoral artery aneurysm, 136
  of hepatic artery aneurysm, 150
  of iliac artery aneurysm, 132, 133f, 134
  of infrainguinal occlusive disease, 192, 193f
  of infrainguinal prosthetic graft infection, 208, 209f
  of lymphedema, 313f, 314
  of popliteal artery aneurysm, 146, 147f, 148
  of popliteal artery disease, 228, 229f
  of pulmonary embolism, 286, 287f
  of renal artery aneurysm, 152
  of renovascular occlusive disease, 238, 238t
  of stroke following carotid endarterectomy, 70, 71f, 72
  of thoracoabdominal aortic aneurysm, 98, 99f, 100
  of vascular trauma
    abdominal, 324, 325, 325f
    brachiocephalic, 318, 319f, 320
Computed tomography angiography
  of carotid body tumors, 67f, 68
  of carotid fibromuscular dysplasia, 62
  of endovascular abdominal aortic aneurysm repair, 120, 121f, 122–123
Congenital lymphedema, familial, 312
Congenital venous malformation(s) (CVM), 350–352, 351f
  Hamburg classification of, 350–351, 351f
  hemangioma vs., 350, 351f
  varicosities with, 290, 350, 351f
Congestive heart failure, perioperative risks with, 2, 3f
Connective tissue disease, in Raynaud's syndrome, 342
Contralateral stroke, with carotid artery stenosis, 30, 35–36, 35f
Coronary artery bypass grafting
  in carotid plus coronary disease, 84, 85f, 86
  in subclavian artery occlusive disease, 76, 77f, 78
  perioperative vascular surgery risks with, 2, 3f
  vertebral artery disease with, 74, 75f
Coronary artery disease
  carotid stenosis plus, 84, 85f, 86
  clinical markers for, 84, 85f
  perioperative risks with, 2–4, 3f, 12
Coronary steal syndrome, with subclavian artery occlusive disease, 76, 77f, 78
Cranial nerves, in carotid body tumors, 66, 67f
  resection cautions with, 68–69
Crawford classification, of thoracoabdominal aortic aneurysms, 98
Critical limb ischemia (CLI)
  acute, 168–170, 169f
  amputation level and, 218, 219f, 220
  chronic, 162, 163f, 164
  leg pain while walking vs., 156, 157f
  with aortic graft limb thrombosis, 180, 181f
  with femoral artery aneurysm, 136, 137
  with infrainguinal graft thrombosis, 204, 205f
  with infrainguinal prosthetic graft infection, 208
  with popliteal artery aneurysm, 147f, 148

Critical limb ischemia (CLI) (Continued)
  with ruptured abdominal aortic aneurysm, 105f, 106
Cross-femoral graft, for iliac vein obstruction, 299f, 302
Crossmatching, for transfusions, 15f, 16
CRPS (complex regional pain syndrome), 336, 337f
Crush injuries, pelvic, with abdominal vascular trauma, 328–329
Cryoamputation, dry-ice, 218, 219f
Cryoprecipitate transfusions
  for intraoperative hemorrhage, 365f, 366, 368
  guidelines for, 14, 16
Culture(s)
  of heparin-induced skin necrosis, 372, 373f
  of infrainguinal prosthetic graft infection, 208, 209f
CVM. See Congenital venous malformation(s) (CVM).
Cyclophosphamide, for Takayasu's disease, 360
Cystectomy, for popliteal artery disease, 230, 231f
Cytotoxic agents, for Takayasu's disease, 360, 361f

Danaparoid, for lower extremity deep vein thrombosis, 278
DDAVP (desmopressin acetate), for intraoperative hemorrhage, 364, 365f, 366
Débridement
  for extremity vascular trauma, 333f, 334
  of diabetic foot infections, 213f, 214, 216
  of infrainguinal prosthetic graft, 208, 209f, 210
  of ulcers, with deep vein insufficiency, 294, 295f
  of wet gangrene of foot, 218, 219f
Debulking procedures, for lymphedema, 313f, 314
Decompression
  portosystemic, for portal hypertension, 306, 307, 307f, 308–310
  surgical. See Fasciotomy.
Deep vein insufficiency
  conservative management of, 295–296, 295f
  evaluation of, 294–295, 295f
  lymphedema vs., 294, 295f
  surgical treatment of, 298–302, 299f
Deep vein obstruction, as congenital venous malformation, 351f, 352
Deep vein thrombosis (DVT)
  hypercoagulable syndrome with, 8, 9f, 10
  iliofemoral, 282, 283f, 284
  of hemodialysis vascular access, 358, 359f
  of leg. See Lower extremity.
  varicose veins from, 290
Deep venous reconstruction
  for deep vein insufficiency, 298–302, 299f
  for varicose veins, 291f, 292
Dermatitis, stasis, with deep vein insufficiency, 294, 295f, 296
Desmopressin acetate (DDAVP), for intraoperative hemorrhage, 364, 365f, 366
Diabetes mellitus
  arteriosclerotic renovascular occlusive disease with, 246, 247f

Diabetes mellitus *(Continued)*
  erectile dysfunction and, 346, 348
  foot infections with, 212, 213f, 214, 216
  hyperlipidemia management in, 6, 7f
  leg pain while walking due to, 156, 157f, 158
  perioperative risks with, 2, 3f
Diaphragm, in abdominal vascular trauma, 326
DIC (disseminated intravascular coagulation), intraoperative, 364, 366
Diet therapy, for hyperlipidemia, 6, 7f
Digital artery occlusion, 342, 343f, 344
Digital ischemia, 342, 343f, 344
Dilatation, open, for carotid fibromuscular dysplasia, 62–63, 63f
D-Dimer tests, serial, for lower extremity deep vein thrombosis, 272, 273f, 278–279
Dipyridamole thallium stress testing, for carotid plus coronary disease, 84
Directed donation, transfusion-associated risks with, 16
Disability, with neurogenic thoracic outlet syndrome, 341, 341f
Disseminated intravascular coagulation (DIC), intraoperative, 364, 366
Diuretics, for renovascular occlusive disease, 240
Dobutamine echocardiography, for preoperative cardiac risk assessment, 3, 4
Doppler studies
  of acute limb ischemia, 168, 169f
  of acute mesenteric ischemia, 250, 251f, 252
  of amputation level, 218, 219f, 220
  of atheroembolism, 172, 173
  of carotid artery dissection, 58
  of carotid endarterectomy, 40
    with postoperative stroke, 70, 71f
  of congenital venous malformation, 350
  of endovascular abdominal aortic aneurysm repair, 124
  of erectile dysfunction, 347f, 348
  of extremity vascular trauma, 332, 333f
  of femoral artery pseudoaneurysm, 142, 143f
  of infrainguinal graft surveillance, 200
  of leg pain while walking, 156, 157f, 158
  of popliteal artery disease, 228, 229f
  of upper extremity ischemia, 232, 233f
  of varicose veins, 290, 291, 291f
  of vertebral artery, with acute stroke, 51f, 52
Drains, surgical, for carotid endarterectomy, 39f, 42
Duplex ultrasonography
  of aortic graft limb thrombosis, 180, 181f
  of aortoiliac occlusive disease, 176, 178
  of aortovenous fistula, 108, 109f
  of atheroembolism, 173, 173f
  of carotid artery. *See* Carotid artery(ies).
  of compartment syndromes, 224
  of congenital venous malformation, 350, 351f, 352
  of deep vein insufficiency, 295, 295f, 300
  of endovascular abdominal aortic aneurysm repair, 123, 124–125
  of femoral artery aneurysm, 138

Duplex ultrasonography *(Continued)*
  of femoral artery pseudoaneurysm, 142, 143, 143f
  of hemodialysis vascular access
    failed, 358, 359, 359f
    new, 354, 355, 355f, 356
  of infrainguinal graft surveillance, 198, 199f, 200, 202
  of infrainguinal graft thrombosis, 204, 205f, 206
  of infrainguinal occlusive disease, 192, 193f
  of lower extremity deep vein thrombosis, 272, 273f, 274, 278, 280
  of lymphedema, 312, 313f
  of mesenteric ischemia, 252, 256, 257f, 259
  of popliteal artery aneurysm, 146, 147f, 148
  of popliteal artery disease, 228, 229f, 230
  of renovascular occlusive disease, 238, 238t, 239f
  of stroke
    acute ischemic, 50–52, 51f
    following carotid endarterectomy, 70, 71f
  of subclavian artery occlusive disease, 76
  of subclavian-axillary venous thrombosis, 262, 263f
  of superficial phlebitis, 269, 269f
  of varicose veins, 290, 291f
  of vascular trauma
    brachiocephalic, 318, 319f
    extremity, 332, 333, 333f
  stenosis correlation with arteriography, 202
  surveillance
    of asymptomatic carotid artery stenosis, 34–36, 35f
    of extracranial cerebrovascular disease, 22, 23f, 24
  with flow imaging. *See* Doppler studies.
DVT. *See* Deep vein thrombosis (DVT).

Echocardiography
  dobutamine, for preoperative cardiac risk assessment, 3, 4
  for acute stroke, 51–52, 51f
  for brachiocephalic vascular trauma, 320
  stress, for carotid plus coronary disease, 84
  transesophageal, 23f, 24, 128, 286, 287f
ECLT (euglobulin clot lysis time), 364, 365f, 366
Edema
  cerebral, 50, 51f, 52
  venous, in lymphedema, 312, 313f
  with aortovenous fistula, 108, 109f
  with compartment syndrome, 222, 224, 226
  with deep vein insufficiency, 294, 295f
  with iliofemoral deep vein thrombosis, 282, 283f
  with lower extremity deep vein thrombosis, 272, 274
  with post-traumatic pain syndrome, 336
  with subclavian-axillary vein thrombosis, 262, 263f
  with varicose veins, 290, 291, 291f
EDV (end-diastolic velocity), in chronic mesenteric ischemia, 256
"Effort thrombosis," in subclavian-axillary venous thrombosis, 262, 263f
EGD (esophagogastroduodenoscopy), for portal hypertension, 306

Electrocardiogram
  for brachiocephalic vascular trauma, 319f, 320
  for ruptured abdominal aortic aneurysm, 104, 105f
Electromyogram
  for compartment syndromes, 224
  for neurogenic thoracic outlet syndrome, 340, 341f
ELISA (enzyme-linked immunosorbent assay), 272, 286, 287f, 370
Embolectomy
  for acute mesenteric ischemia, 251f, 252
  for aortic graft limb thrombosis, 180, 181f
  for pulmonary embolism, 286–288, 287f
  for subclavian artery occlusive disease, 76, 77f
  for upper extremity ischemia, 233f, 234
Emboli. *See also specific type.*
  acute stroke from, 50–51, 51f
  in abdominal aortic aneurysm, 90, 96
  in acute limb ischemia, 168–170, 169f
  in acute mesenteric ischemia, 250, 251f, 252
  in aortovenous fistula repair, 110
  in carotid artery stenosis, 28, 29f, 32
    recurrent, 48
  in extracranial cerebrovascular disease, 23f, 24
  in hypercoagulable syndrome, 8, 9f, 10
  in renal artery aneurysm, 152, 153f
  in stroke following carotid endarterectomy, 70, 71f
  in subclavian artery occlusive disease, 76, 77f
  in transient ischemic attacks, 74, 75f
  in upper extremity ischemia, 233f, 234
Embolization
  for iliac artery aneurysm, 133–134, 133f
  for vascular trauma
    abdominal, 324–325, 325f, 328, 328f
    extremity, 332, 333f
  preoperative, for carotid body tumors, 67f, 68
Embolotherapy, for congenital vascular malformations, 351, 351f
Encephalopathy, with portal hypertension, 308, 310
Endarterectomy
  aortic, for aortoiliac occlusive disease, 177f, 178
  aortorenal, for renovascular occlusive disease, 246, 247f, 248
  carotid. *See* Carotid endarterectomy.
  for aortic graft limb thrombosis, 182
  for atheroembolism, 174
  for infrainguinal occlusive disease, 194
  for mesenteric ischemia, 251f, 252, 258
  innominate, 80–81, 81f
End-diastolic velocity (EDV), in chronic mesenteric ischemia, 256
Endoscopy
  diagnostic. *See specific type.*
  therapeutic
    for esophageal varices, from portal hypertension, 306, 307f
    for portal hypertension, 309, 309f
Endovascular intervention(s). *See also specific technique.*
  for abdominal aortic aneurysm, 91f, 94, 120–125, 121f

Endovascular intervention(s) *(Continued)*
  for abdominal vascular trauma, 325, 325f, 328, 328f, 329, 329f
  for acute limb ischemia, 168, 169f, 170
  for aortic dissection, 128, 129f
  for aortic graft limb thrombosis, 180, 181f, 182, 184
  for aortoiliac occlusive disease, 176, 177f, 178
  for aortovenous fistula, 110
  for carotid artery aneurysm, 55f, 56
    with dissections, 59f, 60
  for hemodialysis vascular access, 358, 359f
  for hepatic artery aneurysm, 150, 151f
  for iliac artery aneurysm, 133f, 134
  for iliac vein obstruction, 299f, 301, 302
  for renal artery aneurysm, 153
  for renovascular occlusive disease, 239f, 240
  for subclavian artery occlusive disease, 76–77, 77f
  learning curve for systems of, 124
Endpoint management techniques, in carotid endarterectomy, 38, 39f, 40
Enoxaparin, for heparin-induced thrombosis, 370, 371f
Entrapment syndrome(s)
  of nerves, post-traumatic, 336–337, 337f
  of popliteal artery, 228, 229f, 230, 231f
Enzyme-linked immunosorbent assay (ELISA), 272, 286, 287f, 370
Eosinophilia, heparin-induced, 372, 373f
Epidural cooling, in thoracoabdominal aortic aneurysm repair, 99f, 102
Erectile dysfunction, 346, 347f, 348
Esophageal devascularization, for portal hypertension, 307, 307f, 308
Esophageal varices, from portal hypertension, 306–307
Esophagogastroduodenoscopy (EGD), for portal hypertension, 306
Ethanol injections, for congenital vascular malformations, 351–352, 351f
Euglobulin clot lysis time (ECLT), 364, 365f, 366
Evisceration, of small bowel, with abdominal vascular trauma, 326, 326f, 327f, 328, 329
Excision, surgical. *See* Resection, surgical.
Exercise program
  for leg pain while walking, 157f, 158, 160
  for neurogenic thoracic outlet syndrome, 340, 341f
Exercise testing. *See* Stress testing.
Exsanguination, fatal, with abdominal vascular trauma, 328, 329, 330
External carotid artery
  bypass
    for carotid artery aneurysm, 55f, 56
    for carotid artery dissection, 59f, 60
    for internal carotid artery stenosis, 29f, 32
  in carotid body tumor resection, 67f
  in carotid endarterectomy, 39f, 40, 42
External fixation, for extremity vascular trauma, 333–334, 333f
Extra-anatomic bypass grafts
  for abdominal vascular trauma, 326f, 327

Extra-anatomic bypass grafts *(Continued)*
  for aortic graft infection, 187f, 188, 190
  for aortoenteric fistula, 113f, 114, 116
  for brachiocephalic artery occlusive disease, 81f, 82
  for femoral artery aneurysm, 140
  for iliac artery aneurysm, 132, 133f
Extremity vascular trauma, 332–334, 333f

Factor V Leiden, in hypercoagulable syndrome, 8, 10
Familial syndrome(s)
  carotid body tumors as, 66
  hypercoagulation as, 8, 9f, 10
Fasciectomy, for compartment syndromes, 223f, 224, 226
Fasciotomy
  for compartment syndromes, 223f, 224, 226
  for iliofemoral deep vein thrombosis, 283f, 284
  for neurogenic thoracic outlet syndrome, 340, 341f
  for vascular trauma
    abdominal, 327, 329
    extremity, 333, 333f
FDPs. *See* Fibrin degradation products (FDPs).
Fecal contamination, with abdominal vascular trauma, 326, 329
Femoral access, for hemodialysis, 355, 356
Femoral artery(ies)
  in aortic graft infection, 188
  in infrainguinal occlusive disease, 192, 193f, 194
  pressure measurement of, for infrainguinal graft thrombosis, 204, 205f
Femoral artery aneurysm, 136–140, 137f
  from trauma, 136, 137f, 138
  infections with, 137, 137f, 139–140
  lower extremity ischemia with, 136, 137
  true vs. false, 136, 137f
  repair techniques for, 137–140, 137f
Femoral artery pseudoaneurysm
  from trauma, 137f, 138, 142–144, 143f
  hematoma vs., 138, 142, 143f
  infections with, 140, 143, 143f
  repair techniques for, 137–170, 137f, 143f
  true aneurysm vs., 136, 137f
Femoral vein(s)
  in deep vein insufficiency, 299, 299f, 300, 302
  in infrainguinal occlusive disease, 194
  in venous reconstruction, for deep vein insufficiency, 298, 299f, 300
Femorofemoral bypass
  for aortic dissection, 130
  for aortic graft limb thrombosis, 181f, 184
  for aortoiliac occlusive disease, 176, 177f, 178
Femoropopliteal lesion, focal, in infrainguinal occlusive disease, 192, 193f, 194
Femoropopliteal vein(s), for aortic graft infection, 186, 187f, 188
Fetal warfarin syndrome, 276
FFP transfusions. *See* Fresh frozen plasma (FFP) transfusions.

Fibrate agents, for hyperlipidemia, 6
Fibrin degradation products (FDPs)
  in intraoperative hemorrhage, 364, 365f, 366
  in lower extremity deep vein thrombosis, 272, 278–279
  in superficial phlebitis, 268
Fibrinogen, in intraoperative hemorrhage, 364, 365f, 366
Fibrinolysis, primary, in intraoperative hemorrhage, 365f, 366
Fibromuscular dysplasia (FMD), of carotid artery, 62–64, 63f
  dissections with, 58
Fistula(s)
  aorta to left renal vein, 108–110, 109f
  aortoenteric, 112, 113f, 114, 116
  aortovenous, 108–111, 109f
  arteriovenous. *See* Arteriovenous fistula (AVF).
  autogenous fistula, as hemodialysis vascular access, 354, 355–356, 355f
    failed, 354, 355–356, 355f
Fluid resuscitation
  for acute mesenteric ischemia, 250, 251f, 254
  for portal hypertension, 306, 307f
  for pulmonary embolism, 286, 287f
  for ruptured abdominal aortic aneurysm, 104, 105f
  for vascular trauma
    abdominal, 324, 325f, 327f
    brachiocephalic, 318, 319f
Fluphenazine (Prolixin), for post-traumatic pain syndrome, 338
FMD (fibromuscular dysplasia), of carotid artery, 62–64, 63f
  dissections with, 58
Foley catheter, in ruptured abdominal aortic aneurysm repair, 105–106
Foot care, for diabetic foot infections, 213f, 214
Foot infections, with diabetes mellitus, 212, 213f, 214, 216
Forearm, hemodialysis vascular access in, 355–356, 355f
Forefoot amputation, 218, 219f, 220
Fresh frozen plasma (FFP) transfusions
  for intraoperative hemorrhage, 364, 365f, 366, 368
  for ruptured abdominal aortic aneurysm, 104
  guidelines for, 14, 18
Functional capacity, in preoperative assessment of cardiac risk, 2
Fungal infections, carotid artery aneurysm from, 54–56, 55f

Gangrene
  management of, 218, 219f
  with acute mesenteric ischemia, 250, 251f, 254
  with critical limb ischemia, 162, 163f
  with diabetic foot infections, 213f, 214
  with leg pain while walking, 156, 157f
Gastrointestinal bleeding
  with aortoenteric fistula, 112, 113f, 114
  with portal hypertension, 306, 307, 307f
Gemfibrozil, for hyperlipidemia, 6
Gene-induced angiogenesis, for critical limb ischemia, 164
Glycoproteins
  in lower extremity deep vein thrombosis, 278

Glycoproteins *(Continued)*
   in superficial phlebitis, 268
Graft excision
   for aortic graft infection, 186, 187f, 188, 190
   for aortoenteric fistula, 113f, 114, 116
   for femoral artery aneurysm, 140
   for infrainguinal prosthetic graft infection, 208–210, 209f
Graft velocity spectra, in infrainguinal graft surveillance, 198, 199f, 200, 202
Grafts and grafting
   postoperative thrombosis of, hypercoagulable syndrome in, 8, 9f, 11f
   techniques for. *See specific anatomy or pathology.*
Great vessels, injuries of, with brachiocephalic vascular trauma, 319f, 320

HAAbs (heparin-associated antiplatelet antibodies), 370, 371f, 372, 373f
Hamburg classification, of congenital venous malformations, 350–351, 351f
Hand ischemia, 232, 233f
Healing potential. *See also* Salvage procedures.
   in amputation level determination, 218, 219f, 220
   of diabetic foot infections, 213f, 216
   with chronic critical limb ischemia, 162, 163f, 164
Heart. *See* Cardiac entries.
Hemangioma, congenital venous malformation *vs.*, 350, 351f
Hematologic studies
   for hypercoagulable syndrome, 8, 9f, 10
   normal ranges for, 14, 15f
Hematoma(s)
   femoral artery pseudoaneurysm *vs.*, 138, 142, 143f
   with infrainguinal prosthetic graft infection, 208, 209f
   with vascular trauma
      abdominal, 324, 325f–327f, 326–328, 329f
      extremity, 332, 333f
Hematuria, with abdominal vascular trauma, 324, 325f
Hemodialysis, vascular access for, 354–356, 355f
   failed, 358–359, 359f
Hemodynamics
   in acute mesenteric ischemia, 250, 251f, 254
   in infrainguinal prosthetic graft complications, 204, 208, 209f
   in pulmonary embolism, 286–288, 287f
   in ruptured abdominal aortic aneurysm, 104, 105f
   in transient ischemic attacks, 74
   in vascular trauma
      abdominal, 324–326, 325f–327f, 329–330, 329f
      brachiocephalic, 318, 319f, 320, 322
Hemorrhage
   gastrointestinal
      with aortoenteric fistula, 112, 113f, 114
      with portal hypertension, 306, 307, 307f
   heparin-induced, 372, 373f
   intracranial, 50, 51f, 52

Hemorrhage *(Continued)*
   in stroke following carotid endarterectomy, 70, 71f, 72
   intraoperative
      assessment of, 16, 18
      management of, 364, 365f, 366, 368
   with infrainguinal prosthetic graft infection, 208, 209, 209f, 210
   with vascular trauma
      abdominal, 324–326, 325f–327f, 328–330, 329f
      brachiocephalic, 318, 319f, 320
      extremity, 332, 333f
Heparin
   allergic reactions to, 372, 373f
   complications with, 370, 371f, 372, 373f
   for acute limb ischemia, 168, 169f
   for acute mesenteric ischemia, 250, 251f
   for acute stroke, 50, 51f
   for aortic graft limb thrombosis, 180, 181f
   for carotid artery dissection, 58, 59f
   for deep vein thrombosis, in lower extremity, 272, 273f, 274, 276, 278
   for extremity vascular trauma, 334
   for hypercoagulable syndrome, 10
   for infrainguinal graft thrombosis, 204, 205f
   for pulmonary embolism, 286–288, 287f
   for ruptured abdominal aortic aneurysm repair, 106
   for vertebral artery disease, 74, 75f
   reversal of, 18
      contraindication to, with carotid endarterectomy, 39f, 42
      in intraoperative hemorrhage, 364, 365f, 366
      routine indication for, 14, 18
Heparin-associated antiplatelet antibodies (HAAbs), 370, 371f, 372, 373f
Heparin-induced thrombocytopenia (HIT), 370, 371f
Hepatic artery aneurysm, 150, 151f
Hepatocellular function, in portal hypertension, 307, 308, 310
Hepatorenal bypass, for renovascular occlusive disease
   adult fibrodysplastic, 244, 245f
   arteriosclerotic, 246, 247
"Herald bleed"
   in aortoenteric fistula, 112, 113f, 114, 116
   in femoral artery pseudoaneurysm, 143, 143f
High-risk procedures, 3
Hirudin, recombinant, for lower extremity deep vein thrombosis, 278
HIT (heparin-induced thrombocytopenia), 370, 371f
Hormone therapy, for erectile dysfunction, 346, 347f
Horner's syndrome
   in brachiocephalic vascular trauma, 318
   in carotid artery aneurysm, 54–55
   in carotid artery dissection, 58
Hypercoagulable syndrome, 8, 9f, 10
   in heparin-induced thrombosis, 370, 371f
   in infrainguinal graft thrombosis, 204
   in lower extremity deep vein thrombosis, 272, 273f, 274
   in portal vein patency, 308
   in superficial phlebitis, 269

Hyperesthesia, with post-traumatic pain syndrome, 336, 337
Hyperkalemia, heparin-induced, 372, 373f
Hyperlipidemia, management of, 6, 7f
Hypertension
   in leg pain while walking, 156, 157f, 158
   portal, 306–310, 307f
   with aortic dissection, control of, 128, 129f, 130
   with carotid body tumors, 66
   with carotid fibromuscular dysplasia, 62, 63f, 64
   with renal artery aneurysm, 152, 153f
   with renovascular occlusive disease
      adult fibrodysplastic, 244, 245f
      arteriosclerotic, 246, 247f, 248
      evaluation of, 238, 238t, 239f, 240, 240t
      pediatric, 242, 243f
   with Takayasu's disease, 362
Hyponatremia, heparin-induced, 372, 373f
Hypoperfusion, global intraoperative, 364, 365f
Hypoplastic kidney, in renovascular occlusive disease
   adult fibrodysplastic, 244, 254f
   pediatric, 242, 243f
Hypothermia, intraoperative, 364, 365f
Hypothermic challenge, digital, for Raynaud's syndrome, 342
Hypothermic circulatory arrest, in thoracoabdominal aortic aneurysm repair, 99f, 102

IAA. *See* Iliac artery aneurysm (IAA).
IADSA (intra-arterial digital subtraction angiography), for renovascular occlusive disease, 238, 238t
Iatrogenic trauma
   femoral artery pseudoaneurysm from, 137f, 138, 142–144, 143f
   subclavian-axillary venous thrombosis from, 262, 263f
   superficial phlebitis from, 268, 269f
ICI (intracavernous injection), for erectile dysfunction, 346, 347f, 348
Ileostomy, for sigmoid ischemia, 118
Iliac artery(ies)
   as graft, for renovascular occlusive disease, 242, 243f, 244, 245f
   atheroembolism of, 173f, 174
   in abdominal vascular trauma, 328–329
   in endovascular abdominal aortic aneurysm repair, 120, 122, 124
Iliac artery aneurysm (IAA), 132–134, 133f
   abdominal aortic aneurysm repair with, 132, 133f
   infections with, 133–134, 133f
   internal *vs.* external repair procedures for, 133f, 134
   isolated, 132, 133f
   rupture risk with, 132, 133f, 134
Iliac vein(s)
   in iliofemoral deep vein thrombosis, 282, 283f, 284
   obstruction of, 299f, 300, 301, 302
Iliocavagram, for iliofemoral deep vein thrombosis, 282, 283f
Iliofemoral bypass, for aortoiliac occlusive disease, 176, 177f
Iliofemoral deep vein insufficiency, 298, 299f, 300, 301, 302

Iliofemoral deep vein thrombosis, 282, 283f, 284
Iliorenal bypass, for renovascular occlusive disease
　adult fibrodysplastic, 244, 245f
　arteriosclerotic, 246, 247
Impotence, 346, 347f, 348
Indium-labeled cellular scanning
　for aortic graft infection, 186, 208, 209f
　for aortoenteric fistula, 112, 113f
　for diabetic foot infections, 214
Indwelling catheters
　subclavian-axillary venous thrombosis from, 262, 263f
　superficial phlebitis from, 268, 269f
Infection(s)
　aortoenteric fistula from, 112, 114
　carotid artery aneurysm vs., 54
　of aortic graft, 186, 187f, 188, 190
　of feet, with diabetes mellitus, 212, 213f, 214, 216
　of infrainguinal prosthetic graft, 208–210, 209f
　with deep vein insufficiency, 294, 295, 295f
　with femoral artery aneurysm, 137, 137f, 139–140
　with femoral artery pseudoaneurysm, 143, 143f
　with iliac artery aneurysm, 133, 133f
　with superficial phlebitis, 268, 269–270, 269f
Infectious aneurysm(s)
　of carotid artery, 54–56, 55f
　of femoral artery, 140, 143, 143f
Inferior vena cava
　filters for. See Vena caval filters.
　in aortovenous fistula, 108–110, 109f
　injuries of, with abdominal vascular trauma, 326, 327, 329–330, 329f
Inflammatory phases, in Takayasu's disease, 360, 361f
Infrainguinal grafting
　prosthetic, infection of, 208–210, 209f
　surveillance of, 198, 199f, 200, 202
　thrombosis of, 204, 205f, 206
Infrainguinal occlusive disease, 192–194, 193f
　in leg pain while walking, 157f, 158
Injury. See Trauma; specific anatomy.
Innominate artery, in Takayasu's disease, 362
Innominate artery occlusive disease, 80–82, 81f
Innominate artery reconstruction, in brachiocephalic artery occlusive disease, 80, 81f, 82
Innominate endarterectomy, for brachiocephalic artery occlusive disease, 80–81, 81f
INR (International Normalized Ratio), in hypercoagulable syndrome, 8, 10
Intercostal reconstruction, in thoracoabdominal aortic aneurysm repair, 99f, 102, 130
Intermediate-risk procedures, 3
Internal carotid artery
　aneurysms of, 54, 55f, 56
　bilateral occlusion of, with vertebral artery disease, 74, 75f
　bypass. See External carotid artery.
　carotid shunting of, 38, 39f
　dissections of, 58, 60
　fibromuscular dysplasia of, 62–63
　in carotid body tumor resection, 67f
　in carotid endarterectomy, 38, 39f, 40

Internal carotid artery (Continued)
　stenosis of
　　acute stroke from, 50, 51f
　　external carotid artery bypass for, 29f, 32
　　progression of, to occlusion, 29f, 30, 32
　　symptomatic, 28, 29f
　ultrasound surveillance of
　　with asymptomatic stenosis, 34–36, 35f
　　with cerebrovascular symptoms, 22, 23f, 24
International Normalized Ratio (INR), in hypercoagulable syndrome, 8, 10
Interphalangeal joints (IPs), in diabetic foot infections, 216
Interposition bypass grafting
　for carotid artery aneurysm, 55f, 56
　for carotid artery dissection, 59f, 60
　for carotid endarterectomy, 38, 39f
　　redo, 44, 45f, 46
　for femoral artery aneurysm, 136, 137f, 139
　for hemodialysis vascular access, 358
　for iliac artery aneurysm, 133f, 134
　for infrainguinal graft surveillance, 200
　for infrainguinal graft thrombosis, 205f, 206
　for infrainguinal prosthetic graft infection, 209f, 210
　for popliteal artery disease, 230, 231f
　for upper extremity ischemia, 234
　for vascular trauma
　　brachiocephalic, 320
　　extremity, 332, 333f
Intra-arterial digital subtraction angiography (IADSA), for renovascular occlusive disease, 238, 238t
Intracavernous injection (ICI), for erectile dysfunction, 346, 347f, 348
Intracranial hemorrhage, 50, 51f, 52
　in stroke following carotid endarterectomy, 70, 71f, 72
Intrarenal webs, in pediatric renovascular occlusive disease, 242, 243f
Intravascular shunt, for extremity vascular trauma, 333–334, 333f
Intravenous digital subtraction angiography (IVDSA), for renovascular occlusive disease, 238, 238t
Intravenous drug abuse (IVDA)
　femoral artery aneurysm from, 137, 137f
　femoral artery pseudoaneurysm from, 143, 143f
　superficial phlebitis from, 268
Intravenous pyelogram, for abdominal vascular trauma, 324
Invasive monitoring, indications for, 4, 12, 13f
IPs (interphalangeal joints), in diabetic foot infections, 216
Ipsilateral stroke, with carotid artery stenosis
　asymptomatic, 34–35
　recurrent after endarterectomy, 44, 45f, 48
　symptomatic, 30, 32
Ischemia. See specific anatomy or pathology.
IVDA. See Intravenous drug abuse (IVDA).
IVDSA (intravenous digital subtraction angiography), for renovascular occlusive disease, 238, 238t

Jehovah's Witnesses, transfusions and, 16
Jugular vein, internal
　for hemodialysis vascular access, 355, 356

Jugular vein (Continued)
　turndown/transposition of, for subclavian-axillary venous thrombosis, 266

Kidney. See Renal entries.
Klippel-Trenaunay syndrome, 350
Kocher maneuver, for abdominal vascular trauma, 327, 327f, 329, 329f, 330

Laminectomy, for vertebral artery decompression, 74
Laparotomy
　for abdominal vascular trauma, 325–326, 325f, 328, 330
　for acute mesenteric ischemia, 250, 251f, 254
　for sigmoid ischemia, 118, 119f
Left ventricular function, in preoperative cardiac risk assessment, 4, 12
Leg. See Lower extremity.
Leg pain
　while walking, 156, 157f, 158, 160
　with infrainguinal prosthetic graft infection, 208
Lepirudin, for heparin-induced thrombocytopenia, 370
Life expectancy, in asymptomatic carotid artery stenosis, 35–36, 35f
Ligation
　in deep vein insufficiency, 295f, 296
　of carotid artery aneurysm, 55f, 56
　of carotid artery dissection, 59f, 60
　of congenital vascular malformations, 351, 351f
　of femoral artery pseudoaneurysm, 143f, 144
　of hepatic artery aneurysm, 150
　of varicose veins, 291f, 292
　of vascular trauma
　　abdominal, 326, 326f, 327, 327f, 328f, 329, 329f, 330
　　brachiocephalic, 322
Limb elevation
　for congenital venous malformation, 351f, 352
　for deep vein insufficiency, 294, 295, 295f
　for iliofemoral deep vein thrombosis, 282, 283f
　for lymphedema, 313f, 314
　for varicose veins, 290, 291f
Limb ischemia, acute, 168–170, 169f. See also Critical limb ischemia (CLI); specific extremity.
Limb length, in congenital venous malformations, 350, 351f, 352
Lipoproteins, management of, 6, 7f
Liver. See also Hepat- entries.
　in abdominal vascular trauma, 329, 329f
Liver transplantation, orthotopic, for portal hypertension, 307–308, 307f, 310
Lower extremity
　compartment syndrome of, 224
　deep vein thrombosis of

Lower extremity (Continued)
  during pregnancy, 273f, 276
  evaluation of, 272, 273f, 274
  recurrent, 273f, 276, 278, 280
  risk factors for, 272, 273f
  superficial phlebitis with, 268–269, 269f
  treatment of, 273f, 274, 276, 278
 in hemodialysis vascular access, 355f, 356
 in Takayasu's disease, 361f, 362
Lower extremity ischemia
 acute. See Critical limb ischemia (CLI).
 subcritical, 162
 with aortic dissection, 128, 129f, 130
 with aortoenteric fistula, 113f, 114, 116
 with leg pain while walking, 156, 157f, 158
Low-risk procedures, 3
Lung. See Pulmonary entries.
Lymphangiography, for lymphedema, 313f, 314, 316
Lymphatic defect(s), congenital venous malformations as, 350, 351
Lymphatic drainage, manual, for lymphedema, 313f, 314
Lymphatic grafting, for lymphedema, 313f, 316
Lymphatic reconstruction, for lymphedema, 313f, 316
Lymphedema, 312, 313f, 314, 316
 deep vein insufficiency vs., 294, 295f
Lymphoscintigraphy, for lymphedema, 313f, 314
Lymphovenous anastomosis, for lymphedema, 313f, 316

Macrofistulous congenital venous malformations, localized, 351–352, 351f
Mafenide acetate (Sulfamylon) cream, for diabetic foot infections, 216
Magnetic resonance angiography
 for abdominal aortic aneurysm, 91f, 94
  in endovascular repair, 120, 121f, 123, 125
 for acute stroke, 51f, 52
 for aortoiliac occlusive disease, 176
 for atheroembolism, 173–174, 173f
 for carotid artery dissection, 58, 59f, 60
 for carotid artery stenosis
  asymptomatic, 36
  recurrent after endarterectomy, 44, 45f, 46, 48
 for carotid fibromuscular dysplasia, 62
 for chronic mesenteric ischemia, 256
 for critical limb ischemia, 162, 163f
 for evaluating cerebrovascular symptoms, 23f, 24
 for femoral artery aneurysm, 136
 for hepatic artery aneurysm, 150
 for infrainguinal occlusive disease, 192, 193f
 for popliteal artery aneurysm, 147f, 148
 for popliteal artery disease, 228, 229f, 230
 for renal artery aneurysm, 152
 for renovascular occlusive disease, 238, 238t, 239f
 for Takayasu's disease, 360
 for thoracoabdominal aortic aneurysm, 99f, 100
Magnetic resonance imaging
 for acute stroke, 50, 51f, 52

Magnetic resonance imaging (Continued)
 for aortic graft infection, 186, 187f
 for aortoenteric fistula, 112, 113f
 for aortovenous fistula, 108, 109f
 for atheroembolism, 173–174, 173f
 for carotid artery aneurysm, 54, 55f
 for carotid artery dissection, 58, 59f, 60
 for carotid body tumors, 66, 67f, 68
 for carotid fibromuscular dysplasia, 62
 for compartment syndromes, 224
 for congenital vascular malformations, 351, 351f, 352
 for diabetic foot infections, 213f, 214, 216
 for evaluating cerebrovascular symptoms, 22, 23f, 24, 28
 for hepatic artery aneurysm, 150
 for lymphedema, 313f, 314
 for neurogenic thoracic outlet syndrome, 340, 341f
 for popliteal artery aneurysm, 146, 148
 for popliteal artery disease, 228, 229f
 for pulmonary embolism, 286, 287f
 for renovascular occlusive disease, 238, 238t, 239f
 for thoracoabdominal aortic aneurysm, 100
Malignancies
 lower extremity deep vein thrombosis from, 272, 273f, 274, 278
 lymphedema with, 313–314
Mammary artery, internal
 in abdominal aortic aneurysm, 91f, 96
  endovascular repair of, 120, 122
 in subclavian artery occlusive disease, 76, 77f
Mandible, subluxation of
 in brachiocephalic vascular trauma, 322
 in carotid body tumor resection, 67f, 68
Marfan's syndrome
 aortic dissection with, 128, 130
 thoracoabdominal aortic aneurysm with, 98, 100
Markov decision analysis model, for aneurysm repair, 120, 146
Massage therapy, for lymphedema, 313f, 314
Maximal surgical blood order schedule (MSBOS), 16
Median arcuate ligament syndrome, in chronic mesenteric ischemia, 256
Mesenteric artery(ies)
 in abdominal vascular trauma, 324, 326, 327, 327f, 328
 in aortic aneurysm repair, 100, 120, 122
Mesenteric bridge procedure, for lymphedema, 314, 316
Mesenteric endarterectomy, 251f, 252, 258
Mesenteric ischemia
 acute, 250, 251f, 252, 254
 chronic, 256–259, 257f
Mesenteric vein, superior
 in acute mesenteric ischemia, 250, 251f, 254
 injuries of, with abdominal vascular trauma, 327
Mesentery, bases of, in abdominal vascular trauma, 326
Mesocaval shunt, for portal hypertension, 307f, 308
Metabolic acidosis
 heparin-induced, 372, 373f
 intraoperative, 364, 365f
Metatarsophalangeal joints (MPs), in diabetic foot infections, 216

Metronidazole, for diabetic foot infections, 212
Microfistulous congenital venous malformations, localized, 351f, 352
Milroy's disease, 312
MPs (metatarsophalangeal joints), in diabetic foot infections, 216
MSBOS (maximal surgical blood order schedule), 16
Muscle flap coverage, for infrainguinal prosthetic graft infection, 209f, 210
Mycotic aneurysm, of carotid artery, 54–56, 55f
Myocardial infarction
 acute, perioperative risks with, 2, 3f
 in carotid plus coronary disease, 84, 85f
Myotomy, for popliteal artery entrapment syndrome, 230, 231f

NAIS (Neo-aortoiliac system), for aortic graft infection, 187f, 188, 190
Nasogastric tube, in ruptured abdominal aortic aneurysm repair, 105–106
Neck wounds
 brachiocephalic vascular trauma with, 318, 319f, 322
 zones of, 318, 320
Neo-aortoiliac system (NAIS), for aortic graft infection, 187f, 188, 190
Nephrectomy
 for abdominal vascular trauma, 328
 for renal artery aneurysm, 153
 for renovascular occlusive disease, 239f, 240
  adult fibrodysplastic, 244, 245f
  arteriosclerotic, 247f, 248
  pediatric, 242, 243f
Nerve(s). See also named nerve, e.g., Ulnar nerve.
 in post-traumatic pain syndrome, 336–337, 337f
Nerve conduction tests
 for compartment syndromes, 224
 for neurogenic thoracic outlet syndrome, 340, 341f
Neuroendocrine secretion, with carotid body tumors, 66, 67f
Neurologic deficit(s)
 patients at high risk for, 12, 13f
 with acute limb ischemia, 168
 with brachiocephalic artery occlusive disease, 80
 with carotid artery aneurysm, 54, 55f, 56
 with carotid artery dissection, 58, 59f
 with carotid artery stenosis, 28, 29f, 30, 32
  recurrent after endarterectomy, 44, 45f, 46, 48
 with carotid fibromuscular dysplasia, 62–64, 63f
 with carotid plus coronary disease, 84, 85f, 86
 with erectile dysfunction, 346, 348
 with iliac artery aneurysm, 132, 133f
 with infrainguinal graft thrombosis, 204
 with stroke following carotid endarterectomy, 70, 71f, 72
 with vascular trauma
  brachiocephalic, 318, 319f, 322
  extremity, 333f, 334
Neurologic risk assessment, preoperative, 12, 29f, 30, 32

Niacin, for hyperlipidemia, 6
Nielsen test, for Raynaud's syndrome, 342
Nifedipine, for Raynaud's syndrome, 342
Normovolemic hemodilution transfusions, 15f, 16, 18

Ophthalmologic deficits, with carotid artery dissection, 58
Orthotic inserts, diabetic foot infections and, 213f, 214
Osteomyelitis, with diabetic foot infections, 214
Ostial stenosis, aortic spillover, in renovascular occlusive disease
   arteriosclerotic, 246, 247f
   pediatric, 242, 243f
Oxygen tension, transcutaneous (Tco_2)
   for amputation level, 218, 219f, 220
   with diabetic foot infections, 212

PAES (popliteal artery entrapment syndrome), 228, 229f, 230, 231f
Pain
   post-traumatic syndrome of, 336–338, 337f
   with abdominal aortic aneurysm, 140
   with aortic dissection, 128, 130
Panel grafts, for abdominal vascular trauma, 329f, 330
Papaverine
   for acute mesenteric ischemia, 251f, 254
   for erectile dysfunction, 346
   for infrainguinal graft surveillance, 198, 199f, 200
Parkes Weber syndrome, 350
Partial thromboplastin time (PTT)
   in iliofemoral deep vein thrombosis, 282
   normal range for, 14
Patch angioplasty. See Vein patch angioplasty.
PCAD (popliteal cystic adventitial disease), 228, 229f, 230, 231f
Peak systolic velocity (PSV)
   in chronic mesenteric ischemia, 256
   in infrainguinal graft surveillance, 198, 199f, 200, 202
Pedal pulses/perfusion
   with atheroembolism, 172, 173f
   with diabetic foot infections, 212
   with popliteal artery disease, 228, 229f
   with ruptured abdominal aortic aneurysm, 105f, 106
Pelvic artery aneurysm, 132
Pelvic crush injuries, with abdominal vascular trauma, 328–329
Pelvic hematomas, with abdominal vascular trauma, 328–329, 328f
Pelvic ischemia, with iliac artery aneurysm, 134
Penetrating trauma
   abdominal vascular, 324, 325f, 326, 327, 329
   extremity vascular, 33f, 332
Penicillin, for diabetic foot infections, 212
Penile implants, for erectile dysfunction, 347f, 348
Penile pressures, for erectile dysfunction, 346, 347f

Pentoxifylline, for leg pain while walking, 158
Percutaneous transluminal angioplasty (PTA). See also Stents and stenting.
   for acute limb ischemia, 169f, 170
   for aortoiliac occlusive disease, 176, 177f, 178, 198
   for brachiocephalic artery occlusive disease, 80, 81f
   for carotid artery dissection, 59f, 60
   for carotid artery stenosis, 28, 29f, 30
   for carotid fibromuscular dysplasia, 63f, 64
   for carotid plus coronary disease, 84, 85f
   for chronic mesenteric ischemia, 257–258, 257f
   for coronary artery disease, 4
   for critical limb ischemia, 163f, 164
   for infrainguinal graft surveillance, 199f, 200, 202
   for infrainguinal graft thrombosis, 205f, 206
   for infrainguinal occlusive disease, 192, 193f, 194
   for renal fibromuscular dysplasia, 62, 63f, 64
   for renovascular occlusive disease, 239f, 240
      adult fibrodysplastic, 244, 245f
      arteriosclerotic, 246, 247f
      pediatric, 242, 243f
   for subclavian artery occlusive disease, 77, 77f
   for subclavian-axillary venous thrombosis, 263f, 264
   for Takayasu's disease, 361f, 362
Perioperative assessment
   of cardiac risk, 2–4, 3f, 12
   of neurologic risk, 12, 29f, 30, 32
Perioperative care, 12–13, 13f
Peritoneal cavity, in abdominal vascular trauma, 324, 325f, 327f
Peritoneal lavage, diagnostic, for abdominal vascular trauma, 324, 325f
Peritonitis
   with acute mesenteric ischemia, 250, 251f, 254
   with sigmoid ischemia, 118, 119f
Pharmacotherapy
   for critical limb ischemia, 163f, 164
   for erectile dysfunction, 346, 347f, 348
   for hyperlipidemia, 6, 7f
   for infrainguinal graft surveillance, 198, 199f, 200
   for leg pain while walking, 157f, 158
   for portal hypertension, 309, 309f
   for post-traumatic pain syndrome, 337
   for Raynaud's syndrome, 342
   for renovascular occlusive disease, 239f, 240, 240t
Phenoxybenzamine (Dibenzyline), for post-traumatic pain syndrome, 338
Phentolamine, for erectile dysfunction, 346
Phenytoin, for post-traumatic pain syndrome, 337
Phlebitis, superficial, 268–270, 269f
Phlebography. See Venography.
Physical therapy
   for compartment syndromes, 223f, 224
   for neurogenic thoracic outlet syndrome, 340, 341f
   for post-traumatic pain syndrome, 337, 337f, 338
Plasmin renin, in renovascular occlusive disease, 239f, 240, 240t
Platelet transfusions
   for intraoperative hemorrhage, 364, 365f, 366

Platelet transfusions (Continued)
   for ruptured abdominal aortic aneurysm, 104
   guidelines for, 14, 18
Platelets and platelet count
   in hypercoagulable syndrome, 8
   in intraoperative hemorrhage, 364, 365f, 366
   in lower extremity deep vein thrombosis treatment, 276, 278
   normal range for, 14
   with heparin therapy, 370, 371f, 373f
Plethysmography
   for amputation level, 218, 219f, 220
   for compartment syndromes, 224
   for congenital venous malformations, 350
   for deep vein insufficiency, 294, 295f
      for reflux vs. obstruction determination, 298–299, 299f
   for diabetic foot infections, 212
   for lymphedema, 313f, 314
   for Raynaud's syndrome, 342
   for varicose veins, 291
Podiatry evaluation, for diabetic foot infections, 213f, 214
Popliteal artery, injuries of, with extremity vascular trauma, 332
Popliteal artery aneurysm, 146, 147f, 148
   occlusive disease vs., 230, 231f
Popliteal artery entrapment syndrome (PAES), 228, 229f, 230, 231f
Popliteal artery occlusive disease, with entrapment syndrome, 230, 231f
Popliteal cystic adventitial disease (PCAD), 228, 229f, 230, 231f
Popliteal vein
   in deep vein insufficiency, 299, 300, 302
   injuries of, with extremity vascular trauma, 334
Popliteotibial vein, in deep vein insufficiency, 300
Portacaval shunt, for portal hypertension, 307, 307f, 308
Portal decompression, for hypertension, 306, 307f, 308–310
Portal hypertension, 306–310, 307f
Portal vein
   injuries of, with abdominal vascular trauma, 329–330, 329f
   patency of, for shunt placement, 307f, 308
Portosystemic decompression, for portal hypertension, 306, 307, 307f, 308–310
Portosystemic encephalopathy (PSE), with portacaval shunt, 308
Postoperative complications, patients at high risk for, 12–13, 13f
Post-thrombotic syndrome (PTS)
   in deep vein insufficiency, 298, 302
   in lower extremity deep vein thrombosis, 274, 278
Post-traumatic pain syndrome (PTPS), 336–338, 337f
Prednisone, for Takayasu's disease, 360
Pregnancy
   lower extremity deep vein thrombosis during, 273f, 276
   renal artery aneurysm during, 152
   varicose veins from, 290

Profunda femoris artery, in aortic graft limb thrombosis, 182
Profunda femoris vein, in deep vein insufficiency, 299f, 300, 302
Prolactinemia, in erectile dysfunction, 346, 347f
Prostaglandin E_1, for erectile dysfunction, 346, 348
Prostanoid agents, for critical limb ischemia, 164
Prosthetic grafts
  bridging, for hemodialysis vascular access, 354, 355f, 356
    failed, 358, 359f
  for aortic graft infection, 187f, 188, 190
  for arteriosclerotic renovascular occlusive disease, 246, 247f
  for carotid endarterectomy, 38, 39f, 40
    redo, 46
  for chronic mesenteric ischemia, 258
  for deep vein insufficiency, 301, 302
  for femoral artery aneurysm, 137
  for hepatic artery aneurysm, 150
  for popliteal artery aneurysm, 148
  for vascular trauma
    abdominal, 326, 329
    brachiocephalic, 320, 322
    extremity, 332, 333f
  infrainguinal
    for occlusive disease, 193, 193f, 194
    infection of, 208–210, 209f
    thrombosis and, 204, 205f, 206
Prosthetic implants, for erectile dysfunction, 347f, 348
Protamine sulfate, for heparin reversal, 18
  contraindication to, with carotid endarterectomy, 39f, 42
  in intraoperative hemorrhage, 364, 365f, 366, 368
Prothrombin time (PT)
  in hypercoagulable syndrome, 8, 9f, 10
  in intraoperative hemorrhage, 364, 365f, 366
  normal range for, 14
PSE (portosystemic encephalopathy), with portacaval shunt, 308
Pseudoaneurysm
  of carotid artery, 54, 55f, 56
  of femoral artery. *See* Femoral artery pseudoaneurysm.
  of infrainguinal prosthetic graft, 209f, 210
Pseudomonas
  in graft infections, 188, 209f, 210
  in superficial phlebitis, 268
PSV (peak systolic velocity)
  in chronic mesenteric ischemia, 256
  in infrainguinal graft surveillance, 198, 199f, 200, 202
PT. *See* Prothrombin time (PT).
PTA. *See* Percutaneous transluminal angioplasty (PTA).
PTPS (post-traumatic pain syndrome), 336–338, 337f
PTS (post-thrombotic syndrome)
  in deep vein insufficiency, 298, 302
  in lower extremity deep vein thrombosis, 274, 278
PTT (partial thromboplastin time)
  activated. *See* Activated partial thromboplastin time (aPTT).
  in iliofemoral deep vein thrombosis, 282
  normal range for, 14
Pulmonary artery catheter, 12, 13f, 18

Pulmonary complications
  patients at high risk for, 12–13, 13f
  with carotid artery aneurysm, 54, 55f
  with thoracoabdominal aortic aneurysm repair, 98, 99f
Pulmonary embolism, 286–288, 287f
  with deep vein thrombosis, 272, 274
  with subclavian-axillary venous thrombosis, 262
Pulsatile neck mass, as carotid artery aneurysm, 54, 55f
Pulse deficits
  in erectile dysfunction, 346
  in Takayasu's disease, 360, 361f
  pedal. *See* Pedal pulses/perfusion.
  with vascular trauma
    brachiocephalic, 318, 319f, 320, 322
    extremity, 332, 333, 333f
Pulse volume recording
  for congenital venous malformation, 350
  for erectile dysfunction, 346, 347f

Questionnaires, for leg pain while walking, 157f, 158
Quinolones, for diabetic foot infections, 212

Radiation therapy
  for carotid body tumors, 66, 67f, 69
  great vessel occlusive disease from, 80–81
Radioactive cellular scanning
  for aortic graft infection, 186, 208, 209f
  for aortoenteric fistula, 112, 113f
  for diabetic foot infections, 214
  for femoral artery aneurysm, 139
Radiography
  for diabetic foot infections, 212, 214
  for neurogenic thoracic outlet syndrome, 340, 341f
  for post-traumatic pain syndrome, 336, 337f
  for vascular trauma
    abdominal, 324, 325f
    brachiocephalic, 318, 319f
Radionuclide microsphere study, for congenital vascular malformations, 350, 351f
Radiopharmaceuticals, for lower extremity deep vein thrombosis, 280
Raynaud's syndrome, 342, 343f, 344
  in upper extremity ischemia, 232, 233f
Reconstruction. *See* Revascularization; *specific anatomy or pathology.*
Red blood cells
  normal ranges for, 14
  substitutes for, in experimental transfusion, 15f, 18
  transfusions of, guidelines for, 14, 15f, 18
Reflex sympathetic dystrophy, 336, 337f
Rehabilitation, for compartment syndromes, 223f, 224
Renal artery(ies)
  arteriography of
    for aneurysm, 152

Renal artery(ies) *(Continued)*
    for carotid fibromuscular dysplasia, 62
  fibromuscular dysplasia of, 62, 63f, 64
  in abdominal aortic aneurysm repair, 91f, 94, 96
  injuries of, with abdominal vascular trauma, 324–325, 325f
  ischemic atrophy of
    in adult fibrodysplastic occlusive disease, 244, 245f
    in arteriosclerotic occlusive disease, 246, 247f, 248
    in pediatric occlusive disease, 242, 243f
  reimplantation of, for pediatric occlusive disease, 242, 243f
  retroperitoneal hematomas and, 327–328, 327f
Renal artery aneurysm, 152–153, 153f
Renal artery stenosis
  in arteriosclerotic occlusive disease, 246, 247f
  in pediatric occlusive disease, 242, 243f
  in Takayasu's disease, 361f, 362
Renal emboli, in renal artery aneurysm, 152, 153f
Renal function
  high-risk complications and, 12, 13f
  in aortic aneurysm repair
    ruptured abdominal, 105–106, 105f
    thoracoabdominal, 98, 99f, 100, 102
  with renal artery aneurysm, 152
Renal injuries, with abdominal vascular trauma, 327–328, 327f
Renal ischemia, in aortic dissection, 128, 129f, 130
Renal vein(s)
  in aortovenous fistula, 108–110, 109f
  retroperitoneal hematomas and, 327–328, 327f
Renal vein renin assay (RVRA), for renovascular occlusive disease, 238, 239f, 240, 240t
Renography, captopril, for renovascular occlusive disease, 239f, 240, 240t
Renovascular occlusive disease
  evaluation of, 238, 238t, 239f, 240, 240t
  treatment of
    adult fibrodysplastic, 244, 245f
    arteriosclerotic, 246, 247f, 248
    pediatric, 242, 243f
Reperfusion injury
  stroke following carotid endarterectomy as, 70
  with extremity vascular trauma, 333
Resection, surgical
  of bowel, for acute mesenteric ischemia, 250, 251f, 254
  of carotid artery aneurysm, 55f, 56
  of carotid artery dissection, 59f, 60
  of carotid body tumors, 66, 67f, 68
  of congenital vascular malformations, 351, 351f, 352
  of femoral artery aneurysm, 137f, 138–139
  of femoral artery pseudoaneurysm, 143f, 144
  of great vessels, for brachiocephalic vascular trauma, 319f, 320, 322
  of hemodialysis vascular access, 358, 359f
  of iliac artery aneurysm, 133, 133f
  of soft tissue, for lymphedema, 313f, 314

Rest pain, with critical limb ischemia, 162, 163f
Resuscitation. See Fluid resuscitation.
Retroperitoneal approach, for abdominal aortic aneurysm repair, 91f, 94, 96
Retroperitoneum, in abdominal vascular trauma, 324, 325f, 326, 329
  hematomas of, 327–328, 327f
Revascularization
  for abdominal aortic aneurysm, 91f, 96
  for abdominal vascular trauma, 327, 327f
  for acute limb ischemia, 168, 169f
  for aortic graft infection, 186, 187f, 188, 190
  for aortoenteric fistula repair, 113f, 114, 116
  for aortoiliac occlusive disease, 176, 177f, 178
  for brachiocephalic artery occlusive disease, 81f, 82
  for carotid plus coronary disease, 84, 85f, 86
  for critical limb ischemia, 163f, 164
  for diabetic foot infections, 213f, 214
  for erectile dysfunction, 347f, 348
  for femoral artery aneurysm, 137, 137f, 138, 140
  for femoral artery pseudoaneurysm, 143f, 144
  for iliac artery aneurysm, 133, 133f
  for infrainguinal graft thrombosis, 204, 205f
  for infrainguinal occlusive disease, 192–194, 193f
  for infrainguinal prosthetic graft infection, 208–210, 209f
  for mesenteric ischemia
    acute, 251f, 252
    chronic, 257, 257f, 258–259
  for popliteal artery aneurysm, 147f, 148
  for Raynaud's syndrome, 343f, 344
  for renovascular occlusive disease
    adult fibrodysplastic, 244, 245f
    arteriosclerotic, 246, 247f, 248
    pediatric, 242, 243f
  for subclavian artery occlusive disease, 77–78, 77f
  for subclavian-axillary venous thrombosis, 263f, 266
  for Takayasu's disease, 361f, 362, 363
  for upper extremity ischemia, 233f, 234
Reversible ischemic neurologic deficit (RIND), with carotid artery stenosis, 28, 29f
Rib resection
  for neurogenic thoracic outlet syndrome, 340, 341f
  for subclavian-axillary venous thrombosis, 264
  for upper extremity ischemia, 234
RIND (reversible ischemic neurologic deficit), with carotid artery stenosis, 28, 29f
Risk assessment, preoperative
  of cardiac status, 2–4
  of neurologic status, 12, 29f, 30, 32
Risk level, of surgical procedures, 3
Rose criteria, for arteriogenic claudication, 156, 157f
RVRA (renal vein renin assay), for renovascular occlusive disease, 238, 239f, 240, 240t

Salvage procedures
  for critical limb ischemia, 162, 163f, 164, 169, 169f

Salvage procedures (Continued)
  for diabetic foot infections, 214
  for extremity vascular trauma, 332, 333f, 334
  for hemodialysis vascular access, 358–359, 359f
  for infrainguinal prosthetic graft infection, 208–210, 209f
Saphenopopliteal bypass, for deep vein insufficiency, 299f, 302
Saphenous vein(s)
  as varicose veins, 290, 291–292, 291f
  in deep vein insufficiency, 299f, 300, 302
Saphenous vein graft/patch
  for abdominal vascular trauma, 326, 326f, 327
  for carotid artery dissection, 60, 68
  for carotid endarterectomy, 40
  for hepatic artery aneurysm, 150
  for infrainguinal graft thrombosis, 206
  for infrainguinal occlusive disease, 193, 193f, 194
  for mesenteric ischemia, 252, 258
  for popliteal artery disease, 230, 231f
  for renal artery aneurysm, 15–153
SAVT (subclavian-axillary venous thrombosis), 262, 263f, 264, 266
Scalene muscle block, for neurogenic thoracic outlet syndrome, 340, 341f
Sciatic artery, anomalies of, 352
Sclerotherapy
  for congenital vascular malformations, 351–352, 351f
  for esophageal varices, from portal hypertension, 306
  for portal hypertension, 309
  for varicose veins, 291f, 292
Segmental limb pressures
  for amputation level, 218, 219f, 220
  with compartment syndromes, 224
  with congenital venous malformation, 350
  with diabetic foot infections, 212
  with upper extremity ischemia, 232, 233f
Sepsis
  amputation level and, 218, 219f
  intraoperative dynamics of, 364, 366
  with diabetic foot infections, 212, 214
  with femoral artery pseudoaneurysm, 143, 143f, 144
  with infrainguinal prosthetic graft infection, 208, 209, 209f, 210
  with superficial phlebitis, 269–270
Septotomy, balloon vs. surgical, for aortic dissection, 128, 130
Shock
  heparin-induced, 372, 373f
  resuscitation of. See Fluid resuscitation.
Short-gut syndrome, in acute mesenteric ischemia, 254
Shunts and shunting
  carotid, for carotid endarterectomy, 38, 39f
  for portal hypertension, 306, 307f, 308, 309–310
  intravascular, for extremity vascular trauma, 333–334, 333f
Sigmoid ischemia, after aortic surgery, 118–119, 119f
  for ruptured abdominal aortic aneurysm, 105f, 106
Sildenafil (Viagra)
  contraindications to, 346

Sildenafil (Viagra) (Continued)
  for erectile dysfunction, 346, 347f
Sinogram, for infrainguinal prosthetic graft infection, 208, 209f
Skin changes
  with deep vein insufficiency, 294, 295f
  with diabetic foot infections, 212, 213f, 214, 216
  with lower extremity deep vein thrombosis, 272
  with lymphedema, 312
  with post-traumatic pain syndrome, 336
  with Raynaud's syndrome, 342, 343f
  with superficial phlebitis, 268, 269, 269f
  with varicose veins, 290, 291, 291f
Skin grafts
  for compartment syndromes, 226
  for diabetic foot infections, 213f, 216
Skin necrosis, heparin-induced, 372, 373f
Skin substitutes, for deep vein insufficiency, 295f, 296
Skull base, carotid artery aneurysms relationship to, 55f, 56
Small vessel occlusive disease, in erectile dysfunction, 348
Smoking
  leg pain on walking due to, 156, 157f, 158
  upper extremity ischemia from, 234
Smooth muscle dysfunction, in erectile dysfunction, 346, 347f
Soap-and-water scrubs
  for Raynaud's syndrome, 344
  for ulcers, with deep vein insufficiency, 294, 295–296, 295f
Sodium nitroprusside, for aortic dissection, 128
Sodium restriction, for renovascular occlusive disease, 240
Soft tissue injury, with extremity vascular trauma, 332, 333, 333f, 334
Spinal cord, protection of, in thoracoabdominal aortic aneurysm repair, 99f, 102
Splanchnic aneurysm, 150, 151f
Splenectomy, for abdominal vascular trauma, 326, 327
Splenic artery, in abdominal vascular trauma, 326, 327
Splenorenal bypass, for renovascular occlusive disease
  adult fibrodysplastic, 244, 245f
  arteriosclerotic, 246, 247
Splenorenal shunt, for portal hypertension, 307f, 308
Staphylococcus
  carotid artery aneurysm from, 54, 55
  femoral artery aneurysm from, 140, 143
  in aortic graft infection, 186, 187f
  in infrainguinal prosthetic graft infection, 209f, 210
  in superficial phlebitis, 268
Stasis dermatitis, with deep vein insufficiency, 294, 295f, 296
Statin agents, for hyperlipidemia, 6
Steal syndrome(s)
  coronary, with subclavian artery occlusive disease, 76, 77f, 78
  in congenital venous malformation, 350, 352
  in Takayasu's disease, 362
  in upper extremity ischemia, 232, 234
Stenosis. See also *specific vessel*.
  correlation of, with duplex scan and arteriography, 202

Stents and stenting
    for abdominal aortic aneurysm, 120–125, 121f
    for aortic dissection, 128, 130
    for aortoiliac occlusive disease, 176, 177f, 198
    for atheroembolism, 173f, 174
    for brachiocephalic artery occlusive disease, 80, 81f
    for carotid artery dissection, 59f, 60
    for carotid artery stenosis, 29f, 30, 44
        recurrent, 44, 45f, 46, 48
    for coronary artery disease, 4
    for critical limb ischemia, 163f, 164
    for iliac vein obstruction, 299f, 301
    for renovascular occlusive disease, 239f, 240, 246, 247f
    for subclavian artery occlusive disease, 77, 77f
    for subclavian-axillary venous thrombosis, 263f, 264
    for upper extremity ischemia, 234
    for vascular trauma
        abdominal, 324–325, 325f, 328, 328f
        extremity, 332, 333f
Sternotomy
    for brachiocephalic artery occlusive disease, 80, 81f, 82
    for vascular trauma
        abdominal, 329
        brachiocephalic, 320
Steroid therapy
    for heparin-induced reactions, 372, 373f
    for post-traumatic pain syndrome, 338
    for Takayasu's disease, 360, 361f
    for upper extremity ischemia, 234
Streptokinase, for pulmonary embolism, 287
Stress maneuvers, for perfusion assessment, in popliteal artery disease, 228, 229f
Stress testing
    for carotid plus coronary disease, 84, 85f
    for compartment syndromes, 223f, 224
    for leg pain while walking, 156, 157f, 158
    for preoperative cardiac risk assessment, 2, 3–4, 3f
Stroke, acute ischemic, 50–52, 51f
    from carotid artery stenosis
        asymptomatic, 34–36, 35f
        contralateral vs. ipsilateral, 30, 35f, 32, 34–36
        following carotid endarterectomy, 70, 71f, 72
        plus coronary disease, 84, 85f, 86
        recurrent, after endarterectomy, 44, 45f, 46, 48
        symptomatic, 28, 29f, 30, 32
    from carotid fibromuscular dysplasia, 62–63
    transient ischemic attack vs., 50
    with Takayasu's disease, 361f, 362
Subclavian artery, transposition of
    for occlusive disease, 77f, 78
    for upper extremity ischemia, 234
Subclavian artery occlusive disease, 76–78, 77f
Subclavian vein, in hemodialysis vascular access, 355, 356
Subclavian-axillary venous thrombosis (SAVT), 262, 263f, 264, 266
Subclavian-carotid artery bypass, for brachiocephalic artery occlusive disease, 81f, 82
Superficial phlebitis, 268–270, 269f

Support stockings. See Compression stockings.
Sympathectomy
    cervicothoracic, for Raynaud's syndrome, 344
    for post-traumatic pain syndrome, 336, 337f, 338
    for upper extremity ischemia, 233f, 234
Sympathetic block, for post-traumatic pain syndrome, 336, 337, 337f, 338
Systemic risk factors
    of critical limb ischemia, 162, 163f
    of infrainguinal graft thrombosis, 204, 205f
    of leg pain while walking, 156, 157f, 158
    of lymphedema, 312, 313f
    of upper extremity ischemia, 232, 233f, 234

TAA. See Thoracoabdominal aortic aneurysm (TAA).
Takayasu's disease, 360, 361f, 362–363
    in brachiocephalic artery occlusive disease, 80, 82
Tco_2 (transcutaneous oxygen tension)
    for amputation level, 218, 219f, 220
    with diabetic foot infections, 212
Technetium Tc 99m apcitide, in lower extremity deep vein thrombosis, 280
Temperature control, in ruptured abdominal aortic aneurysm repair, 105, 105f
TENS (transcutaneous electrical nerve stimulation), for post-traumatic pain syndrome, 338
Teratogen, warfarin as, 276
Thallium stress testing
    adenosine, for preoperative cardiac risk assessment, 3–4
    dipyridamole, for carotid plus coronary disease, 84
Thoracic outlet decompression, for subclavian-axillary venous thrombosis, 262, 263f, 264, 266
Thoracic outlet syndrome (TOS)
    in upper extremity ischemia, 232, 233f, 234
    neurogenic, 340–341, 341f
Thoracoabdominal aortic aneurysm (TAA), 98–102, 99f
    Crawford classification of, 98
    operative risk with, 98, 99f, 100
    rupture of, risk factors for, 98, 99f, 100
    size/extent determination of, 98, 99f
    type I–III repair procedures for, 99f, 100, 102
    type IV repair procedures for, 99f, 100
    with aortic dissection, 129f, 130
Thoracotomy, for vascular trauma
    abdominal, 325, 325f
    brachiocephalic, 320
3-D reconstruction, for endovascular abdominal aortic aneurysm repair, 121f, 122–125
Thrombectomy
    for acute limb ischemia, 169f, 170
    for aortic graft limb thrombosis, 180, 181f, 182
    for hemodialysis vascular access, 358, 359f
    for heparin-induced thrombosis, 370, 371f
    for iliofemoral deep vein thrombosis, 282, 283f, 284
    for infrainguinal graft thrombosis, 204, 205f, 206
    for popliteal artery aneurysm, 147f, 148

Thrombectomy (Continued)
    for popliteal artery occlusive disease, with entrapment syndrome, 230, 231f
    for portal hypertension, 306, 307, 307f, 308–310
    for stroke following carotid endarterectomy, 70, 71f
    for subclavian-axillary venous thrombosis, 262, 263f, 264
Thrombin injections, ultrasound-guided, for femoral artery pseudoaneurysm, 138, 143, 143f
Thrombin time (TT), in intraoperative hemorrhage, 364, 365f, 366
Thrombocytopenia, heparin-induced, 14, 370, 371f
Thromboemboli
    acute stroke from, 50–51, 51f
    in acute limb ischemia, 168–170, 169f
    in aortic fistula repair, 110, 112
    in carotid artery stenosis, 29f, 32
    in femoral artery aneurysm, 136, 137f
    in heparin-induced thrombosis, 370, 371f
    in hypercoagulable syndrome, 8, 9f, 10
    in popliteal artery aneurysm, 146, 147f, 148
    in stroke following carotid endarterectomy, 70, 71f
    in vertebral artery disease, 74, 75f
Thrombolytic therapy
    catheter-directed
        for acute limb ischemia, 168–170, 169f
        for deep vein thrombosis, in lower extremity, 273f, 274
        for iliofemoral deep vein thrombosis, 282, 283f, 284
        for infrainguinal graft thrombosis, 204, 205f, 206
        for subclavian artery occlusive disease, 76, 77f
        for subclavian-axillary venous thrombosis, 262, 263f, 264, 266
    for acute mesenteric ischemia, 251f, 254
    for acute stroke, 50, 51f
    for aortic graft limb thrombosis, 181f, 182, 184
    for deep vein insufficiency, 299f, 301
    for hemodialysis vascular access, 358, 359f
    for heparin-induced thrombosis, 370, 371f
    for iliac vein obstruction, 299f, 301
    for infrainguinal graft thrombosis, 204, 205f, 206
    for popliteal artery aneurysm, 147f, 148
    for pulmonary embolism, 286–288, 287f
    for stroke following carotid endarterectomy, 70, 71f
    for superficial phlebitis, 268, 269f
    for upper extremity ischemia, 233f, 234
Thrombosis. See also Thromboemboli.
    aortic graft and, 180, 181f, 182, 184
    deep vein. See Deep vein thrombosis (DVT).
    heparin-induced, 370, 371f
    in acute mesenteric ischemia, 250, 251f, 252, 254
    in hypercoagulable syndrome, 8, 9f, 10
    in upper extremity ischemia, 233f, 234
    infrainguinal graft and, 204, 205f, 206
    isolated calf vein, 273f, 274, 278
    subclavian-axillary vein, 262, 263f, 264, 266
TIA. See Transient ischemic attack (TIA).
Ticlopidine
    for atheroembolism, 172
    for carotid artery dissection, 60

Ticlopidine (Continued)
    for carotid artery stenosis, 28
TIPS (transjugular intrahepatic portosystemic shunt), for portal hypertension, 306, 307f, 308, 309–310
Tissue plasminogen activator, 282, 287, 366
Toe amputation
    indications for, 218, 219f, 220
    with diabetic foot infections, 213f, 214, 216
Toe pressures, with diabetic foot infections, 212
TOS (thoracic outlet syndrome)
    in upper extremity ischemia, 232, 233f, 234
    neurogenic, 340–341, 341f
Transcutaneous electrical nerve stimulation (TENS), for post-traumatic pain syndrome, 338
Transcutaneous oxygen tension (Tco_2)
    for amputation level, 218, 219f, 220
    with diabetic foot infections, 212
Transesophageal echocardiography
    for aortic dissection, 128
    for evaluating cerebrovascular symptoms, 23f, 24
    for pulmonary embolism, 286, 287f
Transfusion strategies, 14, 15f, 16, 18
    for abdominal aortic aneurysm repair, 91f, 96
    ruptured, 104
Transient ischemic attack (TIA)
    acute stroke vs., 50
    embolic, 74, 75f
    evaluating symptoms of, 22, 23f, 24
    low-flow hemodynamics in, 74
    medical therapy for, 28, 29f
    with carotid artery aneurysm, 54, 55f
    with carotid artery dissection, 58, 59f
    with carotid artery stenosis
        asymptomatic, 34, 36
        plus coronary disease, 84, 85f
        symptomatic, 28, 29f, 30, 32
        with redo endarterectomy, 46
Transjugular intrahepatic portosystemic shunt (TIPS), for portal hypertension, 306, 307f, 308, 309–310
Transperitoneal approach, for abdominal aortic aneurysm repair, 91f, 94
Transthoracic repair
    of brachiocephalic artery occlusive disease, 80, 81f
    of subclavian artery occlusive disease, 77f, 78
Transurethral therapy, for erectile dysfunction, 347f, 348
Trauma
    abdominal vascular, 324–330, 325f–327f, 329f
    brachiocephalic vascular, 318, 319f, 320, 322
    carotid artery aneurysm from, 54, 55f
    carotid artery dissection from, 58, 59f
    deep vein thrombosis from, 272
    extremity vascular, 332–334, 333f
    femoral artery aneurysm from, 136, 137f, 138
    femoral artery pseudoaneurysm from, 137f, 138, 142–144, 143f
    neck wound zones with, 318
    neurogenic thoracic outlet syndrome from, 340, 341f
Treadmill testing. See Stress testing.

Trendelenburg test
    for deep vein insufficiency, 294
    for varicose veins, 290–291, 291f
Triglycerides, management of, 6, 7f
Truncal venous lesion, as congenital venous malformation, 351f, 352
TT (thrombin time), in intraoperative hemorrhage, 364, 365f, 366
Tube graft, for abdominal aortic aneurysm repair, 132, 133f
Tumor(s)
    of carotid body, 66–69, 67f
    preoperative embolization of, 68

Ulcer(s)
    ischemic
        with atheroembolism, 172
        with critical limb ischemia, 162, 163f
        with leg pain while walking, 156, 157f
        with Raynaud's syndrome, 343f, 344
    venous, with deep vein insufficiency, 294, 295–296, 295f
    with diabetic foot infections, 212, 213f, 214, 216
    with varicose veins, 290, 291f
Ulnar artery aneurysm, in upper extremity ischemia, 234
Ulnar artery obstruction, in Raynaud's syndrome, 344
Ulnar nerve, in thoracic outlet syndrome, 340, 341f
Ultrasonography
    duplex. See Duplex ultrasonography.
    for abdominal aortic aneurysm, 90, 91f, 94
        ruptured, 104, 105f
    for femoral artery aneurysm, 136
        with compression therapy, 138, 142–143, 143f
Upper extremity
    compartment syndrome of, 224
    hemodialysis vascular access in, 355–356, 355f
    in Takayasu's disease, 361f, 362
Upper extremity ischemia, 232, 233f, 234
    with brachiocephalic artery occlusive disease, 80
    with subclavian artery occlusive disease, 76, 77f, 78
Upper gastrointestinal endoscopy
    for aortoenteric fistula, 112, 113f
    for portal hypertension, 306, 307f
Urokinase
    for hemodialysis vascular access, 358
    for iliofemoral deep vein thrombosis, 282
    for pulmonary embolism, 287
Urticaria, heparin-induced, 372, 373f

Vacuum constrictor devices, for erectile dysfunction, 347f, 348
Valve substitution procedure, for deep vein insufficiency, 298, 299f, 300
Valve transplantation, for deep vein insufficiency, 299f, 300
Valve transposition, for deep vein insufficiency, 299f, 300
Valvuloplasty, for deep vein insufficiency, 298, 299f, 300

Variceal banding, for esophageal varices, from portal hypertension, 306, 309
Varices, esophageal, from portal hypertension, 306–307
Varicose veins, 290–292, 291f
    congenital venous malformation and, 290, 350, 351f
    in superficial phlebitis, 268–269
Vascular access, for hemodialysis, 354–356, 355f
    failed, 358–359, 359f
Vascular trauma
    abdominal, 324–330, 325f–327f, 329f
    brachiocephalic, 318, 319f, 320, 322
    extremity, 332–334, 333f
Vasoactive agents, for erectile dysfunction, 346, 347f, 348
Vasodilators, for upper extremity ischemia, 234
Vasomotor phenomena, in post-traumatic pain syndrome, 336, 337
Vasospasm, in Raynaud's syndrome, 342, 343f, 344
VBI (vertebrobasilar insufficiency)
    evaluating symptoms of, 22, 23f, 24
    with subclavian artery occlusive disease, 76, 77f, 78
Vein(s). See also named vein, e.g., Subclavian vein.
    anomaly(ies) of
        as congenital venous malformation, 351f, 352
        with aortovenous fistula, 108–110, 109f
    injuries of, with abdominal vascular trauma, 324, 329–330, 329f
    varicosities of. See Varicose veins.
Vein cuffs, with prosthetic grafts
    for infrainguinal graft thrombosis, 206
    for infrainguinal occlusive disease, 193f, 194
Vein excision, for superficial phlebitis, 269–270, 269f
Vein grafts
    for angioplasty. See Vein patch angioplasty.
    saphenous. See Saphenous vein graft/patch.
Vein interruption
    for deep vein insufficiency, 295f, 296
    for varicose veins, 291f, 292
Vein patch angioplasty
    for acute limb ischemia, 169f, 170, 234
    for aortic graft infection, 186, 187f, 188
    for carotid artery aneurysm, 55f, 56
    for carotid artery dissection, 60, 68
    for carotid endarterectomy, 38, 39f, 40, 46
        complications of, 39f, 40, 42
        redo, 44, 45f, 46
    for critical limb ischemia, 164
    for hemodialysis vascular access, 358, 359f
    for iliac vein obstruction, 299f, 301, 302
    for infrainguinal graft thrombosis, 204, 205f, 206
    for infrainguinal occlusive disease, 192–194, 193f
        surveillance of, 198, 199f, 200, 202
    for mesenteric ischemia
        acute, 251f, 252
        chronic, 257f, 258
    for popliteal artery aneurysm, 147f, 148
    for renal artery aneurysm, 15–153
    for renovascular occlusive disease
        adult fibrodysplastic, 244, 245f

Vein patch angioplasty *(Continued)*
   arteriosclerotic, 246, 247f
   for subclavian-axillary venous thrombosis, 263f, 264
   for vascular trauma
      abdominal, 326, 326f, 327, 329
      brachiocephalic, 322
      extremity, 332, 333f, 334
Vein stripping
   for deep vein insufficiency, 295f, 296
   for varicose veins, 291f, 292
Velocity ratio, in infrainguinal graft surveillance, 199f, 200, 202
Vena caval filters
   for deep vein thrombosis, 273f, 274
   for iliofemoral deep vein thrombosis, 282, 283f
   for pulmonary embolism, 287f, 288
Venography
   for deep vein insufficiency, 295f, 296
      with surgical treatment, 298, 299, 299f, 300
   for deep vein thrombosis
      iliofemoral, 282, 284
      lower extremity, 272, 273f, 274, 278
   for hemodialysis vascular access, 358
   for subclavian-axillary venous thrombosis, 263f, 264, 266
Venorrhaphy, for abdominal vascular trauma, 327, 327f, 328f, 329, 330
Venous angiomata, as congenital venous malformation, 351f, 352
Venous edema, in lymphedema, 312, 313f
Venous filling index (VFI), for deep vein insufficiency, 294, 298–299
Venous flow augmentation, in compartment syndromes, 222, 224
Venous incompetence, in varicose veins, 291, 291f, 292
Venous insufficiency
   in varicose veins, 291, 291f

Venous insufficiency *(Continued)*
   of deep veins (chronic)
      conservative management of, 295–296, 295f
      evaluation of, 294–295, 295f
      surgical treatment of, 298–302, 299f
   primary *vs.* congenital *vs.* secondary, 298, 299f
   with leg pain while walking, 156, 157f, 158
Venous reflux
   in deep vein insufficiency, 298–300, 299f
   in lymphedema, 313f, 314
Venous return timing (VRT), for varicose veins, 291
Venous thrombosis. *See* Deep vein thrombosis (DVT).
Ventilation-perfusion (V/Q) scan, for pulmonary embolism, 286, 287f
Ventilatory support, for pulmonary embolism, 286, 287f
Vertebral artery(ies)
   arteriography of, for carotid artery aneurysm, 55, 55f
   ultrasonography of, for acute stroke, 50, 51f
Vertebral artery disease, 74, 75f
   acute stroke from, 50–52, 51f
   fibromuscular dysplasia as, 64
Vertebral artery stenosis, 74, 75f
Vertebrobasilar insufficiency (VBI)
   evaluating symptoms of, 22, 23f, 24
   with subclavian artery occlusive disease, 76, 77f, 78
Vessel shortening, in carotid endarterectomy, 38, 39f, 40
VFI (venous filling index), for deep vein insufficiency, 294, 298–299
Visceral ischemia
   in aortic dissection, 128, 129f, 130
   in ruptured abdominal aortic aneurysm repair, 105f, 106
Vitamin K
   clotting factors dependent on, 8, 366
   for warfarin reversal, 14

V/Q (ventilation-perfusion) scan, for pulmonary embolism, 286, 287f
VRT (venous return timing), for varicose veins, 291

Walking, leg pain while, 156, 157f, 158, 160
Warfarin (Coumadin)
   as teratogen, 276
   for atheroembolism, 172
   for atrial fibrillation, 51
   for carotid artery dissection, 58, 59f, 60
   for carotid artery thromboembolism, 29f, 32
   for deep vein thrombosis, in lower extremity, 273f, 274, 276
   for heparin-induced thrombosis, 370, 371f
   for hypercoagulable syndrome, 10
   for infrainguinal graft surveillance, 198, 199f, 200
   for infrainguinal graft thrombosis, 205f, 206
   for pulmonary embolism, 287f, 288
   for recurrent carotid stenosis, 45f, 46
   for vertebral artery disease, 74, 75f
   hematology disorders with, 14
   reversal of, 14
Warm compresses, for superficial phlebitis, 269
Weight reduction, for hyperlipidemia, 6, 7f
White blood cell scan. *See* Radioactive cellular scanning.
Wound management
   for amputations, 218, 219f
   for diabetic foot infections, 213f, 214, 216
   for femoral artery pseudoaneurysm, 143f, 144
   for infrainguinal prosthetic graft infection, 209f, 210
   for ischemic limb ulcers, 162, 163f
   in deep vein insufficiency, 294, 295f, 296
   in Raynaud's syndrome, 343f, 344
   transcutaneous oxygen tension in, 212, 218, 219f, 220
Wrist-brachial index, in extremity vascular trauma, 332, 333f

ISBN 0-7216-8684-2